# GLAUCOMA - BASIC AND CLINICAL CONCEPTS

Edited by **Shimon Rumelt**

**Glaucoma - Basic and Clinical Concepts**
Edited by Shimon Rumelt

**Published by InTech**
Janeza Trdine 9, 51000 Rijeka, Croatia



**Publishing Process Manager** Davor Vidic

**Technical Editor** Teodora Smiljanic

**Cover Designer** InTech Design Team

Additional hard copies can be obtained from orders@intechopen.com

Glaucoma - Basic and Clinical Concepts, Edited by Shimon Rumelt
p. cm.
ISBN 978-953-307-591-4

For EU product safety concerns:
IN TECH d.o.o., Prolaz Marije Krucifikse Kozulić 3, 51000 Rijeka, Croatia,
info@intechopen.com or visit our website at intechopen.com.

# Meet the editor

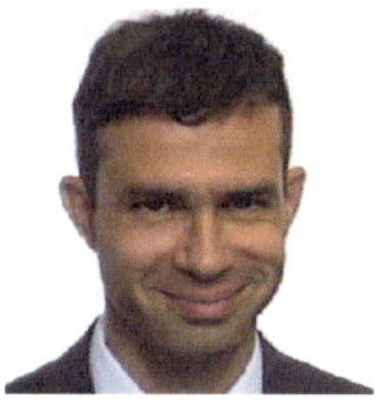

Dr. Shimon Rumelt received his medical degree and a diploma in ophthalmology from Tel Aviv University, Israel. He completed his ophthalmology residency program at Western Galilee - Nahariya Medical Center in Nahariya, Israel,an oculoplastics fellowship at Massachusetts Eye and Ear Infirmary, Boston, Massachusetts, and vitreoretinal fellowship at Boston University. He earned a master degree in Public Administration (Health Systems) from Clark University, Worcester, MA. Dr. Rumelt is a senior ophthalmologist at the Western Galilee - Nahariya Medical Center and is engaged with various fields in ophthalmology. He is engaged with clinical activities, surgery, research and teaching medical students, residents and fellows. Dr. Rumelt edited three books and is the author and co-author of approximately 100 scientific articles and book chapters. He is a member of the editorial board of Evidence - Based Ophthalmology and a reviewer for multiple professional journals.

# Contents

# Preface

The glaucoma specialty underwent an enormous change in the last two decades and a book that is published now is different from one that was published even two years ago. It just reflects this change. We are evident to better understanding the genetics and pathogenesis of different types of glaucomas that will enable us to develop novel approaches for treatment, new imaging techniques such as anterior segment OCT, GDx, or HRT, application of new devices such as the ExPress shunt, iStent and Solx Gold shunt and new procedures such as canaloplasty and deep sclerostomy to minimize postoperative complications of the traditional trabeculectomy without compromising the success of the procedure.

The book is arranged in a systematic approach discussing first the basic concepts of glaucomas, including the final offenders, the retinal ganglion cells and many other topics. The clinical concepts include evaluation and management of glaucoma and the different types of glaucomas, their features, evaluation, differential diagnosis and specific approaches for treatment. The book covers most but not all of the field. It is a product of a balance between expedited publishing process and encompassing the entire field.

The book is intended for the general ophthalmologists, glaucoma specialists, and researchers in the field, residents and fellows. It covers both basic and clinical concepts of glaucoma and all authors incorporated their perspectives on each topic adding their own theories, future trends and research. Therefore, the book should enable researches and clinicians to adopt new ideas for further basic and clinical research.

"Glaucoma - Basic and Clinical Concepts" is a result of contributions from multi-national glaucoma specialists worldwide with a common characteristic of taking care of patients. Some of the authors have been engaged for many years in this field, some are just at their beginning. Some authors are researches, other clinicians. Some are world leaders in glaucoma research, others will be. We hope that our readers will be of wide variety just as our authors are.

The book is accessed online to allow free access to as many readers worldwide as possible and is also available on print for those who do not have online access or are interested in having their own hard copy. This will definitely contribute to distributing the knowledge on glaucoma among researchers and clinicians.

I would like to acknowledge each and every one of the contributors for their excellent work on each chapter. Each of them devoted time and effort to write a chapter and to contribute to the success of this book and for the advancement of glaucoma research.

I would like to thank Mr. Davor Vidic, the book Publishing Process Manager for his tremendous efforts to publish an excellent book and his endless support, Ms. Ana Nikolic, the Head of Editorial Consultants at InTech for her useful assistance and for choosing me to be the Editor of the book. Many thanks to the technical editors for their arranging the book in a uniform format and to InTech – Open Access publisher - without this initiative, the book would have never been published. Lastly, to my family, teachers and students from whom I studied throughout the years.

I hope that this book will be the first in a series of books in all the different specialties within ophthalmology. I wish you, the reader, an enjoyable journey through glaucoma, one of the most interesting and challenging specialties in medicine in general and, in ophthalmology, in particular.

The book is a product of global cooperation for the benefit of physicians and patients all over the world. I hope that it will serve as an example for others to follow.

**Shimon Rumelt, MD, MPA**
Department of Ophthalmology,
Western Galilee – Nahariya Medical Center,
Nahariya,
Israel

# Part 1

## Basic Concepts

# 1

# Mechanism of Aqueous Humor Secretion, Its Regulation and Relevance to Glaucoma

Mohammad Shahidullah[1],
Waleed Hassan Al-Malki[2] and Nicholas A. Delamere[1]
[1]*Department of Physiology, University of Arizona, Tucson, AZ 85724*
[2]*College of Pharmacy, Department of Pharmacology and Toxicology, Umm Al-Qura University, Makkah,*
[1]*USA*
[2]*KSA*

## 1. Introduction

The principal function of the eye is to receive the light signal from the environment and transmit it to the brain to create vision. This requires that the structures of the eye involved in light transmission, such as the cornea and the lens, must be transparent. Unlike other tissues of the body, nutrients and oxygen supply to these structures must be accomplished without blood interference in transmission of light, i.e., these structures must be avascular. Apart from this, the eye must also maintain optimum pressure within the globe, which is important to give the rigidity necessary for optical alignment of the cornea, lens and the retina. The eye achieves this by the production, accumulation and circulation of a clear fluid called aqueous humor (AH). AH is produced by selective transfer of solutes and water from the blood plasma by a complex ocular epithelium, the ciliary epithelium. The fluid then accumulates in the two special compartments within the eye, and the excess leaves the globe to enter the blood through complex pressure dependent outflow pathways. This complex arrangement of production, accumulation and drainage of aqueous humor contributes to the nutrition and survival of the avascular tissues as well as to good optical properties of the eye. However, this also poses a problem in that any imbalance in the production and drainage of aqueous humor inevitably causes abnormal intraocular pressure (IOP). For example, in case of insufficient drainage, excess accumulation of fluid within the globe will raise the IOP to higher than the physiological level; a clinical condition called glaucoma. Abnormally high pressure causes death or degeneration of the light sensitive and signal transmitting tissues of the eye leading progressively to partial or complete blindness. Understanding the mechanism of AH secretion and its regulation is important to develop rational and target specific drugs for the treatment of glaucoma. In this chapter we will try to present the readers with a comprehensive and up to date description of the relevant ocular anatomy, physiology, biochemistry and pharmacology of AH secretion and its relevance to pathophysiology of ocular hypertension or glaucoma.

## 2. Gross structures of the eye

The two eyes together with the appendages (extraocular muscles, lacrimal glands) are situated within the conical or four-sided pyramidal cavities of the skull called the orbits. The eyeball is a sphere, with the segment of a smaller sphere, the cornea, in front. It is composed of three layers or tunics. The outermost protective layer is made up of the sclera posteriorly and the cornea anteriorly. The middle layer is mainly vascular, consisting of the choroid, ciliary body and iris. The innermost coat is the retina, containing the essential sensory elements responsible for vision - the rods and cones, bipolar and ganglion cells. Within the three layers are the refractory media - namely, the AH, the crystalline lens and a clear jelly, the vitreous humor (Fig. 1).

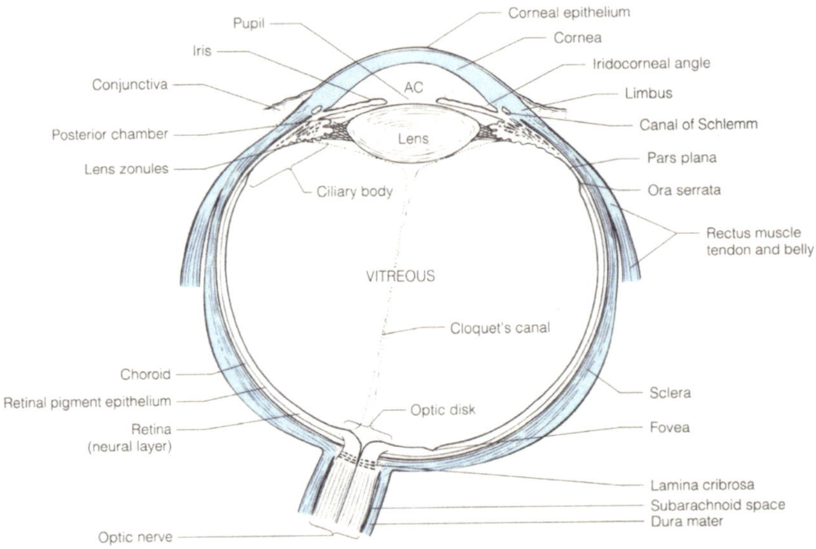


Fig. 1. Diagram of the human eye in horizontal section showing major structures and the arrangement of the three layers (Forrester et al., 1996) (used with permission)

The cornea, the first and the most powerful refracting surface of the optical system of the eye, occupies the anterior sixth of the outermost coat. The crystalline lens is a double convex, transparent body positioned between the iris and AH in front and the vitreous humor behind, and is supported by an elastic capsule and the ciliary zonules (the suspensory ligaments). The ciliary zonules attach the lens to the ciliary body. The iris, a pigmented structure, is the most anterior portion of the vascular tunic of the eye. It is composed of a flat bar of circular muscle fibers surrounding the pupil and a thin layer of smooth muscle fibers by which the pupil is dilated. Relaxation and contraction of the iris regulates the size of the pupil and hence the amount of light entering the eye. It is covered by two layers of epithelia, which are continuous extensions of the pigmented and nonpigmented layers of the ciliary body (CB) epithelium. The CB is the middle thickened portion of the vascular tunic anterior to the ora serrata (the terminating point of the retina at the CB), connecting the choroid with the iris. It is composed of corona ciliaris (the ciliary processes and folds), ciliary ring, ciliary muscle and a basal lamina. The ciliary processes are finger like projections that extend into the posterior chamber, approximately 70 in number in man and 90 to 110 in bovine (Prince et al., 1960). These are composed of capillaries, which are covered by a double layer of epithelium, called the ciliary epithelium (CE). The CE is the key structure responsible for AH production. The choroid is the thin portion of the vascular coat extending from the ora serrata to the optic nerve. It supplies blood to the retina and conducts arteries and nerves to the anterior structures of the eye. The retina is the innermost layer of the three tunics of the eyeball surrounding the vitreous body and continuous posteriorly with the optic nerve. Grossly, the retina is composed of an outer single layer of pigmented epithelial cells (pars pigmentosa), and an inner transparent layer (pars nervosa), which is part of the optical component. The neural retina has many cell types, arranged in distinct layers, including the essential neurons to receive and carry light signal to the brain. The rod and cone (photoreceptor) layer of the neural retina forms the percipient element of the retina (i.e., the element that responds to visual stimuli by a photochemical reaction) and is connected via the bipolar cells to the nerve fiber layer, the ganglion cell layer. The axons of the ganglion cells bundle together to form the optic nerve. The optic nerve in turn extends and carries the light-induced impulse to the brain.

The AH and vitreous body are contained in the three spaces within the eyeball. The largest space is situated between the lens and retina and contains the vitreous humor. The smaller two spaces are called the aqueous chambers (anterior and posterior). The anterior chamber contains most of the aqueous and is the space between the anterior surface of the iris and the internal surface of the cornea. The posterior chamber is the name given to the smaller space surrounded by the lens, the iris and the CB.

The vitreous is a clear hydrophilic mass and physiologically a hydrogel that occupies more than two thirds of the intraocular volume. Forward extensions of the hyaloid membrane form the suspensory ligaments supporting the lens, known as the zonules. The vitreous is probably not a tissue in proper sense, but rather a highly specialized extracellular fluid containing connective tissue-specific elements, such as collagen fibers, hyaluronic acid (hyaluronan) and some other soluble proteins and glycoproteins. Its density, refractive index and pH is slightly higher than those of pure water (Gloor, 1987; Redslob, 1932) and its water content is extremely high, between 98% (Leone et al., 2010; Redslob, 1932) and 99.7% (Sullmann, 1951). The mechanical stability and optical transparency of the vitreous comes from the specific organization of the collagen-hyaluronan network. The vitreous allows light to reach the retina and nutrients to diffuse from the CB to the retina.

### 2.1 Ocular blood supply

The blood vessels of the choroid supply many of the internal structures of the eye. The choroid, CB and iris are supplied by the ciliary system of arteries, comprising the medial and lateral long posterior ciliary arteries, the short ciliary and the anterior ciliary arteries. These are often referred to as the uveal vessels. They emanate from the main arterial supply to the eye, the ophthalmic artery, which is derived from a branch of the internal carotid artery in the human. The venous blood from the uvea drains into the episcleral veins. These are fine veins running through the sclera and from there into the four vortex veins, finally leaving the eye by the superior and inferior ophthalmic veins. The neural retina is supplied from the central retinal artery, a branch of the ophthalmic artery arising proximal to the ciliary arteries. The venous blood from the retina drains into the retinal veins and then into the ophthalmic veins. Fig. 2 shows the physiological plan of ocular blood supply in human.

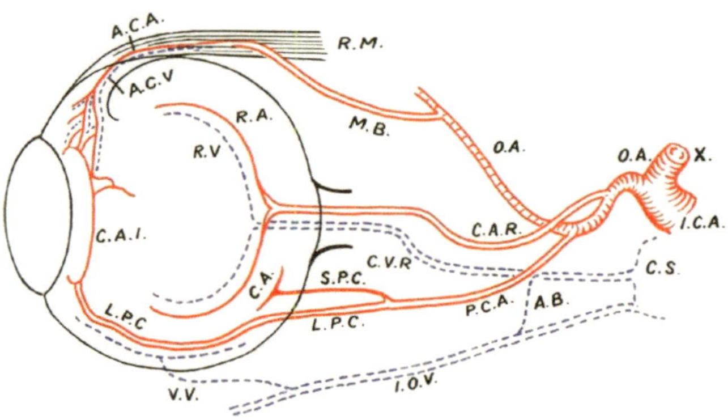


Fig. 2. Diagram showing physiological plan of the circulation in human eye (Duke-Elder, 1926). CA, carotid artery; OA, ophthalmic artery; MB, muscular branch; CAR, central artery of the retina; PCA, posterior ciliary artery; ACA, anterior ciliary artery; LPC, long posterior ciliary artery; SPC, short posterior ciliary artery; ACA, anterior ciliary artery; ACV, anterior ciliary vein; VV, vortex vein, IOV, inferior orbital vein (used with permission)

## 3. Aqueous humor

AH is a transparent fluid contained in the anterior and posterior chambers of the eye and is formed by the ciliary epithelium (CE) of the ciliary processes projecting from the CB. AH is formed by selective transfer of solutes (ions, glucose, ascorbate, amino acids and other solutes) and water from the blood across the CE. The fluid is continuously secreted by the CE and enters first into the posterior chamber. It then seeps forward through the narrow space between the lens and the iris and enters the anterior chamber through the pupil. From the anterior chamber it leaves the eye, mostly by bulk flow (a pressure dependent flow), through the two outflow pathways at the anterior chamber angle, i.e., the angle formed by the cornea and the root of the iris.

### 3.1 Functions of aqueous humor

AH is a nutritive fluid that serves as a blood substitute for the avascular cornea, lens, anterior vitreous and also the trabecular meshwork (TM) of the outflow pathway. AH supplies nutrients and oxygen to these avascular tissues through diffusion. It also removes metabolic wastes of the avascular tissues through its continuous formation, sojourn through the ocular chambers and drainage from the eye to the venous blood. Hydrostatic pressure due to AH establishes the IOP, which inflates the eye to maintain proper alignment of the optical structures. AH also serves to transport ascorbate, an anti-oxidant agent in the anterior segment. Presence of immunoglobulins in the AH indicates a role in immune response to defend against invading pathogens.

### 3.2 Anatomical and structural features of the aqueous secreting tissue

The ciliary body is the tissue responsible for AH secretion. The CB is a musculoepithelial structure, composed of the ciliary muscles and the ciliary processes. The ciliary muscles are responsible for accommodation and the ciliary processes are responsible for AH production. The bulk of the CB consists of three sets of ciliary muscles, the longitudinal, radial, and circular muscles. It is attached to the lens by connective tissue called the zonules of Zinn or simply ciliary zonules. The ciliary muscles, by relaxation or contraction, increase or decrease the thickness of the crystalline lens to focus light on the retina to produce near or distance vision. This process of shaping the lens is called accommodation.

The inner surface of the CB, i.e., the surface facing the posterior chamber, is covered with a double layer epithelium. AH is formed by this epithelium. There are two distinct regions: the anterior third consists of undulated surface and is termed the pars plicata, while the smooth posterior two thirds is termed the pars plana. Projecting inwards from the pars plicata region into the posterior chamber are approximately 70 radial ridges called the ciliary processes (Fig. 3). Each process is 1mm high, 2mm long antero-posteriorly and 0.5mm wide. In the bovine eye these processes are particularly well developed. The ciliary processes have a rich blood supply and are probably the most heavily vascularized part of the eye. The connective stroma in the interior of each process contains a mass of capillaries, arranged that each comes into close relationship, at some point in its course, with the CE covering the ciliary processes. A histological section of a porcine ciliary process are shown (Fig. 4).

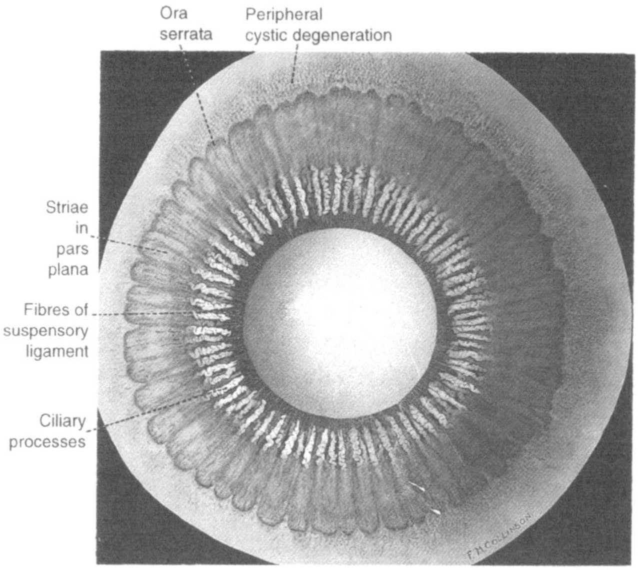


Fig. 3. Posterior view of the ciliary body showing ciliary processes and part plana (Bron et al., 1997) (used with kind permission from Springer Science+Business Media B.V)

The CE consists of an inner layer of nonpigmented epithelium (NPE) and an outer layer of pigmented epithelium (PE). The endothelium of the ciliary capillaries is highly fenestrated so a blood ultrafiltrate fills the stroma. This contains almost all components of the plasma except the blood cells. It is now generally believed that AH is formed mostly by active transport of ions and solutes across the CE. Selective transport of solutes takes place from the stromal fluid across the bilayer into the posterior chamber and this causes a subsequent osmotic flux of water, producing the AH. The exact contribution of each cell type to the secretion of AH is not known. Most recent studies, however, suggest that both cell types function together as a syncytium to produce AH (Civan, 1998; Edelman et al., 1994; Raviola and Raviola, 1978). The contemporary view is that ions and other solutes driven inward from the blood side by the PE cells readily pass through the gap junctions into the NPE cells.

From the NPE, ions and solutes are then secreted across the basolateral membrane into the posterior chamber (Avila et al., 2002; Civan and Macknight, 2004; Do and To, 2000; Jacob and Civan, 1996; To et al., 2002). The situation is complex, however, because NPE cells also may reabsorb some of the solute and water from the aqueous humor back into the stroma (Hu et al., 2011; McLaughlin et al., 2007). The algebraic sum of these secretion and reabsorption processes determines the net secretion rate of AH into the posterior chamber.

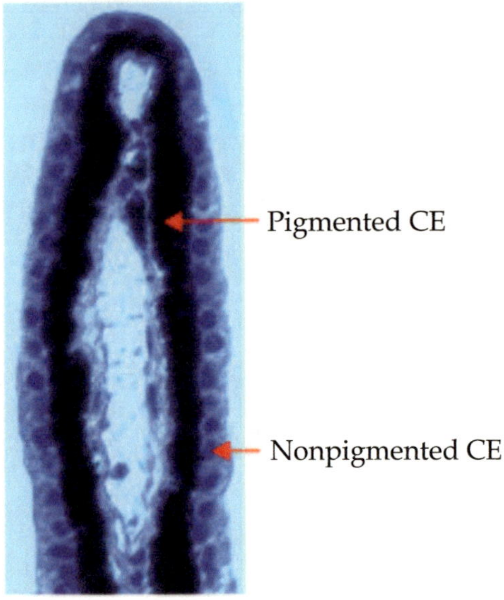


Fig. 4. A histological section of a porcine ciliary process (Shahidullah, 2010, unpublished data) showing pigmented and nonpigmented ciliary epithelial cells.

### 3.2.1 Special features of the CE

The bilayer CE consists of the columnar non-pigmented (NPE) and the cuboidal pigmented epithelial cells (PE). The basal surface of the NPE cells lines the posterior chamber whereas the basal surface of the PE cells rests on the ciliary body stroma (Fig. 5). The apices of the PE and NPE cells are in contact with each other and are connected via gap junctions. This unusual arrangement is the result of the invagination of the neuroepithelial layer during embryogenesis. Despite this arrangement, the secretory process is directed from apex to the base of the NPE cells along the lateral intercellular canals, which are 'closed' at the apical ends by dense junctional complexes, the tight junctions (Cole, 1977; Raviola and Raviola, 1978). The PE represents the forward continuation of the retinal pigment epithelium whilst the NPE layer is the forward continuation of the neuroepithelium from which the retinal cells are derived. Under electron microscopy, the cells of this epithelium display characteristics typical of secretory epithelia, i.e. interdigitations on the lateral surfaces of adjacent cells and basal infoldings (Pappas and Smelter, 1958; Pappas and Smelter, 1961). The coordinated function of the two epithelial cell layers is of importance, since the secreted aqueous must be derived from the blood contained in the capillaries of the ciliary stroma and secretion must occur across both layers. Fig. 6 shows an electron microscopy image of PE and NPE.

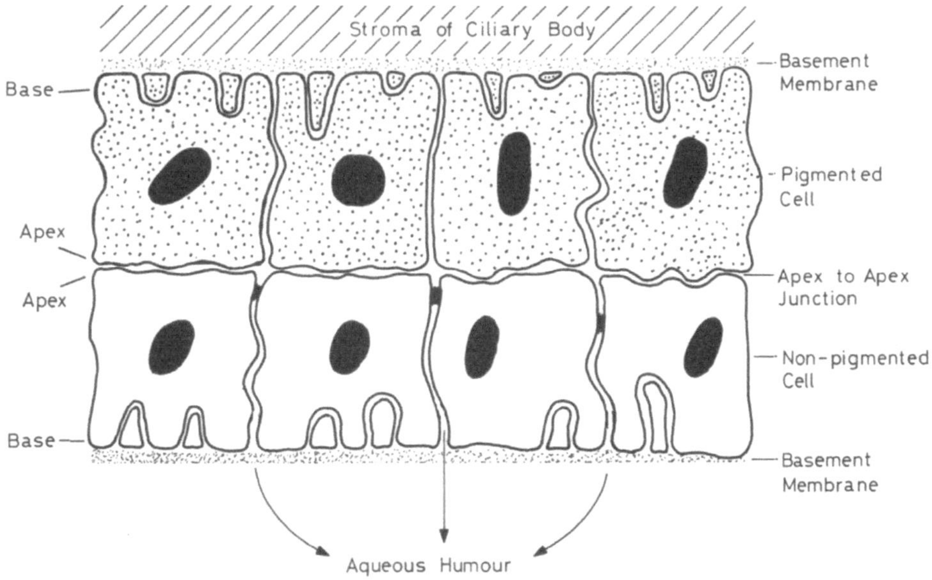


Fig. 5. Schematic diagram of ciliary epithelium bilayer showing apex to apex arrangement of pigmented and non-pigmented ciliary epithelium (Davson, 1990) (used with permission)

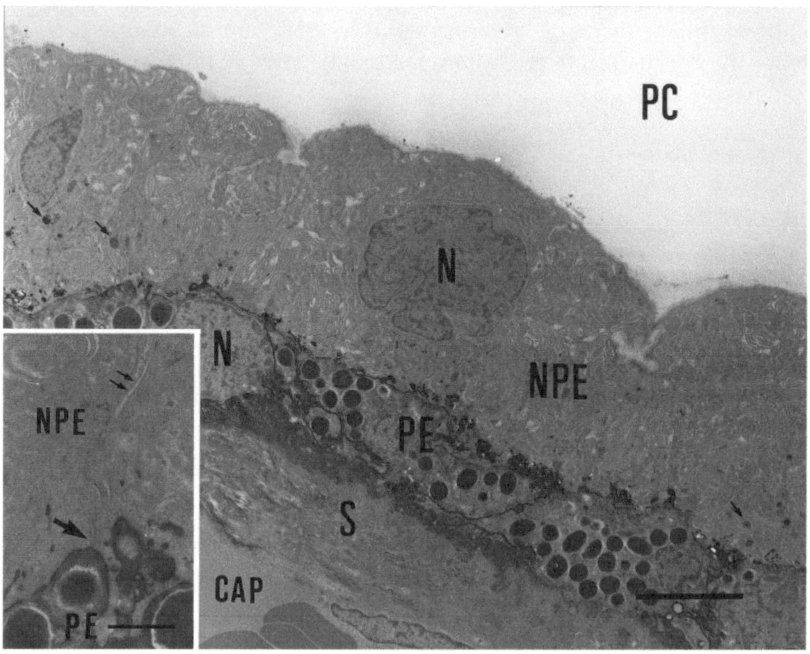


Fig. 6. Transmission electron microscopy image of CE showing PE and NPE cells. CE, ciliary epithelium; PE, pigmented ciliary epithelium; NPE, nonpigmented ciliary epithelium; PC, posterior chamber; N, nucleus; S, stroma; CAP, capillary. Bar = 5 μm (inset bar = 1 μm) (Chen et al., 1996) (used with permission)

The CB epithelium represents a significant barrier to the movement of substances from the blood into the eye (Cunha-Vaz, 1979; Freddo, 2001). The vasculature perfusing the CB is highly fenestrated, and large molecular weight tracers (e.g., horseradish peroxidase) readily leak out into the surrounding interstitium following intravenous administration (Freddo et al., 1990; Vegge, 1971). Since there are no tight junctions between the pigmented cells, the aforementioned tracers have been shown to infiltrate the paracellular space between the PE and NPE cell layers (Smith and Rudt, 1975). However, the tight junctions between NPE cells act as a permeability barrier and prevent diffusion of blood-borne macromolecules (e.g. proteins) into the AH (Cunha-Vaz, 1979; Freddo, 2001). The tight junctions (Vegge, 1971) exclude large molecules from the AH (Green, 1984; Novack and Leopold, 1988). Thus, these specialized junctions constitute the most important part of the blood-aqueous barrier.

Many gap junctions usually are found between the lateral surfaces of the PE cells and less frequently between the lateral surfaces of the NPE cells. Gap junctions and puncta adherentia are located between the PE and NPE cells and between each type of cells (Fig. 7). Each gap junction channel comprises two hemichannels (connexons), each of which is composed of six radially-arranged connexins around a central pore (Scemes et al., 2007). This highly integrated epithelium in addition to the secretion of AH, affords attachment to the ciliary zonules (Fig. 1). All ancillary functions to maintain proper transport activity, diffusion characteristics, mechanical stability of the epithelium, etc. depend upon the properties of these specialized intercellular junctions (Raviola and Raviola, 1978). AH production is only possible if the transport activity of the epithelial cells is precisely coordinated and solute gradients are not dissipated by free diffusion of water and solutes along the intercellular clefts of the epithelium. Mechanical stability is an essential prerequisite for the epithelium to withstand the tensile force of the elastic zonular fibers.

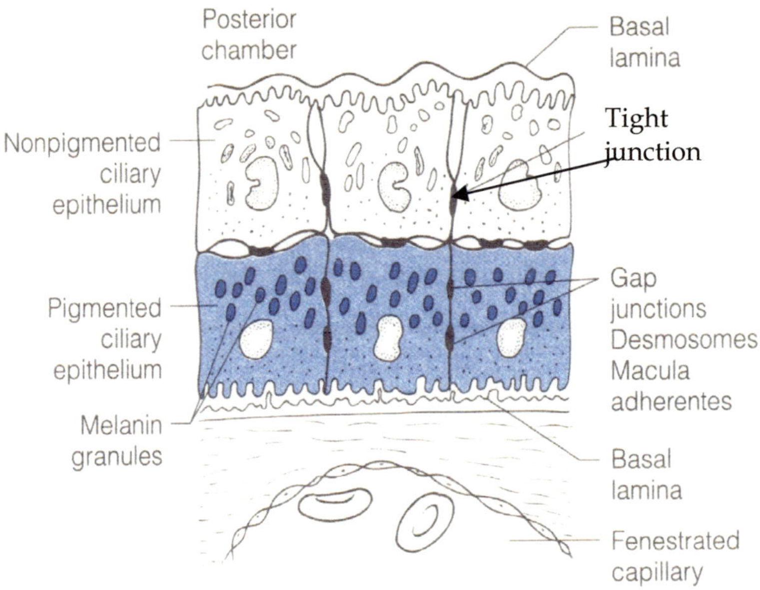


Fig. 7. Diagram of double layer ciliary epithelium showing tight and gap junctions (Forrester et al., 1996) (used with permission)

A large number of gap junctions between both the NPE and PE cells with greater concentration at the interface between the two epithelial layers constitute a striking morphological feature of the CE. These junctions, less commonly referred to as nexuses or macula communicans, are specialized membrane proteins (connexins) that are able to form channels, which permit movement of molecules up to ~1,000 daltons (Kondo et al., 2000; Saez et al., 1993). In electron micrographs of thin sections, they appear as regions of intercellular contact where apposed plasma membranes of adjacent cells are separated by a gap junction of 2 - 3nm (Saez et al., 1993). Gap junctions mediate both electrical and metabolic coupling between cells (Gilula et al., 1972; Wang et al., 2010).

### 3.2.2 The blood-ocular barriers

The striking differences between the composition of plasma and the AH means that substances encounter difficulty in passing from one fluid to the other. In addition, there is no barrier between the posterior chamber and the vitreous body and between the vitreous humor and the retina. Horseradish peroxidase and even Thorotrast particles can pass from the vitreous into the intercellular spaces of the retina (Smelser et al., 1965). The movement of horseradish peroxidase is halted at the tight junctions of the pigment epithelium of retina (Peyman and Apple, 1972; Peyman and Bok, 1972). Thus, to maintain the normal composition of AH, which is distinct from the plasma, some kind of barrier must exist in all the associated structures separating the AH, vitreous and the retina from the plasma. All such structures have either endothelial and/or epithelial barriers. In the mammalian eye, endothelial barriers are localized in the vessels of the retina, optic nerve, ciliary muscle and the iris. Epithelial barriers are present in the pigment epithelium of retina, the NPE of the ciliary body and the iridal epithelium (Raviola, 1977). These structures constitute the two important barrier systems, namely the blood-vitreous or the blood-retinal barrier and the blood-aqueous barrier. The barriers prevent almost all protein movement and they are effective even to low molecular weight solutes, such as sucrose and fluorescein (Bill, 1975).

### 3.2.3 Blood-vitreous or blood-retinal barrier

The endothelial cells of the retinal capillaries and the tight junctions between the retinal pigment epithelial cells (RPE) represent respectively the endothelial and epithelial parts of the blood-retinal barrier. They prevent both outward and inward movement of horseradish peroxidase as examined by injecting intravenously and into the vitreous (Peyman and Apple, 1972; Peyman and Bok, 1972). The epithelial part of the barrier, i. e., the RPE separates the choroidal fluid from the retinal tissue fluid and is very important because choroidal tissue fluid is likely to be very similar to plasma.

### 3.2.4 The blood-aqueous barrier

The ciliary and the iridial epithelia constitute the epithelial part of the blood-aqueous barrier and protect the posterior chamber from circulating macromolecules. The other part of the barrier is constituted by the endothelium of the iris capillaries. The endothelial cells of iris capillaries are joined by tight junctions, making the capillaries non-fenestrated. This prevents movement of macromolecules from the lumen of the iris vessels into the stroma. Horseradish peroxidase does not pass through the walls of these vessels (Vegge, 1971).

### 3.3 Molecular entities involved in AH secretion

The molecules that are involved in AH secretion include transport proteins, enzymes and ion channels. Since the blood-ocular barriers are largely impermeable even to small water soluble substances, such as glucose and amino acids, important metabolic substrates have to be transported to the AH through these barriers by carrier-mediated transport systems. The carrier-mediated transport systems are specialized membrane proteins having the ability of transporting their substrates across the cell membrane either actively against their concentration gradient or passively along the electrochemical gradient. The ionic solutes, which are largely membrane impermeable, must also be transported either by different active or carrier mediated transport systems or by ion channels. Ion channels are specialized proteins spanning the cell membrane that constitute a pathway for movement of a specific ion or ions, e.g., $Na^+$ channel, $Ca^{++}$ channel, $Cl^-$ channel, $K^+$ channel, etc. When a particular ion channel opens it allows the ion to cross the membrane in the direction of its electrochemical gradient.

Intense research in the field of AH secretion over the last several decades has identified many transporter proteins/ion channels and their role in AH production. Most animals produce AH in a similar fashion, although some species differences exist, particularly in $Cl^-$ and $HCO_3^-$ secretion (Do and Civan, 2009). Three $\alpha$ subunits isoforms ($\alpha 1$, $\alpha 2$, $\alpha 3$) of the primary active transport system, Na,K-ATPase, have been shown to be expressed in the NPE (Ghosh et al., 1991; Shahidullah et al., 2007) with the $\alpha 1$ isoform in the PE (Ghosh et al., 1990). Na,K-ATPase is localized mainly along the basolateral infoldings and interdigitations of both the PE and NPE cells (Mori et al., 1991; Usukura et al., 1988) and higher activities were found on the NPE cells (Riley and Kishida, 1986; Usukura et al., 1988). The $Na^+$,$K^+$-ATPase of PE cells probably differs functionally from that of NPE cells as reflected by the different isoforms shown in these two cell types (Ghosh et al., 1991). Pharmacological inhibition of Na,K-ATPase by ouabain caused 62% inhibition of aqueous humor secretion in an arterially perfused bovine eye indicating the major role played by this primary active transport system (Shahidullah et al., 2003). Transport systems for glucose, several amino acids (DiMattio et al., 1981; Hu et al., 2011; Reddy, 1979) and ascorbate (Chu and Candia, 1988) have been identified in the NPE. Potassium channels, chloride channels, bicarbonate transporters and chloride-bicarbonate anion exchanger have also been identified and characterized in the NPE (Edelman et al., 1995; Shahidullah et al., 2009). PE has been shown to express important transport proteins, such as sodium bicarbonate co-transporter (Helbig et al., 1989a), $Cl^-/HCO_3^-$ exchange (Helbig et al., 1988a), $Na^+/H^+$ exchange (Helbig et al., 1988b). The $Na^+$-$K^+$-$2Cl^-$-cotransporter that transports $Na^+$, $K^+$ and $Cl^-$ into and out of cells in an electrically neutral manner, in most cases with a stoichiometry of 1 $Na^+$, 1 $K^+$ and 2 $Cl^-$ (Haas, 1994), has been shown to express at the basolateral membrane of bovine PE (Dunn et al., 2001). In addition functional evidence of this transporter has been identified in the NPE (Crook and Polansky, 1994; Dong and Delamere, 1994). We published immunohistochemical data showing two carbonic anhydrase isoforms (CA II and CAIV) (Fig. 8) enriched in the NPE layer but sparse or absent in the PE layer (Shahidullah et al., 2009). CA II was cytoplasmic but CA IV was localized to the NPE surface, CA II and IV also were abundant in cultured NPE. Carbonic anhydrase inhibitors (CAIs) are highly effective in reducing aqueous inflow. Interestingly, transport systems for glucose (Alm, 1984; Alm et al., 1981; Dollery et al., 1971), amino acids (Miller and Steinberg, 1976), lactate (Alm and Tornquist, 1985) and choline (Karlsson et al., 1984) have also been identified in the cells constituting the blood-retinal barrier.

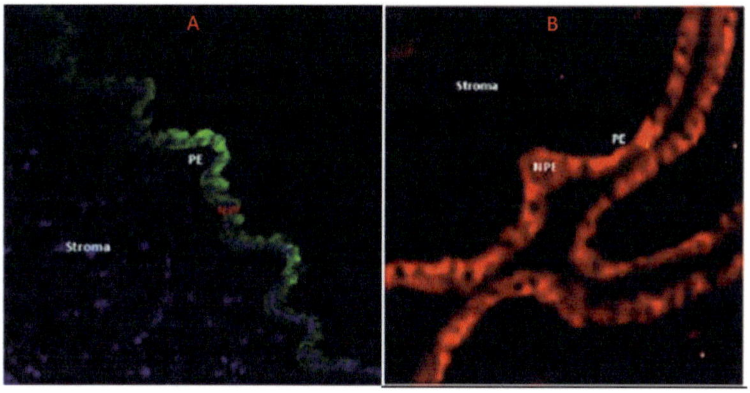


Fig. 8. Immuolocalization of CAII (A) and CAIV in porcine ciliary body (Shahidullah et al., 2009). Note that CAII is localized in the NPE cytoplasm and CAIV on the NPE membrane. (used with permission)

### 3.4 Mechanism of AH secretion

There is now general agreement that AH is produced by the double-layered CE. Three basic mechanisms, ultrafiltration, active transport and diffusion are involved, at one step or other, in the process of AH secretion. AH formation is a complex process and it can be subdivided into three steps:

1. In the first step, an ultrafiltrate is passed through the fenestrated capillaries of the ciliary processes into the ciliary stroma. Due to the fenestrated nature of the ciliary capillaries this ultrafiltrate contains a high percentage of plasma proteins. The capillary wall is a considerable barrier for some of the plasma proteins. Studies on the dynamics of extravascular plasma proteins in the ciliary processes indicate that the net filtrate from the capillaries contain about 4% of the albumin and 3% of the γ-globulin in the plasma (Bill, 1968a). The protein content in the ciliary stroma may be extremely high in some species, e.g. in rabbit it is about 75% of that in the plasma (Bill, 1968b). The high protein concentration in the ciliary stroma reduces the transcapillary difference in the oncotic pressure, which is important for filtration from the capillaries.
2. In the second step, a number of solutes are transported from the ultrafiltrate to the posterior chamber across the CE bilayer. This step is considered as the extraction of materials (electrolytes and other substances, such as glucose, amino acids, ascorbate, etc.) by the CE bilayer, against a concentration gradient, by means of diffusion, active or carrier-mediated secretion of solutes (Cole, 1977). Blood-borne large molecules, such as proteins cannot pass the blood-aqueous barrier (Green, 1984; Novack and Leopold, 1988). The ocular barriers are effective even with respect to low molecular weight solutes, such as sucrose and fluorescein (Bill, 1975).
3. In the third step the osmotic gradient established by the active transfer and accumulation of ions and other solutes into the posterior chamber (step 2) facilitates the passive flow of water into the posterior chamber by osmosis (Bill, 1975; Brubaker, 1991).

#### 3.4.1 Ions and solutes transport across the CE

Transfer of ions and solutes from the ciliary stroma to the posterior chamber requires that the solutes will pass across both the PE and NPE layers. There are still unanswered questions about the functions of each specific cell layers and their interactions. The presence of a large number of gap junctions between the PE and NPE suggests a coupling of these two layers in transepithelial transport (Coca-Prados et al., 1992; Helbig et al., 1989b; Wang et al., 2010). One of the characteristics of the CE is the asymmetric distribution of ion transporters on the membranes of PE and NPE cells, which is essential for mediating the vectorial ion and solute transport. Several models have been suggested for ion and solute movement (Avila et al., 2002; Civan and Macknight, 2004; Do and To, 2000; Jacob and Civan, 1996; To et al., 2002). No unified model has been proposed. However, the consensus is that there are at least three transport steps involved in transferring ion and/or solute across the CE:

1. Loading of ions and/or solutes from the ciliary stroma (blood) into the PE cells across its basolateral border
2. Translocation of ions and/or solutes through the gap junctions into the NPE cells
3. Shifting of ions and/or solutes from the NPE cells to the posterior chamber driven by an electrochemical gradient and/or by active or carrier-mediated transport.

Loading of major ions through the PE basolateral membrane has been proposed to occur through Na-K-2Cl cotransporter (Edelman et al., 1994; Kong et al., 2006), sodium bicarbonate cotransporter (Helbig et al., 1989a) and paired activity of $Na^+/H^+$ and $Cl^-/HCO_3^-$ antiports (Civan and Macknight, 2004; Counillon et al., 2000). Gap junctions both within each of PE and NPE and between PE and NPE layers allow free exchange of metabolites and ions and provide direct electrical coupling between these cells (Raviola and Raviola, 1978). In accordance, gap junction dye coupling between the two cell layers has been demonstrated using intra injection of the fluorescent dye, Lucifer yellow (Oh et al., 1994; Wang et al., 2010). In addition, the fact that there is no difference in membrane potential (Carre et al., 1992; Wiederholt and Zadunaisky, 1986) and intracellular ion contents (Bowler et al., 1996) between PE and NPE cells indicates that the gap junctions allow direct intercellular communication that facilitates the two cell layers functioning as a syncytium. Thus, active transport in AH secretion applies largely to NPE. Secretion by the NPE is accomplished by the active/carrier-and channel mediated transport of one or more ions, such as $Na^+$, $Cl^-$, $HCO_3^-$, and low molecular weight solutes, such as amino acids, glucose, inositol, ascorbic acid, etc. The concentration of ascorbic acid in the aqueous is about 20 times that in the plasma and there is evidence that it is transported actively to the AH (Becker, 1967; Chu and Candia, 1988). A schematic diagram of demonstrating the different junctions, transporters and pump located within the PE and NPE membrane is shown (Fig. 9)

## 4. Composition of the aqueous humor

AH has a unique composition that differs from plasma in several important aspects. Several laboratory studies confirm that AH is not simply a filtrate. It is an intraocular fluid, homeostatically controlled and some of which individual components are in rapid turnover. The AH is composed of ions ($Na^+$, $K^+$, $Ca^{2+}$, $Mg^{2+}$, $Cl^-$, $HCO_3^-$), crystalloid or low molecular weight substances (glucose, ascorbate, lactate, pyruvate, urea, H2O2, amino acids, etc.), colloidal or high molecular weight substances, such as proteins (Borazan et al., 2010; Browne et al., 2011; Ghanem et al., 2011; Lim et al., 2010), lipids (Jahn et al., 1983), biologically active substances (catecholamines, eicosanoids, hormones, etc.) as well as some miscellaneous substances such as hyaluronic acid, hyaluronidase, etc.). These components derive from a number of sources, the principal ones being the plasma (by passive diffusion) and the CE (by active secretion). Specific substances also enter the AH by diffusion or secretion from

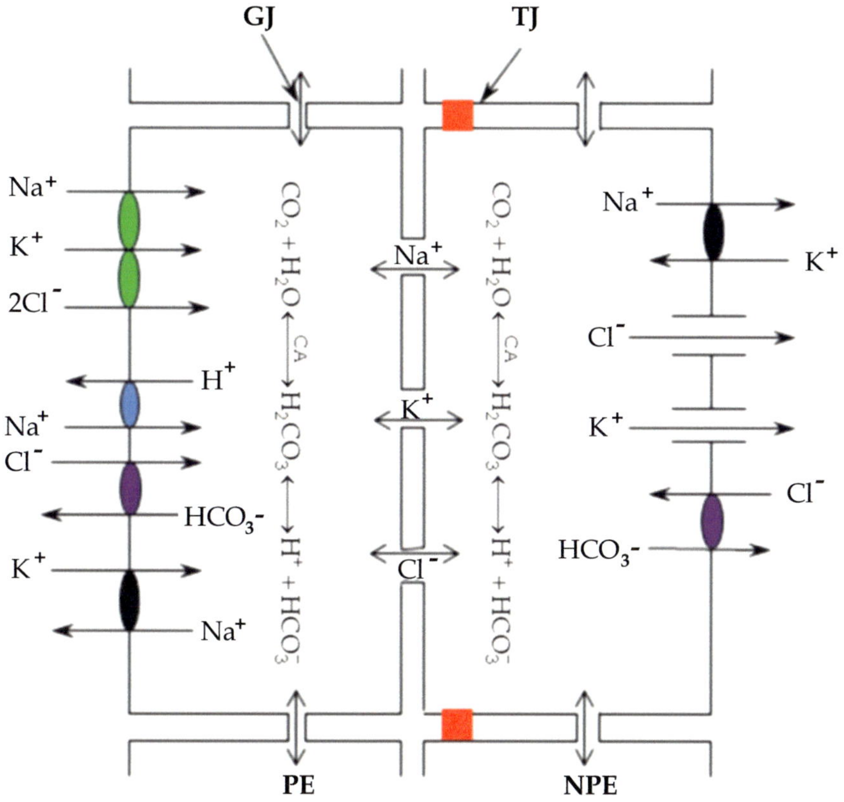


Fig. 9. Schematic diagram of a PE and NPE duplet showing locations of gap junctions, tight junctions, major transporters and ion channels on the membrane, together with the direction of transport of their substrates. PE, pigmented ciliary epithelium; NPE, nonpigmented ciliary epithelium; GJ, gap junction; TJ, tight junction. Note that the gap junctions between the PE and NPE as well as between each type of cells allow free passage of ions and other solutes (double-headed arrows)

surrounding tissues: corneal endothelium, crystalline lens, trabecular meshwork, iris and vitreous. These tissues utilize a number of nutrients present in the AH, e.g. the main source of glucose for the cornea and the lens is the AH. Thus, the composition of AH depends on the nature of the secreted fluid from the CE plus the subsequent passive and active exchange across adjacent tissues. The rate of turnover of AH also contributes to modulation of the composition by accumulating waste products from the surrounding tissues. Alterations of the AH occur continually. For example the lens alters the AH by using glucose, amino acids and other solutes and releasing metabolic wastes, such as lactic acid. It may also act as homeostatic reservoir for amino acids. The normal composition of AH reflects the normality of all the associated structures contributing in AH production and drainage.

The composition of AH can be modulated by many factors. The imbalances in the carefully tuned chemical composition of AH are thought to be both the cause and consequences of pathological conditions in the anterior segment. Biochemical analysis of AH has identified high molecular weight lens proteins as a cause of elevated IOP in phacolytic glaucoma, i.e., sudden onset of open-angle glaucoma caused by a leaking mature or hypermature (rarely immature) cataract (Epstein et al., 1978) and ascorbic acid concentration in AH differs in normal subjects and in Chronic Open Angle Glaucoma (COAG) patients (Lam and Lee, 1975). Several studies have shown that AH can promote proliferation of cells in tissue culture (Albrink and Wallace, 1951; Benezra and Sachs, 1974; Herschler et al., 1980; Herschler and Tucson, 1983) or inhibit cellular growth (Kornblueth and Tenenbaum, 1956). While these opposing findings may perhaps be explained by the different experimental conditions and procedures, the possibility of AH being a growth modulator is a real possibility since a number of growth factors are present in the AH (Borazan et al., 2010; Browne et al., 2011; Ghanem et al., 2011; Lim et al., 2010). AH may be thought of as a growth medium in which stimulatory agents and cytotoxic factors act to affect changes in cell number, morphology and function. Understanding the nature of these cell growth modulators and their functions may provide a clue to solving certain problems in glaucoma. It is possible that derangement of such a modulator system in the AH may lead to changes in the proliferative capacity, biosynthetic properties and ultimately the survival of the cells of the trabecular meshwork resulting in an increased resistance to outflow. Tables 1, 2 and 3 show normal concentration of some of the important components of AH and plasma.

| Components | Aqueous Humor ($ng.ml^{-1}$) | Plasma ($ng.ml^{-1}$) |
|---|---|---|
| Prostaglandins | 2 | — |
| Cyclic AMP | 8 | — |
| Catecholamines | | |
| Noradrenaline | [a]0.8 - 1.14 | 0.311 |
| Adrenaline | 0 - 0.13 | 0.097 |
| Dopamine | 0.12 | 0.037 |

Adapted from: (Cooper et al., 1984) ; [a](Trope and Rumley, 1985).

Table 1. Biologically active substances in AH and plasma

| Components | AH ($\mu g.ml^{-1}$) | Plasma ($\mu g.ml^{-1}$) |
|---|---|---|
| Protein (total) | [a]12.4 ± 2.0 | 7000 |
| Albumin | [b]5.5 - 6.5 | 3400 |
| Transferrin | [b]1.3 - 1.7 | — |
| Prealbumin | [b]0.3 - 0.4 | — |
| Fibronectin | [c]0.25 | 29 |
| Immunoglobulins | | |
| IgG | [c]3.0 | 1270 |
| IgE ($Iu.ml^{-1}$) | [c]<0.75 | 16 - 218 |

Sources: [a](Tripathi et al., 1989); [b](Inada et al., 1984); [c](Berman, 1991)

Table 2. Protein composition of AH in comparison to plasma

| Components | Aqueous Humor (mM) | Plasma (mM) |
|---|---|---|
| $Na^+$ | 142 | 130 - 145 |
| $K^+$ | 4 | 3.5 - 5.0 |
| $Ca^{2+}$ | 1.2 | 2.0 - 2.6 |
| $Mg^{2+}$ | 1 | 0.7 - 1.1 |
| $Cl^+$ | 131 | 92 - 125 |
| $HCO^{-3}$ | 20 | 24 - 30 |
| Ascorbate | 1.1 | 0.04 - 0.06 |
| Lactate | 4.5 | 0.5 - 0.8 |
| Citrate | 0.1 | 0.1 |
| Glucose | 2.7 - 3.9 | 5.6 - 6.4 |
| Urea | 4.1 | 3.3 - 6.5 |
| Glutathione | 0.001 - 0.01 | — |
| [a]$H_2O_2$ | 0.024 - 0.069 | — |
| [b]Amino acids (total) | 0.17 | 0.12 |

Adapted from: (Riley, 1983); [a](Spector and Garner, 1981); [b](Davson, 1969)

Table 3. Electrolytes and low molecular weight solutes in human AH and plasma

## 5. Regulation of AH secretion

The rate of AH flow varies according to a circadian rhythm with different rates of flow during day time and night (Koskela and Brubaker, 1991; McCannel et al., 1992; Reiss et al., 1984; Topper and Brubaker, 1985). In healthy human volunteers it has been shown that the night time seated rate of AH flow, fluorophotometric outflow and seated IOP was reduced by 49, 45 and 16% respectively (Liu et al., 2011). The night time flow rate can be increased by administration of exogenous epinephrine (Topper and Brubaker, 1985) but cannot be reduced by administration of timolol (McCannel et al., 1992; Topper and Brubaker, 1985) even though it can further be reduced by acetazolamide, a CA inhibitor (McCannel et al., 1992; Topper and Brubaker, 1985). These seminal findings indicate that the AH flow is under adrenergic control. Current opinion on the regulation of AH dynamics has been stated as follows: "the pharmacotherapy of glaucoma is based mainly on neuro-hormonal processes controlling aqueous humor dynamics. Systemic hormones as well as local hormones and autonomic nervous system mediators are involved in the processes of aqueous humor formation and drainage. Anti-glaucoma medications act mainly through activation or inhibition of these systems' receptors, assisting to decrease aqueous humor production or improve aqueous humor outflow" (Terelak-Borys and Liberek, 2007a; Terelak-Borys and Liberek, 2007b). The presence of β-adrenergic receptors in the ciliary process of rabbit (Bromberg et al., 1980), ox (Polansky et al., 1985) and human has been demonstrated (Wax and Molinoff, 1987). Other studies have revealed that the β-adrenergic receptors are predominantly β2-subtype (Crook and Riese, 1996; Elena et al., 1984; Nathanson, 1980; Wax and Molinoff, 1987). The administration of timolol, a β-adrenergic antagonist, either systemically or topically reduces AH formation and lowers IOP in normal human subjects (Coakes and Brubaker, 1978; Dailey et al., 1982; Katz et al., 1976) and animals (Shahidullah et al., 1995; Watanabe and Chiou, 1983). Clinical treatment of glaucoma has been most successfully directed towards reducing AH formation with β-blockers.

## 6. Drainage of aqueous humor

AH enters the posterior chamber from the ciliary process and flows around the lens and through the pupil into the anterior chamber (Fig. 1). From the anterior chamber AH leaves the eye and enters the general venous circulation by bulk flow by two exit pathways, both commencing at the anterior chamber angle (Johnson, 2005; Lei et al., 2011; Nilsson, 1997; Sihota, 2011).

### 6.1 The anterior, trabecular or conventional route

This pathway employs through the trabecular meshwork across the inner wall of Schlemm's Canal and then into collector channels, aqueous veins and the anterior ciliary veins. Schlemm's Canal, also known as Canal of Schlemm or the scleral venous sinus, is a circular channel. The canal is essentially an endothelium-lined circular space, resembling a lymphatic vessel and located at the limbus, i.e., the joining point of the cornea and sclera. The inner side of the canal is formed by 3 layers of the trabecular meshwork. The first layer is the uveal meshwork, which is the forward extension of the ciliary muscle inserting in the cornea (Bill and Svedbergh, 1972). The second layer is constituted by several sheets of connective tissue extending between the scleral spur and the peripheral cornea. The third layer, called the juxtacanalicular tissue, is an endothelial meshwork and the inner wall of Schlemm's Canal. It is composed of collagen and elastic fibers, a ground substance and several layers of endothelium enmeshed in a matrix of glycosaminoglycans, proteoglycans and other macromolecules. The major resistance site to outflow is thought to be at the juxtacanalicular tissue (also called cribriform plexus) and the inner wall of Schlemm's Canal.

### 6.2 The posterior, uveoscleral or unconventional route

The second pathway of AH outflow is the posterior, uveoscleral or unconventional route (Johnson, 2005; Nilsson, 1997). Aqueous flows from the chamber angle across the iris root and the anterior face of the ciliary muscle, through the connective tissue spaces between the muscle bundles of the ciliary body. These spaces open into the suprachoroid from which fluid can pass through the sclera or the perivascular spaces into the episcleral tissue and then into the venous circulation. The pressure in the suprachoroid space is lower than in the anterior chamber by at least a few mmHg under normal conditions, thus, favoring this flow. In primates most of the drainage occurs through the trabecular route and a small portion is drained via the uveoscleral route. A small part of the aqueous humor flows into the vitreous to be absorbed into the posterior part of the eye; some of the aqueous apparently is absorbed by the ciliary body (Moses, 1990). In lower animals the Canal of Schlemm is absent but they have a sinus structure with the same function (Bill, 1975). In human eyes, the uveoscleral outflow accounts for about 5 to 20 percent of total outflow (Bill, 1975; Bill and Phillips, 1971), while in monkey, the outflow is fairly equally distributed between the two routes (Bill, 1966a; Bill and Phillips, 1971). In rabbit and cat, there is comparatively little uveoscleral drainage (Bill, 1966b; Cole and Monro, 1976).

The flow of aqueous through the different compartments and outflow pathways is a typical hydraulic flow, where the source of energy is the pressure difference at the ends of the passage; the pressure at the upstream end is greater. The difference of upstream and downstream pressure is called pressure head ($\Delta P$). The rate of hydraulic flow is related to Poiseuille's law. It has been incorporated into the Goldman equation:

$$F = C\ (P - P_e) \text{ or } F = \Delta P.C$$

This equation relates aqueous flow (F) to facility of outflow (C) and $\Delta P$, the pressure head is the difference between IOP (P) and the episcleral venous pressure ($P_e$), i.e. the pressure in the vessels into which AH drains. The mean normal value for outflow facility in human is estimated to be 0.25 $\mu l.min^{-1}.mmHg^{-1}$ of the applied pressure (Davson, 1990)

## 7. The intraocular pressure

The intraocular pressure (IOP) is the hydrostatic pressure exerted by the AH. The mean normal IOP in man is about 15 mmHg with the highest and lowest accepted values of 21 mmHg and 10.5 mmHg respectively (Davson, 1990; Hurvitz et al., 1991). IOP can vary between species, individual and even between eyes of the same individual. This pressure is governed by several factors, such as the rate of secretion of AH, resistance to outflow (by at least 2 pathways) and episcleral venous pressure. Despite the fact that IOP is the most important risk factor of glaucoma and that control for IOP, either by pharmacological agents or by surgery, remains the only effective glaucoma treatment, our mechanistic understanding of IOP regulation in the eye is limited. Proper functioning of the outflow pathways plays an important role in the regulation of IOP. Some of the important factors, identified or proposed, include age, alterations of extracellular matrix, oxidative stress and abnormal function of certain genes.

## 8. Glaucoma

Glaucoma is a multi-factorial ocular disease/syndrome with characterised by progressive damage or degeneration to the optic nerve and visual field loss. Although increased intraocular pressure is usually present, patients with normal range IOP can also develop glaucoma. The definition published by the international consensus panel in 2002 has now been widely accepted (Foster et al., 2002; Quigley, 2011). It is defined as optic neuropathy characterized by damage to the optic nerve and visual field loss. The vision loss is progressive and irreversible and results from retinal ganglion cell (RGC) death. The disease progression is expressed by gradual deformation of the optic nerve head (optic disc), the site where ganglion cell axons exit the eye.

### 8.1 Classification of glaucoma

Currently, glaucoma is classified into primary and secondary. In primary glaucoma, the optic neuropathy is the consequence of primary defects in the circulating pathway of AH or within the neural retina or the ganglion cells themselves, i.e., a glaucoma not caused by another eye or medical condition. In secondary glaucoma, the optic neuropathy or glaucomatous symptoms occur due to some other ocular or systemic disease or defects.
Major types of primary glaucoma:

1. Primary open angle glaucoma (POAG)/chronic open angle glaucoma (COAG): Currently the idea that high IOP is the exclusive cause of optic neuropathy has been almost discarded, since in many patients optic neuropathy occurs at normal IOP (Foster et al., 2002; Quigley, 2011). POAG is now defined as significant optic nerve damage in an eye, which does not have evidence of angle closure on gonioscopy, and where there is no identifiable secondary cause. POAG is the most prevalent type of glaucoma.
2. Primary closed angle glaucoma (PCAG): Patients having narrow or closed anterior chamber angle associated with significant obstruction of trabecular meshwork and glaucomatous optic neuropathy. PCAG can be subdivided into subacute, acute, chronic, symptomatic or asymptomatic according to the nature and severity of the onset. The worldwide prevalence of PCAG is about one third of the rest (Quigley and Broman, 2006)

Secondary glaucoma may occur under many ocular or systemic conditions including:

1. Uveitis
2. Ocular trauma
3. Ocular neovascularization
4. Thyroid orbitopathy

In addition, there are several forms of congenital or hereditary glaucoma, which can be either primary or secondary. Moreover, there are cases where glaucomatous damage occurs without any increase in IOP, the so-called normal tension or low tension glaucoma.

### 8.2 Causes of glaucoma

Glaucoma is an age-related condition. There may be no single cause of glaucoma. Some important risk factors have so far been identified. Elevated intraocular pressure is the most important risk factor. Glaucoma is commonly, but not exclusively, associated with an increase in intraocular pressure (IOP) and optic nerve damage may be a response to chronically elevated IOP and mechanical deformation (Hernandez, 2000; Johnson et al., 1996). Treatments that lower IOP either delay or prevent progression of glaucoma (Leske et al., 2003). There is a correlation between IOP and the likelihood of development of glaucoma and its progression (Boland and Quigley, 2007). Other risk factors are age (Tschumper and Johnson, 1990); family history, ethnicity or genetic variation (Jiao et al., 2009; Rao et al., 2011); other ocular or systemic disease, such as myopia, uveitis, decreased corneal or choroidal thickness, thyroid abnormality, sleep apnea, migraine (Boland and Quigley, 2007; Foster et al., 2002); vacular factors (Yanagi et al., 2011) and others. Age plays an important role in the development of glaucoma. The phagocytosis of the trabecular meshwork is decreased or lost in older individual leading to accumulation of toxic molecules within the drainage channels causing interference with AH flow (Tschumper and Johnson, 1990).

### 8.3 Pathogenesis of glaucoma

The principal pathology of glaucoma is the atrophy of the optic nerve and visual field loss. The exact mechanism of death of ganglion cells is not known. There are a number of hypotheses on the mechanism of ganglion cell injury in glaucoma. One hypothesis is the compromised blood supply to the optic nerve due to mechanical compression exerted by high IOP. There is evidences that suggests tissue hypoxia in the retina may affect the survival ganglion cells (He et al., 2011; Tezel and Wax, 2004). Other hypothesis includes oxidative or nitrative stress, both at the level of trabecular meshwork (Sacca et al., 2007) and retinal ganglion cells (Aslan et al., 2008; Tezel, 2006); autoimmune reactions in which an individual's immune system facilitate somatic/axonal degeneration of retinal ganglion cells (Wax and Tezel, 2009); glutamate toxicity (Vorwerk et al., 1999); loss of neurotrophic factors (Pease et al., 2000), etc. However, a various combination of these factors may be involved.The glial cells in the optic nerve head region (lamina cribrosa cells) (Quill et al., 2011), and in particular the astrocytes, the principal glial cells, have been proposed to play an important role in the glaucomatous change in the extracellular matrix in around the ganglion cells (Hernandez, 2000; Hernandez et al., 2008). In primates, alterations in the expression of metalloproteinases (MMPs) and their inhibitors (TIMPs) occur in the optic nerve head of experimental glaucoma (Agapova et al., 2003a). These changes, which are likely to contribute to remodeling of the glaucomatous optic nerve head, are particularly prominent in the optic nerve head astrocytes (Agapova et al., 2001). Altered protein expression, such as MMP1 and MT1-MMP, was also reported in human glaucomatous optic nerve head astrocytes (Agapova et al., 2003b). In the CNS, injury or stress causes normally quiescent astrocytes to become reactive, displaying altered morphology and protein expression, most notably increased glial fibrillary acidic protein (GFAP) (Gadea et al., 2008). Astrocytes are known to respond to a number of different stresses including injury (Laird et al., 2008), endothelin-1 (He et al., 2007), oxygen-glucose deprivation (Gao et al., 2008) and it is possible that such stress factors cause astrocytes to become reactive.

### 8.4 Medical treatment of glaucoma

Although the history of medical treatments dates back to 1862, all the effective treatments were developed only in the last several decades (Realini, 2011). Until now, five major classes of drugs have been used. Some of these drugs reduce IOP by reducing the secretion of AH and others increasing the outflow. Some have a dual effect. All the preparations are available for topical use. Greater details of these drugs have been given in two recent reviews (Lee and Goldberg, 2011; Realini, 2011). The five classes of drugs are:

1. Adrenergic agonists: The two important drugs in this group are the $\alpha$-2 adrenergic receptor agonists apraclonidine and brimonidine. These two drugs are still available in the market and are used by many patients. Brimonidine is preferable to aprachlonidine because it is a more specific agonist to $\alpha$2 adrenoceptor. Brimonidine has been shown to produce initial reduction in AH secretion and in chronic administration an increase in uveoscleral outflow (Wax and Tezel, 2009). A neuroprotective effect of brimonidine has also been suggested (Wheeler et al., 2003). The use of brimonidine in children is contraindicated due to its systemic side effect and its use in adults is limited by its ocular side effects such as allergy (Rahman et al., 2010). The relatively specific $\alpha$2 adrenergic agonist, apraclonidine, is reported to reduce both AH formation and outflow resistance (Gharagozloo et al., 1988; Robin, 1988).
2. Beta-adrenergic antagonists: Important drugs in this group include timolol, levobunolol, metipranolol, cartiolol and betaxolol. These drugs works by reduce AH secretion (Brooks and Gillies, 1992; Dailey et al., 1982; Hurvitz et al., 1991; Shahidullah et al., 1995). Although these drugs have been largely replaced as first line therapy by prostaglandin analogs, they are still used in many cases. Timolol and metipranolol have been claimed to be neuroprotective (Wood et al., 2003).
3. Parasympathomimetics: Important drugs in this group include pilocarpine, carbachol and echothiphate iodide. Parasympathomimetics increase the outflow of aqueous

humor through the trabecular meshwork. They produce contraction of the iris sphincter and ciliary muscle, which opens the trabecular lamellae. Pilocarpine and carbachol interact directly with the muscarinic receptors of the ciliary muscle whereas echthiophate iodide interacts indirectly by inhibiting cholinesterase (Harris et al., 1973).

4. Carbonic anhydrase inhibitors: Carbonic anhydrase (CA) inhibitors reduce AH secretion rate (Larsson and Alm, 1998; Maren, 2000; Maren and Conroy, 1993; Maus et al., 1997; Vanlandingham et al., 1998; Wang et al., 1991). Acetazolamide was the first systemic CA inhibitors appeared in the early 50's. Useful topical CA inhibitors used extensively in the past and are still in use includes dorzolamide (marketed as Trusopt by Merck) and brinzolamide (marketed as Azopt by Alcon Laboratories). CA inhibitors are very effective drugs in reducing AH secretion but their mechanism is poorly understood. CA inhibitors reduce the availability of substrate ($HCO_3^-$) for anion exchanger-2 (AE2)-mediated blood-to-aqueous bicarbonate transport. Acetazolamide reduces the rate of blood-to-aqueous $^{14}C$-labelled bicarbonate movement (Zimmerman et al., 1976). This is in accordance with their ability to reduce AH formation in dogs (Maren, 1976) and rabbits (Caprioli and Sears, 1984; Kodama et al., 1985), species in which the CE concentrates bicarbonate from blood to aqueous and the AH is bicarbonate-rich. Curiously, however, the CAIs reduce aqueous formation equally efficiently in eyes where the concentration of bicarbonate in plasma and aqueous is similar in human (Dailey et al., 1982; Toris et al., 2004), monkey (Wang et al., 1991), bovine (Shahidullah et al., 2003) and pig (Shahidullah et al., 2009). There is no apparent net bicarbonate movement across the CE in these species, yet the CAIs reduce fluid formation. Thus, the mechanism of CAI is still unknown.
5. Prostaglandins: Prostaglandin F2α analogs are the newest class of drugs and are most effective drugs discovered so far. Among the available drugs in this group, the most effective ones include latanoprost (marketed as Xalatan by Pharmacia in 1996, later acquired by Pfizer), travoprost (Travatan, Alcon) and bimatoprost (Lumigan, Allergan). The effects on IOP and AH dynamics of these drugs are similar. They consistently produce substantial increase uveoscleral outflow and a less consistent finding is an increase in trabecular outflow (Toris et al., 2008).

## 9. Conclusion and future direction

The principal pathological lesion in glaucoma is the degeneration of ganglion cell axons and eventually the ganglion cell bodies. The proven treatments available are effective only in lowering the IOP, one of the most important risk factors of glaucoma. However, glaucoma damage also presents in patients displaying normal IOP (low tension or normal tension glaucoma). It must be recognized that IOP lowering drugs are not curative, even though they delay or in some cases prevent progression of the disease. Thus, future research should be directed towards exploring the exact causes of optic nerve damage or ganglion cell death. Recent studies have suggested some role of the glial cells, such as, lamina cribrosa cells (Quill et al., 2011) and astrocytes (Hernandez, 2000; Hernandez et al., 2008), in the remodeling of the extracellular matrix in the optic nerve head. How these cells and remodeling of the region plays role in causing ganglion cell death is unclear. Better mechanistic understanding of the optic nerve damage and ganglion cell death is crucial to development of curative treatment of glaucoma based on neuroregeneration rather than neuroprotection.

## 10. References

Agapova OA, Kaufman PL, Lucarelli MJ, Gabelt BAT, Hernandez MR. 2003a. Differential expression of matrix metalloproteinases in monkey eyes with experimental glaucoma or optic nerve transection. Brain Research 967(1-2):132-143.

Agapova OA, Ricard C, S. , Salvador-Silva M, Hernandez MR. 2001. Expression of matrix metalloproteinases and tissue inhibitors of metalloproteinases in human optic nerve head astrocytes. Glia 33(3):205-216.

Agapova OA, Yang P, Wang WH, Lane DA, Clark AF, Weinstein BI, Hernandez MR. 2003b. Altered expression of 3 alpha-hydroxysteroid dehydrogenases in human glaucomatous optic nerve head astrocytes. Neurobiology of Disease 14(1):63-73.

Alm A. 1984. Kinetics of glucose transport across the blood-retinal barrier. Investigative Ophthalmology & Visual Science 25(4):491-493.

Alm A., Tornquist P. 1985. Lactate transport through the blood-retinal and the blood-brain barrier in rats. Ophthalmic Research 17(3):181-184.

Alm A., Tornquist P, Maepea O. 1981. The uptake index method applied to studies on the blood-retinal barrier. II. Transport of several hexoses by a common carrier. Acta Physiologica Scandinavica 113(1):81-84.

Aslan M, Cort A, Yucel I. 2008. Oxidative and nitrative stress markers in glaucoma. Free Radical Biology & Medicine 45(4):367-376.

Avila MY, Seidler RW, Stone RA, Civan MM. 2002. Inhibitors of NHE-1 Na+/H+ exchange reduce mouse intraocular pressure. Investigative Ophthalmology & Visual Science 43(6):1897-1902.

Becker B. 1967. Ascorbate transfer in guinea pig eyes. Invest Ophthalmol Vis Sci 6:410.

Berman ER. 1991. Aqueous, Iris-ciliary Body and Trabeculum: In Biochemistry of the Eye. New York, London: Plenum. 151-200 p.

Bill A. 1966a. Conventional and uveo-scleral drainage of aqueous humour in the cynomolgus monkey (Macaca irus) at normal and high intraocular pressures. Experimental Eye Research 5(1):45-54.

Bill A. 1966b. The routes for bulk drainage of aqueous humour in rabbits with and without cyclodialysis. Documenta Ophthalmologica 20(4):157-169.

Bill A. 1968a. Capillary permeability to and extravascular dynamics of myoglobin, albumin and gammaglobulin in the uvea. Acta Physiologica Scandinavica 73(1):204-219.

Bill A. 1968b. A method to determine osmotically effective albumin and gammaglobulin concentrations in tissue fluids, its application to the uvea and a note on the effects of capillary "leaks" on tissue fluid dynamics. Acta Physiologica Scandinavica 73(4):511-522.

Bill A. 1975. Blood circulation and fluid dynamics in the eye. Physiological Reviews 55(3):383-417.

Bill A., Phillips CI. 1971. Uveoscleral drainage of aqueous humour in human eyes. Experimental Eye Research 12(3):275-281.

Bill A., Svedbergh B. 1972. Scanning electron microscopic studies of the trabecular meshwork and the canal of Schlemm--an attempt to localize the main resistance to outflow of aqueous humor in man. Acta Ophthalmologica 50(3):295-320.

Boland MV, Quigley HA. 2007. Risk factors and open-angle glaucoma: classification and application. Journal of Glaucoma 16(4):406-418.

Borazan M, Karalezli A, Kucukerdonmez C, Bayraktar N, Kulaksizoglu S, Akman A, Akova YA. 2010. Aqueous humor and plasma levels of vascular endothelial growth factor and nitric oxide in patients with pseudoexfoliation syndrome and pseudoexfoliation glaucoma. Journal of Glaucoma 19(3):207-211.

Bowler JM, Peart D, Purves RD, Carre DA, Macknight AD, Civan MM. 1996. Electron probe X-ray microanalysis of rabbit ciliary epithelium. Experimental Eye Research 62(2):131-139.

Bromberg BB, Gregory DS, Sears ML. 1980. Beta-adrenergic receptors in ciliary processes of the rabbit. Investigative Ophthalmology & Visual Science 19(2):203-207.

Bron AJ, Tripathi RC, Tripathi BJ, editors. 1997. Wolff's Anatomy of the Eye and Orbit. Eight ed. London, Whwinheim, New York, Tokyo, Melbourne, Madras: Chapman and Hall Medical. 736 p.

Brooks AM, Gillies WE. 1992. Ocular beta-blockers in glaucoma management. Clinical pharmacological aspects. Drugs & Aging 2(3):208-221.

Browne JG, Ho SL, Kane R, Oliver N, Clark AF, O'Brien CJ, Crean JK. 2011. Connective tissue growth factor is increased in pseudoexfoliation glaucoma. Investigative Ophthalmology & Visual Science 52(6):3660-3666.

Brubaker RF. 1991. Flow of aqueous humor in humans [The Friedenwald Lecture]. Investigative Ophthalmology & Visual Science 32(13):3145-3166.

Caprioli J, Sears M. 1984. Combined effect of forskolin and acetazolamide on intraocular pressure and aqueous flow in rabbit eyes. Experimental Eye Research 39(1):47-50.

Carre DA, Tang CS, Krupin T, Civan MM. 1992. Effect of bicarbonate on intracellular potential of rabbit ciliary epithelium. Current Eye Research 11(7):609-624.

Chen H-B, Yamabayashi S, Ou BO, Tsukahara S. 1996. Morphological Changes in Rabbit Ciliary Epithelium and Blood-Aqueous Barriers after Intravitreal 10-5Endothelin-1. Experimental Eye Research 62(6):605-612.

Chu TC, Candia OA. 1988. Active transport of ascorbate across the isolated rabbit ciliary epithelium. Investigative Ophthalmology & Visual Science 29(4):594-599.

Civan MM. 1998. Transport components of net secretion of the aqueous humour and their integrated regulation. The Eye's Aqueous Humor: From secretion to glaucoma. San Diego, London, Boston, New York, Sydney, Tokyo, Toronto: Academic Press. p 1-24.

Civan MM, Macknight AD. 2004. The ins and outs of aqueous humour secretion. Experimental Eye Research 78(3):625-631.

Coakes RL, Brubaker RF. 1978. The mechanism of timolol in lowering intraocular pressure. In the normal eye. Archives of Ophthalmology 96(11):2045-2048.

Coca-Prados M, Ghosh S, Gilula NB, Kumar NM. 1992. Expression and cellular distribution of the alpha 1 gap junction gene product in the ocular pigmented ciliary epithelium. Current Eye Research 11(2):113-122.

Cole DF. 1977. Secretion of the aqueous humour. Experimental Eye Research 25 Suppl:161-176.

Cole DF, Monro PA. 1976. The use of fluorescein-labelled dextrans in investigation of aqueous humour outflow in the rabbit. Experimental Eye Research 23(6):571-585.

Cooper RL, Constable IJ, Davidson L. 1984. Catecholamines in aqueous humour of glaucoma patients. Australian Journal of Ophthalmology 12(4):345-349.

Counillon L, Touret N, Bidet M, Peterson-Yantorno K, Coca-Prados M, Stuart-Tilley A, Wilhelm S, Alper SL, Civan MM. 2000. Na+/H+ and Cl-/HCO3-antiporters of bovine pigmented ciliary epithelial cells. Pflugers Archiv - European Journal of Physiology 440(5):667-678.

Crook RB, Riese K. 1996. Beta-adrenergic stimulation of Na+, K+, Cl- cotransport in fetal nonpigmented ciliary epithelial cells. Investigative Ophthalmology & Visual Science 37(6):1047-1057.

Cunha-Vaz J. 1979. The blood-ocular barriers. Survey of Ophthalmology 23(5):279-296.

Dailey RA, Brubaker RF, Bourne WM. 1982. The effects of timolol maleate and acetazolamide on the rate of aqueous formation in normal human subjects. American Journal of Ophthalmology 93(2):232-237.

Davson H. 1969. The intraocular fluids. Davson H, editor. London: Academic press. 67-72 p.

Davson H. 1990. Physiology of the Eye. New york, Oxford, Beijing, Frankfurt, Sao Paulo, Sydney, Tokyo, Toronto: Pergamon Press. 3-95 p.

DiMattio J, Altszuler N, Ellis S, Zadunaisky JA. 1981. Glucose transport across ocular barriers of the streptozotocin-diabetic rat. Diabetes 30(11):903-906.

Do CW, Civan MM. 2009. Species variation in biology and physiology of the ciliary epithelium: similarities and differences. Experimental Eye Research 88(4):631-640.

Do CW, To CH. 2000. Chloride secretion by bovine ciliary epithelium: a model of aqueous humor formation. Investigative Ophthalmology & Visual Science 41(7):1853-1860.

Dollery CT, Henkind P, Orme ML. 1971. Assimilation of D and L I-C-14 glucose into the retina, brain and other tissues. Diabetes 20(8):519-521.

Duke-Elder WS. 1926. The ocular circulation: Its normal pressure relationships and their physiological significance. British Journal of Ophthalmology 10(10):513-572.

Dunn JJ, Lytle C, Crook RB. 2001. Immunolocalization of the Na-K-Cl cotransporter in bovine ciliary epithelium. Investigative Ophthalmology & Visual Science 42(2):343-353.

Edelman JL, Loo DD, Sachs G. 1995. Characterization of potassium and chloride channels in the basolateral membrane of bovine nonpigmented ciliary epithelial cells
Investigative Ophthalmology & Visual Science 36(13):2706-2716.

Edelman JL, Sachs G, Adorante JS. 1994. Ion transport asymmetry and functional coupling in bovine pigmented and nonpigmented ciliary epithelial cells. American Journal of Physiology 266(5 Pt 1):C1210-1221.

Elena PP, Fredj-Reygrobellet D, Moulin G, Lapalus P. 1984. Pharmacological characteristics of beta-adrenergic-sensitive adenylate cyclase in non pigmented and in pigmented cells of bovine ciliary process. Current Eye Research 3(12):1383-1389.

Epstein DL, Jedziniak JA, Grant WM. 1978. Identification of heavy-molecular-weight soluble protein in aqueous humor in human phacolytic glaucoma. Investigative Ophthalmology & Visual Science 17(5):398-402.

Forrester J, Dick A, McMenamin P, Lee W. 1996. The Eye: Basic Sciences in Practice. London, Philadelphia, Toronto, Sydney, Tokyo: WB Saunders. 13 p.

Foster PJ, Buhrmann R, Quigley HA, Johnson GJ. 2002. The definition and classification of glaucoma in prevalence surveys. British Journal of Ophthalmology 86(2):238-242.

Freddo TF. 2001. Shifting the paradigm of the blood-aqueous barrier. Experimental Eye Research 73(5):581-592.

Freddo TF, Bartels SP, Barsotti MF, Kamm RD. 1990. The source of proteins in the aqueous humor of the normal rabbit. Investigative Ophthalmology & Visual Science 31(1):125-137.

Gadea A, Schinelli S, Gallo V. 2008. Endothelin-1 Regulates Astrocyte Proliferation and Reactive Gliosis via a JNK/c-Jun Signaling Pathway. J Neurosci 28(10):2394-2408.

Gao Q, Li Y, Shen L, Zhang J, Zheng X, Qu R, Liu Z, Chopp M. 2008. Bone marrow stromal cells reduce ischemia-induced astrocytic activation in vitro. Neuroscience 152(3):646-655.

Ghanem AA, Arafa LF, El-Baz A. 2011. Connective tissue growth factor and tissue inhibitor of matrix metalloproteinase-2 in patients with exfoliative glaucoma. Current Eye Research 36(6):540-545.

Gharagozloo NZ, Relf SJ, Brubaker RF. 1988. Aqueous flow is reduced by the alpha-adrenergic agonist, apraclonidine hydrochloride (ALO 2145). Ophthalmology 95(9):1217-1220.

Ghosh S, Freitag AC, Martin-Vasallo P, Coca-Prados M. 1990. Cellular distribution and differential gene expression of the three alpha subunit isoforms of the Na,K-ATPase in the ocular ciliary epithelium. Journal of Biological Chemistry 265(5):2935-29340.

Ghosh S, Hernando N, Martin-Alonso JM, Martin-Vasallo P, Coca-Prados M. 1991. Expression of multiple Na+,K(+)-ATPase genes reveals a gradient of isoforms along the nonpigmented ciliary epithelium: functional implications in aqueous humor secretion. Journal of Cellular Physiology 149(2):184-194.

Gilula NB, Reeves OR, Steinbach A. 1972. Metabolic coupling, ionic coupling and cell contacts. Nature 235(5336):262-265.

Gloor BP. 1987. "The Vitreous," Adler's Physiology of the Eye. Moses RA, Hart WM, editors. Saint Louis: The C. V. Mosby Co. 246-267 p.

Green K. 1984. Physiology and pharmacology of aqueous humor inflow. Survey of Ophthalmology 29(3):208-214.

Haas M. 1994. The Na-K-Cl cotransporters. American Journal of Physiology 267(4 Pt 1):C869-885.

Harris LS, Shimmyo M, Mittag TW. 1973. Cholinesterases and contractility of cat irides. Effect of echothiophate iodide. Archives of Ophthalmology 89(1):49-51.

He S, Prasanna G, Yorio T. 2007. Endothelin-1-Mediated Signaling in the Expression of Matrix Metalloproteinases and Tissue Inhibitors of Metalloproteinases in Astrocytes. Invest Ophthalmol Vis Sci 48(8):3737-3745.

He Z, Vingrys AJ, Armitage JA, Bui BV. 2011. The role of blood pressure in glaucoma. Clinical & Experimental Optometry 94(2):133-149.

Helbig H, Korbmacher C, Kuhner D, Berweck S, Wiederholt M. 1988a. Characterization of Cl-/HCO3- exchange in cultured bovine pigmented ciliary epithelium.[erratum appears in Exp Eye Res 1989 Feb;48(2):319]. Experimental Eye Research 47(4):515-523.

Helbig H, Korbmacher C, Nawrath M, Erb C, Wiederholt M. 1989a. Sodium bicarbonate cotransport in cultured pigmented ciliary epithelial cells. Current Eye Research 8(6):595-598.

Helbig H, Korbmacher C, Stumpff F, Coca-Prados M, Wiederholt M. 1988b. Na+/H+ exchange regulates intracellular pH in a cell clone derived from bovine pigmented ciliary epithelium. Journal of Cellular Physiology 137(2):384-389.

Helbig H, Korbmacher C, Wohlfarth J, Coca-Prados M, Wiederholt M. 1989b. Electrical membrane properties of a cell clone derived from human nonpigmented ciliary epithelium. Investigative Ophthalmology & Visual Science 30(5):882-889.

Hernandez MR. 2000. The optic nerve head in glaucoma: role of astrocytes in tissue remodeling. Progress in Retinal and Eye Research 19(3):297-321.

Hernandez MR, Miao H, Lukas T. 2008. Astrocytes in glaucomatous optic neuropathy. Progress in Brain Research 173:353-373.

Hu RG, Lim JC, Kalloniatis M, Donaldson PJ. 2011. Cellular localization of glutamate and glutamine metabolism and transport pathways in the rat ciliary epithelium. Investigative Ophthalmology & Visual Science 52(6):3345-3353.

Hurvitz LM, Kaufman PL, Robin AL, Weinreb RN, Crawford K, Shaw B. 1991. New developments in the drug treatment of glaucoma. Drugs 41(4):514-532.

Inada K, Baba H, Okamura R. 1984. Quantitative determination of human aqueous proteins by crossed immunoelectrophoresis. Japanese Journal of Ophthalmology 28(1):1-8.

Jacob TJ, Civan MM. 1996. Role of ion channels in aqueous humor formation. American Journal of Physiology 271(3 Pt 1):C703-720.

Jahn CE, Leiss O, von Bergmann K. 1983. Lipid composition of human aqueous humor. Ophthalmic Research 15(4):220-224.

Jiao X, Yang Z, Yang X, Chen Y, Tong Z, Zhao C, Zeng J, Chen H, Gibbs D, Sun X, Li B, Wakins WS, Meyer C, Wang X, Kasuga D, Bedell M, Pearson E, Weinreb RN, Leske MC, Hennis A, DeWan A, Nemesure B, Jorde LB, Hoh J, Hejtmancik JF, Zhang K. 2009. Common variants on chromosome 2 and risk of primary open-angle glaucoma in the Afro-Caribbean population of Barbados. Proceedings of the National Academy of Sciences of the United States of America 106(40):17105-17110.

Johnson DH. 2005. Trabecular meshwork and uveoscleral outflow models. Journal of Glaucoma 14(4):308-310.

Johnson EC, Morrison JC, Farrell S, Deppmeier L, Moore CG, McGinty MR. 1996. The Effect of Chronically Elevated Intraocular Pressure on the Rat Optic Nerve Head Extracellular Matrix. Experimental Eye Research 62(6):663-674.

Karlsson C, Maepea O, Alm A. 1984. Choline transport through the blood-retinal and the blood-brain barrier in vivo. Acta Ophthalmologica 62(5):763-766.

Katz IM, Hubbard WA, Getson AJ, Gould AL. 1976. Intraocular pressure decrease in normal volunteers following timolol ophthalmic solution. Investigative Ophthalmology 15(6):489-492.

Kodama T, Reddy VN, Macri FJ. 1985. Pharmacological study on the effects of some ocular hypotensive drugs on aqueous humor formation in the arterially perfused enucleated rabbit eye. Ophthalmic Research 17(2):120-124.

Kondo RP, Wang S-Y, John SA, Weiss JN, Goldhaber JI. 2000. Metabolic Inhibition Activates a Non-selective Current Through Connexin Hemichannels in Isolated Ventricular Myocytes. Journal of Molecular and Cellular Cardiology 32(10):1859-1872.

Kong C-W, Li K-K, To C-H. 2006. Chloride secretion by porcine ciliary epithelium: New insight into species similarities and differences in aqueous humor formation. Investigative Ophthalmology & Visual Science 47(12):5428-5436.

Koskela T, Brubaker RF. 1991. The nocturnal suppression of aqueous humor flow in humans is not blocked by bright light. Investigative Ophthalmology & Visual Science 32(9):2504-2506.

Laird MD, Vender JR, Dhandapani KM. 2008. Opposing roles for reactive astrocytes following traumatic brain injury. NeuroSignals 16(2-3):154-164.

Lam KW, Lee PF. 1975. Analysis of ascorbate concentration in the aqueous humor by high-pressure liquid chromatography. Investigative Ophthalmology 14(12):947-950.

Larsson LI, Alm A. 1998. Aqueous humor flow in human eyes treated with dorzolamide and different doses of acetazolamide. Archives of Ophthalmology 116(1):19-24.

Lee AJ, Goldberg I. 2011. Emerging drugs for ocular hypertension. Expert Opinion on Emerging Drugs 16(1):137-161.

Lei Y, Overby DR, Boussommier-Calleja A, Stamer WD, Ethier CR. 2011. Outflow physiology of the mouse eye: pressure dependence and washout. Investigative Ophthalmology & Visual Science 52(3):1865-1871.

Leone G, Consumi M, Aggravi M, Donati A, Lamponi S, Magnani A. 2010. PVA/STMP based hydrogels as potential substitutes of human vitreous. Journal of Materials Science: Materials in Medicine 21(8):2491-2500.

Leske MC, Heijl A, Hussein M, Bengtsson B, Hyman L, Komaroff E, Early Manifest Glaucoma Trial G. 2003. Factors for glaucoma progression and the effect of treatment: the early manifest glaucoma trial. Archives of Ophthalmology 121(1):48-56.

Lim JW, Kim MU, Shin M-C. 2010. Aqueous humor and plasma levels of vascular endothelial growth factor and interleukin-8 in patients with central serous chorioretinopathy. Retina 30(9):1465-1471.

Liu H, Fan S, Gulati V, Camras LJ, Zhan G, Ghate D, Camras CB, Toris CB. 2011. Aqueous humor dynamics during the day and night in healthy mature volunteers. Archives of Ophthalmology 129(3):269-275.

Maren TH. 1976. The rates of movement of Na+, Cl-, and HCO-3 from plasma to posterior chamber: effect of acetazolamide and relation to the treatment of glaucoma. Investigative Ophthalmology 15(5):356-364.

Maren TH. 2000. Carbonic anhydrase inhibition in ophthalmology: aqueous humor secretion and the development of sulfonamide inhibitors. EXS(90):425-435.

Maren TH, Conroy CW. 1993. A new class of carbonic anhydrase inhibitor. Journal of Biological Chemistry 268(35):26233-26239.

Maus TL, Larsson LI, McLaren JW, Brubaker RF. 1997. Comparison of dorzolamide and acetazolamide as suppressors of aqueous humor flow in humans. Archives of Ophthalmology 115(1):45-49.

McCannel CA, Heinrich SR, Brubaker RF. 1992. Acetazolamide but not timolol lowers aqueous humor flow in sleeping humans. Graefes Archive for Clinical & Experimental Ophthalmology 230(6):518-520.

McLaughlin CW, Zellhuber-McMillan S, Macknight ADC, Civan MM. 2007. Electron microprobe analysis of rabbit ciliary epithelium indicates enhanced secretion posteriorly and enhanced absorption anteriorly. Am J Physiol Cell Physiol 293(5):C1455-1466.

Miller S, Steinberg RH. 1976. Transport of taurine, L-methionine and 3-o-methyl-D-glucose across frog retinal pigment epithelium. Experimental Eye Research 23(2):177-189.

Mori N, Yamada E, Sears ML. 1991. Immunocytochemical localization of Na/K-ATPase in the isolated ciliary epithelial bilayer of the rabbit. Archives of Histology & Cytology 54(3):259-265.

Moses RA. 1990. Intraocular pressure. Adler's Physiology of the Eye. p 223-245.
Nathanson JA. 1980. Adrenergic regulation of intraocular pressure: identification of beta 2-adrenergic-stimulated adenylate cyclase in ciliary process epithelium. Proceedings of the National Academy of Sciences of the United States of America 77(12):7420-7424.
Nilsson SF. 1997. The uveoscleral outflow routes. Eye 11(Pt 2):149-154.
Novack GD, Leopold IH. 1988. The blood-aqueous and blood-brain barriers to permeability. American Journal of Ophthalmology 105(4):412-416.
Oh J, Krupin T, Tang LQ, Sveen J, Lahlum RA. 1994. Dye coupling of rabbit ciliary epithelial cells in vitro. Investigative Ophthalmology & Visual Science 35(5):2509-2514.
Pappas GD, Smelter GK. 1958. Studies on the ciliary epithelium and zonule. Am J Ophthalmology 46:299-318.
Pappas GD, Smelter GK. 1961. The fine structure of the ciliary epithelium in relation to aqueous humor secretion. In the Structure of the Eye. Smelter GK, editor. New York: Academic Press. 453-467 p.
Pease ME, McKinnon SJ, Quigley HA, Kerrigan-Baumrind LA, Zack DJ. 2000. Obstructed axonal transport of BDNF and its receptor TrkB in experimental glaucoma. Investigative Ophthalmology & Visual Science 41(3):764-774.
Peyman GA, Apple D. 1972. Peroxidase diffusion processes in the optic nerve. Archives of Ophthalmology 88(6):650-654.
Peyman GA, Bok D. 1972. Peroxidase diffusion in the normal and laser-coagulated primate retina. Investigative Ophthalmology 11(1):35-45.
Polansky JR, Zlock D, Brasier A, Bloom E. 1985. Adrenergic and cholinergic receptors in isolated non-pigmented ciliary epithelial cells. Current Eye Research 4(4):517-522.
Prince JH, Diesem CD, Eglitis I, Ruskell GL. 1960. Cattle. In "Anatomy and Hiostology of the Eye and Orbit in Domestic Animals." Illianois: Thomas Springfield. 171-175 p.
Quigley HA. 2011. Glaucoma. Lancet 377(9774):1367-1377.
Quigley HA, Broman AT. 2006. The number of people with glaucoma worldwide in 2010 and 2020. British Journal of Ophthalmology 90(3):262-267.
Quill B, Docherty NG, Clark AF, O'Brien CJ. 2011. The effect of graded cyclic stretching on extracellular matrix-related gene expression profiles in cultured primary human lamina cribrosa cells. Investigative Ophthalmology & Visual Science 52(3):1908-1915.
Rahman MQ, Ramaesh K, Montgomery DMI. 2010. Brimonidine for glaucoma. Expert Opinion on Drug Safety 9(3):483-491.
Rao KN, Nagireddy S, Chakrabarti S. 2011. Complex genetic mechanisms in glaucoma: an overview. Indian Journal of Ophthalmology 59 Suppl:S31-42.
Raviola G. 1977. The structural basis of the blood-ocular barriers. Experimental Eye Research 25 Suppl:27-63.
Raviola G, Raviola E. 1978. Intercellular junctions in the ciliary epithelium. Investigative Ophthalmology & Visual Science 17(10):958-981.
Realini T. 2011. A history of glaucoma pharmacology. Optometry & Vision Science 88(1):36-38.
Reddy VN. 1979. Dynamics of transport systems in the eye. Friedenwald Lecture. Investigative Ophthalmology & Visual Science 18(10):1000-1018.
Redslob E. 1932. Le Corps Vitre. Paris: Masson & Cie. pp218-306 p.

Reiss GR, Lee DA, Topper JE, Brubaker RF. 1984. Aqueous humor flow during sleep. Investigative Ophthalmology & Visual Science 25(6):776-778.

Riley MV. 1983. The Chemistry of aqueous humor. In: Anderson RE, editor. Biochemistry of the Eye. Sanfrancisco: American Academy of Ophthalmology. p 79-95.

Riley MV, Kishida K. 1986. ATPases of ciliary epithelium: cellular and subcellular distribution and probable role in secretion of aqueous humor. Experimental Eye Research 42(6):559-568.

Robin AL. 1988. Short-term effects of unilateral 1% apraclonidine therapy. Archives of Ophthalmology 106(7):912-915.

Sacca SC, Izzotti A, Rossi P, Traverso C. 2007. Glaucomatous outflow pathway and oxidative stress. Experimental Eye Research 84(3):389-399.

Saez JC, Berthound VM, Moreno AP, Spray DC. 1993. Gap junctions: mulplicity of controls in differentiated and undiffrentiated cells and possible functional implications. . In: Shenolikar S, Nairn AC, editors. Advances in Cyclic Nucleotide and Phosphoprotein Res Vol 27. New York: Raven Press. p 163-198.

Scemes E, Suadicani SO, Dahl G, Spray DC. 2007. Connexin and pannexin mediated cell-cell communication. Neuron GLIA Biology 3(3):199-208.

Shahidullah M, Tamiya S, Delamere NA. 2007. Primary culture of porcine nonpigmented ciliary epithelium. Current Eye Research 32(6):511-522.

Shahidullah M, To C-H, Pelis RM, Delamere NA. 2009. Studies on bicarbonate transporters and carbonic anhydrase in porcine nonpigmented ciliary epithelium. Investigative Ophthalmology & Visual Science 50(4):1791-1800.

Shahidullah M, Wilson WS, Millar C. 1995. Effects of timolol, terbutaline and forskolin on IOP, aqueous humour formation and ciliary cyclic AMP levels in the bovine eye. Current Eye Research 14(7):519-528.

Shahidullah M, Wilson WS, Yap M, To CH. 2003. Effects of ion transport and channel-blocking drugs on aqueous humor formation in isolated bovine eye. Investigative Ophthalmology & Visual Science 44(3):1185-1191.

Sihota R. 2011. Classification of primary angle closure disease. Current Opinion in Ophthalmology 22(2):87-95.

Smelser GK, Ishikawa T, F. PY. 1965. Electron microscope studies on intra-retinal spaces: diffusion of particle material. . In: Rohen JW, editor. Structure of the Eye, II Symp. p 109-120.

Smith RS, Rudt LA. 1975. Ocular vascular and epithelial barriers to microperoxidase. Investigative Ophthalmology 14(7):556-560.

Spector A, Garner WH. 1981. Hydrogen peroxide and human cataract. Experimental Eye Research 33(6):673-681.

Sullmann H. 1951. Chemis des Auges. Tabul Biol 22:79.

Terelak-Borys B, Liberek I. 2007a. Neuro-hormonal regulation of aqueous humor dynamics as the basis of glaucoma pharmacotherapy. Part I. Aqueous humor secretion]. Klinika Oczna 109(1-3):60-63.

Terelak-Borys B, Liberek I. 2007b. Neuro-hormonal regulation of aqueous humor dynamics as the basis of glaucoma pharmacotherapy. Part II - Aqueous humor outflow. Klinika Oczna 109(1-3):64-67.

Tezel G. 2006. Oxidative stress in glaucomatous neurodegeneration: mechanisms and consequences. Progress in Retinal & Eye Research 25(5):490-513.

Tezel G, Wax MB. 2004. Hypoxia-inducible factor 1alpha in the glaucomatous retina and optic nerve head. Archives of Ophthalmology 122(9):1348-1356.

To CH, Kong CW, Chan CY, Shahidullah M, Do CW. 2002. The mechanism of aqueous humour formation. Clinical & Experimental Optometry 85(6):335-349.

Topper JE, Brubaker RF. 1985. Effects of timolol, epinephrine, and acetazolamide on aqueous flow during sleep. Investigative Ophthalmology & Visual Science 26(10):1315-1319.

Toris CB, Gabelt BAT, Kaufman PL. 2008. Update on the mechanism of action of topical prostaglandins for intraocular pressure reduction. Survey of Ophthalmology 53 Suppl1:S107-120.

Toris CB, Zhan GL, Yablonski ME, Camras CB. 2004. Effects on aqueous flow of dorzolamide combined with either timolol or acetazolamide. Journal of Glaucoma 13(3):210-215.

Tripathi RC, Millard CB, Tripathi BJ. 1989. Protein composition of human aqueous humor: SDS-PAGE analysis of surgical and post-mortem samples. Experimental Eye Research 48(1):117-130.

Trope GE, Rumley AG. 1985. Catecholamines in human aqueous humor. Investigative Ophthalmology & Visual Science 26(3):399-401.

Tschumper RC, Johnson DH. 1990. Trabecular meshwork cellularity. Differences between fellow eyes. Investigative Ophthalmology & Visual Science 31(7):1327-1331.

Usukura J, Fain GL, Bok D. 1988. [3H]ouabain localization of Na-K ATPase in the epithelium of rabbit ciliary body pars plicata. Investigative Ophthalmology & Visual Science 29(4):606-614.

Vanlandingham BD, Maus TL, Brubaker RF. 1998. The effect of dorzolamide on aqueous humor dynamics in normal human subjects during sleep. Ophthalmology 105(8):1537-1540.

Vegge T. 1971. An electron microscopic study of the permeability of iris capillaries to horseradish peroxidase in the vervet monkey (Cercopithecus aethiops). Ptschrift Fur Zellforschung Und Mikroskopische Anatomielexus 121(1):74-81.

Vorwerk CK, Naskar R, Dreyer EB. 1999. The excitotoxicity theory of glaucoma. Klinische Monatsblatter fur Augenheilkunde 214(1):2-11.

Wang RF, Serle JB, Podos SM, Sugrue MF. 1991. MK-507 (L-671,152), a topically active carbonic anhydrase inhibitor, reduces aqueous humor production in monkeys. Archives of Ophthalmology 109(9):1297-1299.

Wang Z, Do CW, Valiunas V, Leung CT, Cheng AKW, Clark AF, Wax MB, Chatterton JE, Civan MM. 2010. Regulation of gap junction coupling in bovine ciliary epithelium. American Journal of Physiology - Cell Physiology 298(4):C798-806.

Watanabe K, Chiou GC. 1983. Action mechanism of timolol to lower the intraocular pressure in rabbits. Ophthalmic Research 15(3):160-167.

Wax MB, Molinoff PB. 1987. Distribution and properties of beta-adrenergic receptors in human iris-ciliary body. Investigative Ophthalmology & Visual Science 28(3):420-430.

Wax MB, Tezel G. 2009. Immunoregulation of retinal ganglion cell fate in glaucoma. Experimental Eye Research 88(4):825-830.

Wheeler L, WoldeMussie E, Lai R. 2003. Role of alpha-2 agonists in neuroprotection. Survey of Ophthalmology 48(Suppl 1):S47-S51.

Wiederholt M, Zadunaisky JA. 1986. Membrane potentials and intracellular chloride activity in the ciliary body of the shark. Pflugers Archiv - European Journal of Physiology 407(Suppl 2):S112-115.

Wood JP, Schmidt KG, Melena J, Chidlow G, Allmeier H, Osborne NN. 2003. The beta-adrenoceptor antagonists metipranolol and timolol are retinal neuroprotectants: comparison with betaxolol. Experimental Eye Research 76(4):505-516.

Yanagi M, Kawasaki R, Wang JJ, Wong TY, Crowston J, Kiuchi Y. 2011. Vascular risk factors in glaucoma: a review. Clinical & Experimental Ophthalmology 39(3):252-258.

Zimmerman TJ, Garg LC, Vogh BP, Maren TH. 1976. The effect of acetazolamide on the movements of anions into the posterior chamber of the dog eye. Journal of Pharmacology & Experimental Therapeutics 196(2):510-516.

# 2

# Retinal Ganglion Cell Death

Yasemin Budak and Müberra Akdoğan
*Şevket Yılmaz Research and Education Hospital*
*Bursa, Turkey*

## 1. Introduction

### 1.1 Topographic and cellular organization of the retina

The retina is the thin (0.2 mm) lining of the back of the eye that gathers light focused on it by the cornea and lens. The retina has a complex laminar organization; cells are organized into layers (Fig. 1). These layers are named by reference to the middle of the eyeball; the innermost layers are located nearest the vitreous chamber, whereas the outermost lie adjacent to the retinal pigment epithelium and choroid. The most important layers, progressing from the inner to the outer, are: **(1) the inner limiting membrane** (formed by astrocytes and the conical end-feet of Müller cells); **(2) the nerve fiber layer**, composed of the axons of ganglion cells; **(3) the ganglion layer**, containing the cell bodies of ganglion cells; **(4) the inner plexiform layer**, composed of synapses formed between bipolar, amacrine, and ganglion cells; **(5) the inner nuclear layer**, containing the cell bodies and nuclei of horizontal, bipolar, and amacrine cells; **(6) the outer plexiform layer**, composed of synapses connecting photoreceptor cells from the outer nuclear layer with bipolar and horizontal cells from the inner nuclear layer; **(7) the outer nuclear layer**, containing the synapses and cell bodies of two classes of photoreceptors, namely the rods and cones; **(8) the outer limiting membrane**, a junction line between photoreceptor cells and Müller cells; **(9) the photoreceptor layer**, which contains the light-sensitive outer segments of the photoreceptors; and **(10) the retinal pigment epithelium (RPE)**, which is a monolayer of melanin-containing cells forming part of the blood/retina barrier. Although the RPE is not a component of the neural retina, this layer provides critical metabolic support to photoreceptors and the integrity thereof is fundamental in terms of proper retinal function [Bok, 1993; Krstić, 1997].

Retinal tissue contains both neuronal and non-neuronal elements, which work together to enable vision and to maintain retinal homeostasis

Neurons: The retina contains five types of neurons: (1) photoreceptors (cone and rod cells); (2) bipolar cells (of the flat, midget, and rod types); (3) horizontal cells; (4) amacrine cells; and, (5) ganglion cells [Krstić, 1997]. Photoreceptors are photosensitive neurons that absorb photons from the field of view and, using a specific complex biochemical pathway, turn this information into electrical signals via the process termed phototransduction [Sung & Chuang, 2010] to bipolar cells. Horizontal cells connect rods and cones that horizontally convey information within the retina. The horizontal cells receive input from one or more photoreceptors and transmit information to other photoreceptors and to bipolar cells [Poche & Reese, 2009]. Amacrine cells modulate signaling between bipolar and ganglion cells. The amacrine cells receive inputs from one or more bipolar cells and contact ganglion cells that in turn accept inputs from other bipolar cells. As with the horizontal cells, amacrine cells release inhibitory neurotransmitters in a graded manner, hyperpolarizing ganglion cells with which they are they contact, rendering it less likely that such cells will fire action potentials [Forrester, 2002]. Bipolar cells transmit signals from photoreceptors or horizontal cells, and pass such signals on to ganglion cells either directly or indirectly (via amacrine cells). Ganglion cells are the only retinal cells that produce action potentials; the release of glutamate by (a) bipolar cell(s) in contact with such cells is sufficient to depolarize the ganglion cells to threshold levels. These action potentials are transmitted to the brain via the fibers of the optic nerve.

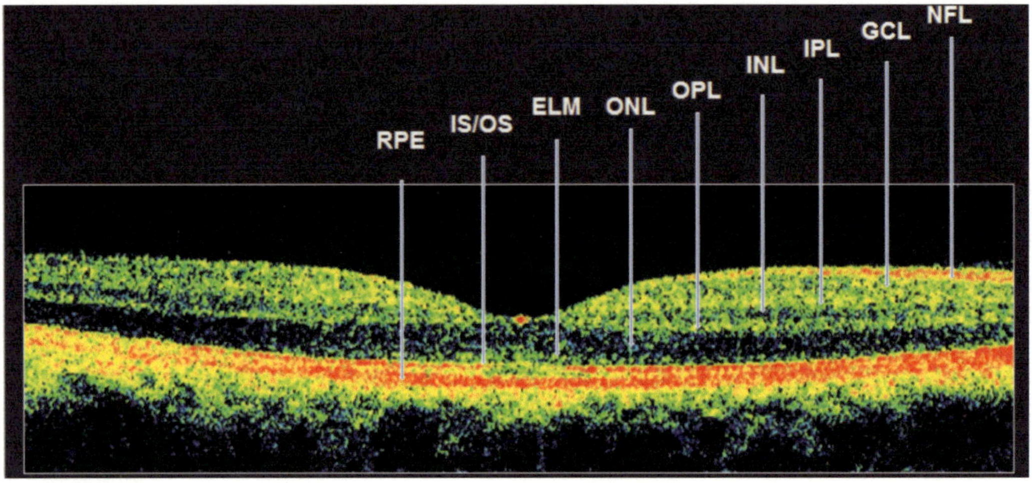


Fig. 1. Several layers can be resolved and have been labeled in the optical coherence tomography image of a normal human retina: Retinal pigment epithelium (RPE), inner segment/outer segment intersection of photoreceptors (IS/OS), external limiting layer (ELM), outer nuclear layer (ONL), outer plexiform layer (ONL), nerve fiber layer (NFL), ganglion cell layer (GCL), inner plexiform layer (IPL), inner nuclear layer (INL)

**Some retinal cells have regulatory, nutritional, and immunomodulatory functions**

**Glial cells (Müller cells and astrocytes)** are non neuronal cells that serve as an interface between neurons and the vasculature and provide support and nutrition, maintain homeostasis of the retinal extracellular milleu [Bringman *et al.*, 2006]. **Müller cells** form the majority of glial cells within the retina, and are arranged in a parallel manner. These cells span the entire thickness of the retina, projecting from the vitreous humor (the viscous fluid in the back of the eye) to the rear of the retina. These tubular cells wrap all retinal neurons and act as living optical fibers within the eye, funneling light to rod and cone cells [Franze *et al.*, 2007]. **Astrocytes** are confined principally to the retinal fiber layer, wherein they wrap ganglion cell axons and axon bundles that ultimately form the optic nerve. Other astrocytes line the inner surface of the retina and surround the blood vessels. Astrocytes vary in morphology, depending on their precise retinal location and their interaction with surrounding cells [Trivino *et al.*, 1992; Chang & Stone, 1991].

**Retinal pigment epithelium cells** (also termed melanosomes) are cuboidal cells that are arranged in a monolayer, and are easily recognized because they are pigmented [Bok, 1993]. **Microglial cells** are phagocytic cells within the retina that play important roles in defense against invading microorganisms, in immunoregulation, and in tissue repair [Chen *et al.*, 2002]. **Vascular endothelial cells and pericytes** provide nutritional support to, and aid in waste product removal from, the inner retina [Hosoya & Tomi, 2005].

**Retinal topography**

The retina may be divided into several regions that differ in structure; these regions contain neurons of different types. The **macula lutea** is in the center of the retina, and includes the fovea and surrounding tissue. The **fovea** is a small depression within the retina. In the fovea, the retina is thinner than elsewhere, consisting only of cones that are longer and thinner than the other cones of the eye. All **neurons** and **capillaries** originating elsewhere become compacted around the edges of the fovea. In the region surrounding the fovea, a gradual decrease in cone density is apparent, whereas rod density gradually rises. Finally, the eye contains a region in which there are no receptors, but rather an accumulation of ganglion cell axons, forming the optic nerve. This region, termed the **optic disc**, contains the point where the optic nerve emerges from the retina. Because no photoreceptors are present in this region, a break in the visual field (the so-called blind spot) may be noted. The optic disk is also the point of entry of the major blood vessels that supply the retina [Forrester, 2002].

## 2. Glaucoma and retinal ganglion cell death

Glaucoma is a neurodegenerative disease characterized by progressive, irreversible loss of vision [Gupta & Yücel, 2007]. Retinal ganglion cells are the only neurons affected in glaucoma; cells of other regions of the inner and outer retina remain unaffected, as confirmed by electroretinographic tests and histopathological studies [Aldebasi *et al.*, 2004; Glovinsky *et al.*, 1991; North *et al.*, 2010; Quigley *et al.*, 1998].

Retinal ganglion cells (RGCs) are the output neurons of the retina. The dendrites of these cells receive synapses from bipolar and amacrine cells in the inner plexiform layer. The cell somata reside in a narrow ganglion cell layer, and the axons of the cells travel through the optic nerve to retinorecipient structures in the brain, wherein the axons form glutamatergic synapses [Masland, 2001; Mu & Klein, 2004; Nassi & Callaway, 2009; Wassle, 2004]. Although RGCs share many features with other neurons, the former cell type vary significantly in terms of size, interconnections, and responses to visual stimulation. More than 12 types of ganglion cells have been distinguished in the mammalian retina studies [Rockhill, 2002]. It remains unclear whether some ganglion cells are more susceptible to apoptosis than are others, under glaucomatous conditions [Quigley, 1999]. Early studies indicated that large ganglion cells (magnocellular ganglion cells) and nerve fibers were selectively lost in experimental glaucoma models in nonhuman primates, and in human glaucoma patients [Quigley *et al.*, 1988]. In support of these observations, another work found selective loss of anterograde axonal transport to the magnocellular layer of the dorsal lateral geniculate nucleus, which is the region containing the largest RGCs [Dandone *et al.*, 1991]. There are also observations that doesnot support the hypothesis that selective loss of RGC occurs in glaucoma [Morgan *et al.*, 2000].

The axons of RGCs are non-myelinated from the retina to the lamina cribrosa, but become myelinated thereafter. In unmyelinated axons, action potentials propagate by depolarization along the membrane; this process consumes more energy than does the saltatory conduction of myelinated axons [Wang *et al.*, 2003]. Therefore as an adaptive process to the increased energy need, the axons of RGCs are characterized by many varicosities filled with mitochondria [Wang *et al.*, 2003].

RGCs have very long axons, thus increasing cell vulnerability to various disorders. Axon regions are likely to encounter metabolic stress such as hypoxia, and to be exposed to free radicals and mechanical compression (e.g., in the lamina cribrosa). These insults induce RGC death [Schmidt *et al.*, 2008]. To deal with these stressors, RGCs have a high antioxidant capacity (attributable to endogenous antioxidant defenses including expression of all of catalase, superoxide dismutase, glutathione peroxidase, and peroxiredoxins) compared with other neurons [Fatma *et al.*, 2008; Kortuem *et al.*, 2000], but the cells remain more vulnerable to stressors than, for example, Müller or vascular cells. [Schmit *et al.*, 2008].

## 2.1 In glaucoma, the mechanisms of cell death differ in retinal ganglion cell bodies and axons

### 2.1.1 Cell body death

RGC cell body death occurs via apoptosis or necrosis [Farkas & Grosskreutz, 2001; Kuehn *et al.*, 2005; Tatton *et al.*, 2001]. **Apoptosis** is an active genetic process whereby a cell undergoes an organized series of events culminating in self-destruction. All animal cells are programmed to self-destruct when they are not further required, or when damaged. Because cells play an active role in their own death, apoptosis is often termed "cell suicide". Apoptosis is in play during development and neurodegeneration, facilitating cell destruction without affecting neighboring cells that are destined to survive.

Whatever the initiating insult, actual cell death (the last step in apoptosis) features a final common pathway characterized by an orderly pattern of inter-nucleosomal DNA fragmentation, chromosomal clumping, cell shrinkage, and membrane blebbing. Eventually, the cell dies and marks itself for phagocytosis by nearby macrophages [Mace & Riedl, 2010].

**Necrosis** is another mechanism of cell body death. It is accidental in nature, and serves to eliminate cells that have been severely damaged. Unlike apoptosis, necrosis is a passive process during which the cell membrane is rapidly destroyed and toxic cellular components spill into the extracellular space, potentially injuring nearby cells [Dawson, 2005]. A low ATP concentration or impaired ATP generation predisposes cells to necrosis [Nicotera *et al.*, 1998]. The cell membrane becomes permeable early during this process. Organelles may become dilated, and ribosomes dissociate from the endoplasmic reticulum. The nucleus disintegrates later. Proteases play major roles in cell degradation during necrosis. As a consequence, cellular contents are libareted into the intracellular space and evoke an inflammatory response (Fig. 2). Although a growing body of evidence supports the idea that apoptosis serves as the primary mechanism of ganglion cell death in glaucoma patients, necrosis contributes to cell death in the late phase of the disease, as observed in rats subjected to optic nerve transection [Bien *et al.*, 1999]. RGC necrosis also has been reported to occur immediately after ischemic injury induced by imposition of high-level intraocular pressure [Joo *et al.*, 1998] and under intense excitotoxic conditions [Bonfocco *et al.*, 1995].

### 2.1.2 Axon death

Axon death occurs via either of two basic mechanisms: Wallerian degeneration and die-back [Borgens, 1988; Coleman & Freeman, 2010].

**Wallerian degeneration**, classically defined as degeneration of axons distal to an injury, is generally noted in severely damaged axons, and results in atrophy and rapid loss of structure throughout the entire length of the axon. At the cellular level, initial segmentation of the myelin sheath is apparent, followed by swelling of the axolemma, disorganization of neurofilaments and microtubules, and mitochondrial swelling. The remaining axonal fragments then undergo phagocytosis by glial cells and macrophages. The cell body can live for a number of days, but ultimately undergoes apoptosis [Saxena & Caroni, 2007].

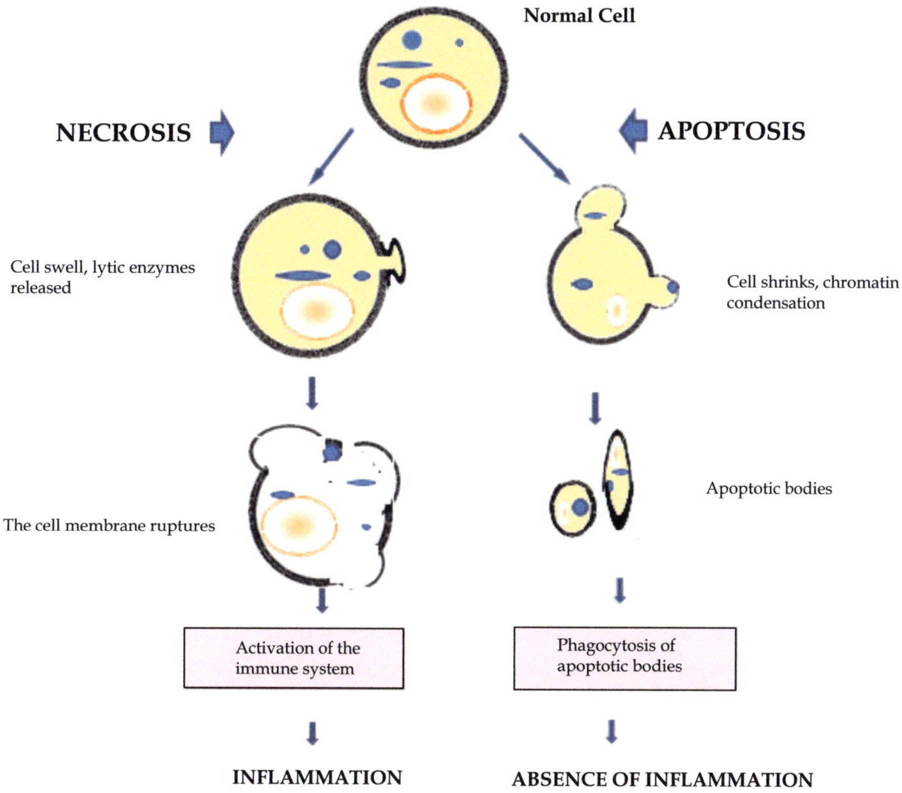


Fig. 2. Scheme representing necrosis and apoptosis

**Die-back** occurs in axons that experience more moderate injury, and is characterized by slower retrograde degeneration with a distal-to-proximal progression (thus from the synapse to the soma) [Seif *et al.*, 2007]. Milder insults may allow greater functional connectivity between the soma, proximal and distal axonal segments and die-back death can occur over several months.

### 2.2 Morphological features of apoptosis and apoptotic process in RGCs

Examination of apoptotic cells by light microscopy allows evaluation of morphological features including condensation of chromatin and cytoplasm, cell fragmentation, and apoptotic body formation [Kerr *et al.*, 1972].

**Electron microscopy** has shown that the earliest detectable ultrastructural change of apoptosis is chromatin condensation, which commences peripherally along the nuclear membrane and leads to the formation of a crescent or ringlike structure [Cummings *et al.*, 1997]. This is followed by nuclear changes including convolution of the nuclear outlines and peripheral nuclear chromatin breakdown. Early in apoptosis, and contemporaneously with the described nuclear changes, cells cease to contact neighboring cells, usually accompanied by loss of special membrane structures such as microvilli and desmosomes, and apoptotic cells begin to exhibit protrusions of the plasma membrane [Wyllie,1997].

Apoptosis is accompanied by cell volume decreases, cell density increases, more compact cytoplasmic organelles, and convolution of both cellular and nuclear outlines [Cummings *et al.*, 1997; Kerr *et al.*, 1994]. Concommitantly, cytoplasmic changes may be detected, including aggregation of cytoskeletal filaments, clumping of ribosomal particles, and rearrangement of the rough endoplasmic reticulum. Cytoplasmic and nuclear condensation is followed by production of numerous membrane protuberances, resulting in development of membrane-bound apoptotic bodies with well-preserved cytoplasmic organelles [Cummings *et al.* 1997; Kerr *et al.*, 1994; Wyllie, 1997]. Finally, the protrusions detach from the cells, forming apoptotic bodies densely packed with cellular organelles and nuclear fragments, which are phagocytosed by neighboring cells in the absence any inflammatory reaction. The latter feature is crucial, because it allows cell death to occur without damage to adjacent cells [Cummings *et al.*, 1997; Kerr *et al.*, 1994; Wyllie 1997].

**Biochemical features of apoptosis**

Cleavage of chromosomal DNA into oligonucleosomes is a biochemical hallmark of apoptosis. During the early stage of the process, DNA is broken into large fragments (50-300 kb in size) [Bortner *et al.*, 1995], which are subsequently cleaved into nucleosomal units (180 bp in size) [Zhang *et al.*, 2010].

Another biochemical feature of apoptosis is expression of cell surface markers that result in recognition and eventual phagocytosis of apoptotic cells, but with minimal damage to surrounding tissue. This is achieved by externalization of phosphatidylserine from the normal location on the inner leaf of the plasma membrane lipid bilayer to the outer leaf [Bratton *et al.*, 1997]. Normally, viable cells show asymmetric distributions of particular phospholipids between the inner and outer leaflets of the plasma membrane. Early in apoptosis, however, loss of such plasma membrane asymmetry, accompanied by phosphatidylserine externalization, occurs in all cell types [van Engeland *et al.*, 1998].

Condensation of the cytoplasmic space resulting in cell shrinkage is a universal characteristic of apoptosis [Wyllie, 1986]. Apoptotic cell shrinkage is associated with a decrease in $[Na+]i$ and $[K+]i$ which occurs after chromatin condensation and internucleosomal DNA fragmentation, and prior to apoptotic body formation [Mc Carthy & Cotter, 1997]. Coupled with this loss of intracellular ions, the cell may also lose the ability to take up ions, as exemplified by an early inhibition of the $Na^+/K^+$-ATPase in certain model systems [Bortner *et al.*, 2007]. This dramatic decrease in intracellular ions results in a cellular ionic environment permitting the activation of various cell death enzymes including caspases and apoptotic nucleases. The presence of high extracellular potassium prevents cell shrinkage by inhibiting the efflux of this ion, indicating that the normal intracellular ionic environment has a repressive effect on the apoptotic process [Bortner *et al.*, 2007].

### 2.3 The apoptotic process

Apoptosis is an active, energy-requiring process which can be separated into three distinct phases: (a) signaling, (b) commitment, and (c) execution.

**In the signaling phase** pro-apoptotic stimuli (ligand-induced activation of the death receptors, cellular stress signals *etc*..) initiate the sequence of events that leads to cell death.

**The commitment phase** is the step by which the cell either commits to apoptosis or activates mechanisms stopping the signaling cascade initiated during the signaling phase. **The**

**execution phase** begins after the cell fully commits to apoptosis. This is the point of no return for the cell, which is now irreversibly committed to die. Enzyme systems become activated; these actions result in the biochemical and morphological features of apoptosis. The enzyme systems cleave proteins, externalize phosphatidylserine, and degrade DNA. During this phase, the cell membrane begins to bleb, forming vesicles that contain high concentrations of cellular components that were formerly distributed in a more widespread manner with the cell [Mills, 2001; Hengartner, 2000]. At the end of the execution phase, vital cell structures and functions are destroyed. Externalization of phosphatidylserine serves as an "eat-me" signal to phagocytosing cells, which ingest newly dead cells without causing inflammation.

**Apoptosis occurs via two major pathways: the intrinsic and extrinsic pathways**

The **intrinsic pathway** is initiated from within the cell when intracellular stress is sensed. This pathway is controlled by the balance of activity of pro- and anti-apoptotic members of the *Bcl2* gene family and involves regulation of mitochondrial membrane permeability. In response to pro-apoptotic signals, cytochrome c, apoptotic protease activating factor 1 (APAF-1), and caspase-9 are released from the mitochondrial membrane and form apoptosomes [Hengartner, 2000], which in turn activate caspase cascades. In contrast, the **extrinsic pathway** is initiated by cell surface signaling following binding of an extracellular ligand to a "death receptor". Formation of the death-induced signaling complex (DISC) directly stimulates the caspase cascade via activation of caspase-8, without any mitochondrial involvement. Caspase-8 acts on pro-caspase-3, generating active caspase-3, which in turn cleaves the DNA fragmentation factor (DFF) [Hengartner, 2000]. The active (cleaved) form of the latter factor induces internucleosomal DNA strand cleavage at 200 bp intervals, a hallmark of apoptosis [Nagata, 2000].

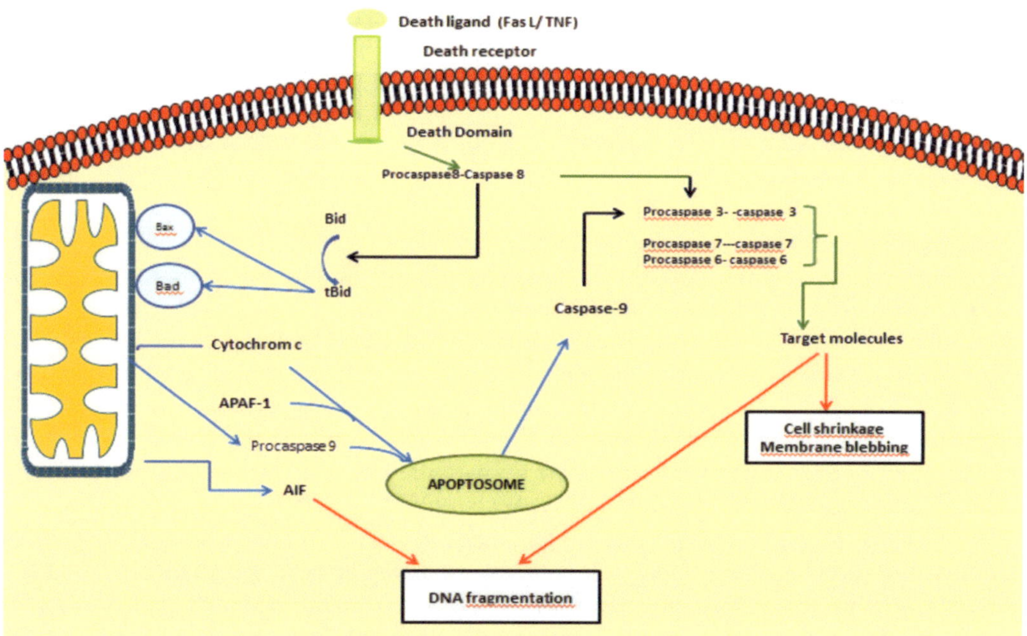


Fig. 3. Intrinsic and extrinsic pathways of apoptosis

Links between the extrinsic and the intrinsic pathway exist at several levels (Fig 3). Upon death receptor triggering, activation of caspase-8 may result in cleavage of Bcl-2 interacting domain (BID), which in turn translocates to the mitochondria to release cytochrome c [Cory & Adams, 2002; Yin, 2000]. In addition, cleavage of caspase-6 (a downstream component of the mitochondrial pathway) may generate feedback to the receptor pathway, via cleavage of caspase-8 [Cowling & Downward, 2002]. The extrinsic and intrinsic pathways share a common endpoint at the level of caspase-3 activation [Guerin *et al.*, 2006].

### 2.3.1 Direct signal transduction (death receptors)

Death receptors are cell surface molecules that transmit apoptotic signals initiated by specific death ligands from the extra- to the intra-cellular environment, and play central roles in initiation of apoptosis. In addition, all death receptors contain a homologous cytoplasmic aminoacid sequence termed the "death domain" [Itoh & Nagata, 1993; Tartaglia *et al.*, 1993]. Death receptors belong to the tumor necrosis factor **(TNF)** receptor family. Eight members of the death receptor family sharing homologous cytoplasmic death domains have been characterized to date; these are Fas/Apo-1/CD95, TNF-R1 [tumor necrosis factor (TNF) receptor 1], DR3 (death receptor 3), TRAIL-R1 (TNF-related apoptosis-inducing ligand receptor 1), TRAIL-R2, DR6, p75-NGFR (p75-nerve growth factor receptor), and EDAR (ectodermal dysplasia receptor) [Lavrik *et al.*, 2005].

Binding of a death-inducing ligand to the appropriate receptor can result in release of ceramide, typically produced by the action of acid sphingomyelinase [Gulbins, 2003], that in turn rapidly forms ceramide-enriched signaling platforms within the cell membrane [Zhang *et al.*, 2009]. Such platforms result in clustering of receptor molecules, which greatly enhances apoptotic signaling. Indeed, this effect is so marked that death receptor signaling in the absence of receptor clustering is rarely able to activate the full apoptotic process. Binding of the appropriate ligand to a death receptor typically causes a conformational change in the intracellular region of the receptor that in turn results in the death domain motif becoming accessible [Zimmermann *et al.*, 2001]. Such exposure allows various adaptor proteins to bind to the receptor to form a death-inducing signalling complex (DISC). The adaptor proteins, such as FADD (Fas-associated death domain) contain motifs described as death effector domains, which permit recruitment of pro-caspases, typically pro-caspase 8, to the DISC [Kaufmann *et al.*, 2002]. Activation of caspase 8 follows, and apoptosis is initiated within seconds after ligand binding.

TNF receptor-1, a death receptor, has recently been identified to be one mediator of the RGC death evident in patients with various neurodegenerative injuries [Tezel *et al.*, 2004]. Immunohistochemical studies and in situ hybridization have shown that the level of TNF receptor-1 is greater in glaucomatous eyes than in age-matched control eyes [Tezel *et al.*, 2001]. RGCs of glaucoma patients were usually positive when immunostained for TNF-$\alpha$ receptor-1. It is tempting to speculate that the relatively selective expression of this receptor in RGCs may in part explain the increased vulnerability of such cells to apoptosis during glaucomatous optic nerve degeneration [Tezel *et al.*, 2001].

Fas is a transmembrane protein expressed by numerous cells. Components of the FAS/FAS-ligand system represent the prototypical receptor-mediated apoptosis pathway [Love, 2003]. Fas-Associated protein with death domain (FADD) is an adaptor molecule that bridges the Fas death receptor, to caspase-8. In rats with elevated intraocular pressure, FADD immunoreactivity was evident in Müller glial cells and RGCs [Ju *et al.*, 2006].

### 2.3.2 Mitochondrial abnormalities

Mitochondrial dysfunction leads to RGC death via caspase-dependent and -independent pathways, initiated by the loss of mitochondrial membrane potential, release of cell death mediators, and/or oxidative stress [Tezel *et al.*, 2004]. Members of the Bcl-2 protein family regulate the mitochondrial pathway. This protein family is subdivided into two protein groups: anti-apoptotic proteins, such as Bcl-2 and Bcl-XL; and pro-apoptotic multidomain proteins, such as BAX and "BH3 domain-only" proteins [Antonnsson, 2001]. Mitochondrial membrane integrity is maintained by the actions of the anti-apoptotic group members. Internal stimuli from cell damage sensors (e.g., p53) can stimulate mitochondrion-driven apoptosis by activation of the pro-apoptotic proteins. Protein p53 and members of the Bcl-2 family are active in retinal ganglion cells in glaucoma [Nichells, 1999].

Protein localization studies suggest that, upon activation of cell death, Bcl-2-associated X protein (BAX) is recruited from the cytoplasm to the mitochondrial outer membrane [Nichells, 1999]. The transition to membrane permeability and the release of cytochrome c are critical events in terms of the subsequent steps taken toward apoptosis. Release of cytochrome c activates the caspase cascade via protein association with pro-caspase 9 and apoptosis protease activating factor-1 (Apaf-1) [Adams & Cory, 2007; Danial & Korsmeyer, 2004].

Several studies have found that BAX is a major effector of apoptotic ganglion cell death in the retina after exposure to ischemia, excitotoxicity, or axotomy; and during retinal degeneration [Chen *et al.*, 2003; Isenmann *et al.*, 1997; Isenmann *et al.*, 1999; Zhang *et al.*, 2002]. Complete BAX deficiency of the DBA/2J mouse line prevented RGC somal death during glaucoma development [Libby et al., 2005].

**Mitochondrial permeability transition pores (MPTPs)**

The mitochondrial permeability transition pore (MPTP) is a pore protein that spans the inner and outer mitochondrial membranes, allowing the passage of any molecule <1,500 Da in size [Crompton *et al.*, 1987]. MPTP induction can lead to mitochondrial swelling and cell death, and plays an important role in some types of apoptosis. Mitochondrial calcium overload, oxidative stress, adenine nucleotide depletion, depolarization, and/or elevated phosphate concentration, results in opening of the MPTP. This leads to osmotic swelling of the mitochondrial matrix as water influx is followed by compression of the intercristal space. It is presumed that cytochrome c and other apoptogenic factors, including apoptosis-inducing factor (AIF), are released through the pores, [Zoratti *et al.*, 2005] although the mechanism of mitochondrial membrane permeabilization remains unclear.

**Release of cytochrome c**

**Cytochrome c** is an electron carrier of the respiratory chain, normally located in the space between the inner and outer mitochondrial membranes. The protein is released by the mitochondria to the cytosol in response to pro-apoptotic stimuli. Such release activates the caspase-dependent apoptotic pathway. Once in the cytosol, cytochrome c forms a complex with apoptotic protease-activating factor 1 (APAF-1) and caspase-9 to form the apoptosome [Cain *et al.*, 2002], which initiates a cascade of proteolytic cleavages.

### 2.4 Signaling mechanisms protecting RGCs from apoptosis

**Bcl-2**, an anti-apoptotic protein of mitochondria, has been shown to inhibit cytochrome c release and to protect against oxidative stress-induced apoptosis [Takahashi *et al.*, 2004]. The actions of members of the Bcl-2 protein family thus counterbalance the effects of proapoptotic BAX proteins [Antonnsson, 2001]. When BAX species are predominant, apoptosis occurs. However, if Bcl-2 levels are higher, cell survival is favored. For example, if a rise in intraocular pressure leads to neurotrophin insufficiency, this will in turn cause downregulation of Bcl-2 and upregulation of BAX, resulting in apoptosis.

### 2.5 Killing of RGCs by activated proteolytic caspases

Many signals and pathways cause apoptosis, but the only cell killing mechanism is the organized degradation of cellular organelles by activated proteolytic caspases. The enzymes belong to the cysteine proteases that upon activation through the intrinsic and/or extrinsic pathways destroy essential cellular proteins. In a healthy cell, caspases are held in inactive zymogenic states, thus as pro-caspases, and do not become functional until proteolytically processed. Caspases can be divided into two groups; the initiator (e.g., caspases 8 and 9) and effector (e.g., caspases 3, 4, and 7) caspases [Alenzi *et al.*, 2010]. Initiator caspases activate effector caspases in response to specific cell death signals, and effector caspases in turn cleave other protein substrates within the cell resulting in apoptotic process [Chang & Yang, 2000].

Caspase activation in mammalian cells is mediated via two main routes, often referred to as 'the intrinsic pathway and 'the extrinsic pathway [Hengartner, 2000]. Enzymes at the upper end of the cascade include caspase-8, 10 and caspase-9. Caspase-8 is the initial caspase of the extrinsic pathway, thus representing the cellular response to triggering of receptors with death domains. While caspases 8 and 10 act as initiator caspases of the extrinsic apoptosis pathway, caspase 9 acts as an initiator caspase of the intrinsic apoptosis pathway [Kuida K. 2000]. The intrinsic pathway commences with release of cytochrome c from mitochondria, which then interacts with apoptosis protease activating factor-1 (Apaf-1), resulting in self-cleavage and activation of caspase-9. Caspase 3 is considered to be the main effector caspase involved in both intrinsic and extrinsic pathways. Caspases-3, -6, and -7 are downstream enzymes that are activated by upstream proteases, and act to cleave cellular targets. These caspases are responsible for destruction of key cytoskeletal proteins, causing the morphological changes typically observed in cells undergoing apoptosis. Caspases activate DNAses, inhibit DNA repair enzymes, and break down nuclear structural proteins [Kitazumi & Tsukahara 2011].

To prevent unnecessary cell death, cells synthesize inhibitors of apoptosis proteins (IAPs); these proteins are grouped into a family that modulates initiator and effector caspase activity.

Several studies have found that caspase-3 is involved in the apoptotic death of RGCs induced by ischemia [Lam *et al.*, 1999; Tezel & Wax, 1999], excitotoxicity [Tezel & Wax, 1999], and chronic ocular hypertension [McKinnon *et al.*, 2003]. Inhibition of caspase-3 activity reduced the level of apoptotic cell death induced in retinal cells by either excitotoxicity or ischemia [Lam *et al.*, 1999, Chen *et al.*, 2001].

## 3. Mechanisms of RGC death

### 3.1 Mechanical stress

Optic nerve axons exit the eye at the lamina cribrosa. At this site, the glial-wrapped axon bundles are confined within the rigid pores of the laminar cribriform plates, termed the lamina cribrosa pores. Axon bundles are thought to be vulnerable to mechanical stress in the region of passage through the laminar pores. It has been suggested that compression at the level of the lamina cribrosa (often caused by elevated intraocular pressure) damages RGC axons [Quigley & Addicks, 1981]. Although differences in lamina cribrosa pore shape in glaucomatous eyes have been observed in glaucoma patients, it remains unknown whether such alterations precede the onset of RGC loss [Tezel *et al*, 2004].

It is hypothesized that the force exerted by extrinsic intraocular pressure on the optic nerve results in backward bowing of laminar support tissues, distortion of laminar plates, misalignment of laminar pores, and nerve cell damage caused by direct mechanical compression or interruption of axoplasmic flow [Quigley *et al.*, 1980]. It is also possible that mechanical distortion of extracellular matrix plates contributes to glaucoma, as blood vessels are thereby affected [Quigley & Addicks, 1981]. Importantly, the extracellular matrix plates of the lamina are covered by astrocytes that provide the axons with support that is both neurotrophic in nature and otherwise.

Elevated intraocular pressure may obstruct the retrograde transport that is thought to inhibit delivery of neurotrophic substances to RGCs, thereby triggering apoptosis [Quigley, 1999]. An alternative hypothesis is that intraocular pressure elevation alters glial cells in some manner, resulting in damage to RGC axons [Hernandez *et al.*, 2000]. Loss of glial support functions may also be important in terms of neuronal compromise [Lappe & Siefke, 2003].

In addition, RGC death induced by elevated intraocular pressure involves caspase activation (including that of caspases-3,8 and -9) in experimental rat models of glaucoma [Hanninen et al., 2002; Huang et al., 2005; McKinnon et al., 2002;].

### 3.2 Hypoxia-ischemia

Dysregulation of blood flow, causing tissue hypoxia, either secondary to or independent of intraocular pressure elevation, has been suggested to cause retinal damage in glaucoma patients [Cioffi,2001; Flammer et al., 2002; Osborne et al., 2001]. The structural and functional integrity of the retina depends on a regular supply of oxygen. The inner retinal layers exhibit the highest sensitivity to hypoxic challenge, whereas the outer retina is more resistant to hypoxic stress [Kaur et al., 2008].

RGCs have been reported to be particularly sensitive to acute, transient, and mild systemic hypoxic challenge [Kergoat et al., 2006]. RGC death has been found to occur in many different models of induced retinal ischemia [Adachi et al., 1996, Lafuente et al., 2002]. Analysis of the expression of a hypoxia-induced transcription factor, HIF-1$\alpha$, the synthesis of which is tightly regulated by cellular oxygen concentration, has provided direct evidence that hypoxia occurs in the retina and optic nerve head of glaucomatous eyes, and hypoxic signaling is likely to be one pathogenic mechanism involved in glaucomatous neurodegeneration [Tezel & Wax, 2004]. Hypoxia induces HIF-1$\alpha$ synthesis; the target genes of this transcription factor include those encoding vascular endothelial growth factor (VEGF) and nitric oxide synthase (NOS) [Levy et al., 1995]. NOS is the the enzyme responsible for production of nitric oxide (NO), an important cellular signaling molecule.

Upregulated expression of VEGF and NOS in the retina has been reported following hypoxic injury [Kaur et al., 2006], as well as in the glaucomatous retina [Tezel & Wax, 2004]. NO synthesis by NOS contributes to the cytotoxicity that culminates in cell death and axonal damage. In addition to generating free radicals, NO induces the pro-apoptotic cascade by enhancing phosphorylation of Bcl-2 [Mishra et al., 2004; Seminara et al., 2007], which in turn results in the loss of anti-apoptotic potential.

Hypoxia-ischemia causes accumulation of reactive oxygen species (ROS), which have been shown to be cytotoxic to RGCs [Tezel & Yang, 2004]. ROS are chemically-reactive molecules containing oxygen. ROS cause necrotic cell death via direct oxidative damage to cellular constituents. ROS also trigger apoptotic death, as they participate in the signal transduction pathway characteristic of apoptosis [Kortuem et al., 2000, Levkovitch-Verbin et al., 2000, Lieven *et al.*, 2003]. Hypoxia activates microglia, the immune effector cells of the retina, resulting in release of TNF-$\alpha$ (an inflammatory cytokine) [Kaur *et al.*, 2008].
Abnormally high-level release of the excitatory amino acid glutamate under hypoxic-ischemic conditions has been implicated in hypoxic and ischemic neuronal death [Benveniste et al., 1984], and glaucoma [Sucher *et al.*, 1997]. RGCs are very sensitive to the toxic effects of elevated glutamate, but the mechanism by which this response is mediated remains unclear. Upon hyperstimulation of one or more glutamate receptors, neuronal cell death is induced by excitotoxins; the process is complex and is not yet fully understood. Several studies have found that both the apoptotic and necrotic pathways of cell death can be activated under such conditions [Ankarcrona *et al.*, 1995].

### 3.3 Free radical-induced damage

The source of reactive oxygen species (ROS) may be either exogenous (the extracellular fluid) or endogenous. ROS are created in the eye by sunlight, mitochondrial respiration, and intra- and extra-cellular metabolic reactions [Roth, 1997]. The major producers of ROS in RGCs are mitochondria. The lamina cribrosa contains more mitochondria than are present in other regions of the RGC axon. As the number of mitochondria increases, more oxygen is consumed, and ROS synthesis rises. ROS initiate many metabolic cascades that have a wide variety of downstream effects. In vitro studies with RGC-5 cells (RGC-5 is a clonal rat RGC line) showed that oxidative stress perturbs calcium homeostasis, activates pro-apoptotic caspases, depletes glutathione levels, and increases the extent of DNA fragmentation, suggesting that a final common pathway of oxidative stress-induced cell death may exist [Maher & Hanneken 2005a, Maher & Hanneken 2005b].

### 3.4 Excessive glutamate stimulation

Glutamate, the excitatory neurotransmitter of the retina, is released by photoreceptors, bipolar cells, and ganglion cells, and mediates the transfer of visual signs from the retina to the brain [Wong *et al.*, 2007]. However, when glutamate levels are elevated, neuronal death can occur via either apoptosis or necrosis [Ankarcrona *et al.*, 1995]. Thus, appropriate clearance of synaptic glutamate is required if retinal excitatory synapses are to function normally, and to prevent neurotoxicity. Glial cells surround glutamatergic synapses; such cells express glutamate transporters and the glutamate-metabolizing enzyme glutamine synthetase. Together, these enzymes convert glutamate to the non-toxic amino acid glutamine [Bringmann *et al.*, 2009].
Glutamate interacts with numerous receptor subtypes; these fall into two major classes. One class is coupled to G-proteins (the metabotropic class), the other class connect directly to transmembrane channels (the ionotropic class, including the amino-methyl-propionic-acid [APMA], NMDA, and kainate glutamate receptors). The toxic effects of elevated glutamate levels are predominantly mediated by overstimulation of receptors for the glutamate analog N-methyl-D-aspartate (NMDA). Activation of NMDA receptors by glutamate results in overloading of intracellular $Ca^{2+}$, which in turn activates calcium-dependent enzymes and

leads to principally necrotic cell death [Shen *et al.*, 2006]. Excess glutamate, which may result from ischemia, can trigger apoptosis. It has been shown that glutamate, acting via the ionotropic receptors, significantly elevates the levels of neuronal nitric oxide synthase (nNOS), TNF-α, and interleukin-1β [Kaur *et al.*, 2009]. This results in influx of $Na^+$ and $Cl^-$ ions, in turn inducing osmotic swelling and glutathione depletion.

Glutamate release has been implicated as a mechanism of RGC death in glaucoma [Levin & Peeples 2008, Osborne *et al.*, 1999, Levkovitch-Verbin *et al.*, 2001]. Although numerous studies have examined the role played by glutamate in acute ischemia, the relevance of glutamate excitotoxicity in glaucoma remains doubtful.

### 3.5 Activated glial cells

Microglial and macroglial cells (Müller cells and astrocytes) have important immunoregulatory functions and control the extracellular environment of the optic nerve head and retina. In the optic nerve, glial cells include astrocytes, oligodendrocytes (located behind the lamina cribrosa), and microglia [Johnson & Morrison, 2009]. In the retina, Müller cells and astrocytes are predominant. Under normal conditions, glial cells support neuronal function via a variety of mechanisms including structural and nutritional roles as well as the removal of ions and neurotransmitters from the extracellular space [Johnson & Morrison, 2009].

It is possible that activation of glial cells in glaucomatous eyes serves primarily to support neuronal function. However, at some point, triggered by the prolonged stress associated with glaucoma, a shift in cell function seems to occur; the cells are no longer supportive but rather damage neuronal tissue. The injury involves both mechanical insult and changes in the microenvironment. In addition, a growing body of evidence suggests that, under glaucomatous stress conditions, glial cells may even become neurodestructive, releasing increased amounts of neurotoxic substances including TNF-α and nitric oxide (NO) [Tezel, 2006].

Astrocytes become reactive in response to various stimuli, including elevated intraocular pressure, excitotoxicity, and retinal ischemia [Neufeld & Liu 2003, Hernandez et al., 2008]. Reactive astrocytes in glaucomatous optic nerve heads apparently play important roles in the development of local neurotoxicity, confined to the retinal ganglion cell axons, by producing excessive levels of NO in patients with glaucomatous optic neuropathy [Liu & Neufeld 2000]. The use of inhibitors of nitric oxide synthase, such as 3-aminoguanidine, reduced RGC loss in rat eyes with elevated intraocular pressure [Neufeld et al., 1999].

Chronic activation of retinal and optic nerve head glia in glaucomatous eyes also involves activation of the antigen-presenting abilities of such cells, thereby facilitating initiation of an autoimmune process via antigen presentation [Tezel et al., 2007].

In glaucoma patients, microglia become activated and redistributed within the optic nerve head [Neufald et al., 1999], after which cytokines and chemokines are synthesized [Block 2007, Kim 2005]. However, the influence of microglial factors on other retinal cells, including RGCs, is unclear, although such interactions may be relevant to glaucoma pathology. This aspect of the field merits further study.

### 3.6 Inflammatory cytokines (tumor necrosis factor-α and NO)

Glial production of **tumor necrosis factor- α** (TNF-α) is increased, and the level of TNF receptor-1 upregulated, in RGCs and their axons in glaucomatous donor eyes [Tezel G, 2008]. The two main subgroups of the TNF receptor superfamily, TNF-R1 and TNF-R2, recognize both the membrane-bound and soluble forms of TNF-α. The current view of TNF-α-mediated signaling is that binding of the factor to TNF-R1 promotes neuronal cell death whereas messages from TNF-R2 trigger proliferative and regulatory signals promoting cell survival. Establishment of a critical balance between the considerable variety of intracellular signaling pathways determines whether an RGC will die or will survive exposure to TNF-α. This factor, secreted by stressed glial cells within glaucomatous tissues, can induce RGC death via induction of a receptor-mediated caspase cascade, mitochondrial dysfunction, and/or oxidative damage. In addition to direct neurotoxic effects on RGCs and axons thereof, TNF-α signaling is likelyto contribute to secondary degeneration of primarily uninjured RGCs [Tezel G, 2008].

TNF-α can induce glial NO production thus the extent of excitotoxic injury. NO induces the proapoptotic cascade in hypoxic neural tissues by enhancing phosphorylation of Bcl-2 [Mishra et al. 2004]. The anti-apoptotic potential of Bcl-2 is lost because the protein can no longer heterodimerize with the pro-apoptotic protein BAX, resulting in BAX-mediated activation of caspases and initiation of apoptosis. Other mechanisms by which NO may contribute to cytotoxicity include peroxynitrite-mediated oxidative injury, DNA damage, and energy failure [StClair et al., 1997].

Involvement of TNF-α in the innate immune response may also have implications in terms of axonal degeneration in glaucomatous eyes. TNF-α signaling may be associated with axonal dysfunction and Wallerian degeneration. One function of TNF-α during the latter type of degeneration has been suggested to be induction of macrophage recruitment for debris removal [Tezel G, 2008].

TNF- α also activates matrix metalloproteinases, which are involved in tissue remodeling within the glaucomatous optic nerve head. The matrix metalloproteinases are a family of proteolytic enzymes secreted by glial cells, and are capable of degrading almost all components of the extracellular matrix. The intensity of immunostaining for matrix metalloproteinases (MMP-1, MMP-2, and MMP-3), was greater in glaucomatous optic nerve heads compared with controls [Yan X *et al.*, 2000]. TNF-α induced matrix metalloproteinase activity has also been shown to facilitate macrophage recruitment by nerves injured during delayed axonal degeneration [Tezel G, 2008].

TNF- α stimulates endothelin-1 synthesis and secretion in optic nerve head astrocytes [Tezel G, 2008]. Endothelin-1 is a vasoconstrictor peptide and along with nitric oxide (NO) regulate optic nerve head, retinal, and choroidal blood flow. Exposure of retinal ganglion cells (RGCs) or RGC-5 cells, a transformed cell line, to endothelin-1 causes apoptic cell death [ Salvatore & Vingolo, 2010]

## 4. Axonal compromise

The human RGC axon travels a distance of approximately 50 mm from the cell body to the target synapse. On leaving the eye, axons turn through 90° to enter the optic nerve head and then traverse the lamina cribrosa to enter the retrobulbar optic nerve [Morgen, 2004]. The lamina cribrosa provides structural and functional support to the RGC axons as they pass from the relatively high-pressure environment in the eye to a low-pressure region in the retrobulbar cerebrospinal space. Within the lamina cribrosa, axonal viability requires adequate delivery of nutrients (assessed in terms of lamellar capillary volume flow) and sufficient diffusion of such nutrients (from lamellar capillaries across endothelial cell basement membranes, through the trabecular extracellular matrix, and across astrocyte basement membranes) to the centers of axon bundles. The route taken by individual axons can place them at increased risk of damage [Morgen, 2004].

Specifically, compartmental degeneration of axons, synapses, and dendrites can occur independently of somal loss [Whitmore et al., 2005]. Using a murine model of inherited glaucoma, Libby et al [2005] showed that axonal loss occurred independently of somal loss, not just in a spatial sense but via a distinct molecular pathway. The cited authors also found that distinct degeneration pathways were activated in different regions of retinal nerve cells. It was noted that appropriate biochemical function of the nerve cell body, which resides in the retina, required the pro-apoptotic protein BAX (the Bcl2-associated X protein). In contrast, metabolic pathway function in the part of the cell (the axon) that connects the cell body to the brain did not require BAX. In addition, work in a primate model of experimental glaucoma showed that retinal ganglion cells undergo a pattern of degeneration that originates in the dendritic arbor and concludes with shrinkage of the cell soma. In DBA/2J mice, in which intraocular pressure rises spontaneously, axons degenerate before cell bodies, and distal axons appear to be first affected [Schlamp *et al.*, 2006].

The mechanism of vision loss in glaucoma is not understood, but various lines of evidence indicate that RGC axons are critical sites for early pathological changes, including retention of intraretinal RGC axons concomitant with axon loss in the optic nerve [Soto *et al.*, 2008], retrograde degeneration as assessed via axon quantification [Schlamp *et al.*, 2006], and maintenance of RGC somata under circumstances in which retrograde label is lost [Buckingham *et al.*, 2008].

These findings indicate the need to understand axon-specific degeneration pathways in glaucoma, suggesting, first, that distinct somal and axonal degeneration pathways may exist and, second, that both pathways must be to targeted to save vision.

### 4.1 Axoplasmic flow

RGCs are long projecting neurons, the axons of which form the optic nerve. As with other neurons, ganglion cells must possess a mechanism whereby the cell body remains informed of conditions along the axon and at the synapse, to allow axon size and functions to be maintained. This is accomplished via active axonal transport, a complex energy-driven process that moves molecules from the cell body to the axon terminus (anterograde transport) and also toward the cell body (retrograde transport). Anterograde transport can be divided into fast (50–400 mm/day) and slow (less than 10mm/day) transport. Fast anterograde transport is related to the transport of synaptic vesicles proteins, kinesins, and enzymes involved in the metabolism of neurotransmitters. Slow anterograde transport is given over to the transport of neuronally synthesised proteins that include cytoskeletal components, polymers, and protein complexes that are to be delivered to the axon and its terminal regions. Retrograde transport is classified as fast (200–400 mm/day) and is concerned with the movement of endosomes and lysosomes containing internalised membrane receptors and neurotrophins towards the cell body [Morgan, 2004].

Both anterograde and retrograde transport require integrity of the axonal cytoskeleton, which is composed of microtubules, neurofilaments, and microfilaments. Active axonal transport refers to the process whereby vesicles are transported along microtubules by the dynein and kinesin motor molecules; the kinesins drive anterograde transport and the dyneins retrograde transport. Kinesins typically contain two heavy chains with motor heads which move along microtubules via a pseudo-processive asymmetric walking motion. In comparison with kinesin, the size of a dynein is much larger. Dyneins don't seem to follow paths that are parallel to protofilament direction but they move across the microtubule surface [Ross *et al.*, 2008]. The dynein and kinesin motor molecules acquire energy by hydrolysis of ATP produced by mitochondria. Active axonal transport is essential to ensure communication along axons and interruption thereof is potentially fatal to cells.

Obstruction of axonal transport in RGCs compromises cell viability by preventing delivery of substrates, such as neurotrophic factors, that are necessary for somal survival. Such small growth-enhancing peptides include brain-derived neurotrophic factors (BDNFs), nerve growth factors (NGFs), and neurotrophin-3 (NT-3) and -4 (NT-4) [Funakoshi *et al.*, 1993].

Brain-derived neurotrophin factor (BDNF) is one mediator known to be vital for the buildup and preservation of neurons. BDNF is transported to retinal ganglion cell bodies via retrograde axonal transportation, using synaptic connections within these cells. BDNF has a specific receptor, termed TrkB, which exists in all retinal layers except those of the photoreceptors and the optic nerve. Activation of TrkB directly elicits pro-survival signals during glaucoma progression, and rescues RGCs from death in the context of optic nerve axotomy or glaucoma [Bai, 2010]. Mechanical stress at the level of the lamina cribrosa impairs the retrograde transport of neurotrophins, including BDNF. Thus, retinal ganglion cell somae are deprived of the mediator and the apoptotic cascade is activated [Wong *et al.*, 2011].

### 4.2 Retrograde degeneration

Wallerian degeneration generally occurs in severely damaged axons and is characterized by a rapid loss of axonal structure throughout the length of the axon. Die-back occurs in axons with more moderate injury and is characterized by a slower retrograde degeneration that proceeds from the synapse to the soma [Levin & Albert 2010]. Although it is not known how axons in a glaucomatous human eye degenerate, clues to this process have come from recent studies in (Wld(S)) mutant rats; suggesting that axonal degeneration in glaucoma follows a Wallerian-like mechanism [Beirowski *et al.*, 2008].

Damage to the optic nerve in mammals induces retrograde degeneration and apoptosis of the retinal ganglion cell (RGC) bodies. The molecular mechanisms responsible for transforming the repellent guidance cue from the damaged axon into a death signal that may affect the cell body are yet to be discovered.

## 5. References

Adachi M, Takahashi K, Nishikawa M, Miki H, Uyama M. (1996). High intraocular pressure-induced ischemia and reperfusion injury in the optic nerve and retina in rats. *Graefes Arch Clin Exp Ophthalmol*, Vol. 234, No.7, pp. (445-451).

Adams JM, Cory S. (2007). The Bcl-2 apoptotic switch in cancer development and therapy. *Oncogene*, Vol. 26, No.9, pp. (1324–1337).

Aldebasi YH, Drasdo N, Morgan JE, North RV. (2004). S-cone, L + M-cone, and pattern, electroretinograms in ocular hypertension and glaucoma. *Vision Res*, Vol. 44, No 24, pp. (2749-2756).

Alenzi FQ, Lotfy M, Wyse R. (2010) Swords of cell death: caspase activation and regulation. *Asian Pac J Cancer Prev*, Vol.11, No 2, pp. (271-280).

Ankarcrona M, Dypbukt JM, Bonfoco E, Zhivotovsky B, Orrenius S, Lipton SA, Nicotera P. (1995). Glutamate- induced neuronal death: a succession of necrosis or apoptosis depending on mitochondrial function. *Neuron*, Vol. 15, No.4, pp. (961-973).

Antonsson B. (2001). Bax and other pro-apoptotic Bcl-2 family "killer-proteins" and their victim the mitochondrion. *Cell Tissue Res*, Vol. 306, No 3, pp. (347-361).

Artal-Sanz M, Tavernarakis N. (2005). Proteolytic mechanisms in necrotic cell death and neurodegeneration. *FEBS Letters*, Vol. 579, No. 15, pp.(3287-3296).

Benveniste H, Drejer J, Schousboe A, Diemer NH. (1984). Elevation of the extracellular concentrations of glutamate and aspartate in rat hippocampus during transient cerebral ischemia monitored by intracerebral microdialysis. *J Neurochem*, Vol. 43, No. 5, pp. (1369-1374).

Beirowski B, Babetto E, Coleman MP, Martin KR. (2008) The WldS gene delays axonal but not somatic degeneration in a rat glaucoma model. *Eur J Neurosci*, Vol (28) No.,(6), pp. (1166-1179).

Bien A, Seidenbecher CI, Böckers TM, Sabel BA, Kreutz MR.( 1999) Apoptotic versus necrotic characteristics of retinal ganglion cell death after partial optic nerve injury. *J Neurotrauma*, Vol. 16, No. 2, pp. (153-163).

Bok D. (1993) The retinal pigment epithelium: a versatile partner in vision. *J Cell Sci*, Vol.17, pp (189-195).

Bonfocco E, Krainic D, Ankarcrina M, Nicotera P, Lipton SA. (1995). Apoptosis and necrosis: two distinct events induced, respectively, by mild and intense insults with N-methyl-D-aspartate or nitric oxide/superoxide in cortical cell cultures. *Neurobiology*, Vol. 92, pp. (7162–7166).

Borgens RB. (1988) Voltage gradients and ionic currents in injured and regenerating axons. *Adv Neurol*, Vol 47, pp. (51-66).

Bortner CD, Oldenburg NBE, Cidlowski JA. (1995). The role of DNA fragmentation in apoptosis. *Trends Cell Biol*, Vol. 5, No. 1, pp ( 21-26).

Bratton DL, Fadok VA, Richter DA, Kailey JM, Gutrie LA Henson PM. (1997). Appearance of Phosphatidylserine on Apoptotic Cells Requires Calcium-mediated Nonspecific Flip-Flop and Is Enhanced by Loss of the Aminophospholipid Translocase. Vol. 17, No. 272, pp . (26159–26165).

Bringmann A, Pannicke T, Biedermann B, Francke M, Iandiev I, Grosche J, Wiedemann P, Albrecht J, Reichenbach A. (2009). Role of retinal glial cells in neurotransmitter uptake and metabolism. *Neurochem Int*, Vol *54*, No *3-4*, pp. (143-160).

Bringmann A, Pannicke T, Grosche J, Francke M, Wiedemann P, Skatchkov SN, Osborne NN, Reichenbach A. (2006). Muller cells in the healthy and diseased retina. *Prog Retin Eye Res*, Vol.25, No.4, pp.(397–424).

Bringmann A, Pannicke T, Grosche J, Francke M, Wiedemann P, Skatchkov SN, Osborn NN, Bortner CD, Cidlowski JA. (2007). Cell shrinkage and monovalent cation fluxes: role in apoptosis. *Arch Biochem Biophys*, Vol 15, No 462 (2): pp. (176-188).

Cain K, Bratton SB, Cohen GM. (2002). The Apaf-1 apoptosome: a large caspase-activating complex. *Biochimie*, Vol. 84, No 2-3, pp. (203-214).

Chang L.T, Stone J. (1991). Factors determining the morphology and distribution of astrocytes in the cat retina: a 'contact-spacing' model of astrocyte interaction. *J Comp Neurol*, Vol 15, No.303(3), pp. (387-399).

Chang HY , Yang X. (2000). Proteases for Cell Suicide: Functions and Regulation of Caspases. *Microbiol Mol Biol Rev*, Vol 64, No 4, pp. (821–846).

Chen L, Yang P, Kijlstra A. (2002). Distribution, markers, and functions of retinal microglia. *Ocul Immunol Inflamm*, Vol.10, No.1, pp. (27-39).

Chen ST, Hsu JR, Hsu PC, Chuang JI. (2003). The retina as a novel in vivo model for studying the role of molecules of the Bcl-2 family in relation to MPTP neurotoxicity. *Neurochem Res*, Vol. 28, No.6, pp. (805–814).

Chen TA, Yang F, Cole GM, Chan So. (2001). Inhibition of caspase-3-like activity reduces glutamate induced cell death in adult rat retina. *Brain Res Vol*, 904, No.1 pp. (177–188).

Cioffi GA. (2001). Three common assumptions about ocular blood flow and glaucoma. *Surv Ophthalmol*, Vol.45 No (suppl 3), pp.(325–331)

Coleman MP, Freeman MR. (2010). Wallerian degeneration, wld(s), and nmnat. *Annu Rev Neurosci*, Vol.33, pp. (245-267).

Cory S, Adams JM. ( 2002). The Bcl2 family: regulators of the cellular life-or-death switch. *Nat Rev Cancer*, Vol. 2, No.9, pp. (647-656).

Cowling V, Downward J. (2002). Caspase-6 is the direct activator of caspase-8 in the cytochrome c-induced apoptosis pathway: absolute requirement for removal of caspase-6 prodomain. *Cell Death Differ*, Vol. 9, No.10, pp. (1046-1056).

Crompton M, Costi A, Hayat L. (1987). Evidence for the presence of a reversible Ca2+-dependent pore activated by oxidative stress in heart mitochondria. *Biochem J*, Vol. 245, No. 3, pp. (915-918).

Cummings MC, Winterford CM, Walker NI. (1997). Apoptosis. *Am J Surg Pathol*, Vol.21, No.1, pp.(88-101)

Dandona L, Hendrickson A, Quigley HA. (1991). Selective effects of experimental glaucoma on axonal transport by retinal ganglion cells to the dorsal lateral geniculate nucleus. Invest Ophthalmol Vis Sci, Vol. 32, No. 5, pp. (1593-1599).

Danial NN, Korsmeyer SJ. (2004). Cell death: critical control points. Cell. 116:205–219.

Dawson VL. 2005 Molecular mechanisms in neuronal and axonal apoptosis and necrosis. *Adv Stud Med*, Vol. 5, No.4, pp. (387-391).

Fatma N, Kubo E, Sen M, Agarwal N, Thoreson WB, Camras CB, Singh DP. (2008). Peroxiredoxin 6 delivery attenuates TNF-α-and glutamate-induced retinal ganglion cell death by limiting ROS levels and maintaining $Ca^{2+}$ homeostasis. *Brain Research*, Vol. 1233, No 3: pp. (63-78).

Farkas RH, Grosskreutz CL. (2001). Apoptosis, neuroprotection, and retinal ganglion cell death: an overview. *Int Ophthalmol Clin*,. Vol.41, No 1, pp. (111-130).

Flammer J, Orgül S, Costa VP, Orzalesi N, Krieglstein GK, Serra LM, Renard JP, Stefennsson E .(2002) The impact of ocular blood flow in glaucoma. *Prog Retin Eye Res*, Vol. 21, No 4, pp. (359–393).

Franze K, Grosche J, Skatchkov SN, Schinkinger S, Foja C, Schild D, Uckermann O, Travis K, Reichenbach A, Guck J. (2007). Muller cells are living optical fibers in the vertebrate retina. *Proc Natl Acad Sci USA*, Vol. 104 No. 20, pp. (8287-8292).

Forrester JV. (2002) The eye: basic sciences in practice

Funakoshi H, Frisen J, Barbany G, et al. (1993). Differential expression of mRNAs for neurotrophins and their receptors after axotomy of the sciatic nerve. *J Cell Biol*, Vol (123) pp. (455-465).

Glovinsky Y, Quigley HA, Dunkelberger GR. (1991). Retinal ganglion cell loss is size dependent in experimental glaucoma. *Invest Ophthalmol Vis Sci*, Vol. 32, No . 3, pp. (484–491).

Guerin MB, McKernan DP, O'Brien CJ, Cotter TG. (2006). Retinal ganglion cells:dying to survive. *Int J Dev Biol*, Vol.50, No 8, pp. (665-674).

Gulbins E. (2003). Regulation of death receptor signaling and apoptosis by ceramide. *Pharmacol Res*, Vol. 47, No 5, pp. (393-399).

Gupta N, Yücel YH. (2007). Glaucoma as a neurodegenerative disease *Current Opinion in Ophthalmology*, Vol. 18, No 2, pp.(110-114).

Hanninen VA, Pantcheva MB, Freeman EE, Poulin NR, Grosskreutz CL. (2002). Activation of caspase 9 in a rat model of experimental glaucoma.*Curr Eye Res*, Vol. 25, No 6, pp. (389-395).

Hengartner MO. (2000). The biochemistry of apoptosis. *Nature* Vol. 407, No 12 pp. (770-776).

Hernandez MR, Miao H, Lukas T (2008). Astrocytes in glaucomatous optic neuropathy. *Prog Brain Res*, Vol. 173, pp. (353–373).

Hernandez MR, Pena JD, Selvidge JA, Salvador- Silva M, Yang P. (2000) Hydrostatic pressure stimulates synthesis of elastin in cultured optic nerve head astrocytes.*Glia*, Vol. 32, No 2 pp. (122-136).

Hosoya K, Tomi M. (2005) Advances in the Cell Biology of Transport *via* the Inner Blood-Retinal Barrier: Establishment of Cell Lines and Transport Functions. *Biol Pharm Bull*, Vol. 28,No.1, pp.(1-8 ).

Huang W, Dobberfuhl A, Filippopoulos T, Ingelssson M, Fileta JB, Poulin NR, Grosskreutz CL. (2005) Transcriptional up-regulation and activation of initiating caspases in experimental glaucoma. *Am J Pathol*, Vol. 167, No 3, pp. (673-681).

Krstić RV. (1997) Human microscopic anatomy: an atlas for students of medicine and biology.

Kuida K. (2000) Caspase-9. *Int J Biochem Cell Biol*, Vol. 32, No 2, pp. (121-124).

Isenmann S, Wahl C, Krajewski S, Reed JC, Bähr M. (1997) Up-regulation of Bax protein in degenerating retinal ganglion cells precedes apoptotic cell death after optic nerve lesion in the rat. *Eur J Neurosci*, Vol. 9, No 8, pp. (1763–1772).

Isenmann S, Engel S, Gillardon F, Bahr M. (1999) Bax antisense oligonucleotides reduce axotomy-induced retinal ganglion cell death in vivo by reduction of Bax protein. *Cell Death Differ*, Vol. 6, No.7, pp. (673–682).

Itoh N, Nagata S. (1993). A novel protein domain required for apoptosis: mutational analysis of human Fas antigen. *J Biol Chem*, Vol.268, No 15, pp. (10932–10937).

Johnson EC, Morrison JC. (2009) Friend or Foe? Resolving the Impact of Glial Responses in Glaucoma. *Glaucoma*, Vol.18, No 5, pp. (341-353).

Joo C, Choi JS, Ko HW, Park KY, Sohn S, Chun MH, Oh YJ, Gwag BJ. (1998) Necrosis and apoptosis after retinal ischemia: involvement of NMDA-mediated excitotoxicity and p53. *Invest Ophthalmol Vis Sci*, Vol. 40, No 3 pp. (713–720).

Ju KR, Kim HS, Kim JH, Lee NY, Park CK. (2006) Retinal glial cell responses and Fas/FasL activation in rats with chronic ocular hypertension. *Brain Res*, Vol.1122, No. 1, pp. (209-221).

Kaufmann M, Bozic D,Briand C, Bodmer JL,Zerbe O,Kohl A, Tschopp J, Grütter MG. (2002) Identification of a basic surface area of the FADD death effector domain critical for apoptotic signaling. *FEBS Lett*, Vol. 527, No. 1-3, pp. (250-254).

Kaur C, Foulds WS Ling EA. (2008) Hypoxia-ischemia and retinal ganglion cell damage. *Clin Ophthalmol*, Vol.2 No4, pp. (879–889).

Kergoat H, Hérard ME, Lemay M. (2006) RGC sensitivity to mild systemic hypoxia. *Invest Ophthalmol Vis Sci*, Vol. 47 No. 12, pp. (5423-5427).

Kerr JF, Wyllie AH, Currie AR. (1972) Apoptosis: a basic biological phenomenon with wide-ranging implications in tissue kinetics. *Br J Cancer*, Vol. 26, No. 4, pp.(239-257).

Kerr JF, Winterford CM, Harmon BV. (1994) Apoptosis. Its significance in cancer and cancer therapy. *Cancer,* Vol. 73, No. 8, pp. (2013-2026).

Kim Kortuem, Geiger LK, Levin LA. (2000) Differential Susceptibility of Retinal Ganglion Cells to Reactive Oxygen Species. *IOVS,* Vol. 41, No 10, pp. (3176-3186).

Kitazumi I, Tsukahara M. (2011) Regulation of DNA fragmentation: the role of caspases and phosphorylation. *FEBS J.* Vol. 278, No.3, pp. (427-441).

Kortuem K, Geiger LK, Levin LA. (2000) Differential susceptibility of retinal ganglion cells to reactive oxygen species. *Invest Ophthalmol Vis Sci,* Vol.41, No.10, pp. (3176-3182).

Kuehn MH, Fingert JH, Kwon YH. (2005) Retinal Ganglion Cell Death in Glaucoma: Mechanisms and Neuroprotective Strategies. *Ophthalmol Clin N Am,* Vol.18, No 3, pp.(383 - 395).

Lam TT, Abler AS, Tso MO. (1999) Apoptosis and caspases after ischemia-reperfusion injury in rat retina. *Invest Ophthalmol Vis Sci,* Vol. 40, No. 5, pp (967-975)

Lafuente MP, Villegas-Pérez MP, Sellés-Navarro I, Mayor-Torroglosa S, Miralles de Imperial J, Vidal-Sanz M. (2002) Retinal ganglion cell death after acute retinal ischemia is an ongoing process whose severity and duration depends on the duration of the insult. *Neuroscience,* Vol.109, No.1, pp. (157-168).

Lappe-Siefke C, Goebbels S, Gravel M, Lee J, Braun PE, Griffiths IR, Nave KA. (2003). Disruption of Cnp1 uncouples oligodendroglial functions in axonal support and myelination. *Nat Genet,* Vol. 33, No. 3, pp. (366–374).

Lavrik I, Golks A, Krammer PH. (2005). Death receptor signaling. *J Cell Sci,* Vol.118, No. 2, pp.(265-267).Leist M, Nicotera P. (1998) Apoptosis versus necrosis: the shape of neuronal cell death. *Results Probl Cell Differ.* Vol. 24, pp.(105-135).

Levin L, Albert DM. (2010). Ocular Disease: Mechanisms and Management. Elsevier Inc.

Levin LA, Peeples P. (2008). History of neuroprotection and rationale as a therapy for glaucoma. *Am J Manag Care,* Vol.14, No.1 Suppl, pp. (11-14).

Levkovitch-Verbin H, Quigley HA, Kerrigan-Baumrind LA, D' Anna SA, Kerrigan D, Pease ME. (2001). Optic nerve transection in monkeys may result in secondary degeneration of retinal ganglion cells. *Invest Ophthalmol Vis Sci,* Vol.42, No. 5, pp. (975-982).

Levkovitch-Verbin H,Harris-Cerruti C,Groner Y, Wheeler LA, Schwartz M, Yoles E. (2000). RGC death in mice after optic nerve crush injury: oxidative stress and neuroprotection. *Invest Ophthalmol Vis Sci,* Vol. 41, No. 13, pp.(4169-4174).

Levy AP, Levy NS, Wegner S, Goldberg MA. (1995). Transcriptional regulation of the rat vascular endothelial growth factor gene by hypoxia. *J Biol Chem,* Vol. 270, pp.(13333–13337)

Lewin, B. (2000). Genes VII. New York: Oxford University Press.

Libby RT, Li Y, Savinova OV, Barter J, Smith RS, Nickells RW, John SWM. (2005). Susceptibility to neurodegeneration in glaucoma is modified by Bax gene dosage. *PLoS Genet,* Vol.1, No. 1, pp. (17-26).

Lieven CJ, Vrabec JP, Levin LA. (2003) The effects of oxidative stress on mitochondrial transmembrane potential in retinal ganglion cells. *Antioxid Redox Signal,* Vol. 5, No.5, pp. (641-646).

Liu B, Neufeld AH. (2000) Expression of nitric oxide synthase-2 (NOS-2) in reactive astrocytes of the human glaucomatous optic nerve head. *Glia,* Vol. 30, No.2, pp. (178-186).

Love S. (2003) Apoptosis and brain ischaemia. *Prog Neuropsychopharmacol Biol Psych,* Vol. 27, pp. (267–282).

Mace PD, Riedl SJ. (2010) Molecular cell death platforms and assemblies. *Curr Opin Cell Biol,* Vol. 22, No. 6, pp. (828-836).

Maher P, Hanneken A. (2005) The molecular basis of oxidative stress-induced cell death in an immortalized retinal ganglion cell line. *Invest Ophthalmol Vis Sci,* Vol. 46, No. 2, pp.(749-757).

Maher P, Hanneken A. (2005) Flavonoids Protect Retinal Ganglion Cells from Oxidative Stress–Induced Death. *Invest Ophthalmol Vis Sci,* Vol.46, No.12, pp. (4796-4803).

Masland RH. (2001). The fundamental plan of the retina. *Nat Neurosci,* 4 No 9, pp. (877-886).

Masland RH. (2001) Neuronal diversity in the retina. *Curr Opin Neurobiol,* Vol.11, No. 4, pp. (431-436).

McCarthy JV, Cotter TG. (1997) Cell shrinkage and apoptosis: a role for potassium and sodium ion efflux. *Cell Death Differ,*Vol. 4, No 8, pp.(756-770).

McKinnon Sj, Lehman DM, Kerrigan-Baumrind LA,Merges CA, Pease MF, Kerrigan DF, Ransom NL, Tahzib NG, Reitsamer HA, Levkovitch-Verbin H, Quigley HA, Zack DJ. (2002) Caspase activation and amyloid precursor protein cleavage in rat ocular hypertension. *Invest Ophthalmol Vis Sci,*Vol. 43, No 4, pp. (1077-1087)

Mills JC. (2001). Mechanisms underlying the Hallmark features of the execution-phase of apoptosis. *Advances in Cell Aging and Gerontology,* Vol. 5, pp. (1-38).

Mishra OP, Delivoira Papadopoulos M. (2004). Effect of hypoxia on protein tyrosine kinase activity in cortical membranes of newborn piglets--the role of nitric oxide. *Neurosci Lett,* Vol. 372, No. 1-2, pp. (114-118).

Mishra OP, Zubrow AB, Ashraf QM. (2004). Nitric oxide-mediated activation of extracellular signal-regulated kinase (ERK) and c-jun N-terminal kinase (JNK) during hypoxia in cerebral cortical nuclei of newborn piglets. *Neuroscience,* Vol. 123, No. 1, pp. (179- 186).

Morgan JE, Uchida H, Caprioli J. (2000). Retinal ganglion cell death in experimental glaucoma. *Br J Ophthalmol,* Vol. 84, No. 3, pp. (303-310).

Morgan JE. (2004). Circulation and axonal transport in the optic nerve. *Eye,* Vol. 18, pp. (1089-1095).

Mu X, Klein WH. (2004). A gene regulatory hierarchy for retinal ganglion cell specification and differentiation. *Semin Cell Dev Biol,* Vol. 15, No. 1, pp. (115-123)

Nagata S.( 2000) Apoptotic DNA fragmentation. *Exp Cell Res,* Vol. 256, No. 1, pp. 12-18.

Nassi JJ, Callaway EM. (2009). Parallel processing strategies of the primate visual system. *Nat Rev Neurosci,* Vol. 10, No.5, pp. (360-372).

Neufeld AH. (1999) Microglia in the Optic Nerve Head and the Region of Parapapillary Chorioretinal Atrophy in Glaucoma *Arch Ophthalmol.* Vol. 117, No. 8, pp.(1050-1056).

Neufeld AH, Liu B. (2003) Glaucomatous optic neuropathy: when glia misbehave. *Neuroscientist,* Vol. 9, No. 6, pp. (485-495).

Neufeld AH, Sawada A, Becker B. (1999) Inhibition of nitric-oxide synthase 2 by aminoguanidine provides neuroprotection of retinal ganglion cells in a rat model of chronic glaucoma. *Proc Natl Acad Sci USA,.* Vol. 96, No. 17, pp. (9944-9948).

Nicotera P, Leist M, Ferrando-May E. (1998). Intracellular ATP, a switch in the decision between apoptosis and necrosis.*Toxicol Lett,* Vol. 102-103, pp. (139-142).

Nickells RW. (1999) Apoptosis of Retinal Ganglion Cells in Glaucoma: An Update of the Molecular Pathways Involved in Cell Death. *Surv Ophthalm*, Vol. 43 No.1, pp.151-161

North RV, Jones AL, Drasdo N, Wild JM, Morgen JE. (2010). Electrophysiological evidence of early functional damage in glaucoma and ocular hypertension. Invest *Ophthalm Invest Ophthalmol Vis Sci*, Vol. 5, No. 2, pp. (1216-1222).

Osborne NN, Melena J, Chidlow G, Wood JP. (2001). A hypothesis to explain ganglion cell death caused by vascular insults at the optic nerve head: possible implication for the treatment of glaucoma. *Br J Ophthalmol*, Vol. 85, No. 10, pp. (1252–1259).

Osborne NN, Wood JP, Chidlow G, Bae JH, Melena J, Nash MS. (1999) Ganglion cell death in glaucoma: what do we really know *Br J Ophthalmol*,Vol. 83, No.8, pp.(980-986).

Poche RA, Reese BE. (2009). Retinal horizontal cells: challenging paradigms of neural development and cancer biology. Development Vol. 136, No. 13, pp. (2141-2151).

Quigley HA, Flower RW, Addicks EM,McLoad DS. (1980). The mechanism of optic nerve damage in experimental acute intraocular pressure elevation. *Invest Ophthalmol Vis Sci*, Vol. 19, No. 5, pp. (505-517)

Quigley HA, Addicks EM. (1981). Regional differences in the structure of the lamina cribrosa and their relation to glaucomatous optic nerve damage. *Arch Ophthalmol*, Vol. 99, No. 1, pp. (137-143).

Quigley HA, Dunkelberger GR, Green WR. (1988). Chronic human glaucoma causing selectively greater loss of large optic nerve fibers. *Ophthalmol*,Vol. 95, No. 3, pp. (357–363).

Quigley HA. (1999). Neuronal death in glaucoma *Prog Retin Eye Res*, Vol. 18, No. 1, pp. (39-57).

Rockhill RL, Daly FJ, MacNeil MA, Brown SP, Masland RH. (2002). The diversity of ganglion cells in a mammalian retina. *J Neurosci*, Vol. 22, No. 9, pp. (3831-3843).

Ross JL, Shuman H, Holzbaur ELF, Goldman YE. (2008). Kinesin and dynein-dynactin at intersecting microtubules: motor density affects dynein function. *Biophy J*, Vol. 94, No. 8, pp. (3115-3125).

Roth E. (1997). Oxygen free radicals and their clinical implications. *Acta Chir Hung*, Vol. 36, No.1-4, pp. (302–305).

Salvatore S, Vingolo EM. (2010). Endothelin-1 Role in Human Eye: A Review. *J Ophthalmol*, 354645. Saxena S, Caroni P. (2007). Mechanisms of axon degeneration: from development to disease. *Prog Neurobiol*, Vol. 83, No.3, pp. (174-191).

Schmidt KG, Bergert H, Funk RHW. (2008) Neurodegenerative Diseases of the Retina and Potential for Protection and Recovery. *Curr Neuropharmacol*, Vol. 6, No. 2, pp. (164–178).

Schlamp CL, Li Y, Dietz JA, Janssen KT, Nickells RW. (2006). Progressive ganglion cell loss and optic nerve degeneration in DBA/2J mice is variable and asymmetric. *BMC Neurosci*, Vol. 3, No. 7, pp. 66.

Seif GI, Nomura HM, Tator C H. (2007). Retrograde axonal degeneration "dieback" in the corticospinal tract after transection injury of the rat spinal cord: a confocal microscopy study. *J Neurotrauma*, Vol. 24, No. 9, pp. (1513-1528).

Seminara AR, Ruvolo PP, Murad F. (2007). LPS/IFNgamma-induced RAW 264.7 apoptosis is regulated by both nitric oxide-dependent and -independent pathways involving JNK and the Bcl-2 family. *Cell Cycle*, Vol. 6, No. 14, pp. (1772-1778).

Shen Y, Liu XL, Yang XL. (2006) N-methyl-D-aspartate receptors in the retina. Vol. 34, No. 3, pp. (163-179).

St Clair EG, Anderson SJ, Oltvai ZN. (1997). Bcl-2 counters apoptosis by Bax heterodimerization-dependent and -independent mechanisms in the T-cell lineage. *J Biol Chem,* Vol. 272, No. 46, pp. (29347-29355).

Sucher NJ, Lipton SA, Dreyer EB. (1997). Molecular basis of glutamate toxicity in retinal ganglion cells. *Vision Res,* Vol. 37, No. 24, pp. (3483-3493).

Tartaglia LA, Ayres TM , Wong GHW, Goeddel DV. (1993). A novel domain within the 55 kd TNF receptor signals cell death. *Cell,* Vol.74, No. 5, pp.(845–853).

Takahashi A, Masuda A,Sun M, Centonze VE, Herman B. (2004) Oxidative stress-induced apoptosis is associated with alterations in mitochondrial caspase activity and Bcl-2-dependent alterations in mitochondrial pH (pHm). *Brain Res Bull,* Vol. 62, No. 6, pp. (497-504).

Tatton NA, Tezel G, Insolia SA, Nandor SA, Edward PD, Wax MB. (2001). In situ detection of apoptosis in normal pressure glaucoma. a preliminary examination. *Surv Ophthalmol,* Vol. 45, No. 3, pp. (268-272).

Tezel G. (2006). Oxidative Stress in Glaucomatous Neurodegeneration: Mechanisms and Consequences. *Prog Retin Eye Res.* Vol. 25, No. 5, pp. (490–513).

Tezel G. (2008). TNF-α signaling in glaucomatous neurodegeneration. *Prog Brain Res.* Vol.173, pp. (409-421).

Tezel G, Li LY, Patil RV, Wax MB. (2001). TNF-alpha and TNF-alpha receptor-1 in the retina of normal and glaucomatous eyes. *Invest Ophthalmol Vis Sci,* Vol.42,No.8, pp. (1787-1794).

Tezel G, Yang X, Luo C, Peng Y, Sun SL, Sun D. (2007). Mechanisms of Immune System Activation in Glaucoma: Oxidative Stress-Stimulated Antigen Presentation by the Retina and Optic Nerve Head Glia. *Invest Ophthalmol Vis Sci,* Vol. 48, No2 pp. (705-714).

Tezel G, Yang X, Yang1 J, Wax MB. (2004) Role of tumor necrosis factor receptor-1 in the death of retinal ganglion cells following optic nerve crush injury in mice. *Brain Res,*Vol. 996, No.2, pp. (202–212).

Tezel G, Wax MB. (1999) Inhibition of caspase activity in retinal cell apoptosis induced by various stimuli in vitro. *Invest Ophthalmol Vis Sci,* Vol. 40, No.11, pp. (2660-2667).

Tezel G, Wax MB. (2003). Glial modulation of retinal ganglion cell death in glaucoma. *J Glaucoma,* Vol.12, No.1, pp. (63-68).

Tezel G, Wax MB. (2004). Hypoxia-inducible factor 1alpha in the glacomatous retina and optic nerve head. *Arch Ophthalmol,* Vol.122 No. 9, pp.(1348-1356).

Tezel G, Trinkaus K, Wax MB. (2004). Alterations in the morphology of lamina cribrosa pores in glaucomatous eyes. *Br J Ophthalmol,* Vol. 88, No. 2, pp. (251–256).

Tezel G, Yang X. (2004). Caspase-independent component of retinal ganglion cell death, in vitro. *Invest Ophthalm Vis Sci,* Vol.45, No 11, pp. 4049-4059.

John E. (1987)The retina: an approachable part of the brain

Trivino A, Ramirez JM, Ramirez AI, Salazar JJ, Garcia- Sanchez J. (1992) Retinal perivascular astroglia: an immunoperoxidase study. *Vision Res,* Vol. 32, No. 9, pp. (1601-1607).

van Engeland M, Nieland LJ, Ramaekers FC, Schutte B, Reutelingsperger CP. (1998). Annexin V-affinity assay: a review on an apoptosis detection system based on phosphatidylserine exposure. *Cytometry,.* Vol. 31, No.1, pp. (1-9).

Tombran-Tink J, Barnstable CJ. (2008). Visual Transduction and Non-Visual Light Perception.

Wang L, Dong J, Cull G, Fortune B, Cioffi GA. (2003) Varicosities of Intraretinal Ganglion Cell Axons in Human and Nonhuman Primates. *Invest Ophthalmol Vis Sci*, Vol. 44 No. 1, pp. (2-9).

Wässle H. Parallel processing in the mammalian retina. (2004). *Nat Rev Neurosci*, Vol. 5, No.10, pp. (747-757).

Whiteman AL, Klauss G, Miller PE, Dubielzig RR. (2002). Morphologic features of degeneration and cell death in the neurosensory retina in dogs with primary angle-closure glaucoma. *Am J Vet Res*, Vol. 63, No. 2, pp. (257-261).

Whitmore AV, Libby RT, John SWM. (2005). Glaucoma: Thinking in new ways—a rôle for autonomous axonal self-destruction and other compartmentalised processes. *Prog Retin Eye Res*, Vol. 24, No. 6, pp. (639-662).

Wong KW, Dunn FA, Graham DM, Berson DM. (2007) Synaptic influences on rat ganglion-cell photoreceptors. *J Physiol*, Vol.582, No. 1, pp. (279–296).

Wong VH, Bui BV, Vingrys A J. (2011). Clinical and experimental links between diabetes and glaucoma. *Clinical and Experimental Optometry*, Vol. 94, pp. 4–23.

Wyllie AH. (1997). Apoptosis: an overview. *Br Med Bull*, Vol. 53, No. 3, pp. (451-465).

Wyllie AH. (1986). What is apoptosis? *Histopathology*, Vol.10, No. 9, pp. (995-998).

Yan X, Tezel G, Wax MB, Edward DP. (2000) Matrix metalloproteinases and tumor necrosis factor α in glaucomatous optic nerve head. *Arch Ophthalmol*, Vol. 118, pp.(666-673)

Yin XM. (2000) Signal transduction mediated by Bid, a pro-death Bcl-2 family proteins, connects the death receptor and mitochondria apoptosis pathways. *Cell Res*, Vol. 10, No. 3, pp. (161-167).

Zhang C, Rosebaum DM, Shaikh AR, Li Q, Rosebaum PS,Pelham DJ,Roth S. (2002) Ischemic preconditioning attenuates apoptotic cell death in the rat retina. *Invest Ophthalmol Vis Sci*, Vol. 43, No. 9, pp. (3059–3066).

Zhang L, Zhang M, Yang S, Cao Y, Zhang SB, Yin L, et al. (2010). A new biodosimetric method: branched DNA-based quantitative detection of B1 DNA in mouse plasma. *Br J Radiol*, Vol. 83, No. 992, pp. (694 - 701).

Zhang Y, Li X, Becker KA, Gulbins E. (2009). Ceramide-enriched membrane domains-structure and function. *Biochim Biophys Acta*, Vol. 1788, No1, pp.(178-183).

Zimmermann KC, Bonzon C, Green DR. (2001). The machinery of programmed cell death. *Pharmacol Ther*, Vol. 92, No. 1, pp. (57-70).

Zoratti M, Szabo I, De Marchi U. (2005). Mitochondrial permeability transitions: how many doors to the house? *Biochim Biophys Acta*, Vol. 1706, No. 1-2, pp. (40-52).

3

# Adaptive Changes in the Retina and Central Visual Areas in Glaucoma

Sansar C. Sharma[1], Jin Li[2] and Elena Vecino[3]
[1]*Department of Ophthalmology, Cell Biology and Anatomy, New York Medical College, Valhalla, NY 10595*
[2]*Department of Neurology, New York Medical College, Valhalla, NY 10595*
[3]*Faculty of Medicine, Univ. del Pais Vasco, Leoia,*
[1,2]*USA*
[3]*Spain*

## 1. Introduction

Glaucoma with or without elevated intraocular pressure (IOP) leads to the loss of retinal ganglion cells and the visual fields loss. Most studies of glaucomatous conditions have dealt with the pathophysiology within the retina. In many cases, retinal ganglion cell death continues after medical or surgical management of elevated IOP. Relatively little attention has been given to the functional consequences of the remaining retinal ganglion cells following normalized intraocular pressure. Here we review the studies dealing with loss of visual acuities and contrast sensitivities of the glaucomatous retina with changes that follow the dendritic arbors of remaining ganglion cells and compare with the adaptive changes observed in the terminal areas of the optic axons in the brain visual centers.

## 2. Background

Glaucoma is the most common neurodegenerative disease of the eyes, leading to the blindness. The loss of vision in glaucoma has been attributed to the retinal ganglionic cell death (RGCs) and optic nerve axonal loss. In a recent study, advanced glaucoma intervention study, the relationship between intraocular pressure control and the visual field deficits has been established (1). This report has established the role of elevated IOP, in clinical trials, to the initiation of glaucoma and further elaborated that reduction of IOP can reduce the progressive vision loss in glaucomatous patients.

In the pathology of the glaucoma, visual field losses first occur in the peripheral retina and progressively lead to the loss of all vision and complete blindness. The main therapy for the treatment of glaucoma has been the reduction of IOP that stabilizes the vision loss. However, in certain population, the visual loss continues in spite of the reduction of IOP.

The death of RGCs in glaucoma is primarily apoptotic in experimental animals (2, 3) and in Human (4). The exact mechanism, which initiates the cascade of death signals in RGC of glaucomatous eye, is unclear. Similarly, how the elevation of IOP translates or triggers changes in either RGC or its effect to the optic disc and/or the optic axons is uncertain. Actually over the past 20 years, more efforts have been made in searching for the perfect model that replicate human disease yet nothing close to human disease process has emerged in experimental animal models. However, these efforts have led to myriad theories of the initiation of changes in the prelaminar optic axons supporting the assumptions that optic axons are injured first followed by the death of RGCs. Similarly data exist that leads one to believe that RGCs are directly affected by elevated IOP.

Relatively less efforts has been made in deciphering how the pressure triggers changes in cells other than RGCs. In animal models of glaucoma, activation of micoglia leads to proliferation and hypertrophy, visible within hours after the initial insult (5). The mechanisms of activation, proliferation, and hypertrophy are not understood. In glaucomatous eye, either the optic nerve or the retina initiates changes in microglia that have been known to trigger the formation of reactive oxygen species. The reactive oxygen species activate nuclear factor kappa B (NFKβ), which then results in the expression of proinflammatory cytokines. Persistence of these factors leads to the peroxidation of lipid and the activation of apoptotic neuronal death pathways. Speculations regarding such a role for microglia in glaucoma have been made, although no definite answers have yet emerged.

Similarly, other glial cells, such as astrocytes, become hypertrophied and have enlarged end feet at the retinal blood vessels in glaucoma.

It has also been reported that astrocyte migration occurs in response to neuronal injury through the action of myriad growth factors, such as epidermal growth factor (6); cytokines, such as tumor necrosis factor (TNF-α) and interleukin 1 alpha (IL-1α) (7); and other mediators, such as adenosine triphosphate (ATP) (8). This migration is considered an important component in the remodeling of the optic nerve head in glaucoma (9). Reactive astrocytes migrate from the cribriform plates into the nerve bundles and synthesize neurotoxic mediators such as nitric oxide (NO) and TNF-α, which may be released near the axons causing neuronal damage (10, 11). Agents that inhibit the migration of astrocytes by transforming growth factor B (TGFβ) and myosin light chain kinase pathways were suggested for glaucoma treatment (12).

Müller cells have also been shown to respond to growth factors and cytokines (13), though their role in initiating RGC death in glaucoma is unclear.

Recent evidence suggests that metabolic stress to astrocytes releases ATP which leads to the propagation of calcium waves causing axonal loss (14). Reactive microglia then follows the gradient of ATP to remove the axonal debris. The marked activation of microglia in the retina, optic nerve, and tract was postulated to accompany ongoing axonal degeneration. The degree of activation in the optic nerve correlated with axonal damage (14). Interestingly, as microglia is the major cell population in the central nervous system with the potential to act as antigen-presenting cell, upregulated major histocompatibility complex (MHC) antigens were not sufficient to stimulate significant T-cell infiltration in a mouse model of glaucoma (15,16).

The steps of programmed cell death in glaucoma are similar to the steps in other neurodegenerative diseases, such as Alzheimer disease (AD), Parkinson disease, or even Huntington diseases. The agents that cause these diseases may be varied. There are certain common features, for example, the death of RGCs in glaucoma. In a recent article Crish et al. (16) showed that distal axonal injury appears early in mouse glaucoma, similar to the distal changes in AD and other neurodegenerative diseases. These authors showed the changes in axonal transports progress from the distal to the proximal end. The early changes showing the breakdown of optic axonal terminals were seen in superior colliculus followed by changes in the optic axons and finally in the retina. They further elaborated that in addition to the failure or decrease in axonal transport (distal to the proximal area) the axonal terminal persisted in the colliculus. There is absolutely no information regarding this topic in Human glaucoma.

Glaucomatous loss of RGC can cause neurodegeneration in the central visual pathways in animal (17) and in humans (18). Recent advance of functional magnetic resonance imaging (fMRI) provide functional assessment of visual changes in glaucoma patients, which correlated, well with the loss of visual field in the eye (19). Extensive reorganization of visual terminal area was detected in macular degeneration patients (20). In rat glaucoma model, the visual scotoma was not apparent in the tectum two to three weeks after surgery, and larger receptive fields on the periphery represent early signs of altered geometry of the retinal projections (21). It was further assumed that following the death of larger cells on the periphery, the remaining ganglion cells expanded their axonal arbors in the tectum leading to the enlarged receptive fields. The size of the receptive field correlated with the duration and magnitude of intraocular pressure elevation. In primates glaucoma RGC death leads to changes in the lateral geniculate nucleus (LGN) and visual area 1 where cell loss and the shrinkage of lateral geniculate nucleus was noted (23). Similar changes have been shown in the death of specific cell types in the LGN (22,24,28).

In spite of massive literature that has emerged in the past decade regarding glaucoma, we are still uncertain regarding the initiation of RGC death. Relatively little attention has been given regarding the remaining RGC's function following medical or surgical intervention to reduce the IOP and subsequent RGC death. In addition to observed scotoma, do remaining RGCs after glaucoma IOP management adapt to or show changes in their connectivity patterns to the terminal center of the optic axons in the brain?

There are ample scientific evidences suggesting that retinal photoreceptor degeneration can lead to remodeling of the retinal circuitry (for a recent review see Ref. 25). It has been reported that even adult retina shows signs of neuronal plasticity as evidenced by the presence of hypertrophy and axonal sprouting in bipolar, amacrine and photoreceptors.

In monkey retina with elevated IOP, retinal ganglion cells showed shrinkage of dendritic arbors (17). During non-human primate development, plasticity of RGC dendritic arbors and axonal terminals has been observed (25); however, there is a paucity of data supporting such claims in the adult retina. In monkey glaucomatous retina, there was no increase in RGC soma size or dendritic arborization (26); however, a decrease in the dendritic field sizes of the RGC was reported within 3-6 months of induced glaucoma. In monkeys, Smith et al. (27) reported visual deficits in long-term glaucoma as a consequence of RGC loss with no changes in the functional property of the surviving neurons. In addition, loss of some lateral geniculate neurons and reduction in the soma sizes of others were observed.

### 2.1 Evaluation of recent findings

In experimental rat glaucoma, ganglion, amacrine, and rod bipolar cell loss was observed within 5 weeks of elevated intraocular pressure (IOP), suggesting that inner nuclear layer cells of the retina were affected as well (36,37). We previously showed 3-4% RGC death per week in glaucomatous rats (29). The IOP elevation was induced by episcleral venous cauderization. In these animals, IOP usually returned to normal after 10-12 weeks of elevation, possibly due to revascularization. During the period of elevated IOP in the experimental eyes, the remaining ganglion cell soma increased in size of all RGC types. This increase in soma size can be attributed as a precursor to their death. Another possibility is derived from developmental studies on the retina that points to the fact that increase in

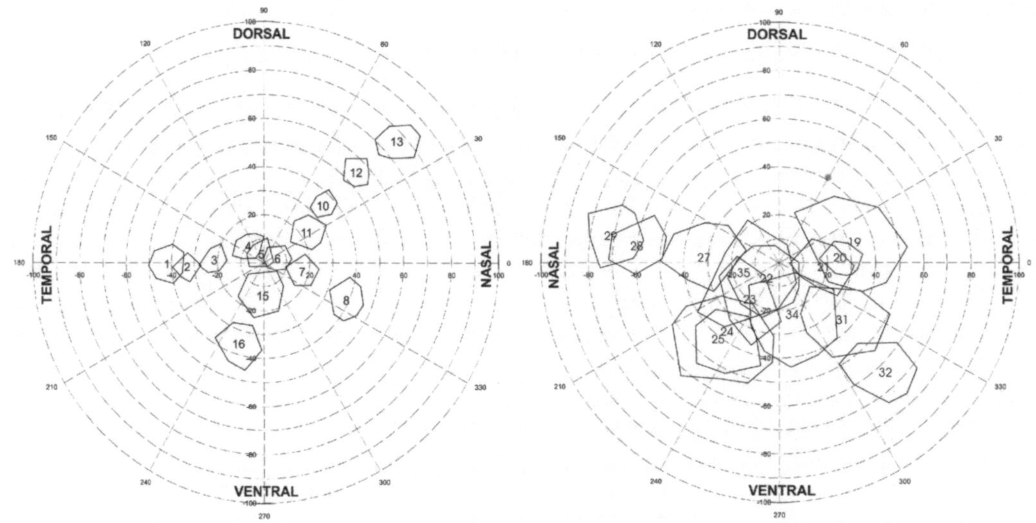


Fig. 1. The retinotopic projective maps in a normal rat when recorded from the electrode positions place on the contralateral superior colliculus. Figure on the left shows numbers 1-16 are representative examples of the visually driven receptive field sizes form the tectum when driven by a normal eye. Receptive field sizes were between 12-25° degrees. The right visual field map shows visually driven receptive field sizes (positions 19-35) in glaucomatous eye that are almost doubled in size when compared to normal. In these topographic mapping there was no overlap of receptive fields in the normal eye mapping, however, experimental glaucomatous eye showed numerous overlapping receptive fields. The normal order of the map was degraded. Many other abnormalities were seen in other maps

soma size of RGC is linked to the soma density. As in glaucomatous RGC, when the cell number decreases, the remaining ganglion cells may hypertrophy. Upon the induction of elevated IOP in pigs using episcleral venous occlusion as in rats (32), Ruitz-Ederra et al. similarly showed an increase in the mean soma area of the remaining RGC (31). A recent study in rat glaucoma showed the neuroprotective effect on retinal ganglion cell survival following systemically administration of bromonidine and it further prevented the increase in soma sizes usually associated with RGC death (38). Additionally, because RGCs are ensheathed by Müller cell processes, these processes must change their milieus to allow the soma to increase in size. These findings stand in contrast to findings in the glaucomatous monkey retina, where all retinal ganglion cells shrink in size, perhaps due to the constraints of very tight Müller cell processes that may not allow expansion (30). Future studies must explore the possibility of ganglion cell dendritic arbor expansion following the breakdown of Müller cell ensheathment.

In addition to soma size increases in rat RGCs, Ahmed et al. also showed the increase in the dendritic arbors of the remaining ganglion cells in glaucomatous eyes (28). Do these changes observed in remaining RGCs have compensatory effects on the target centers as well? Towards this goal visually evoked receptive fields were mapped onto the superior colliculus contralateral to the experimental glaucomatous eyes (21).

Recent evidence from mouse and rat studies showed that the optic axonal terminal synapses degenerate from the distal to proximal direction and precede the degeneration and death of

RGCs (33-35). We theorize that the larger visual receptive fields in the superior colliculus of rats with elevated IOP may be the consequence of expanding terminals of the intact axons into spaces vacated by dying retinal axon terminals (22). Within 6-8 weeks of induced glaucoma, electrophysiological mapping showed no significant changes in receptive field sizes when recorded in the superior colliculus. Dramatic changes were not observed until 4-10 months following IOP elevation (22).
Visual receptive fields measured in the contralateral superior colliculus fall in the range of 15 to 20° (Figure 1A) in normal animals. Receptive fields measured 4 months later in experimental animals with elevated IOP were in the range of 40 to 60° (Figure 1B). These observations indicate some adaptive changes.

### 2.2 Changes in axonal terminal arbors

Anatomical evidences for observed enlargement of receptive fields in experimental glaucoma point to the increase in the axonal terminal arbors of the remaining retinal ganglion cells axons in the contralateral superior colliculus. Figure 2 shows the morphology of RGC axonal terminal in the superior colliculus. The axons at proximal and distal portion of superior colliculus (Figure 2A and 2C) in the normal IOP animal are displayed. With elevation of IOP for 4 months, the axons at the same level were enlarged and more terminal branches were identified (Figure 2B and 2D). This suggests that surviving axons may occupy the territory of the dead axons.

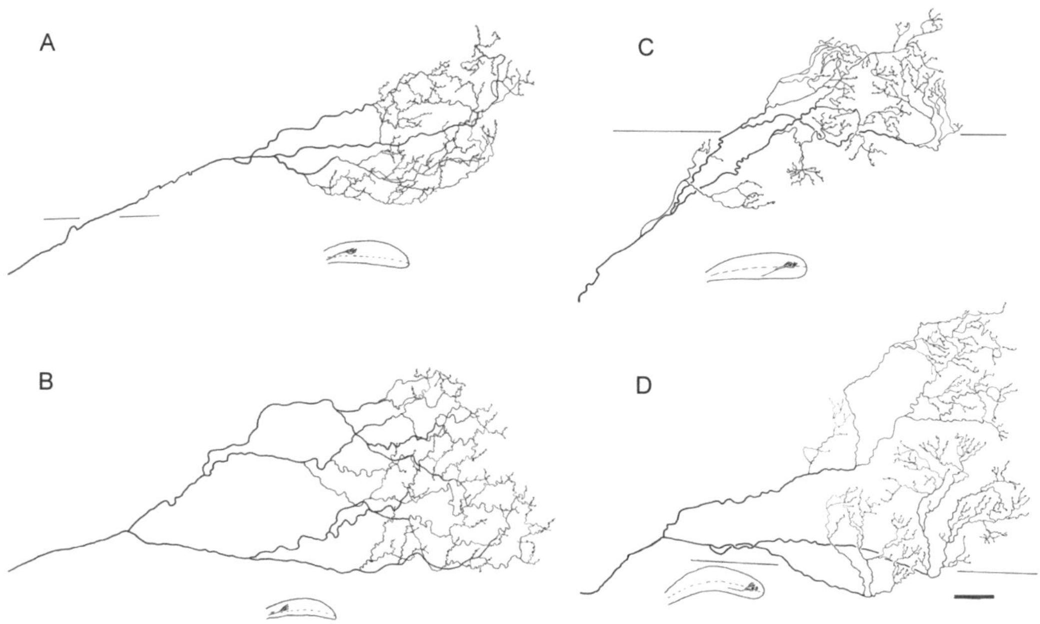


Fig. 2. Camera lucida drawing of the axonal arbor in the mid rostal (Fig. 2A) tectal region of a normal rat, total area of the terminal was 11250 μm². In the glaucomatous animal, the area of terminal axonal arbor at similar location to the normal was 12480 μm² (Fig. 2B). In the caudal tectum of normal rat, the area of the normal optic axonal terminal was 14290 μm² (Fig. 2C) whereas it was 18060 μm² in glaucomatous side (Fig. 2D). It was also noted that these were less vericosities and relatively less dense boutons when compared to the normal

The functional consequences of the changes observed in glaucomatous animals following changes in RGC somas and dendritic arbors of the remaining ganglion cells and the axonal terminal arbors in the contralateral superior colliculus, as described above, were determined psychophysiologically in the experimental animals. Slow horizontal head and body rotation occurs in rats when the visual fields are rotated around them. These optomotor responses can be readily reproduced. When one eye is closed, only motion in the temporal to nasal direction for the contralateral eye evokes the tracking response. In these animals, visual acuity refers to the maximal spatial frequency capable of evoking an optomotor response. In a normal animal, the visual acuity of the right and left eyes is identical in monocular or binocular viewing conditions. In an experimental eye of elevated IOP, the visual acuity was significantly lower when compared to the control eye ($p < 0.0005$). In addition, the contrast sensitivity as a function of spatial frequency was also studied. At all spatial frequencies studied, the contrast sensitivity of the experimental eye was lower than the control eye ($p < 0.0005$) (39).

### 2.3 Future directions

The contrasting changes seen in studies involving rat and those involving human glaucoma are at first unsettling. We strongly believe that the following studies need to be undertaken in human.

a. Longitudinal studies using optical coherence tomography (OCT) with adaptive optics to discern changes in different retinal cell types during the progression of glaucoma.
b. Studies of the progression or regression of scotomas in human patients following management of elevated IOP either surgically and/or medically

If there are documented changes, one can pursue the means to induce adaptive changes. At present one can only partially block the progression of glaucomatous scomota and one assumes that partial vision is better than no vision. We must therefore seek the new avenues to overcome our limitations.

## 3. Acknowledgements

*Supported by grants from Basque Government (IT43710), Red Patologia Oular Retics (RD 07/0062/2004), organization for Spanish Blind People (ONCE) and U.S. N.I.H. N.E.I. grants.*

## 4. References

[1] The AGIS Investigators. The Advanced Glaucoma Intervention Study (AGIS): 7. The relationship between control of intraocular pressure and visual field deterioration. *Am J Ophthalmol.* 2000 Oct;130(4):429-40

[2] Garcia-Valenzuela, E., Shareef, S., Walsh, J., and Sharma, S.C. Programmed cell death of retinal ganglion cells during experimental glaucoma. *Exp. Eye Res.* 1995; 61:33-44.

[3] Quigley, H.A., Nickells, R.W., Kerrigan, L.A., Pease, M.E., Thibault, D.J., and Zack, D.J. Retinal ganglion cell death in experimental glaucoma and after axotomy occurs by apoptosis. *Invest. Ophthalmol. Vis. Sci.* 1995;36:774-786.

[4] Quigley, H.A., Guy, J., and Anderson, D.R. Blockade of rapid axonal transport. Effect of intraocular pressure elevation in primate optic nerve. *Arch. Ophthalmol.* 1999; 97:525-531.

[5] Lam D, Jim J, To E, Rasmussen C, Kaufman PL, Matsubara J. Astrocyte and microglial activation in the lateral geniculate nucleus and visual cortex of glaucomatous and optic nerve transected primates. *Molecular Vision* 2009;15: 2217-2229

[6] Hernandez MR, Miao H, Lukas T. Astrocytes in glaucomatous optic neuropathy. *Prog Brain Res.* 2008:173:353-373

[7] Gavillet M, Allaman I, Magistretti PJ. Modulation of astrocytic metabolic phenotype by proinflammatory cytokines. *Glia.* 2008;56:975-989

[8] Wang M, Long Q, Gonzalez FA, et al. P2Y nucleotide receptor interaction with alpha integrin mediates astrocyte migration. *J Neurochem.* 2005; 95:630-640

[9] Hernandez MR. The optic nerve head in glaucoma: role of astrocytes in tissue remodeling. *Prog Retin Eye Res.* 2000;19:297-321

[10] Liu B, Neufled AH. Expression of nitric oxide syndthase-2 (NOS-2) in reactive astrocytes of the human glaucomatous optic nerve head. *Glia.* 2000. 2000;30:178-186

[11] Liu B, Chen H, Johns TG, Neufeld AH. Epidermal growth factor receptor activation: an upstream signal for transition of quiescent astrocytes into reactive astrocytes after neural injury. *J Neurosci.* 2006;26:7532-7540

[12] Miao H, Crabb AW, Hernandez MR and Lukas TJ. Modulation of factors affecting optic nerve head astrocyte migration. *Invest ophthalmol & Vis Sci.* 2010;51:4096-4103

[13] Johnson CA, Cioffi GA, Liebmann JR, Sample PA, Zangwill LM, Weinreb RN. The relationship between structural and functional alterations in glaucoma: a review. *Semin Ophthalmol.* 2000 Dec;15(4):221-33.

[14] Johnson EC, Deppmeier LM, Wentzien SK, et al. Chronology of optic nerve head and retinal responses to elevated intraocular pressure. *Invest Ophthalmol Vis Sci.* 2000;41:431-442

[15] Ebneter A, Casson RJ, Wood JP, Childlow G. Microglial activation in the visual pathway in experimental glaucoma: spatiotemporal characterization and correlation with axonal injury. *Invest Ophthalmol Vis Sci.* 2010;51:6448-6460

[16] Lucin KM, Wyss-Coray T. Immune activation in brain aging and neurodegeneration: too much or too little? *Neuron.* 2009;64:110-122

[17] Crish SD, Sappington RM, Inman DM, Horner PJ, Calkins DJ. Distal axonopathy with structural persistence in glaucomatous neurodegeneration. *Proc Natl Acad Sci U S A.* 2010 Mar 16;107(11):5196-201. Epub 2010 Mar 1.

[18] Weber AJ, Chen H, Hubbard WC, Kaufman PL. Experimental glaucoma and cell size, density, and number in the primate lateral geniculate nucleus. *Invest Ophthalmol Vis Sci* 2000;41:1370-9

[19] Gupta N, Ang LS, Noël de Tilly L, Bidaisee L, Yücel YH. Human glaucoma and neural degeneration in intracranial optic nerve, lateral geniculate nucleus, and visual cortex. *Br J Ophthalmol* 2006;90:674-8

[20] Duncan DO, Sample PA, Weinreb RW, Bowd C, Zangwill LM. Retinotopic organization of primary visual cortex in glaucoma: comparing fMRI measurements of cortical function with visual loss. *Prog Retin Eye Res.* 2007;26:38-56

[21] Baker CI, Peli E, Knouf N, Kanwisher NG. Reorganization of visual processing in macular degeneration. *J Neuroscience.* 2005; 25:614-618

[22] King WM, Sarup V, Sauve Carpenter DO, Sharma SC. Expansion of visual receptive fields in glaucomatous rat. *Visual Neurosci* 2006;23:137-142

[23] Yücel YH, Zhang Q. Weinreb RN, Kaufman PL, Gupta N. Effects of retinal ganglion cell loss on Magno-, Parvo-konicellular pathways in the lateral geniculate nucleus and the visual cortex in glaucoma. *Prog Retin Eye Res* 2003; 22: 465-481

[24] Wang X, Sam-Wah Tay S, Ng YK. Nitric oxide, microglial activities and neuronal cell death in the lateral geniculate nucleus of glaucomatous rats. *Brain Res* 2000;878:136-147.

[25] Marc RE, Jones BW, Watt CB. Retinal remodeling: circuitry revision triggered by photoreceptor degeneration. In Pinaud, Tremere and De-Weerd (Eds.), *Plasticity in the visual system: From Genes to Circuits,* Spring Science, 2006. pp.35-54

[26] Leventhal AG, Ault SJ, Vitek DJ. The nasotemporal division in primate retina: the neural bases of macular sparing and splitting. *Science.* 1988; 40(4848):66-7.

[27] Weber AJ, Harman CD. Structure-function relations of parasol cells in the normal and glaucomatous primate retina. *Invest Ophthalmol Vis Sci.*2005; 46(9):3197-207.

[28] Smith EL, Chino YM, Harwerth RS, Ridder RS, Crawford ML. Retinal imputs to the monkey lateral geniculate nucleus in experimental glaucoma. *Clin.Vis. Sci* 1993;8:113-139

[29] Ahmed FA, Hegazy K, Chaudhary P, Sharma SC. Neuroprotective effect of alpha(2) agonist (brimonidine) on adult rat retinal ganglion cells after increased intraocular pressure. *Brain Res.* 2001; 913(2):133-9.

[30] Weber AJ, Kaufman PL, Hubbard WC. Morphology of single ganglion cells in the glaucomatous primate retina. *Invest Ophthalmol Vis Sci.*1998;39(12):2304-20

[31] Ruiz-Ederra J, García M, Hernández M, Urcola H, Hernández-Barbáchano E, Araiz J, Vecino E. The pig eye as a novel model of glaucoma. *Exp Eye Res.*2005;81(5):561-9

[32] Shareef S, Garcia-Valenzuela E, Salierno A, Walsh J, Sharma SC. Chronic ocular hypertension following episcleral venous occlusion in rats. *Exp Eye Res.*1995; 61:379-382.

[33] Harwerth RS, Crawford ML, Frishman JL, Wiswanathan S. Smith EL III, Carter-Dawson L. Visual field defects and neural losses from experimental glaucoma. *Prog Retin Eye Res.* 2002;21:91-125

[34] Whitmore AV, Libby RT, John SW. Glaucoma: thinking in new ways-a role for autonomous axonal self-destruction and other compartmentalized processes? *Prog Retin Eye Rse.* 2005;24:639-662

[35] Morrison JC, Johnson EC, Cepurna W, Jia L. Understanding mechanisms of pressure-induced optic nerve damage. *Prog Retin Eye Res.* 2005;24:217-240

[36] Fu QL, Li X, Shi J, Xu G, Wen W, Lee DH et al. Synaptic degeneration of retinal ganglion cells in a rat ocular hypertension glaucoma model. *Cell Mol Neurobiol.* 2009; 29: 575-581

[37] Hernandez, M., Rodriguez, F. D., Sharma, S.C., & Vecino, E. Immunohistochemical changes in rat retinas at various time periods of elevated intraocular pressure. 2009; *Molecular Vision,* 15, 2696-2709

[38] Pinar-Suerio, S., Urcola, H., Rivas, M. A., Vecino, E. Prevention of retinal ganglion cell swelling by systemic brimonidine in a rat experimental glaucoma model. 2011; *Clinical and Experimental Ophthalmology (in press)*

[39] Prusky, G.T., West, P.W., and Douglas, D.M. Behavioral assessment of visual acuity in mice and rats. 2000, *Vision Research,* 40, 2201-2209

# 4

# Molecular Control of Retinal Ganglion Cell Specification and Differentiation

Mengqing Xiang[1], Haisong Jiang[1,2], Kangxin Jin[1] and Feng Qiu[1]
[1]*Center for Advanced Biotechnology and Medicine and Department of Pediatrics, UMDNJ-Robert Wood Johnson Medical School, New Jersey;*
[2]*Institute for Cell Engineering, Departments of Neurology and Neuroscience, Johns Hopkins University School of Medicine, Maryland;*
*USA*

## 1. Introduction

The mammalian retina is a laminated sensorineural epithelium composed of six classes of neurons that include the rod, cone, bipolar, horizontal, amacrine, and ganglion cells (RGCs), and one type of glia, the Müller cells. RGCs are the sole output neurons in the retina whose projecting axons form the optic nerve essential for conveying light signals to the higher visual system in the brain. Glaucoma causes degeneration of the optic nerve and RGCs that leads to impaired vision and blindness. Recent advances in stem cell-based therapy to restore functional retinal circuits in the damaged retina have made it promising to develop an effective treatment of glaucoma in the future. It is conceivable that, in the future, RGCs derived through controlled differentiation of stem cells by various retinogenic factors may provide renewable sources of replacement RGCs for glaucoma patients. Because differentiation of stem cells normally recapitulates the events that occur during embryogenesis, it will be important to understand the molecular basis of RGC development and identify intrinsic and extrinsic factors involved in RGC fate determination and differentiation.

In this chapter, we will summarize and discuss recent molecular genetic studies on intrinsic and extrinsic factors required for RGC development, and how they act to establish RGC competence, determine RGC fate and facilitate RGC differentiation (Fig. 1). We will also discuss gene regulatory networks governing RGC development as well as safeguard mechanisms ensuring RGC differentiation from multipotent retinal precursors. Finally, we will discuss how our knowledge about the intrinsic and extrinsic retinogenic factors may contribute to devising efficient means to generate RGCs from stem cells. Some of our own work will be highlighted throughout the chapter.

## 2. Intrinsic factors

### 2.1 Transcription factors involved in RGC fate and differentiation

**Pou4f/Brn3 factors.** Our molecular cloning of the POU-domain transcription factor Pou4f2/Brn3b and demonstration of its expression in RGCs about two decades ago (Xiang et al., 1993) provided an entry point for the ensuing explosion of studies on the genetic

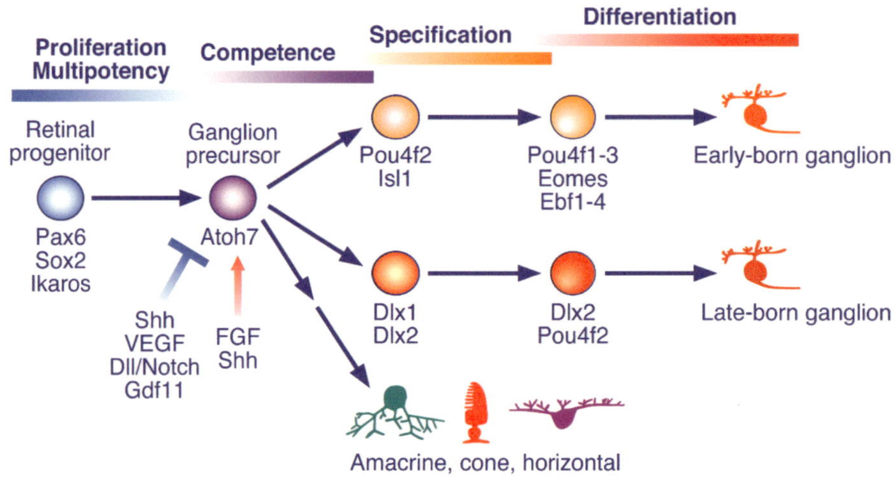


Fig. 1. Schematic illustration of developmental stages and intrinsic and extrinsic factors leading to RGC production from progenitors. Multiple transcription factors and signaling molecules are involved to drive progression from multipotent retinal progenitors to RGC competent precursors and to eventually specified and differentiated RGCs. The Atoh7-expressing RGC precursors are also competent to generate amacrine, horizontal and cone cells

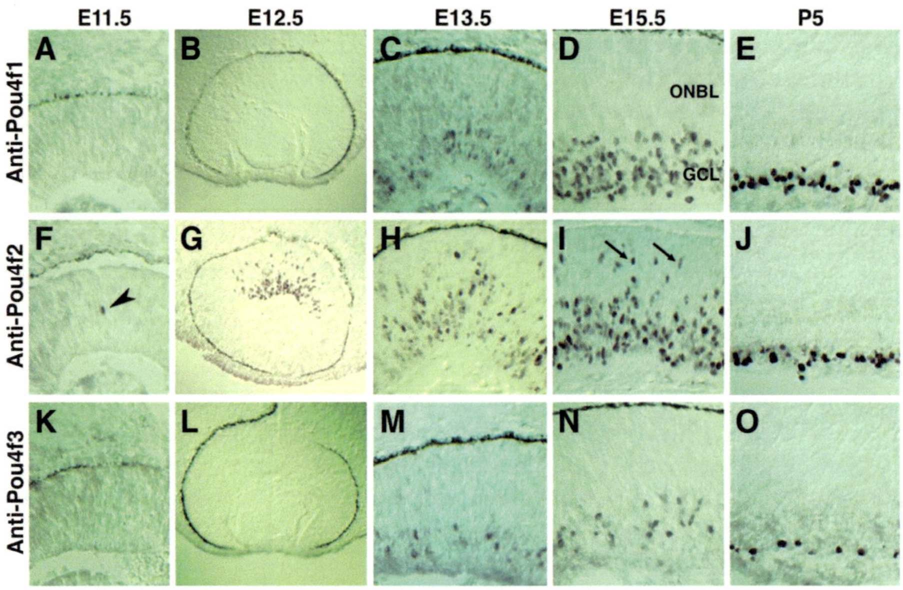


Fig. 2. Expression patterns of Pou4f proteins during mouse retinogenesis. Retinal sections from the indicated stages were immunostained with anti-Pou4f1, anti-Pou4f2 and anti-Pou4f3 antibodies. Pou4f2 commences its expression in occasional cells (indicated by the arrow head) of E11.5 retinas. At E12.5-E18.5, it is localized in a large number of cells in the ganglion cell layer (GCL), as well as in scattered cells (indicated by arrows) within the outer neuroblastic layer (ONBL). In postnatal retinas, Pou4f2 expression is restricted to the RGCs in the GCL. Pou4f1 and 3 are found only in cells of the GCL beginning at E13.5

pathway and gene regulatory network of RGC development. In vertebrates (from zebrafish to human), there exist three family members of Pou4f factors (Pou4f1-3 or Brn3a-c) and within the retina their expression is all confined to RGCs (DeCarvalho et al., 2004; Gerrero et al., 1993; Hutcheson and Vetter, 2001; Turner et al., 1994; Xiang et al., 1995; Xiang et al., 1993). In the adult mouse retina, Pou4f1 and 2 are estimated to be localized in more than 70% of RGCs whereas Pou4f3 in ~ 30% of total RGCs (Xiang et al., 1995). During mouse retinogenesis, the three Pou4f factors exhibit overlapping but spatiotemporally distinct expression patterns, with only Pou4f2 sporting a pattern characteristic of the dynamic profile of RGC genesis (Gan et al., 1996; Xiang, 1998). At prenatal stages, Pou4f2-immunoreactive cells are seen at the time of first RGC birth at embryonic day 11.5 (E11.5) (Young, 1985), and in newborn migrating RGCs in the outer neuroblastic layer (Fig. 2F-J) (Gan et al., 1996; Xiang, 1998). The onset of Pou4f1 and 3 expression occurs two days later only in differentiated RGCs within the ganglion cell layer (Fig. 2A-E, K-O) (Xiang, 1998). Interestingly, there seems to be always one Pou4f factor whose spatiotemporal expression pattern follows closely with the timing of RGC generation in other vertebrates, such as cPou4f3/cBrn3c and XBrn3d, in the case of chicken and *Xenopus*, respectively (Hutcheson and Vetter, 2001; Liu et al., 2000a). This correlative early Pou4f expression suggested to us that Pou4f function might not only be required for RGC differentiation but also for an earlier role (Xiang, 1998), which we later showed to be in RGC fate specification (Qiu et al., 2008).

All three *Pou4f* genes were deleted in mice by gene targeting to study their developmental function (Erkman et al., 1996; Gan et al., 1999; Gan et al., 1996; McEvilly et al., 1996; Xiang et al., 1997; Xiang et al., 1996). *Pou4f2* inactivation leads to optic nerve hypoplasia as well as thinner retinas with reduced thickness of the ganglion cell, nerve fiber and inner plexiform layers (Fig. 3A-C) (Gan et al., 1996). *Pou4f2* mutant optic nerves are diminished in cross-sectional area by approximately 5-fold and have a significantly reduced density of axons (Fig. 3D,E). The mutant retinas lose ~ 70-80% of total RGCs and exhibit a dramatic decrease in the number of Pou4f1- and Pou4f3-positive cells and Thy1- and SMI-32-immunoreactive processes (Fig. 3F-I) (Gan et al., 1996). These RGC defects occur early in development in the mutant (Fig. 3J-Q). Optic nerve hypoplasia, nerve fiber defasciculation, and diminished Pou4f1, Pou4f2, Ebf1, and Pou6f2/RPF-1 expression are visible as early as E12.5 (Gan et al., 1999; Xiang, 1998). RGC axon guidance errors are also present at multiple intraocular and extraocular points along their projection pathways in developing and adult *Pou4f2* null mutant mice (Erkman et al., 2000). Meanwhile, inactivating *Pou4f2* appears to cause many presumptive RGC precursors to switch to amacrine or horizontal cell fates (Qiu et al., 2008). These improperly differentiated cells are likely to degenerate by apoptosis as cell death significantly increases in the mutant retina (Gan et al., 1999; Xiang, 1998). Thus, Pou4f2 plays an essential role in RGC differentiation as well as their fate specification. It was thought that Pou4f2 might be required only for RGC differentiation and survival because in *Pou4f2*$^{lacZ/lacZ}$ knockin retinas, normal number of β-gal(galactosidase)$^{+}$ cells is initially produced that migrate into the inner neuroblastic layer (Gan et al., 1999). All of these β-gal$^{+}$ cells were assumed to be RGCs but they were not confirmed as such using molecular markers. In fact, many cells within the inner neuroblastic layer of *Pou4f2* null retinas extend short, microtubule-rich and nonfasciculated neurites characteristic of dendrites rather than axons (Gan et al., 1999; Wang et al., 2000). This phenotype may manifest a switch from RGCs to dendrite-bearing amacrine and horizontal cells even though a change of RGC cell polarity cannot be completely ruled out.

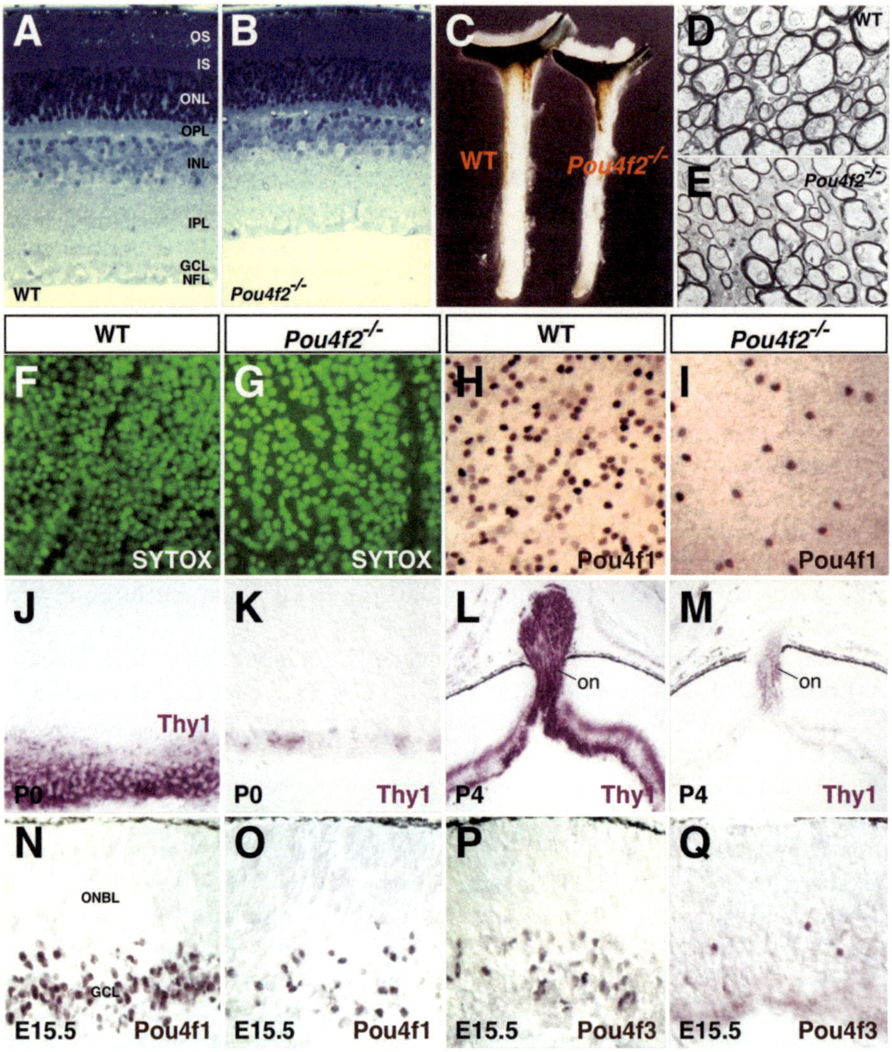


Fig. 3. Loss of RGCs in *Pou4f2-/-* retinas. (A,B) Semi-thin sections of wild-type (WT) and mutant retinas stained with toluidine blue. (C) Optic nerves of the wild-type and mutant mice. (D,E) Electron micrographs of wild-type and mutant optic nerves. (F-I) In wholemount retinas, nuclei in the ganglion cell layer were labeled with SYTOX (F,G) or immunostained with an anti-Pou4f1 antibody (H,I). (J-M) Thy1 immunoreactivity in sections of retinas from the indicated stages. (N-Q) E15.5 retinal sections were immunolabeled with anti-Pou4f1 (N,O) or anti-Pou4f3 (P,Q) antibodies. In the adult *Pou4f2-/-* retina, there is a dramatic loss of RGCs as indicated by the reduced retinal thickness (A,B), diminished optic nerve diameter (C), decreased axon density within the optic nerve (D,E), and reduced cell number in the ganglion cell layer (F-I). The loss of RGCs immunoreactive for Thy1, Pou4f1 or Pou4f3 occur early in development in the mutant retina (J-Q). GCL, ganglion cell layer; INL, inner nuclear layer; IPL, inner plexiform layer; IS, inner segment; NFL, nerve fiber layer; ONBL, outer neuroblastic layer; on, optic nerve; ONL, outer nuclear layer; OPL, outer plexiform layer; OS, outer segment

Given that the three Pou4f factors are 95% identical in protein sequence of the DNA-binding POU domain and have similar DNA-binding specificity and transcriptional activity (Gruber et al., 1997; Liu et al., 2000a; Xiang et al., 1995), it is unsurprising that they display a significant degree of functional redundancy in RGC development. Thus, no obvious RGC defects are found in *Pou4f1* and *3* conventional knockout mice despite the presence of other severe sensory deficiency (Xiang et al., 1997; Xiang et al., 1996). Moreover, there are more severe RGC loss and axon growth defects in *Pou4f2* and *3* compound mutant mice (Wang et al., 2002). We speculate that Pou4f2 can largely take over the function of Pou4f1 and 3 due to its early expression whereas the converse is not true because the belated expression of Pou4f1 and 3 precludes them from compensating an early specification/differentiation role of Pou4f2 (Xiang, 1998). Consistent with this notion, when *Pou4f1* was knocked in the *Pou4f2* locus to ensure its early expression, all phenotypes associated with *Pou4f2* inactivation were apparently completely rescued (Pan et al., 2005). In spite of the extensive overlap in expression and function, however, individual Pou4f factors have distinct roles during RGC development. For instance, conditional deletion of *Pou4f1* changes dendritic morphology and stratification of RGCs, increases the ratio of bistratified to monostratified RGCs, and causes modest RGC loss (Badea et al., 2009; Badea and Nathans, 2011). Although conditional inactivation of *Pou4f2* results in similar defects, it causes no alteration in RGC dendritic stratification but additionally leads to RGC transdifferentitation and central projection defects (Badea et al., 2009; Badea and Nathans, 2011). However, conditional *Pou4f3* mutants lack any of these RGC phenotypes (Badea and Nathans, 2011).

Pou4f2 is not only necessary but also sufficient to promote RGC differentiation from retinal progenitors. In mouse embryonic retinas, misexpressed Pou4f2 dramatically increased Pou4f1-positive RGCs (Qiu et al., 2008). When misexpressed in chick retinal progenitors by the replication-competent RCAS retroviral vector, mouse Pou4f2 increased cells immunoreactive for Isl1 and NF200, two RGC markers, by 20-50% (Fig. 4C,D,L) (Liu et al., 2000a). Forced expression of mouse Pou4f1 and Pou4f3 as well as chicken Pou4f3 (cPou4f3) all similarly promoted RGC differentiation (Fig. 4M,N) (Liu et al., 2000a), suggesting that all Pou4f factors have a similar potential to promote RGC development but this potential may be limited by their order of expression in vivo. Moreover, misexpression of each of the three mouse Pou4f factors induced many cells to express cPou4f3 in the outer neuroblastic layer (Fig. 4G-I) (Liu et al., 2001). No cPou4f3-positive cells were induced when a mutant Pou4f3 protein was ectopically expressed that contained a deletion in the POU-homeodomain (Fig. 4J) (Liu et al., 2001). Therefore, *Pou4f* gene expression may be cross-activated and auto-activated to help maintain their expression necessary for RGC specification and differentiation (Fig. 4O). Nevertheless, other mechanisms must operate to maintain *Pou4f1* and *2* expression since inactivating either gene in mice does not completely abolish the expression the other in RGCs (Badea et al., 2009; Gan et al., 1996; Xiang et al., 1996). In this regard, the Isl1 LIM-homeodomain transcription factor appears to play a role in the maintenance of *Pou4f2* expression (Mu et al., 2008; Pan et al., 2008).

Pou4f2 regulates a large set of downstream genes to fulfill its crucial function in RGC specification and differentiation. Microarray gene expression profiling of *Pou4f2* wild-type and mutant retinas has revealed hundreds of genes whose expression is altered in the mutant (Mu et al., 2004; Qiu et al., 2008). Among the downregulated genes are those encoding transcription factors and proteins involved in morphogenesis, nervous system development, neuronal cell projection, synaptic vesicle, and neurofilament, consistent with the role of Pou4f2 in RGC development. In particular, Pou4f2 activates the expression of Shh

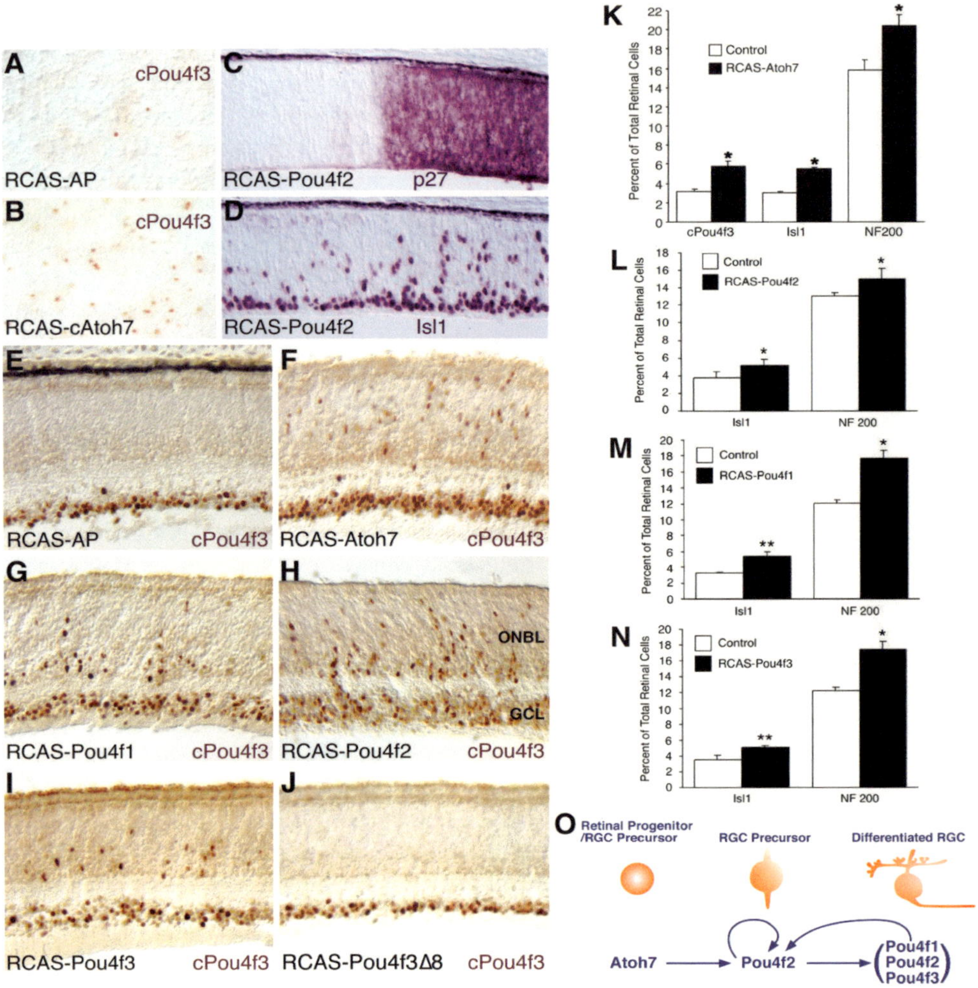


Fig. 4. Regulatory relationship between Atoh7 and Pou4f factors and effects of misexpressed Atoh7 and Pou4f factors on RGC production in the chick retina. (A,B) In the outer neuroblastic layer (ONBL) of E11.5 flat-mount retinas infected with RCAS-cAtoh7 viruses, there was a significant increase of cPou4f3-immunoreactive cells compared to the control (RCAS-AP). (C,D) Adjacent sections from an E7.5 retina infected with RCAS-Pou4f2 viruses were immunostained with anti-p27 gag (C) or anti-Isl1 (D) antibodies. More Isl1-immunoreactive cells were found in the patch stained with the anti-p27 gag antibody than in the patch negative for it. (E-J) Sections from intermediate regions of E11.5 control retinas and retinas infected with RCAS-Atoh7, RCAS-Pou4f1, RCAS-Pou4f2, RCAS-Pou4f3, or RCAS-Pou4f3Δ8 viruses were immunostained with an anti-cPou4f3 antibody. Misexpressed Atoh7, Pou4f1, Pou4f2, and Pou4f3 caused a significant increase of cPou4f3 immunoreactive cells in the ONBL, whereas misexpressed Pou4f3Δ8 had no effect. (K-N) Quantitation of cPou4f3-, Isl1- or NF200-positive RGCs in retinas infected with RCAS-Atoh7, RCAS-Pou4f2, RCAS-Pou4f1, or RCAS-Pou4f3 viruses. (O) Schematic illustrating regulatory relationship between Atoh7 and Pou4f factors during RGC development. Atoh7 may directly activate *Pou4f2* expression which in turn may activate the expression of *Pou4f1* and *Pou4f3*. *Pou4f* gene expression may be cross-activated and auto-activated to help maintain their expression. GCL, ganglion cell layer

(sonic hedgehog) signal pathway genes (Mu et al., 2004). On the other hand, Pou4f2 is also required to repress many genes involved in non-RGC generation to ensure faithful differentiation of RGCs (Qiu et al., 2008).

**Isl1.** Isl1 resembles Pou4f2 in many ways in controlling RGC development. During mouse retinogenesis, it is co-expressed with Pou4f2 in migrating newborn RGCs beginning at E11.5 (Pan et al., 2008). Conditional inactivation of *Isl1* results in optic nerve hypoplasia, a loss of ~70% of RGCs, delayed RGC axon growth, and RGC axon pathfinding errors and fiber defasciculation (Mu et al., 2008; Pan et al., 2008). Further RGC loss is seen in *Pou4f2* and *Isl1* compound null mice (Pan et al., 2008), implicating distinct as well as redundant functions between Pou4f2 and Isl1 during RGC development. Indeed, these two factors regulate overlapping but distinct groups of genes and they co-occupy the promoters of several shared RGC genes (Mu et al., 2008; Pan et al., 2008). Isl1 does not act genetically upstream of Pou4f2 since its absence does not alter *Pou4f2* expression in early embryonic retinas (Mu et al., 2008). However, it is unclear whether Isl1 acts only in parallel with Pou4f2 or additionally downstream of it to control RGC differentiation.

**Dlx1 & Dlx2.** The Dlx1 and 2 homeodomain transcription factors are also co-expressed with Pou4f2 in developing RGCs during mouse retinal development (de Melo et al., 2003). Their compound mutants display a mild optic nerve hypoplasia, a loss of ~ 30-40% of RGCs, and increased apoptosis (de Melo et al., 2005). The RGC loss in double mutants results from decreased generation of late born RGCs, thereby indicating a critical role for Dlx1 and 2 in differentiation of late-born RGCs (de Melo et al., 2005). Because these two factors normally repress the expression of a photoreceptor marker *Crx* (de Melo et al., 2005), it is possible that they may also have a role in specifying late-born RGCs.

**Eomes & Ebf factors.** These factors act as Pou4f2 effectors to mediate part of Pou4f2 function during RGC development. Their genes are among the most downregulated in *Pou4f2* null retinas as determined by microarray analysis (Qiu et al., 2008). Eomes is a T-box transcription factor that similar to Pou4f1 and 3, is expressed in developing RGCs only upon their arrival into the RGC layer (Mao et al., 2008). Its expression is directly activated by Pou4f2 through a 5′ enhancer and is completely downregulated in *Pou4f2* null retinas (Mao et al., 2008). Conditional inactivation of *Eomes* causes a 30% decrease in RGC number and optic nerve size, reduced and disorganized RGC axon myelination, and increased apoptosis (Mao et al., 2008). Ebf1-4 belong to a small family of HLH (helix-loop-helix) transcription factors that are selectively expressed in RGCs in mouse embryonic retinas (Fig. 5A) (Jin et al., 2010). Their RGC expression is dramatically downregulated in *Pou4f2* null mutants (Fig. A-D). It appears that Pou4f2 can bind to the promoter of *Ebf3* to directly activate its expression (Jin et al., 2010). To investigate a possible role for Ebfs during RGC development, we used a replication-incompetent retroviral vector that carries a GFP reporter to misexpress Ebf1 and Ebf-EnR, a dominant-negative form of Ebf constructed by fusing the repressor domain of the *Drosophila*-engrailed protein to the Ebf1 N-terminus. We infected mouse retinal explants with Control-GFP, Ebf1-GFP or Ebf-EnR-GFP viruses at E13.5 when progenitors are still competent for producing RGCs. The infected retinas were harvested after 4 days in culture to analyze RGC production. We found that forced Ebf-EnR expression reduced the proportion of Pou4f1- and Pou4f2-immunoreactive RGCs by ~40-50%, whereas Ebf1 exerted no effect on them (Fig. 5E-K) (Jin et al., 2010). Thus, Ebfs are necessary but insufficient to promote RGC differentiation. It is unknown whether Eomes is sufficient to promote RGC formation as there is yet no report of pertinent gain-of-function analysis.

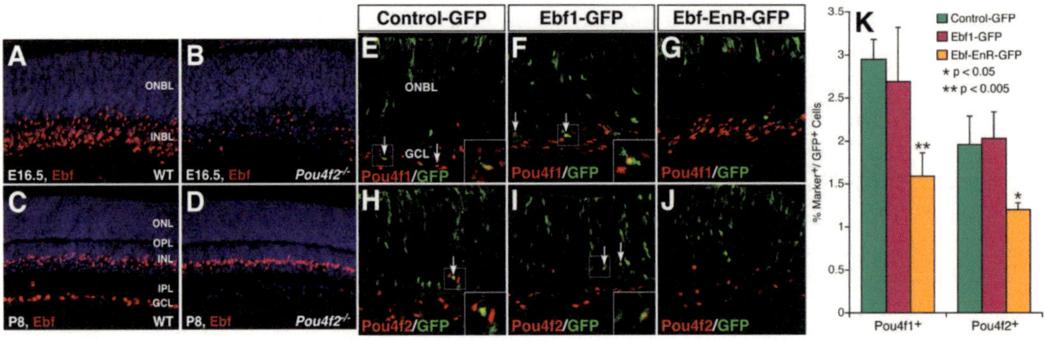


Fig. 5. Requirement for Ebf factors in RGC differentiation. (A-D) Retinal sections from wild-type (WT) and *Pou4f2-/-* mice at the indicated stages were immunostained with a pan-Ebf antibody and weakly counterstained with nuclear DAPI. In the mutant retina, there is a dramatic decrease of Ebf-immunoreactive cells within the INBL or GCL. (E-K) Effect of Ebf1 and a dominant-negative Ebf misexpressed in E13.5 mouse retinal explants on the formation of RGCs. Sections from retinas infected with Control-GFP, Ebf1-GFP or Ebf-EnR-GFP viruses were double immunostained with an anti-GFP antibody and antibodies against Pou4f1 or Pou4f2 (E-J). Virus-transduced retinal cells that became immunoreactive for Pou4f1 or Pou4f2 were then quantified (K, each histogram represents the mean±SD for three retinas). Misexpressed wild-type Ebf1 does not change the number of RGCs immunoreactive for Pou4f1 or Pou4f2; whereas, the dominant-negative form diminishes cells immunoreactive for them. Arrows point to representative colocalized cells, and insets show corresponding outlined regions at a higher magnification. GCL, ganglion cell layer; INL, inner nuclear layer; INBL, inner neuroblastic layer; IPL, inner plexiform layer; ONBL, outer neuroblastic layer; ONL, outer nuclear layer; OPL, outer plexiform layer

### 2.2 Transcription factors involved in RGC competence

Prior to the initiation of retinogenesis, neuroepithelial cells in the optic vesicle must acquire multipotency and establish competence for the generation of the full range of retinal cell types. Pax6, a paired homeodomain transcription factor, and Sox2, a HMG-box transcription factor, appear to coordinately regulate multipotency of retinal progenitor cells including the potency to generate RGCs. Conditional ablation of either gene in mouse retinal progenitors results in a failure to produce RGCs and other non-RGC cell types (Marquardt et al., 2001; Taranova et al., 2006). Retinal progenitors are postulated to undergo a series of successive stages of competence for the ordered generation of different cell types (Cepko, 1999; Cepko et al., 1996; Harris, 1997; Livesey and Cepko, 2001). It has been shown that the Ikaros zinc finger transcription factor plays a key role in establishing the early temporal competence stages responsible for generating early-born cell types including RGCs (Elliott et al., 2008). Inactivating *Ikaros* causes decreased numbers of early-born neurons without affecting late-born cell types whereas its misexpression in postnatal retinal progenitors is sufficient to confer them with prenatal competence to generate early-born cell types (Elliott et al., 2008). Pax6, Sox2 and Ikaros all directly and/or indirectly activate *Atoh7/Math5* expression to confer progenitors with the competence of RGC genesis (Fig. 1), as genetic ablation of any of these three genes leads to loss or decreased *Atoh7* expression (Elliott et al., 2008; Marquardt et al., 2001; Taranova et al., 2006).

Atoh7 is a proneural bHLH (basic helix-loop-helix) transcription factor expressed transiently in a subset of retinal progenitors/precursors (Brown et al., 1998; Kanekar et al., 1997; Liu et al., 2001). Misexpression of *Xenopus* Atoh7 (Xath5) in retinal progenitors promoted RGC differentiation by ~ 3-fold at the expense of amacrine, bipolar and Müller cells (Kanekar et al., 1997). We used the RCAS retroviral vector to overexpress chicken Atoh7 (cAtoh7/Cath5) in chick retinal progenitors and found that forced cAtoh7 expression significantly induced the expression of cPou4f3, a functional equivalent of Pou4f2 in the chick retina (Fig. 4A,B) (Liu et al., 2001). It increased RGCs immunoreactive for cPou4f3, Isl1 or NF200 by ~30-60% (Liu et al., 2001). Similarly, forced expression of mouse Atoh7 induced cPou4f3 expression and significantly promoted the differentiation of RGCs expressing Isl1 and NF200 in the developing chick retina (Fig. 4F,K). Furthermore, Atoh7 from both mouse and chicken was able to activate reporter gene expression through a *Pou4f2* promoter (Liu et al., 2001). Because all Pou4f factors have the ability to promote RGC formation (Liu et al., 2000a), our results demonstrate that Atoh7 can promote RGC differentiation by directly activating *Pou4f2/cPou4f3* expression, and further define an Atoh7-Pou4f2/cPou4f3 pathway underlying the specification and differentiation of RGCs (Fig. 4O) (Liu et al., 2001). This molecular pathway can be confirmed in *Atoh7* knockout mice by the near complete downregulation of *Pou4f2* expression in *Atoh7* mutant retinas (Wang et al., 2001).

Consistent with the gain-of-function studies, loss-of-function analyses in zebrafish and mice have confirmed an essential role for Atoh7 in RGC development. Its mutation in the zebrafish *lakritz* mutant causes a complete loss of RGCs and its deletion in mice results in the absence of optic nerve and a loss of ~95% of RGCs (Brown et al., 2001; Kay et al., 2001; Wang et al., 2001). The virtual absence of Pou4f2-expressing cells in early *Atoh7* mutant retinas suggests that Atoh7 must have an early role during RGC development. However, a role for Atoh7 in RGC fate specification can be ruled out because genetically marked Atoh7-expressing precursors are found to give rise to multiple early-born retinal cell types including RGC, amacrine, horizontal and photoreceptor cells (Yang et al., 2003). Therefore, Atoh7-positive retinal precursors are multipotential and Atoh7 is required only for conferring these precursors with the competence of RGC generation. In agreement with this early function, microarray gene expression profiling analysis has revealed that Atoh7-regulated genes include the two branches of genes controlled by Pou4f2 and Isl1 and additionally contain many more that are not regulated by either factor (Mu et al., 2005). Moreover, *Atoh7* and *Pou4f2* double knockout mice display more severe loss of RGCs (Moshiri et al., 2008). Wt1, a zinc-finger transcription factor encoded by the Wilms' tumor gene, appears to regulate RGC differentiation also by directly activating *Pou4f2* expression (Wagner et al., 2002). However, it is unclear what is the relationship between Wt1 and Atoh7 and whether Wt1 is involved in conferring retinal precursors with RGC competence.

### 2.3 Safeguard mechanism by transcription factors to ensure RGC fidelity

As discussed above, RGC-competent Atoh7$^{+}$ precursors are able to generate RGC, amacrine, horizontal, and cone photoreceptor cells during mouse retinogenesis (Fig. 1) (Feng et al., 2006; Yang et al., 2003). Thus, in order to select the RGC fate from the multiple fates available for an RGC-competent precursor, it is conceivable that the commitment factor must suppress non-RGC fates while promoting the RGC fate to ensure the fidelity of RGC differentiation. In this regard, we have demonstrated that Pou4f2 has the ability to suppress amacrine, horizontal and late-born RGC fates to preferentially specify the early-born RGC fates (Qiu et al., 2008)

In E14.5 *Pou4f2* null retinas, our gene expression profiling study identified a large set of upregulated genes including *Th, Slc32a1/VIAAT, Slc6a1/GAT-1, Slc18a3/VAChT*, and *Gad1/GAD67*, which are normally expressed by amacrine and/or horizontal cells (Qiu et al., 2008). Consistent with this, immunostaining and RNA in situ hybridization revealed a marked increase in the expression of Th, GABA, GAT-1, calbindin D28K, and *Viaat* in the mutant retina (Fig. 6A-F) (Qiu et al., 2008), suggesting that GABAergic amacrine cells abnormally form in early embryonic retinas in the absence of *Pou4f2*. In *Pou4f2*$^{lacZ/lacZ}$ retinas, nearly all Th-immunoreactive cells were co-labeled for β-gal (Fig. 6B), indicating that these cells arise cell-autonomously due to a switch in fate of RGC precursors that would normally express Pou4f2. Double-immunostaining showed a significant increase of cells immunoreactive for both Lim1 and calbindin in *Pou4f2* null retinas (Fig. 6*E,F*), suggesting that loss of *Pou4f2* function causes increased horizontal cell differentiation. These supernumerary horizontal cells also arise cell-autonomously because in *Pou4f2*$^{lacZ/lacZ}$ retinas, many Lim1-immunoreactive cells co-expressed β-gal whereas these double-immunoreactive cells were absent from *Pou4f2*$^{+/lacZ}$ retinas (Qiu et al., 2008). The transcripts of *Dlx1* and *Dlx2* were among the most upregulated in *Pou4f2* null retinas as determined by microarray analysis. At E14.5, scattered in situ hybridization signals for *Dlx1* and *Dlx2* were seen in the outer neuroblastic layer but absent from the inner neuroblastic layer (INBL) of wild-type retinas (Fig. 6*Q,S*). In *Pou4f2*$^{-/-}$ retinas, however, both *Dlx1* and *Dlx2* were aberrantly expressed within the INBL (Fig. 6*R,T*), suggesting the generation of superfluous late-born RGCs within the INBL in the absence of *Pou4f2*. Thus, Pou4f2 has the activity to cell-autonomously inhibit differentiation of amacrine, horizontal and late-born RGCs. This inhibitory activity can be confirmed by overexpression experiments where we showed that misexpressed Pou4f2 suppressed the differentiation of all non-RGC cell types including amacrine and horizontal cells (Qiu et al., 2008).

Pou4f2 acts to inhibit the fates of non-RGCs by repressing the expression of transcription factor genes required for their specification and differentiation. By microarray analysis, in situ hybridization, qRT-PCR, and immunostaining, we were able to show that the expression of *Bhlhb5, Nr4a2/Nurr1, Neurod1, Math3*, and *Ptf1a* all exhibited significant increase in *Pou4f2* null retinas, especially within the INBL (Fig. 6G-L) (Qiu et al., 2008), consistent with the abnormal differentiation of most amacrine cells in this layer of the mutant retina. It has been shown that Neurod1, Math3 and Ptf1a are required for specifying amacrine cells and Bhlhb5 and Nr4a2 for differentiation of GABAergic amacrine cells (Feng et al., 2006; Fujitani et al., 2006; Inoue et al., 2002; Jiang and Xiang, 2009; Nakhai et al., 2007). Similarly, there was a significant increase in expression of *Prox1, Ptf1a, Lim1* and *Ngn2*, all transcription factor genes involved in horizontal cell development (Akagi et al., 2004; Dyer et al., 2003; Fujitani et al., 2006; Liu et al., 2000b; Nakhai et al., 2007; Poche et al., 2007), within the INBL of *Pou4f2* null retinas (Fig. 6E,F,M-P). In addition, we observed in *Pou4f2*$^{-/-}$ retinas a moderate but significant increase in the expression of *Otx2, Crx, Thrb2* and *Prdm1/Blimp1* (Qiu et al., 2008), which are all transcription factor genes involved in photoreceptor cell development (Brzezinski et al., 2010; Furukawa et al., 1997; Furukawa et al., 1999; Ng et al., 2001; Nishida et al., 2003; Wilm and Solnica-Krezel, 2005).These studies have led us to propose that while promoting the differentiation of early-born RGCs, Pou4f2 may actively suppress the differentiation of late-born RGC, amacrine, horizontal, and cone cells by repressing a network of transcription factor genes involved in their commitment and differentiation (Fig. 7*A*) (Qiu et al., 2008). This built-in negative regulatory program may serve as a safeguard mechanism to ensure the differentiation of all Pou4f2-expressing precursors as early-born RGCs, thereby guaranteeing the fidelity of RGC differentiation. In the absence of *Pou4f2,* the release of the safeguard mechanism may cause RGC precursors to change their cell fates and abnormally generate amacrine, horizontal and late-born RGC cells that may ultimately degenerate by apoptosis (Fig. *7B*). In spite of the apparent inhibition of late-born RGC fates, it is still possible that Pou4f2 may be involved in terminal differentiation of late-born RGCs given the crucial role of Pou4f2 in RGC differentiation and the co-expression between Pou4f2 and Dlx1/2 (de Melo et al., 2003).

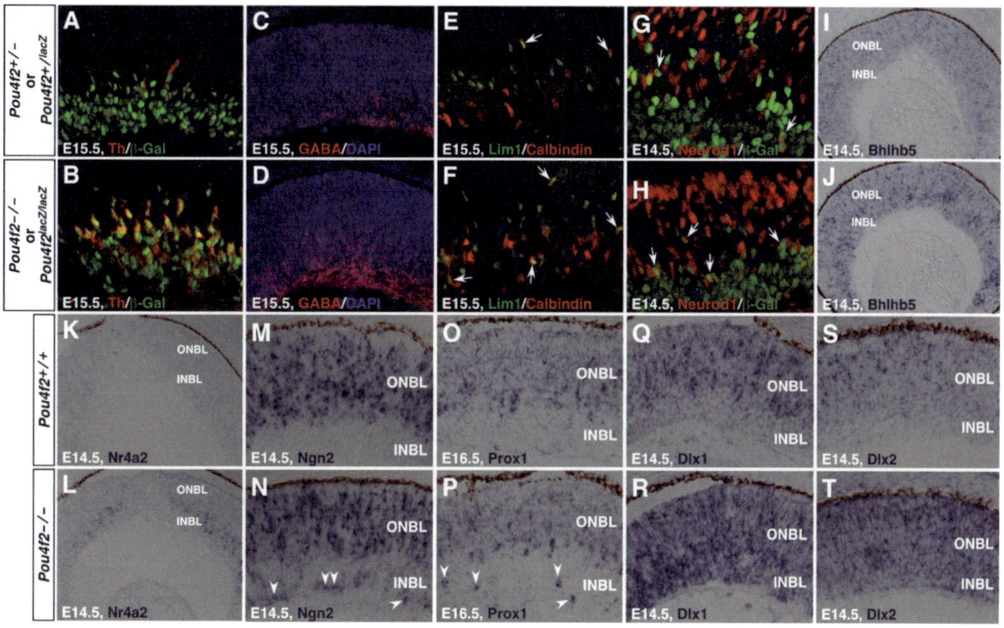


Fig. 6. Aberrant differentiation of amacrine, horizontal and ganglion cells in *Pou4f2* null mutant retinas. (A-H) Retinal sections at the indicated stages from *Pou4f2*$^{+/lacZ}$ (A,E,G), *Pou4f2*$^{lacZ/lacZ}$ (B,F,H), *Pou4f2*$^{+/-}$ (C), and *Pou4f2*$^{-/-}$ (D) embryos were immunostained with the indicated antibodies. Within the INBL of null retinas, there was a significant increase of GABA-immunoreactivity and cells double-immunoreactive for Lim1 and calbindin or β-gal and Th or Neurod1 (indicated by arrows). (I-T) Retinal sections at the indicated stages from *Pou4f2*$^{+/+}$ (K,M,O,Q,S), *Pou4f2*$^{+/-}$ (I), and *Pou4f2*$^{-/-}$ (J,L,N,P,R,T) embryos were in situ hybridized with the indicated RNA probes. Within the INBL of null retinas, there was a significant increase in expression of *Bhlhb5*, *Nr4a2*, *Ngn2* (indicated by arrowheads), *Prox1* (indicated by arrowheads), *Dlx1*, and *Dlx2*. INBL, inner neuroblastic layer; ONBL, outer neuroblastic layer

Despite the comprehensive negative regulatory program, Pou4f2 appears to suppress photoreceptor or glycinergic amacrine cell fates only weakly or not at all (Qiu et al., 2008), raising the possibility that it may have to cooperate with other regulatory factors to inhibit all other alternative cell fates available to a particular RGC precursor. Targeted *Atoh7* inactivation leads to increased cones and cholinergic amacrine cells (Brown et al., 2001; Wang et al., 2001), thereby indicating an inherent activity for Atoh7 to suppress cone and cholinergic amacrine cell fates even though the precursors expressing it are able to produce both cell types (Yang et al., 2003). Conceivably, Pou4f2 may cooperate with Atoh7 to ensure complete suppression of the amacrine and cone differentiation programs in RGC precursors.

Similar to Pou4f2, Atoh7 appears to repress the expression of *Neurod1*, *Math3*, *Bhlhb5*, and *Ngn2* to suppress the amacrine and/or horizontal cell fates (Feng et al., 2006; Mu et al., 2005). Although it remains to be determined whether Atoh7 also represses the expression of photoreceptor transcription factor genes, it seems that Pou4f2 and Atoh7, and likely other RGC transcription factors, may all have built-in safeguard mechanisms that only when working together can ensure the highest fidelity of RGC differentiation.

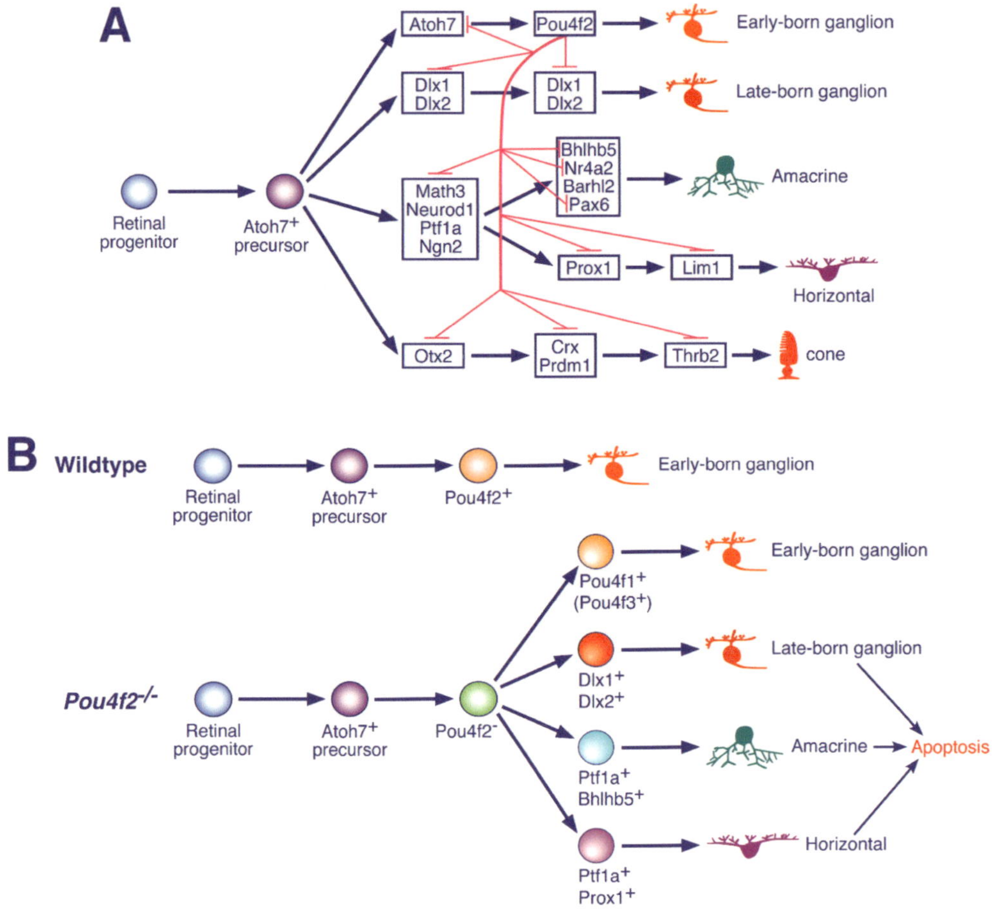


Fig. 7. Schematics illustrating the safeguard mechanism by which Pou4f2 specifies early-born RGCs. (A) RGC-competent Atoh7+ precursors are able to generate early-born and late-born RGCs and amacrine, horizontal and cone cells. When Pou4f2 is expressed in such a multipotential precursor, it commits it to an early-born RGC fate while preventing it from following other differentiation pathways by repressing the expression of a network of retinogenic transcription factor genes involved in fate commitment and differentiation of late-born RGC, amacrine, horizontal, and cone cells. (B) When expressed in RGC-competent precursors, Pou4f2 specifies early-born RGCs and promotes their differentiation in wild-type retinas. In the *Pou4f2* mutant, the safeguard mechanism is compromised and the precursors that would normally express Pou4f2 switch their fates to aberrantly produce late-born RGC, amacrine and horizontal cells that would quickly degenerate by apoptosis. A small portion of early-born RGCs may be produced due to functional compensation by Pou4f1 and Pou4f3

## 3. Extrinsic signaling

During retinal development, RGC generation initiates near the center of the developing retina and then propagates toward the periphery in a wave-like fashion (McCabe et al., 1999; Neumann and Nuesslein-Volhard, 2000). It has been shown that fibroblast growth factor 3 (FGF3) and FGF8 secreted from local organizing centers act together to induce the first wave of RGC differentiation from retinal progenitors (Martinez-Morales et al., 2005). FGF8 released from coated beads promotes *Atoh7* expression and triggers RGC differentiation whereas pharmacological inhibition of FGF signaling blocks *Atoh7* expression and RGC differentiation (Martinez-Morales et al., 2005). In zebrafish deficient for both *Fgf3* and *Fgf8*, *Atoh7* expression fails to initiate in the developing retina (Martinez-Morales et al., 2005). Indeed, FGF signaling activates *Xenopus Atoh7* gene expression through its 5′ regulatory sequence (Willardsen et al., 2009). FGF signaling may cooperate with Shh to coordinate the subsequent spread of RGC differentiation wave front. FGF19, via regulation of the *Pea3* and *Erm* Ets-domain transcription factor genes, together with Shh released from new born RGCs, are required for propagation of Shh own gene expression (McCabe et al., 2006; Vinothkumar et al., 2008). Mutations in Shh signaling components and cyclopamine treatment all disrupt normal propagation of *Shh* and *Atoh7* expression as well as RGC differentiation (Neumann and Nuesslein-Volhard, 2000; Stenkamp and Frey, 2003). FGF and Shh appear to activate the Ras-MAPK pathway to trigger and drive the wave of RGC differentiation (Neumann and Nuesslein-Volhard, 2000). Despite these compelling evidence in support of sequential induction of RGCs, other studies suggest that the progression of RGC differentiation wave may be governed by a dominant intrinsic mechanism pre-programmed into the progenitors (Kay et al., 2005).

In contrast to the crucial requirement of Shh signaling in RGC differentiation progression, Shh secreted by new born RGCs behind the neurogenesis wave front prevents progenitors from generating more RGCs, thereby ensuring a proper number of total RGCs to be produced in the retina. In the chick retina, Shh overexpression decreases RGC production whereas inhibiting endogenous Shh activity increases RGC differentiation (Zhang and Yang, 2001). Similarly, conditional ablation of *Shh* and *Smoothened* (*Smo*) in mice results in Atoh7-dependent overproduction of RGCs (Sakagami et al., 2009). VEGF (vascular endothelial growth factor) is also secreted by RGCs and other postmitotic neurons and can negatively regulate RGC differentiation (Hashimoto et al., 2006). Thus, RGC formation is reduced by enhanced VEGF signals but increased by disrupting VEGF signaling activity (Hashimoto et al., 2006). Besides these diffusible signals, Dll-Notch signaling mediated by cell-cell contacts also limits RGC production. Constitutively activated Notch and elevated Dll signal are shown to decrease RGC generation whereas inhibiting Notch signaling has the opposite effect (Ahmad et al., 1997; Austin et al., 1995; Dorsky et al., 1997; Dorsky et al., 1995; Nelson et al., 2007). Interestingly, both Shh and VEGF signaling activates expression of the Dll-Notch effector gene *Hes1*, which has an activity to suppress RGC differentiation (Hashimoto et al., 2006; Sakagami et al., 2009; Wang et al., 2005). Therefore, these divergent signaling pathways appear to converge on Hes1 to control proper RGC production during retinogenesis (Hashimoto et al., 2006).

In the mouse retina, inactivation of the *Gdf11* gene, which encodes a member of the TGF-β/activin protein family, causes an increase of RGC production from progenitors whereas inactivating the follistatin gene, its antagonist, reduces RGCs (Kim et al., 2005). On the other hand, treating embryonic retinal explants with Gdf11 in culture results in a decrease of

RGCs. Neither Gdf11 nor follistatin exert any effect on the proliferation of retinal progenitors (Kim et al., 2005). Therefore, follistatin appears to increase the number of progenitors competent for RGC generation whereas Gdf11 antagonizes this activity, thereby contributing to a balanced production of RGCs. Gdf11 and follistatin control retinal progenitor competence by shortening and elongating the duration of *Atoh7* expression, respectively (Kim et al., 2005).

## 4. Generation of RGCs from stem cells

As potential renewable sources of replacement cells for cell transplantation/replacement treatment, stem cells offer exciting future possibilities to restore functional retinal circuits in patients inflicted with retinal degeneration such as glaucoma (Dahlmann-Noor et al., 2010; Klassen et al., 2004; Lamba et al., 2008; MacLaren et al., 2006). It appears that the intrinsic and extrinsic mechanisms utilized to generate RGCs during normal development are recruited to stimulate RGC differentiation from stem cells both in vivo and in vitro. In the post-hatch chicken retina, FGF signaling is required to induce *Atoh7* expression and subsequent production of Pou4f1- and Isl1-immunoreactive RGCs from stem cells in the ciliary marginal zone (Fischer et al., 2002). Similarly, mouse embryonic stem (ES) cells can be induced to generate RGC-like cells that express Atoh7, Pou4f2 and Isl1 only when exposed to FGF2, and this RGC-inducing activity by FGF2 is further potentiated by Shh (Jagatha et al., 2009). In rat retinal progenitors, transient expression of the intrinsic factor Atoh7 led to *Pou4f2* upregulation and RGC induction (Yao et al., 2007). Pluripotent stem (iPS) cells induced from mouse fibroblasts can be also directed to form retinal progenitors that are capable of differentiating into RGC-like cells in the presence of suitable extrinsic and intrinsic cues. They produced RGCs expressing a variety of RGC-specific markers when cultured in retinal differentiation medium containing conditioned medium from E14 rat retinal cells (Parameswaran et al., 2010). These induced RGCs were able to extend processes toward superior collicular explants and exhibited typical neuronal activity (Parameswaran et al., 2010). Similarly, overexpression of Atoh7 could direct the iPS-derived retinal progenitors toward a RGC differentiation program, which could be further enhanced by inhibiting Notch signaling activity (Chen et al., 2010). Conceivably, application of a combination of stimulatory intrinsic and extrinsic factors while suppressing negative ones may lead to even greater induction of RGCs from stem cells. Transplanting in vitro induced retinal progenitors and RGCs intravitreally into postnatal rodent eyes resulted in only few cells that integrated into the RGC layer of the host retina (Chen et al., 2010; Jagatha et al., 2009), suggesting that postnatal retinas present a formidable barrier to cell migration and integration.

## 5. Summary and perspectives

Great strides have been made over the past two decades toward understanding both the intrinsic and extrinsic mechanisms of RGC specification and differentiation from retinal progenitors. Molecular genetic studies coupled with bioinformatic approaches have yielded a wealth of information about transcription factors and their regulatory gene networks as well as signaling events that lead to the establishment of RGC competence and eventual differentiation of RGCs (Fig. 1). Significant inroads have also been made toward understanding the molecular basis underlying the fidelity of RGC differentiation and production of proper number of RGCs. Despite these exciting advances, however, there are still many questions remaining to be answered. For instance, how do intrinsic and extrinsic factors interact and cooperate at cellular and transcriptional levels to drive RGC development and ensure proper RGC number? How do Atoh7 and Pou4f2 activate RGC differentiation program genes while repressing non-RGC differentiation program genes at the molecular level and what are their direct targets? What factors are responsible for specifying the extremely diverse RGC subtypes? What factors are required to efficiently induce RGCs from stem cells and what prevents them from migrating and integrating into the intact retina? Progress in these areas will undoubtedly lead to many more exciting discoveries in years to come. Ultimately, understanding the molecular events and factors involved in RGC development may lay the groundwork to improve stem cell-mediated regeneration, leading to eventual development of effective treatments of glaucoma in the future.

## 6. Acknowledgements

We thank Shengguo Li, Kamana Misra and Min Zou for thoughtful comments on the manuscript. This work was supported by the National Institutes of Health.

## 7. References

Ahmad, I., Dooley, C.M., Polk, D.L., 1997. Delta-1 is a regulator of neurogenesis in the vertebrate retina. Dev Biol 185, 92-103.

Akagi, T., Inoue, T., Miyoshi, G., Bessho, Y., Takahashi, M., Lee, J.E., Guillemot, F., Kageyama, R., 2004. Requirement of multiple basic helix-loop-helix genes for retinal neuronal subtype specification. J Biol Chem 279, 28492-28498.

Austin, C.P., Feldman, D.E., Ida, J.A., Jr., Cepko, C.L., 1995. Vertebrate retinal ganglion cells are selected from competent progenitors by the action of Notch. Development 121, 3637-3650.

Badea, T.C., Cahill, H., Ecker, J., Hattar, S., Nathans, J., 2009. Distinct roles of transcription factors Brn3a and Brn3b in controlling the development, morphology, and function of retinal ganglion cells. Neuron 61, 852-864.

Badea, T.C., Nathans, J., 2011. Morphologies of mouse retinal ganglion cells expressing transcription factors Brn3a, Brn3b, and Brn3c: analysis of wild type and mutant cells using genetically-directed sparse labeling. Vision Res 51, 269-279.

Brown, N.L., Kanekar, S., Vetter, M.L., Tucker, P.K., Gemza, D.L., Glaser, T., 1998. Math5 encodes a murine basic helix-loop-helix transcription factor expressed during early stages of retinal neurogenesis. Development 125, 4821-4833.

Brown, N.L., Patel, S., Brzezinski, J., Glaser, T., 2001. Math5 is required for retinal ganglion cell and optic nerve formation. Development 128, 2497-2508.

Brzezinski, J.A.t., Lamba, D.A., Reh, T.A., 2010. Blimp1 controls photoreceptor versus bipolar cell fate choice during retinal development. Development 137, 619-629.

Cepko, C.L., 1999. The roles of intrinsic and extrinsic cues and bHLH genes in the determination of retinal cell fates. Curr Opin Neurobiol 9, 37-46.

Cepko, C.L., Austin, C.P., Yang, X., Alexiades, M., Ezzeddine, D., 1996. Cell fate determination in the vertebrate retina. Proc Natl Acad Sci U S A 93, 589-595.

Chen, M., Chen, Q., Sun, X., Shen, W., Liu, B., Zhong, X., Leng, Y., Li, C., Zhang, W., Chai, F., Huang, B., Gao, Q., Xiang, A.P., Zhuo, Y., Ge, J., 2010. Generation of retinal ganglion-like cells from reprogrammed mouse fibroblasts. Invest Ophthalmol Vis Sci 51, 5970-5978.

Dahlmann-Noor, A., Vijay, S., Jayaram, H., Limb, A., Khaw, P.T., 2010. Current approaches and future prospects for stem cell rescue and regeneration of the retina and optic nerve. Can J Ophthalmol 45, 333-341.

de Melo, J., Du, G., Fonseca, M., Gillespie, L.A., Turk, W.J., Rubenstein, J.L., Eisenstat, D.D., 2005. Dlx1 and Dlx2 function is necessary for terminal differentiation and survival of late-born retinal ganglion cells in the developing mouse retina. Development 132, 311-322.

de Melo, J., Qiu, X., Du, G., Cristante, L., Eisenstat, D.D., 2003. *Dlx1*, *Dlx2*, *Pax6*, *Brn3b*, and *Chx10* homeobox gene expression defines the retinal ganglion and inner nuclear layers of the developing and adult mouse retina. J Comp Neurol 461, 187-204.

DeCarvalho, A.C., Cappendijk, S.L., Fadool, J.M., 2004. Developmental expression of the POU domain transcription factor Brn-3b (Pou4f2) in the lateral line and visual system of zebrafish. Dev Dyn 229, 869-876.

Dorsky, R.I., Chang, W.S., Rapaport, D.H., Harris, W.A., 1997. Regulation of neuronal diversity in the *Xenopus* retina by Delta signalling. Nature 385, 67-70.

Dorsky, R.I., Rapaport, D.H., Harris, W.A., 1995. Xotch inhibits cell differentiation in the *Xenopus* retina. Neuron 14, 487-496.

Dyer, M.A., Livesey, F.J., Cepko, C.L., Oliver, G., 2003. Prox1 function controls progenitor cell proliferation and horizontal cell genesis in the mammalian retina. Nat Genet 34, 53-58.

Elliott, J., Jolicoeur, C., Ramamurthy, V., Cayouette, M., 2008. Ikaros confers early temporal competence to mouse retinal progenitor cells. Neuron 60, 26-39.

Erkman, L., McEvilly, R.J., Luo, L., Ryan, A.K., Hooshmand, F., O'Connell, S.M., Keithley, E.M., Rapaport, D.H., Ryan, A.F., Rosenfeld, M.G., 1996. Role of transcription factors Brn-3.1 and Brn-3.2 in auditory and visual system development. Nature 381, 603-606.

Erkman, L., Yates, P.A., McLaughlin, T., McEvilly, R.J., Whisenhunt, T., O'Connell, S.M., Krones, A.I., Kirby, M.A., Rapaport, D.H., Bermingham, J.R., O'Leary, D.D., Rosenfeld, M.G., 2000. A POU domain transcription factor-dependent program regulates axon pathfinding in the vertebrate visual system. Neuron 28, 779-792.

Feng, L., Xie, X., Joshi, P.S., Yang, Z., Shibasaki, K., Chow, R.L., Gan, L., 2006. Requirement for Bhlhb5 in the specification of amacrine and cone bipolar subtypes in mouse retina. Development 133, 4815-4825.

Fischer, A.J., Dierks, B.D., Reh, T.A., 2002. Exogenous growth factors induce the production of ganglion cells at the retinal margin. Development 129, 2283-2291.

Fujitani, Y., Fujitani, S., Luo, H., Qiu, F., Burlison, J., Long, Q., Kawaguchi, Y., Edlund, H., Macdonald, R.J., Furukawa, T., Fujikado, T., Magnuson, M.A., Xiang, M., Wright, C.V., 2006. Ptf1a determines horizontal and amacrine cell fates during mouse retinal development. Development 133, 4439-4450.

Furukawa, T., Morrow, E.M., Cepko, C.L., 1997. *Crx*, a novel *otx*-like homeobox gene, shows photoreceptor-specific expression and regulates photoreceptor differentiation. Cell 91, 531-541.

Furukawa, T., Morrow, E.M., Li, T., Davis, F.C., Cepko, C.L., 1999. Retinopathy and attenuated circadian entrainment in *Crx*-deficient mice. Nat Genet 23, 466-470.

Gan, L., Wang, S.W., Huang, Z., Klein, W.H., 1999. POU domain factor Brn-3b is essential for retinal ganglion cell differentiation and survival but not for initial cell fate specification. Dev Biol 210, 469-480.

Gan, L., Xiang, M., Zhou, L., Wagner, D.S., Klein, W.H., Nathans, J., 1996. POU domain factor Brn-3b is required for the development of a large set of retinal ganglion cells. Proc Natl Acad Sci U S A 93, 3920-3925.

Gerrero, M.R., McEvilly, R.J., Turner, E., Lin, C.R., O'Connell, S., Jenne, K.J., Hobbs, M.V., Rosenfeld, M.G., 1993. Brn-3.0: a POU-domain protein expressed in the sensory, immune, and endocrine systems that functions on elements distinct from known octamer motifs. Proc Natl Acad Sci U S A 90, 10841-10845.

Gruber, C.A., Rhee, J.M., Gleiberman, A., Turner, E.E., 1997. POU domain factors of the Brn-3 class recognize functional DNA elements which are distinctive, symmetrical, and highly conserved in evolution. Mol Cell Biol 17, 2391-2400.

Harris, W.A., 1997. Cellular diversification in the vertebrate retina. Curr Opin Genet Dev 7, 651-658.

Hashimoto, T., Zhang, X.M., Chen, B.Y., Yang, X.J., 2006. VEGF activates divergent intracellular signaling components to regulate retinal progenitor cell proliferation and neuronal differentiation. Development 133, 2201-2210.

Hutcheson, D.A., Vetter, M.L., 2001. The bHLH factors Xath5 and XNeuroD can upregulate the expression of XBrn3d, a POU-homeodomain transcription factor. Dev Biol 232, 327-338.

Inoue, T., Hojo, M., Bessho, Y., Tano, Y., Lee, J.E., Kageyama, R., 2002. Math3 and NeuroD regulate amacrine cell fate specification in the retina. Development 129, 831-842.

Jagatha, B., Divya, M.S., Sanalkumar, R., Indulekha, C.L., Vidyanand, S., Divya, T.S., Das, A.V., James, J., 2009. In vitro differentiation of retinal ganglion-like cells from embryonic stem cell derived neural progenitors. Biochem Biophys Res Commun 380, 230-235.

Jiang, H., Xiang, M., 2009. Subtype specification of GABAergic amacrine cells by the orphan nuclear receptor Nr4a2/Nurr1. J Neurosci 29, 10449-10459.

Jin, K., Jiang, H., Mo, Z., Xiang, M., 2010. Early B-cell factors are required for specifying multiple retinal cell types and subtypes from postmitotic precursors. J Neurosci 30, 11902-11916.

Kanekar, S., Perron, M., Dorsky, R., Harris, W.A., Jan, L.Y., Jan, Y.N., Vetter, M.L., 1997. *Xath5* participates in a network of bHLH genes in the developing *Xenopus* retina. Neuron 19, 981-994.

Kay, J.N., Finger-Baier, K.C., Roeser, T., Staub, W., Baier, H., 2001. Retinal ganglion cell genesis requires *lakritz*, a zebrafish *atonal* homolog. Neuron 30, 725-736.

Kay, J.N., Link, B.A., Baier, H., 2005. Staggered cell-intrinsic timing of *ath5* expression underlies the wave of ganglion cell neurogenesis in the zebrafish retina. Development 132, 2573-2585.

Kim, J., Wu, H.H., Lander, A.D., Lyons, K.M., Matzuk, M.M., Calof, A.L., 2005. GDF11 controls the timing of progenitor cell competence in developing retina. Science 308, 1927-1930.

Klassen, H., Sakaguchi, D.S., Young, M.J., 2004. Stem cells and retinal repair. Prog Retin Eye Res 23, 149-181.

Lamba, D., Karl, M., Reh, T., 2008. Neural regeneration and cell replacement: a view from the eye. Cell Stem Cell 2, 538-549.

Liu, W., Khare, S.L., Liang, X., Peters, M.A., Liu, X., Cepko, C.L., Xiang, M., 2000a. All Brn3 genes can promote retinal ganglion cell differentiation in the chick. Development 127, 3237-3247.

Liu, W., Mo, Z., Xiang, M., 2001. The Ath5 proneural genes function upstream of Brn3 POU domain transcription factor genes to promote retinal ganglion cell development. Proc Natl Acad Sci U S A 98, 1649-1654.

Liu, W., Wang, J.H., Xiang, M., 2000b. Specific expression of the LIM/homeodomain protein Lim-1 in horizontal cells during retinogenesis. Dev Dyn 217, 320-325.

Livesey, F.J., Cepko, C.L., 2001. Vertebrate neural cell-fate determination: lessons from the retina. Nat Rev Neurosci 2, 109-118.

MacLaren, R.E., Pearson, R.A., MacNeil, A., Douglas, R.H., Salt, T.E., Akimoto, M., Swaroop, A., Sowden, J.C., Ali, R.R., 2006. Retinal repair by transplantation of photoreceptor precursors. Nature 444, 203-207.

Mao, C.A., Kiyama, T., Pan, P., Furuta, Y., Hadjantonakis, A.K., Klein, W.H., 2008. *Eomesodermin*, a target gene of Pou4f2, is required for retinal ganglion cell and optic nerve development in the mouse. Development 135, 271-280.

Marquardt, T., Ashery-Padan, R., Andrejewski, N., Scardigli, R., Guillemot, F., Gruss, P., 2001. Pax6 is required for the multipotent state of retinal progenitor cells. Cell 105, 43-55.

Martinez-Morales, J.R., Del Bene, F., Nica, G., Hammerschmidt, M., Bovolenta, P., Wittbrodt, J., 2005. Differentiation of the vertebrate retina is coordinated by an FGF signaling center. Dev Cell 8, 565-574.

McCabe, K.L., Gunther, E.C., Reh, T.A., 1999. The development of the pattern of retinal ganglion cells in the chick retina: mechanisms that control differentiation. Development 126, 5713-5724.

McCabe, K.L., McGuire, C., Reh, T.A., 2006. *Pea3* expression is regulated by FGF signaling in developing retina. Dev Dyn 235, 327-335.

McEvilly, R.J., Erkman, L., Luo, L., Sawchenko, P.E., Ryan, A.F., Rosenfeld, M.G., 1996. Requirement for *Brn-3.0* in differentiation and survival of sensory and motor neurons. Nature 384, 574-577.

Moshiri, A., Gonzalez, E., Tagawa, K., Maeda, H., Wang, M., Frishman, L.J., Wang, S.W., 2008. Near complete loss of retinal ganglion cells in the *math5/brn3b* double knockout elicits severe reductions of other cell types during retinal development. Dev Biol 316, 214-227.

Mu, X., Beremand, P.D., Zhao, S., Pershad, R., Sun, H., Scarpa, A., Liang, S., Thomas, T.L., Klein, W.H., 2004. Discrete gene sets depend on POU domain transcription factor Brn3b/Brn-3.2/POU4f2 for their expression in the mouse embryonic retina. Development 131, 1197-1210.

Mu, X., Fu, X., Beremand, P.D., Thomas, T.L., Klein, W.H., 2008. Gene regulation logic in retinal ganglion cell development: Isl1 defines a critical branch distinct from but overlapping with Pou4f2. Proc Natl Acad Sci U S A 105, 6942-6947.

Mu, X., Fu, X., Sun, H., Beremand, P.D., Thomas, T.L., Klein, W.H., 2005. A gene network downstream of transcription factor Math5 regulates retinal progenitor cell competence and ganglion cell fate. Dev Biol 280, 467-481.

Nakhai, H., Sel, S., Favor, J., Mendoza-Torres, L., Paulsen, F., Duncker, G.I., Schmid, R.M., 2007. Ptf1a is essential for the differentiation of GABAergic and glycinergic amacrine cells and horizontal cells in the mouse retina. Development 134, 1151-1160.

Nelson, B.R., Hartman, B.H., Georgi, S.A., Lan, M.S., Reh, T.A., 2007. Transient inactivation of Notch signaling synchronizes differentiation of neural progenitor cells. Dev Biol 304, 479-498.

Neumann, C.J., Nuesslein-Volhard, C., 2000. Patterning of the zebrafish retina by a wave of sonic hedgehog activity. Science 289, 2137-2139.

Ng, L., Hurley, J.B., Dierks, B., Srinivas, M., Salto, C., Vennstrom, B., Reh, T.A., Forrest, D., 2001. A thyroid hormone receptor that is required for the development of green cone photoreceptors. Nat Genet 27, 94-98.

Nishida, A., Furukawa, A., Koike, C., Tano, Y., Aizawa, S., Matsuo, I., Furukawa, T., 2003. *Otx2* homeobox gene controls retinal photoreceptor cell fate and pineal gland development. Nat Neurosci 6, 1255-1263.

Pan, L., Deng, M., Xie, X., Gan, L., 2008. ISL1 and BRN3B co-regulate the differentiation of murine retinal ganglion cells. Development 135, 1981-1990.

Pan, L., Yang, Z., Feng, L., Gan, L., 2005. Functional equivalence of Brn3 POU-domain transcription factors in mouse retinal neurogenesis. Development 132, 703-712.

Parameswaran, S., Balasubramanian, S., Babai, N., Qiu, F., Eudy, J.D., Thoreson, W.B., Ahmad, I., 2010. Induced pluripotent stem cells generate both retinal ganglion cells and photoreceptors: therapeutic implications in degenerative changes in glaucoma and age-related macular degeneration. Stem Cells 28, 695-703.

Poche, R.A., Kwan, K.M., Raven, M.A., Furuta, Y., Reese, B.E., Behringer, R.R., 2007. Lim1 is essential for the correct laminar positioning of retinal horizontal cells. J Neurosci 27, 14099-14107.

Qiu, F., Jiang, H., Xiang, M., 2008. A comprehensive negative regulatory program controlled by Brn3b to ensure ganglion cell specification from multipotential retinal precursors. J Neurosci 28, 3392-3403.

Sakagami, K., Gan, L., Yang, X.J., 2009. Distinct effects of Hedgehog signaling on neuronal fate specification and cell cycle progression in the embryonic mouse retina. J Neurosci 29, 6932-6944.

Stenkamp, D.L., Frey, R.A., 2003. Extraretinal and retinal hedgehog signaling sequentially regulate retinal differentiation in zebrafish. Dev Biol 258, 349-363.

Taranova, O.V., Magness, S.T., Fagan, B.M., Wu, Y., Surzenko, N., Hutton, S.R., Pevny, L.H., 2006. SOX2 is a dose-dependent regulator of retinal neural progenitor competence. Genes Dev 20, 1187-1202.

Turner, E.E., Jenne, K.J., Rosenfeld, M.G., 1994. Brn-3.2: a Brn-3-related transcription factor with distinctive central nervous system expression and regulation by retinoic acid. Neuron 12, 205-218.

Vinothkumar, S., Rastegar, S., Takamiya, M., Ertzer, R., Strahle, U., 2008. Sequential and cooperative action of Fgfs and Shh in the zebrafish retina. Dev Biol 314, 200-214.

Wagner, K.D., Wagner, N., Vidal, V.P., Schley, G., Wilhelm, D., Schedl, A., Englert, C., Scholz, H., 2002. The Wilms' tumor gene *Wt1* is required for normal development of the retina. EMBO J 21, 1398-1405.

Wang, S.W., Kim, B.S., Ding, K., Wang, H., Sun, D., Johnson, R.L., Klein, W.H., Gan, L., 2001. Requirement for *math5* in the development of retinal ganglion cells. Genes Dev 15, 24-29.

Wang, S.W., Mu, X., Bowers, W.J., Kim, D.S., Plas, D.J., Crair, M.C., Federoff, H.J., Gan, L., Klein, W.H., 2002. *Brn3b/Brn3c* double knockout mice reveal an unsuspected role for Brn3c in retinal ganglion cell axon outgrowth. Development 129, 467-477.

Wang, Y., Dakubo, G.D., Thurig, S., Mazerolle, C.J., Wallace, V.A., 2005. Retinal ganglion cell-derived sonic hedgehog locally controls proliferation and the timing of RGC development in the embryonic mouse retina. Development 132, 5103-5113.

Willardsen, M.I., Suli, A., Pan, Y., Marsh-Armstrong, N., Chien, C.B., El-Hodiri, H., Brown, N.L., Moore, K.B., Vetter, M.L., 2009. Temporal regulation of *Ath5* gene expression during eye development. Dev Biol 326, 471-481.

Wilm, T.P., Solnica-Krezel, L., 2005. Essential roles of a zebrafish *prdm1/blimp1* homolog in embryo patterning and organogenesis. Development 132, 393-404.

Xiang, M., 1998. Requirement for Brn-3b in early differentiation of postmitotic retinal ganglion cell precursors. Dev Biol 197, 155-169.

Xiang, M., Gan, L., Li, D., Chen, Z.Y., Zhou, L., O'Malley, B.W., Jr., Klein, W., Nathans, J., 1997. Essential role of POU-domain factor Brn-3c in auditory and vestibular hair cell development. Proc Natl Acad Sci U S A 94, 9445-9450.

Xiang, M., Gan, L., Zhou, L., Klein, W.H., Nathans, J., 1996. Targeted deletion of the mouse POU domain gene *Brn-3a* causes selective loss of neurons in the brainstem and trigeminal ganglion, uncoordinated limb movement, and impaired suckling. Proc Natl Acad Sci U S A 93, 11950-11955.

Xiang, M., Zhou, L., Macke, J.P., Yoshioka, T., Hendry, S.H., Eddy, R.L., Shows, T.B., Nathans, J., 1995. The Brn-3 family of POU-domain factors: primary structure, binding specificity, and expression in subsets of retinal ganglion cells and somatosensory neurons. J Neurosci 15, 4762-4785.

Xiang, M., Zhou, L., Peng, Y.W., Eddy, R.L., Shows, T.B., Nathans, J., 1993. *Brn-3b*: a POU domain gene expressed in a subset of retinal ganglion cells. Neuron 11, 689-701.

Yang, Z., Ding, K., Pan, L., Deng, M., Gan, L., 2003. Math5 determines the competence state of retinal ganglion cell progenitors. Dev Biol 264, 240-254.

Yao, J., Sun, X., Wang, Y., Xu, G., Qian, J., 2007. Math5 promotes retinal ganglion cell expression patterns in retinal progenitor cells. Mol Vis 13, 1066-1072.

Young, R.W., 1985. Cell differentiation in the retina of the mouse. Anat Rec 212, 199-205.

Zhang, X.M., Yang, X.J., 2001. Regulation of retinal ganglion cell production by Sonic hedgehog. Development 128, 943-957.

# 5

# The Role of Retinal Oxidative and Nitrative Injury in Glaucomatous Neurodegeneration

Serdar Dogan and Mutay Aslan
*Department of Biochemistry, Akdeniz University School of Medicine. Antalya 07070, Turkey*

## 1. Introduction

The mechanical compression theory explaining the origin of glaucoma considers elevated intraocular pressure as the most important risk factor for the disease. This theory gives support to the essential signs of glaucomatous optic neuropathy, such as increased cupping and neuroretinal rim thinning but does not explain the existence of normal tension glaucoma. Alternatively, the vascular ischemia theory supposes that vascular insufficiency in the optic nerve head results in decreased metabolic activity, which subsequently leads to increased glutamate accumulation and ganglion cell death. Indeed, a large number of studies have shown a high association between glaucomatous optic neuropathy and vascular disorders related to hypertension, diabetes and hypercholesterolemia.

Oxidative stress has been implicated to cause increased intraocular pressure by triggering trabecular meshwork degeneration and thus contributing to alterations in the aqueous outflow pathway. It has also been demonstrated that oxidative DNA damage is significantly greater in trabecular meshwork cells of glaucoma patients compared with controls. Moreover, *in vivo* studies in humans have shown that both intraocular pressure increase and visual field damage are significantly related to the amount of oxidative DNA damage. Similarly, severity of optic nerve damage in eyes with primary open angle glaucoma is correlated with changes in the trabecular meshwork. Retinal oxidative injury occurring in models of elevated intraocular pressure or in normal tension glaucoma also directly damage the retinal ganglion cell layer, leading to glaucomatous optic neuropathy. Free radical injury has been reported to cause caspase independent cell death in retinal ganglion cells *in vitro*. Furthermore, many retinal proteins exhibit oxidative modifications in experimental glaucoma, which may lead to important structural and functional alterations.

Ocular tissues and fluids contain antioxidants that play a key role in protecting against oxidative damage. However, specific activity of a major antioxidant enzyme, superoxide dismutase, demonstrates an age-dependent decline in normal human trabecular meshwork. Similarly, plasma glutathione levels assessed in patients with newly diagnosed primary open angle glaucoma and age- and gender-matched control subjects revealed that glaucoma patients exhibited significantly lower levels of reduced and total glutathione than did control subjects.

Recent studies have also highlighted the role of nitric oxide in glaucoma by reporting the presence of inducible nitric oxide synthase in the iris-ciliary body, retina and in the glaucomatous optic nerve head of experimental rat models. This chapter will discuss the role of reactive oxygen and nitrogen species in the pathogenesis of glaucoma and examine the relevance of antioxidants in neurodegeneration associated with the disease.

Pathophysiological mechanisms leading to glaucomatous optic neuropathy remain uncertain. Mechanical compression and vascular ischemia have been suggested to play a leading role in the observed neuronal damage (Fechtner & Weinreb, 1994). The mechanical compression theory considers elevated intraocular pressure as the most important risk factor for the disease (Yan et al., 1994). The mechanism of elevated intraocular pressure in glaucoma is impaired outflow of aqueous humour resulting from abnormalities within the drainage system of the anterior chamber angle (open-angle glaucoma) or impaired access of aqueous humour to the drainage system (angle-closure glaucoma) (Salmon et al., 2008). Aqueous humour produced by the ciliary body enters the posterior chamber, passes through the pupil into the anterior chamber and then to the trabecular meshwork in the anterior chamber angle. Trabecular meshwork drains the aqueous fluid into the canal of Schlemm (Figure 1) and is composed of beams of collagen and elastic tissue covered by trabecular cells (Salmon et al., 2008). Trabecular cells are endothelial-like cells that have capacities of phagocytosis, and the ability to produce matrix-degrading enzymes, extracellular matrix elements and transforming growth factor-β (Tripathi et al., 1994; Yun et al., 1989).

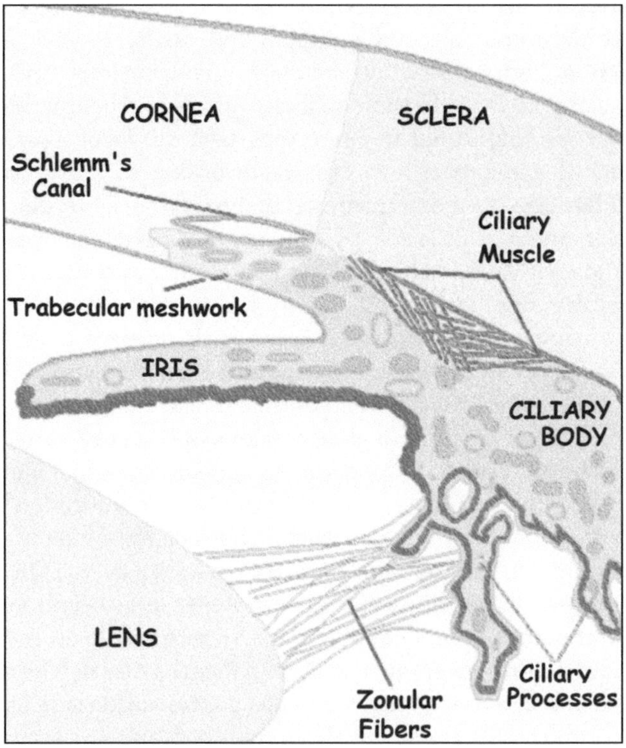


Fig. 1. Anterior segment structures and formation of aqueous humour

Oxidative stress has been implicated to cause increased intraocular pressure by triggering trabecular meshwork degeneration and thus contributing to alterations in the aqueous outflow pathway (Sacca et al., 2007). Indeed, treatment with hydrogen peroxide ($H_2O_2$) impairs trabecular meshwork cell adhesion to the extracellular matrix and causes rearrangement of cytoskeletal structures (Zhou et al., 1999). It has also been demonstrated that oxidative DNA damage is significantly greater in trabecular meshwork cells of glaucoma patients compared with controls (Izzotti et al., 2003). Moreover, *in vivo* studies in humans have shown that both intraocular pressure increase and visual field damage are significantly related to the amount of oxidative DNA damage (Sacca et al., 2005). Similarly, severity of optic nerve damage in eyes with primary open-angle glaucoma is correlated with changes in the trabecular meshwork (Gottanka et al., 1997).

MicroRNA (miRNA) are an abundant class of noncoding small (~22 nucleotides) RNAs that modulate gene expression at the post-transcriptional level and participate in the regulation of many cellular functions (Wu et al, 2006; Filipowicz et al., 2008; Stefani et al., 2008) Specifically, miR-29b has been demonstrated to regulate multiple genes coding for extracellular matrix proteins, including multiple collagens, fibrillins, and elastin (Luna et al., 2009b). The role of microRNA (miRNA) in the trabecular meshwork and the potential involvement on the alterations in extracellular matrix synthesis induced by oxidative stress was studied in human trabecular meshwork cell cultures, which were generated from cadaver eyes with no history of eye disease within 48 h post mortem. These cells were transfected with miR-29b mimic. Chronic oxidative stress was induced by incubation at 40% oxygen for 4–5 days. Control human trabecular meshwork cell cultures were incubated at 5% oxygen. Transfection of human trabecular meshwork cells with miR-29b mimic resulted in downregulation of multiple extracellular matrix components. Chronic oxidative stress induced a significant downregulation of miR-29b in human trabecular meshwork cell lines and increased expression of several extracellular matrix genes known to be regulated by miR-29b. The increase in expression of these genes was inhibited by transfection with miR-29b mimic. MiR-29b increased cell viability under both chronic oxidative stress and physiologic oxygen concentrations. These data suggest that miR-29b negatively regulates the expression of multiple genes involved in the synthesis and deposition of extracellular matrix in trabecular meshwork cells. Downregulation of miR-29b might contribute to increased expression of several extracellular matrix genes under chronic oxidative stress conditions. The balance between the activation of extracellular matrix production induced by oxidative stress and the protective effects of miR-29b could be a relevant factor in understanding how oxidative damage may lead to increased deposition of extracellular matrix in the trabecular meshwork and contribute to the elevation of intraocular pressure via obstruction of the trabeculum by deposition of an extracellular matrix (Luna et al., 2009b).

Oxidative destruction of cellular components usually accompanies ocular tissue injury in animal models of elevated intraocular pressure. Markers of oxidative stress such as protein carbonyl formation and lipid peroxidation products have been documented in experimental models of ocular hypertension. Glyceraldehyde-3-phosphate dehydrogenase, heat shock protein 72 and glutamine synthetase show a significant increase in the relative percentage of carbonyl immunoreactivity in chronic pressure induced rat models of glaucoma as compared with controls (Tezel et al., 2005) Likewise, increased retina lipid oxidation is detected in rats with elevated intraocular pressure (Ko et al., 2005).

Circadian fluctuation of mean ocular perfusion pressure is a consistent risk factor for disease progression in normal-tension glaucoma (Choi et al., 2007). It is hypothesized that unstable ocular blood flow in patients with normal intraocular pressure can lead to reperfusion injury and result in oxidative stress (Mozaffarieh et al., 2008b). Peripheral vascular insufficiency, accompanied by restoration of blood flow, places organs at risk of additional injury by inducing a proinflammatory state reflected by enhanced superoxide ($O_2^{\bullet -}$)and hydrogen peroxide ($H_2O_2$) generation (Henry et al., 1990). These reactive species are usually derived from autoxidation of mitochondrial respiratory chain components (Wallace, 1999), which are also found to be present within the retinal ganglion cells, nerve fiber layer, outer plexiform layer, inner segments of photoreceptors, and the retinal pigment epithelium (Andrews et al., 1999).
A recent study has showed that mice deficient in the glutamate transporters GLAST or EAAC1 demonstrate spontaneous retinal ganglion and optic nerve degeneration without elevated intraocular pressure. In GLAST deficient mice, the glutathione level in Müller glia was found to be decreased and it was concluded that glutamate transporters are necessary both to prevent excitotoxic retinal damage and to synthesize glutathione, a major cellular antioxidant (Harada et al., 2007).
Reported findings also suggest a role for oxidative stress in the pathogenesis and progression of pseudoexfoliation glaucoma. Pseudoexfoliation syndrome is characterized by production and progressive accumulation of fibrillar extracellular material in many ocular tissues, most commonly seen on the pupillary border and anterior lens capsule (Ritch & Schlotzer-Schrehardt, 2001). Accumulation of the exfoliation material or pigment particles in the angle can predispose to both open angle and angle-closure glaucoma (Ritch et al., 2003). The pathogenesis and etiology underlying the development of Pseudoexfoliation syndrome and the subsequent progression from Pseudoexfoliation syndrome to glaucoma remain unclear.
In summary, this review discusses the role of retinal oxidative and nitrative injury in the pathogenesis of glaucomatous neurodegeneration and examines the relevance of antioxidants in altering and/or inhibiting neuronal degeneration associated with the disease

## 2. Reactive oxygen and nitrogen species

### 2.1 Sources of superoxide and reactive oxygen species

The generation of reactive oxygen species is associated with life under aerobic conditions and reactive intermediates are produced under both physiological and pathophysiological conditions (Freeman & Crapo, 1982). Reactive oxygen species are capable of damaging biological macromolecules such as DNA, carbohydrates or proteins. These oxygen metabolites are either radicals, e.g. hydroxyl radical ($OH^{\bullet}$), peroxyl radical ($ROO^{\bullet}$), or reactive non-radical compounds such as singlet oxygen, peroxynitrite ($ONOO^-$) or hydrogen peroxide ($H_2O_2$) (Bergamini et al., 2004). As explained in more detail below, sources of reactive oxygen species in the eye are sunlight, mitochondria respiration, and cellular metabolic reactions.
Superoxide ($O_2^{\bullet -}$) is the primary free radical formed within the cell by the reduction of molecular oxygen (Freeman & Crapo, 1982). The superoxide radical anion ($O_2^{\bullet -}$) appears to play a central role as other reactive intermediates are formed from it. The respiratory chain in mitochondria is a powerful source of reactive oxygen species, primarily superoxide ($O_2^{\bullet -}$) and consequently hydrogen peroxide ($H_2O_2$), as a product of superoxide ($O_2^{\bullet -}$)

dismutation (Chance et al., 1979) figure 2. This is due to the probable 'leak' of single electron at the specific site of the mitochondrial electron transport chain, resulting in inappropriate single electron reduction of oxygen to superoxide ($O_2^{\bullet -}$) (Loschen et al., 1974.) Another significant source of reactive oxygen species is inflammatory reactions, especially chronic inflammation. Inflammatory cells such as activated macrophages and neutrophils release various reactive oxygen species (hydrogen peroxide [$H_2O_2$], nitric oxide [$NO^{\bullet}$], superoxide [$O_2^{\bullet -}$]) and hypochlorite (HOCl) (Fantone & Ward, 1982). Neutrophils possess a membrane-bound multicomponent enzyme complex termed the NADPH oxidase that, when activated, generates large quantities of reactive oxygen species (Babior et al., 2002). This system is responsible for the neutrophil "respiratory burst" (increased respiration of phagocytosis).

The external environment can also generate reactive oxygen species from many sources including heat, UV light, therapeutic drugs, and $\chi$- and $\gamma$- radiation (Nikjoo et al., 1994). In an iron catalyzed Haber-weiss reaction, superoxide ($O_2^{\bullet -}$), ascorbate, thiols and other reductants reduce $Fe^{3+}$ to $Fe^{2+}$, which in turn reduces hydrogen peroxide ($H_2O_2$) to form the hydroxyl radical ($OH^{\bullet}$), a potent oxidant that causes lipid oxidation (Freeman & Crapo, 1982) figure 2. Mitochondria are also a major site for the accumulation of low molecular weight $Fe^{2+}$ complexes, which promote the oxidative damage of membrane lipids, proteins, and mitochondrial DNA.

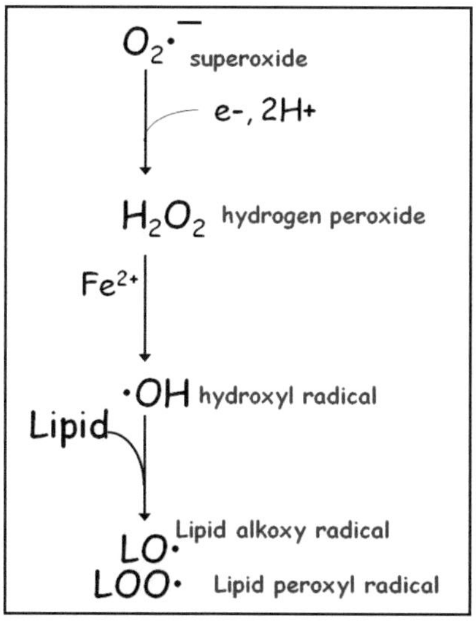


Fig. 2. Formation of reactive oxygen radicals

The hydroxyl radical ($OH^{\bullet}$) is the most reactive oxygen species. Due to its high reactivity, this radical immediately reacts with surrounding target molecules at the site where it is generated. Peroxyl radicals can be generated in the process of lipid peroxidation, which is initiated by the abstraction of a hydrogen atom from polyunsaturated fatty acids (Spiteller, 2006). Peroxyl radicals are relatively long-lived species with a considerable diffusion pathlength in biological systems. Further products generated in lipid peroxidation are aldehydes (Esterbauer et al., 1991).

While lipid peroxidation is not initiated by superoxide ($O_2^{\bullet -}$) and hydrogen peroxide ($H_2O_2$), hydroxyl radical ($OH^{\bullet}$), alkoxy radicals ($RO^{\bullet}$), and peroxyl radical ($ROO^{\bullet}$) result in the initiation of lipid peroxidation (Kanner et al., 1987) figure 2. Lipid peroxy radicals react with other lipids, proteins, and nucleic acids propagating thereby the transfer of electrons and bringing about the oxidation of substrates. Cell membranes, which are structurally made up of large amounts of polyunsaturated fatty acids, are highly susceptible to oxidative attack and, consequent changes result in altered membrane fluidity, permeability, and cellular metabolic dysfunction (Spiteller, 2002).

### 2.2 Sources of nitric oxide and reactive nitrogen species

Nitric oxide ($NO^•$) is a free radical but is believed to be essentially a beneficial metabolite and indeed it may react with lipid peroxides and function as an antioxidant (Hogg et al., 1993). Because nitric oxide ($NO^•$) is a free gas, it easily penetrates through biological membranes (Lancaster, 1997). Nitric oxide synthase (NOS) enzymatically generates nitric oxide ($NO^•$) by catalyzing the oxidation of the terminal guanidino nitrogen of L-arginine, converting the precursor amino acid substrate to L-citrulline (Alderton et al., 2001). Nitric oxide synthase isoforms generally fall into two categories: (i) constitutive nitric oxide synthases (NOS-I and NOS-III) that are dependent on $Ca^{2+}$/calmodulin and (ii) inducible nitric oxide synthase (NOS-II or iNOS), the expression of which is increased by cytokines and other inflammatory stimuli. Inducible nitric oxide synthase binds $Ca^{2+}$/calmodulin at all physiologic $Ca^{2+}$ concentrations and unlike the other two isoforms is not subject to $Ca^{2+}$-dependent regulation (Daff, 2010). There are three nitric oxide synthase isoforms, neuronal (nNOS, NOS-I), inducible (iNOS, NOS-II), and endothelial (eNOS, NOS-III), all of which require NADPH and $O_2$ as co-substrates. Nitric oxide synthases- I and nitric oxide synthases-III isoforms have been cloned from the human retina and retinal vascular endothelial cells, respectively (Park et al., 1994; Chakravarthy et al., 1995). Nitric oxide synthases-I has also been identified in amacrine cells, in the inner nuclear layer and in photoreceptors of the retina from different species by immunohistochemistry (Perez et al., 1995). Nitric oxide synthases-II isoform has been documented in the cornea, iris, ciliary body, neural retina, retinal glial cells, retinal pigmented epithelial cells and optic nerve head under conditions of increased intraocular pressure and uveitis (Becquet et al., 1997; Aslan et al., 2007).

### 2.3 Interaction between nitric oxide and oxygen radicals

Superoxide radical ($O_2^{•-}$) has a high affinity toward nitric oxide ($NO^•$). Reaction between nitric oxide ($NO^•$) and superoxide ($O_2^{•-}$) produces a new molecule, which is called peroxynitrite ($ONOO^-$) (Beckman et al., 1990). Peroxynitrite ($ONOO^-$) is a highly reactive molecule and can cause extensive damage to proteins, lipids, and especially DNA molecules. The reaction of nitric oxide ($NO^•$) with metalloproteins, protein sulfhydryls and oxygen derived free radicals enables nitric oxide ($NO^•$) to modulate inflammation and oxidative stress (Rubbo et al., 1996).

The conjugate acid of peroxynitrite ($ONOO^-$), peroxynitrous acid (ONOOH), reacts by two pathways, with the first pathway yielding nitrate ($NO_3^-$) without forming strong oxidant intermediates. The second pathway forms hydroxyl radical ($OH^•$) and nitrogen dioxide ($NO_2$), a potent oxidant that can initiate fatty acid oxidation and nitration of amino acids (Beckman et al., 1990). Peroxynitrite ($ONOO^-$) reactivity is also influenced by $CO_2$, with the formation of a reactive nitrosoperoxocarbonate ($ONOOCO_2^-$) intermediate. Consequently, $CO_2$ stimulates both peroxynitrite ($ONOO^-$) decay and enhances peroxynitrite ($ONOO^-$)–mediated nitration of molecules by nearly 2-fold (Radi et al., 1999) figure 3.

Oxidases and oxygenases, in particular, are critical sources of oxygen radical production and can lead to an overall impairment of nitric oxide ($NO^•$) signaling, via the metalloprotein and free radical–mediated consumption of this vasoactive molecule. Oxidase and oxygenase activities can thus account for the functional inactivation of nitric oxide ($NO^•$), leading to a prooxidative milieu and chronic inflammation (Aslan & Freeman, 2007).

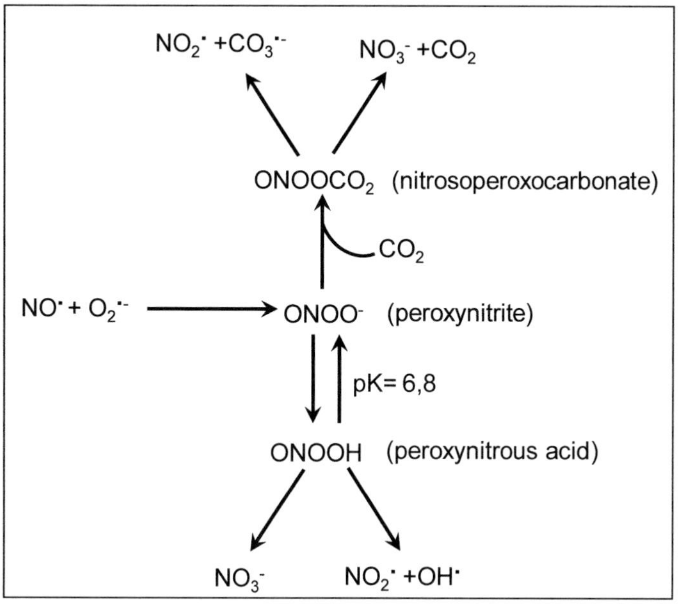


Fig. 3. Pathways of peroxynitrite formation and decay

## 3. Apoptosis in glaucomatous neurodegeneration

The major mechanism of visual loss in glaucoma is retinal ganglion cell apoptosis, leading to thinning of the inner nuclear and nerve fiber layers of the retina and axonal loss in the optic nerve (Fechtner & Weinreb, 1994). Atrophy occuring in neurons located at magno- and parvocellular layers in the lateral geniculate nucleus of the thalamus is also reported in experimental glaucoma (Yücel et al., 2001). The lateral geniculate nucleus is the primary relay center for visual information received from the retina of the eye. (Xu et al., 2001). It is reported that neurons in parvocellular layers undergo significantly more shrinkage than neurons in magnocellular layers (Yücel et al., 2001).

In animal models of ocular hypertension, elevated intraocular pressure augments apoptosis in retinal cells, induces nitric oxide synthases-2 expression and leads to protein nitration (Aslan et al., 2006) suggesting that nitrative stress exacerbates disease progression in clinical conditions accompanied by ocular degeneration. Reported studies also demonstrate the presence of nitric oxide synthases-2 in glaucomatous optic nerve head with consistent staining of nitrotyrosine, indicating that reactive nitrogen species may contribute to retinal ganglion cell death associated with elevated intraocular pressure (Liu & Neufeld, 2000; Shareef et al., 1999). Indeed, pharmacological studies have shown that inhibition of nitric oxide synthases-2 by aminoguanidine provides neuroprotection to retinal ganglion cells in a rat model of chronic glaucoma (Neufeld et al., 1999).

Nitric oxide-mediated cytotoxicity and the capacity of nitric oxide (NO•) to induce apoptosis have been documented in macrophages (Sarih et al., 1993) astrocytes (Hu & Van Eldik, 1996) and neuronal cells (Heneka et al., 1998). Reactive oxygen and nitrogen species are important regulators of apoptosis, which can be induced by two major pathways. The extrinsic pathway involves binding of TNF-α and Fas ligand to membrane receptors leading to caspase-8 activation, while the intrinsic pathway participates in stress-induced mitochondrial cytochrome c release. Released cytochrome c makes a complex with apoptotic protease-activating factor-1 (Apaf-1) and procaspase-9, which induces activation of caspase-9. Both pathways converge on caspase-3 activation, resulting in cellular morphological changes such as blebbing and nuclear degradation (Figure 4) (Reed, 2000).

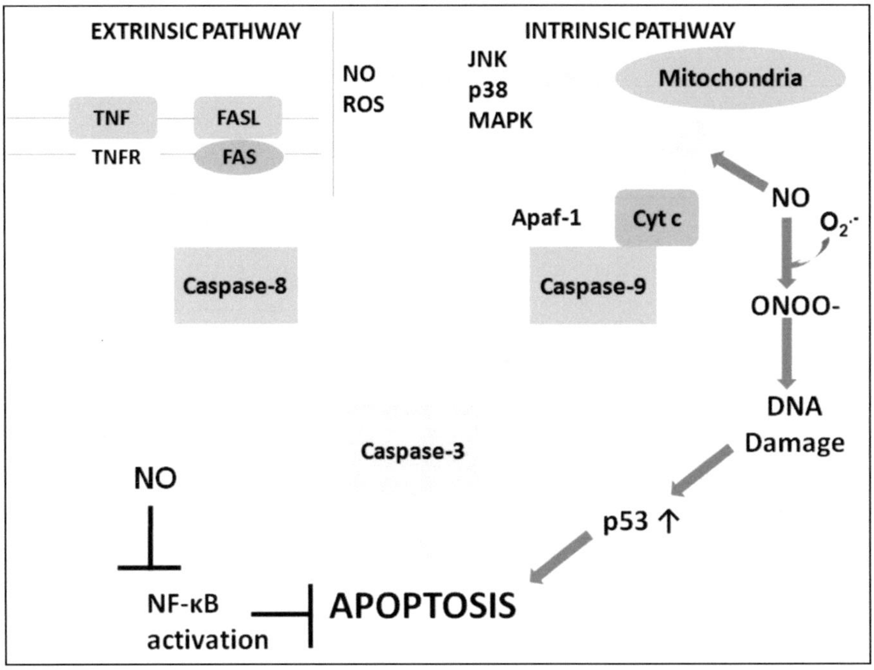


Fig. 4. Extrinsic and intrinsic pathways for apoptosis. The extrinsic pathway can be induced by members of the TNF family receptors such as TNFR and FAS. The intrinsic pathway can be activated by release of cytochrome c from mitochondria. In the cytosol, cytochrome c binds and activates Apaf-1, allowing it to bind and activate caspase-9. Caspase-9 and -8 activate caspase-3. Main signaling components of nitric oxide (NO•)-initiated apoptotic cell death are presented in red. For details, see the text. Apaf-1, apoptotic protease-activating factor-1; Cyt c, cytochrome c; JNK, c-Jun N-terminal kinase; p38 MAPK, p38 mitogen-activated protein kinase

Nitrative and oxidative stress induce apoptotic cell death by the activation of c-Jun N-terminal kinase (JNK; also referred to as stress activated protein kinase or SAPK) and p38 mitogen-activated protein (MAP) kinase leading to caspase 3 activation (Saeki et al., 2002; Jun et al., 1999) . Nitric oxide can also directly induce cytochrome c release from the mitochondria by tyrosine nitration of cytochrome c (Hortelano et al., 1999). High concentrations of nitric oxide (NO•) and peroxynitrite (ONOO−) are reported to cause DNA damage and lead to p53-mediated growth arrest and apoptosis (Kim et al., 1999).

Nuclear factor-κB plays a protective role against apoptosis through the up-regulation of genes encoding anti-apoptotic proteins (Chen et al., 1999). Nitric oxide inhibits nuclear factor-κB activation, by inducing the expression of the nuclear factor-κB inhibitor, and stabilization of the nuclear factor-κB/nuclear factor-κB inhibitor complex (Peng et al., 1995). In contrast to nitric oxide ($NO^{\bullet}$), oxidative stress activates nuclear factor-κB inhibitor kinase, which leads to the phosphorylation of nuclear factor-κB inhibitor and activation of nuclear factor-κB. The activation of nuclear factor-κB inhibitor kinase and phosphorylation of nuclear factor-κB inhibitor can be blocked by antioxidants and nitric oxide ($NO^{\bullet}$) (Chen et al., 1999). With reference to reported studies one can predict that induction of apoptosis requires fine biochemical interplay between oxygen and nitrogen species. The main signaling components of nitric oxide ($NO^{\bullet}$)-initiated apoptotic cell death are illustrated in figure 4.

## 4. Oxidative stress and immune response regulation in glaucomatous neurodegeneration

Oxidative stress is also linked to immunostimulatory signaling on the immunogenic aspects of glaucoma. The regulation of immune response can be in many different ways via oxidative stress in glaucoma (Tezel, 2010). One of these events is oxidative protein modifications as detected by proteomic analysis of the retina in experimental glaucoma (Tezel et al. 2005). Oxidation may change the antigenic features of these proteins, thereby serving as an immunostimulatory signal during glaucomatous neurodegeneration (Tezel, 2010). In addition to increasing antigenity, oxidative modifications may also affect the neurosupportive and immunoregulatory functions of glial cells (Tezel, 2010). Oxidized proteins, lipids, and DNA become para-inflammatory stimuli and signal to resident immune cells, mainly including microglia, to initiate an innate immune response (Xu et al., 2009). With enhanced scavenger functions, microglial cells are able to remove oxidation products by phagocytosis and they may release growth factors and cytokines to promote tissue healing (Schwartz, 2003; Ransohoff & Perry, 2009). This is in the same notion proposed for regulatory T cells (Schwartz & Kipnis, 2002). However, if oxidative stress reaches to a certain level, the physiological homeostasis may be impaired, thereby evolving into an injury process. In this case, initial glial response expands and leads to increased production of pro-inflammatory cytokines (Tezel, 2010).
Complement activation constitutes another important component of the innate immune activities detected in glaucomatous neurodegeneration. The regulation of complement activation was studied in oxidative stress-mediated glaucoma. Human retinal protein samples obtained from donor eyes with or without glaucoma were analyzed by a quantitative proteomic approach using mass spectrometry. Tissue lysates were spiked with recombinant protein standards for spectral count normalization and digested with modified trypsin. Resulting peptides were loaded onto an analytical capillary chromatography column attached to an analytical reverse phase chromatography column. Ionized peptides were eluted into a linear ion trap mass spectrometer. Spectra were acquired and analyzed via tandem mass spectrometry. Cellular localization of protein expression for different complement components and regulators were also determined by immunohistochemical analysis of an additional group of human donor eyes with glaucoma compared with age-matched control eyes without glaucoma. In addition, to determine the regulation of complement factor H by oxidative stress, *in vitro* experiments were performed using rat

retinal cell cultures incubated in the presence and absence of an oxidant treatment. Proteomic and immunohistochemical analysis identified an increase in complement components C1q and C3b and the membrane attack complex C5b-9. In addition, several complement regulatory proteins were detected in the human retinal proteome, and glaucomatous samples exhibited a trend toward downregulation of complement factor H expression. *In vitro* experiments revealed that oxidative stress, which was also prominently detectable in the glaucomatous human retinas, downregulated complement factor H expression in retinal cells. These findings expand the current knowledge of complement activation by presenting new evidence in human glaucoma and support that despite important roles in tissue cleaning and healing, a potential deficiency in intrinsic regulation of complement activation, as is evident in the presence of oxidative stress, may lead to uncontrolled complement attack with neurodestructive consequences (Tezel et al., 2010).

Other consequences of oxidative stress facilitating an aberrant immune activity in glaucoma include the augmented generation of advanced glycation end products through oxidative stress-dependent processes (Tezel et al., 2007). Advanced glycation end products may act as persistent antigenic stimulus and also be immunostimulatory through a specific receptor for advanced glycation end products-mediated signaling that leads to pro-inflammatory cytokine production (Lin, 2006). Oxidative stress provides a common trigger for many downstream pathways compromising the perivascular barrier function (Pun et al., 2009) may similarly affect blood vessels in human glaucoma (Feilchenfeld et al., 2008).

The regulation of immune response through glial toll-like receptor signaling was studied in glaoucumatous oxidative stress (Luo et al., 2010). Retinal protein samples obtained from human donor eyes were analyzed by a quantitative proteomic approach involving mass spectrometry. Cellular localization of toll-like receptor-2, -3, and -4 was also determined by immunohistochemical analysis of an additional group of human donor eyes with glaucoma and control eyes. In addition, in vitro experiments were performed in rat retinal microglia and astrocytes to determine glial toll-like receptor expression and immunoregulatory function after exposure to hydrogen peroxide ($H_2O_2$)-induced oxidative stress. Proteomic analyses of the human retina detected expression and differential regulation of different toll-like receptors in glaucomatous samples. Immunohistochemical analysis supported upregulated expression of toll-like receptors on both microglia and astrocytes in the glaucomatous retina. In vitro experiments provided additional evidence that oxidative stress upregulate glial toll-like receptor and MHC class II expression and cytokine production through toll-like receptor signaling and stimulate proliferation and cytokine secretion of co-cultured T cells during antigen presentation. This study supports the upregulation of toll-like receptor signaling in human glaucoma, which may be associated with innate and adaptive immune responses. In vitro findings showed that oxidative stress-mediated glaucomatous tissue stress and may initiate the immunostimulatory signaling through glial toll-like receptors (Luo et al., 2010).

## 5. The role of retinal oxidative and nitrative injury in glaucomatous neurodegeneration

### 5.1 Protein oxidation in glaucomatous neurodegeneration

Protein carbonyl formation is a widely utilized marker for protein oxidation (Stadtman et al., 1991). The measurement of carbonyl groups is considered to be a good estimation for the extent of oxidative damage to proteins. Carbonyls, formed following reactive oxygen species-mediated oxidation of sugar and membrane lipids, are able to form adducts commonly known as CO-proteins (proteins bearing carbonyl groups) with structural proteins, causing alterations in their biological activity (Shacter, 2000). Reactive carbonyl groups on proteins can also be formed by direct oxidation of protein side-chains (Reznick & Packer, 1994). Reactive oxygen species may oxidize amino acid residue side-chains into ketone or aldehyde derivatives. Histidine, arginine, and lysine are the most susceptible amino acids for reactive oxygen species-mediated protein carbonyl formation (Stadtman & Berlett, 1997).

Most methods detecting protein-bound carbonyls are based on the covalent reaction of the carbonylated protein side chain with 2,4 dinitrophenyl-hydrazine and detection of 2,4-dinitrophenylhydrazone groups with a specific anti-dinitrophenyl antibody. Protein-hydrazone produced via the 2,4 dinitrophenyl-hydrazine reaction can also be quantified spectrophotometrically at an absorbance between 360-385 nm (Reznick & Packer, 1994).

Serum protein carbonyl levels measured in 50 patients with pseudoexfoliation glaucoma and in 55 healthy controls revealed a significant increase in the diseased group (Yagci et al., 2006). Protein carbonyl formation was also identified via proteomic analysis in a chronic pressure induced rat model of glaucoma (Tezel et al., 2005). In the reported study, carbonylated protein side chains present in control and ocular hypertensive retinal protein lysates were reacted with 2,4 dinitrophenyl-hydrazine and the formation of 2,4-dinitrophenyl-hydrazone groups were identified with anti-dinitrophenyl antibody via two-dimensional polyacrylamide gel electrophoresis. Approximately 60 protein spots, detected on 2D-oxyblots exhibited protein carbonyl immunoreactivity in ocular hypertension. Three of these proteins showed a significant increase in the relative percentage of carbonyl immunoreactivity as compared with controls. These spots were excised and in-gel digested prior to identification by matrix-assisted laser desorption ionization time-of flight mass spectrometry. Spectral masses obtained by matrix-assisted laser desorption ionization time-of flight mass spectrometry were analyzed via bioinformatics through the Mascot and Profound search engines. Identified proteins through mass fingerprinting were glyceraldehyde-3-phosphate dehydrogenase, heat shock protein 72 and glutamine synthetase.

Glyceraldehyde-3-phosphate dehydrogenase is a glycolytic enzyme, which catalysis the phosphorylation of glyceraldehyde-3-phosphate. The active site of this enzyme contains reactive SH-groups (Olsen et al., 1975), which can easily be oxidized in the presence of hydrogen peroxide ($H_2O_2$) or in the presence of systems producing superoxide ($O_2^{\bullet -}$) (Schmalhausen et al., 1999). Mild oxidation of glyceraldehyde-3-phosphate dehydrogenase results in the uncoupling of the oxidation and phosphorylation in glycolysis and decreases the content of ATP in the cell (Danshina et al., 2001). Thus, the oxidation of glyceraldehyde-3-phosphate dehydrogenase leading to altered enzyme activity can play a key role in the development of different pathological processes including neuronal cell death associated with glaucoma.

Posttranslational oxidative modification of heat shock protein 72 may have deleterious concequences on protein function. The primary function of heat shock protein 72 is to serve as an intracellular molecular chaperone of naive, aberrantly folded, or mutated proteins (Lindquist & Craig, 1988). Indeed, the expression of heat shock protein 72 in cultured rat retinal ganglion cells has been shown to increase tolerance to hypoxic and excitotoxic injury (Caprioli et al., 1996). Similarly, retinal ganglion cell protection was observed in a rat model of glaucoma treated with a heat shock protein inducer, geranylgeranylacetone (Caprioli et al., 2003). Transient increase of Hsp expression in some regions of the brain has been reported following oxidative injury. Hsp70 is induced in injured neurons, while upregulation of Hsp27 occurs predominantly in glial cells following ischemic stress (Kalmar & Greensmith, 2009).

Glutamine synthetase catalyzes the conversion of glutamate to glutamine and is a key enzyme participating in the metabolism of the major excitatory neurotransmitter, glutamate (Albrecht et al., 2007). Glutamine synthetase expression, also shown in retinal ganglion Müller cells (Linser et al., 1984), thus plays an important protective role against neuronal excitotoxicity. The effect of carbonyl formation on the function of glutamine synthetase remains to be elucidated but may have potential consequences on retinal ganglion cell death associated with glaucoma.

### 5.2 Glyco-oxidation in glaucomatous neurodegeneration

Advanced glycation end products form via non-enzymatic condensation reactions between reducing sugars and ε-amino groups or N-terminal groups. These glycation modifications occur preferentially on lysine and arginine amino acids, although they can occur on free amine containing lipids and DNA and proceed spontaneously via a complex series of chemical rearrangements to yield reactive products with varying crosslinking, pigmentation, and fluorescence properties (Brownlee et al., 1988). If oxidation accompanies glycation then the products formed are known as glyco-oxidation products (Fu et al., 1994). Advanced glycation end products are measured by spectroscopic and fluorimetric methods, exploiting their particular values of absorption (280 mn) and fluorescence (emission at 440 mn, excitation at 370 mn). However, these methods are not very specific and can only give indications on the general trend of the glycation process (Brownlee et al., 1988). More recently, radioimmunoassay and enzyme-linked immunosorbent assay methods have been developed, using polyclonal antibodies raised against advanced glycation end products and obtained *in vitro* from the glycation reaction of glucose with ribonuclease (Lapolla et al., 2005).

Although, nonenzymatic glycation of proteins is an important phenomenon in the development of vascular disease complications like macro- and microangiopathy (Bierhaus et al., 1998) it has also been recently observed in glaucoma (Tezel et al., 2007). Lens capsules of patients with Pseudoexfoliation syndrome and pseudoexfoliation glaucoma were immunostained to investigate the presence carboxymethylysine, a common glyco-oxidation product. In most of the obtained samples carboxymethylysine staining could be detected in epithelial cells of the lens capsules. However, direct correlation between clinical course and immunohistochemical reactivity could not be found (Zoric et al., 2006).

The formation of advanced glycation end products leads to protein cross-linking and causes the destruction of cellular structures (Brownlee et al., 1988). Indeed, advanced glycation end products inhibitors such as aminoguanidine, has been reported to retard the development of vascular disease complications in animal models by preventing the formation of advanced glycation end products in various proteins including collagen (Yucel et al., 2006; Vasan et al., 2003).

In a recent study, immunoperoxidase and double-immunofluorescence labeling were performed to determine advanced glycation end products and their receptor in the retina and optic nerve head obtained from donor eyes with glaucoma and age matched controls. Enhanced accumulation of advanced glycation end products and an up-regulation of receptor for advanced glycation end products were detectable in the glaucomatous retina and optic nerve head compared with controls (Tezel et al., 2007). In the reported study, cellular localization of advanced glycation end products and receptor for advanced glycation end products were determined via double immunolabeling with antibodies against glial fibrillary acidic protein, antivimentin and brn-3, markers of astrocytes, Müller cells, and retinal ganglion cells, respectively. Increased advanced glycation end products immunolabeling in glaucoma was mainly observed in the extracellular compartment and included laminar cribriform plates in the optic nerve head, while immunolocalization of receptors for advanced glycation end products was predominantly associated with astrocytes (Tezel et al., 2007).

### 5.3 Lipid peroxidation in glaucomatous neurodegeneration

Reactive oxygen species, generated during oxidative stress can induce peroxidation of lipids (either cellular membrane lipids or circulating lipoprotein molecules) and generate highly reactive aldehydes (Spiteller, 2006). The resultant end products, malondialdehyde or 4-hydroxynonenal are well-known markers in the pathologic molecular process in oxidative stress (Poli & Schaur, 2000). 4-hydroxynonenal derives from ω-6 polyunsaturated fatty acids like linoleic and arachidonic acid, whose conjugated double bonds are an easy target for species that can extract a hydrogen atom or add to a double bond (Poli et al., 2004).

Although lipid peroxidation has been quantitatively assessed by measuring malondialdehyde levels by the thiobarbituric acid-reacting substances assay, Thiobarbituric acid-reacting substances is considered to be a nonspecific marker of membrane lipid peroxidation, likely due to reaction of thiobarbituric acid with non-lipid moities (Yeo et al., 1994). Free radical-induced oxidation of arachidonic acid (20:4ω6), an unsaturated 20 carbon fatty acid released from membrane phospholipids, results in formation of F2- and D2/E2-isoprostanes (IP) (Pratico, 1999). Recent studies indicate that measurement of IP provides a reliable noninvasive approach to assess lipid peroxidation *in vivo* (Morrow, 2000).

A number of DNA adducts arising from lipid hydroperoxide-derived products have been identified by liquid chromatography-mass spectrometry (Blair, 2008). Malondialdehyde is one of the most studied lipid hydroperoxide-derived product that causes DNA damage (Marnett et al., 2003). However, the cyclic DNA-adduct it forms with dGuo (M1dG) is not a specific marker of lipid hydroperoxide-mediated DNA-adduct formation. M1dG may be a useful biomarker of endogenous DNA damage resulting from oxidative stress (Blair, 2008). Lipid hydroperoxide-DNA adducts, which are repaired and appear in the urine, can be used as surrogate biomarkers of DNA damage. Urinary heptanone-etheno (Hε) dAdo (HεdAdo), HεdGuo, and HεdCyd, which are formed exclusively by lipid hydroperoxide-mediated DNA damage, can be useful urinary biomarkers (Blair, 2008). Heptanone-etheno dCyd is highly mutagenic in cells (Pollack et al., 2006) and thus its quantification in the urine may have a clinical relevance.

UV spectrophotometry and fluorescent analysis were used to study the accumulation of conjugated dienes, end products of lipid peroxidation, in lipid extracts from lenses, aqueous humour and trabecular tissues, obtained from 49 eyes of patients with primary open angle glaucoma. Lipid peroxidation products have been found in significantly higher concentrations in the aqueous humour and trabecular tissue of glaucoma patients compared with control subjects (Babizhayev & Bunin, 1989). Similarly, a 2.5-fold increase in malondialdehyde levels were observed in lens capsule samples of patients with pseudoexfoliation syndrome when compared with normal age-matched control subjects (Gartaganis et al., 2007). Likewise, the mean concentration of 8-isoprostaglandin F2 measured in the aqueous fluid from patients with Pseudoexfoliation syndrome was significantly higher than those of age-matched control patients (Koliakos et al., 2003).

Increased vitreous and retina malondialdehyde levels were also detected in rats with elevated intraocular pressure (Yucel et al., 2005). As mentioned previously, peroxidation of polyunsaturated fatty acids results in the formation of multiple aldehydes including 4-hydroxynonenal, which is capable of inducing apoptosis in neuronal cells (Kruman et al., 1997). The dose and time dependent effects of 4-hydroxynonenal were studied on primary cultures of human optic nerve head astrocytes, generated from normal and glaucomatous human eyes (Malone & Hernandez, 2007). Treatment with 4-hydroxynonenal at concentrations of 50 mM and higher led to a greater than 50% reduction in cell viability of normal optic nerve head astrocytes over 6 h (Malone & Hernandez, 2007).

Glutathione is the most abundant non protein thiol in the cell and a key cellular antioxidant important in the inactivation of 4-hydroxynonenal (Dickinso et al., 2004). A significant depletion of glutathione levels was observed in normal astrocytes after exposure to 4-hydroxynonenal for over an hour (Kruman et al., 1997). Basal levels of glutathione in primary cultures of human optic nerve head astrocytes from glaucomatous eyes were reported to be below the level of detection compared with primary cultures from normal astrocytes (Malone & Hernandez, 2007). This finding suggests the presence of an altered antioxidant defence mechanism in glaucoma. A significant increase in glutathione levels were measured in both normal and glaucomatous astrocytes 24 h after 4-hydroxynonenal removal (Malone & Hernandez, 2007).

Human optic nerve head astrocytes treated with 25 µM 4-hydroxynonenal for over an hour induced expression of glutamate cysteine ligase catalytic subunit (Malone & Hernandez, 2007), leading to an increase in glutathione synthesis thereby enhancing cellular oxidant defense mechanisms (Dickinson et al., 2002). Expression of aldoketo reductase 1C, which metabolizes 4-hydroxynonenal to an inactive metabolite, was also elevated in optic nerve head astrocytes treated with 25 µM 4-hydroxynonenal for over an hour (Malone & Hernandez, 2007). The expression of glutathione S-transferase, which catalyzes the conjugation of 4-hydroxynonenal to glutathione, was similarly induced in optic nerve head astrocytes via 4-hydroxynonenal incubation (Malone & Hernandez, 2007). Induction of the aforementioned enzymes confers a protection mechanism against oxidative damage in optic nerve head neuronal cells in humans.

Increased lipid peroxidation accompanied by altered antioxidant enzyme activities was also observed in rats with glaucoma induced by 6 week injection of hyaluronic acid into the anterior chamber (Moreno et al., 2004). Retina lipid peroxidation, measured as thiobarbituric acid-reacting substances significantly increased in a time and hypertension dependent manner. The observed increase in thiobarbituric acid-reacting substances was accompanied by a decrease in glutathione, catalase and superoxide dismutase enzyme activities suggestive of an altered antioxidant defense mechanism (Moreno et al., 2004).

### 5.4 Protein nitration in glaucomatous neurodegeneration

Aromatic nitration is recognized to be a mediator of pathological conditions and signaling events encompassing nitric oxide ($NO^{\bullet}$) and oxidative stress. Numerous *in vitro* biochemical studies have demonstrated that nitration of protein tyrosine residues can alter protein function (Cassina et al., 2000). It has been shown that 3-nitrotyrosine ($NO_2$Tyr), 3-bromotyrosine and 3-chlorotyrosine, selective markers of protein nitration (MacPherson et

al., 2001). Indeed, the detection of protein $NO_2$Tyr is commonly used as a diagnostic marker of nitric oxide (NO•).-derived oxidants in both human disease states and animal models (Aslan et al., 2003). Various techniques including western blotting, enzyme-linked immunosorbent assay, immunochemistry, HPLC and mass spectrometry are employed to determine the formation of $NO_2$Tyr in a variety of disease states (Aslan et al., 2003).
Elevated intraocular pressure augments nitric oxide synthase-2 expression, retinal protein nitration and apoptosis (Aslan et al., 2006) and suggests that protein nitration and apoptosis exacerbate disease progression in clinical conditions accompanied by ocular degeneration. Thus, selective inhibiton of nitric oxide synthase-2 and appropriate intraocular pressure-lowering may prevent long-term visual loss and lead to improvement in the management of glaucoma. Indeed, pharmacological studies have shown that inhibition of nitric oxide synthases-2 by aminoguanidine provides neuroprotection of retinal ganglion cells in a rat model of chronic glaucoma (Neufeld et al., 1999). Nitric oxide synthase-2 immunostaining observed in glaucomatous optic nerve head suggests that it may contribute to retinal ganglion cell death associated with elevated intraocular pressure (Liu & Neufeld, 2000; Shareef et al., 1999).

### 5.5 DNA oxidation in glaucomatous neurodegeneration

Oxidative DNA damage can lead to DNA-protein cross linking, strand breaks and base modifications. Oxidative DNA damage is assessed by measuring levels of 8-hydroxy-2'-deoxyguanosine (8-OH-dG), an indicator of oxidative DNA damage (Dizdaroglu, 1992). 8-hydroxy-2'-deoxyguanosine (8-OH-dG) can be measured by high pressure liquid chromatography with electrochemical detection or by gas chromatography/mass spectrometry, a technique that combines gas-liquid chromatography and mass spectrometry to identify different substances within a test sample (Shigenaga et al., 1994). DNA strand breaks can be detected in tissues and cells via alkaline elution assay or terminal deoxynucleotide transferase-mediated in situ end-labeling, respectively (Collins & Horvathova, 2001).
Elevated intraocular pressure due to reduction in aqueous outflow facility is a major causal effect in glaucoma (Yan et al., 1994). The eye's outflow system consists of a series of endothelial cell–lined structures in the angle of the anterior chamber, which also include the trabecular meshwork. Levels of 8-hydroxy-2'-deoxyguanosine (8-OH-dG), a marker of oxidative DNA damage, was determined in human trabecular meshwork specimens collected from patients with primary open angle glaucoma (Sacca et al., 2005). The relationship between DNA oxidation, intraocular pressure and visual field damage and disease duration were also evaluated. Eight-hydroxy-2'-deoxyguanosine (8-OH-dG) was measured in extracted DNA samples by using a $^{32}$P-postlabeling procedure (Sacca et al., 2005). A statistically significant correlation was also found among oxidative DNA levels, visual field damage and intraocular pressure. It was concluded that oxidative DNA damage may induce human trabecular meshwork degeneration, leading to increased intraocular pressure.
Glutathione S-transferases are ubiquitous multifunctional enzymes, which play a key role in cellular detoxification. These enzymes protect cells against toxicants by conjugating them to glutathione, thereby neutralizing their electrophilic sites and increasing the products water-solubility (Mannervik et al., 1985). Glutathione S-transferase M1 gene polymorphism was examined in human trabecular meshwork specimens collected from 45 primary open angle

glaucoma patients undergoing therapeutical eye surgery (trabeculectomy) and unaffected controls (Izzotti, 2003). An association was found between Mu-class glutathione S-transferase null allele and primary open angle glaucoma, suggesting a possible genetic predisposition of defective Mu-class glutathione S-transferase null allele in the disease. Primary open angle glaucoma patients having Mu-class glutathione S-transferase null allele deletion had 2.2-fold higher 8-hydroxy-2'-deoxyguanosine (8-OH-dG) amounts than Mu-class glutathione S-transferase null allele positive subjects. In addition, Mu-class glutathione S-transferase null allele deletion was significantly more frequent in primary open angle glaucoma patients than in unaffected controls. 8-hydroxy-2'-deoxyguanosine (8-OH-dG) was increased (3.6-fold) in primary open angle glaucoma patients as compared with controls. Preliminary results from this study indicate that glutathione S-transferase genes are expressed in human trabecular meshwork under physiological conditions and that oxidative DNA damage is associated with primary open angle glaucoma.

## 6. Potential applications of antioxidants in glaucomatous neurodegeneration

As presented herein, chronic oxidative stress is involved in glaucoma pathogenesis, most notably, its age-dependent clinical onset. Ocular tissues and fluids contain antioxidants that play a key role in protecting against oxidative damage. Superoxide ($O_2^{\bullet -}$) is removed either by cytoplasmic, mitochondrial or extracellular superoxide dismutases, which dismutate superoxide ($O_2^{\bullet -}$) to yield hydrogen peroxide ($H_2O_2$) and oxygen ($O_2$) (Fridovich, 1986). Hydrogen peroxide formed in the anterior segment tissues of the eye is removed by the heme-containing enzyme catalase or by glutathione peroxidase (Costarides et al., 1991). The specific activity of superoxide dismutase and catalase can be measured in both normal fresh human cadaver trabecular meshwork (De La Paz & Epstein, 1996) and in the iris and corneal endothelium of rabbits (Riley, 1990). Specific activity of superoxide dismutase, but not catalase, demonstrates an age-dependent decline in normal cadaver human trabecular meshwork. However, age-dependent decline of catalase activity is only observed in the iris and corneal endothelium of rabbits.

A decrease in serum superoxide dismutase and catalase activity was also observed in patients with Pseudoexfoliation syndrome compared with age-matched controls (Zoric et al., 2006). Glutathione and oxidized glutathione levels were also decreased in pseudoexfoliation lens epithelial cells compared with non- pseudoexfoliation controls (Gartaganis et al., 2007). Furthermore, mean ascorbic acid concentration in the aqueous humour of patients pseudoexfoliation syndrome was significantly lower than that found in control patients (Koliakos et al., 2003).

Glutathione and ascorbic acid (Vitamin C) are low molecular weight antioxidants that can be detected in the aqueous humor of humans (Richer & Rose, 1998). Rapid loss of Vitamin E during lipid peroxidation can be diminished by ascorbic acid, which is known to recycle the Vitamin E radical (May, 1999). No significant difference was found in blood levels of ascorbic acid measured in 38 patients with chronic open-angle glaucoma and 12 controls (Asregadoo, 1979). On the contrary, plasma glutathione levels assessed in 21 patients with newly diagnosed primary open angle glaucoma and 34 age- and gender-matched control subjects revealed that glaucoma patients exhibited significantly lower levels of reduced and total glutathione than did control subjects (Gherghel et al., 2005).

Lutein and zeaxanthin are oxygenated carotenoids that form the macular pigment. Of the 10 carotenoids that have been reported in the human serum, only two, zeaxanthin and lutein are found in the human retina (Roberts et al., 2009). Although it is suggested that zeaxanthin and lutein are concentrated in the retina because of their ability to cross the blood brain barrier of the retinal pigment epithelium and scavenge free radicals (Roberts et al., 2009), no strong association was found between dietary intake of lutein and zeaxanthin and the risk for glaucoma (Rhone & Basu, 2008). Conversely, a recent study showed that treatment with astaxanthin, a naturally occurring carotenoid pigment and a powerful biological antioxidant, reduced oxidant-induced protein oxidation, lipid peroxidation and apoptotic cell death in experimental rat models of elevated intraocular pressure (Cort et al., 2010).

Polyphenolic flavonoids (tea, coffee, wine, dark chocolate and ginkgo bilboa), alpha lipoic acid, coenzyme Q10 and melatonin are natural substances with antioxidant activity in glaucomatous neurodegeneration (Mozaffarieh et al., 2008a).

The effects of resveratrol, which is a naturally occurring polyphenol found in berries, nuts, and red wine was studied in primary porcine trabecular meshwork cells subjected to chronic oxidative stress (Luna et al., 2009a). Primary porcine trabecular meshwork cells were submitted to chronic treatment with resveratrol or vehicle every three days for 15 days. Cells under resveratrol or vehicle treatment were incubated under oxidative stress conditions (40% oxygen) and control cultures were treated with vehicle and incubated at physiological oxygen concentration (5%). The level of endogenous reactive oxygen species was significantly decreased by resveratrol treatment (4 fold) compared with cells treated with vehicle. The amount of intracellular reactive oxygen species in resveratrol-treated cells under oxidative stress was similar to that of non-stressed control cells. The induction of mRNA expression of the inflammatory markers interleukin-1α, -6, -8 and endothelial-leukocyte adhesion molecule after chronic oxidative stress was significantly inhibited by chronic treatment with resveratrol. The accumulation of carbonylated proteins induced by oxidative stress was significantly lower in resveratrol-treated samples compared with samples treated with vehicle under oxidative stress. Resveratrol-treated cells showed protection against apoptosis after acute oxidative stress (200, 400, and 800 μM of hydrogen peroxide [$H_2O_2$]), when compared with cells treated with vehicle. Vehicle-treated cells showed a linear correlation between hydrogen peroxide (H2O2) concentration and apoptosis; cells treated with resveratrol exhibited protection against apoptosis in all hydrogen peroxide ($H_2O_2$) concentrations. Resveratrol treatment did not result in significant changes in proliferation and in the amount of DNA damage when compared with cells treated with vehicle. The data suggests that resveratrol could potentially have a role in preventing the trabecular meshwork tissue abnormalities observed in primary open angle glaucoma (Luna et al., 2009).

The antioxidative properties of ginkgo are due to its direct radical scavenging activity. Ginkgo biloba prevents oxidative damage to mitochondria, exhibits neuroprotective properties, inhibits LDL oxidation, has a relaxing effect on vascular walls, and an antagonistic action on platelet activating factor (Mozaffarieh et al., 2008a). Administration of ginkgo increases ocular blood flow velocity in patients (Chung et al., 1999), and improves visual field in normal tension glaucoma patients (Quaranta at al., 2003). The beneficial properties of ginko biloba suggest it to be of major therapeutic value in the treatment of glaucoma (Ritch, 2000).

The water and fat soluble vitamin alpha lipoic acid is found in foods such as red meat, liver, and yeast. Alpha lipoic acid is capable of regenerating several other antioxidants back to their active states, including vitamin C, vitamin E, glutathione and coenzyme Q10 (Mozaffarieh et al., 2008a).

Coenzyme Q10 is a coenzyme for the inner mitochondrial enzyme complexes involved in energy production within the cell (Choi et al., 2005). Coenzyme Q10 has been demonstrated to prevent lipid peroxidation and DNA damage induced by oxidative stress (Tomasetti et al., 2001). Oral administration of ubiquinone was shown to be useful in mitigating cardiovascular side-effects without affecting intraocular pressure in glaucoma patients (Takahashi et al., 1989).

Melatonin reduces the elevation of cGMP by suppressing nitric oxide synthase activity, indicating a neuroprotective role in the retina (Mozaffarieh et al., 2008a; Sa'enz et al., 2002). Findings indicate that melatonin reduces nitric oxide ($NO^{\bullet}$)-induced retinal oxidative damage both *in vitro* and *in vivo*. Furthermore, several of the metabolites that are generated when melatonin inactivates toxic reactants are themselves free radical scavengers (Mozaffarieh et al., 2008a). In addition, melatonin stimulates a number of antioxidative enzymes, which further promote antioxidative protection (Rodriguez et al., 2004).

The role of dorzolamide, which is a topical carbonic anhydrase inhibitor that plays significant intraocular pressure-lowering activity and vasoactive effect, was studied on the oxidative/antioxidant status of aqueous humor in patients with primary open angle glaucoma (Zanon-Moreno et al., 2009). One hundred thirty patients were divided into three groups; patients with primary open angle glaucoma without dorzolamide administration (n=34); patients with primary open angle glaucoma with dorzolamide administration (n=36); and subjects with cataract (comparative group, n=60). Oxidative activity was measured in the aqueous humor by malondialdehyde determination by thiobarbituric acid-reacting substances assay. Antioxidant status was assessed in the aqueous humor samples by measuring the superoxide dismutase activity and the total antioxidant status. Oxidative activity was significantly higher in both glaucoma groups than in the cataract group and was significantly higher in subjects without dorzolamide administration. Superoxide dismutase activity was significantly higher in both glaucoma groups than in the cataract group, and was significantly higher in glaucoma without dorzolamide administration than in glaucoma with dorzolamide treatment. Total antioxidant status was significantly decreased in both glaucoma groups compared with the cataract group, and was more significantly decreased in glaucoma without dorzolamide administration than in glaucoma with dorzolamide administration (Zanon-moreno et al., 2009). The data suggest that topical administration of dorzolamide diminishes oxidative stress in patients with glaucoma.

The protective effects of prostaglandin analogues (bimatoprost, travoprost, and latanoprost) on oxidative stress–induced trabecular meshwork changes in primary open angle glaucoma was studied in primary cell cultures of human trabecular meshwork and furthermore whether these protective effects of prostaglandin analogues could be blocked by pretreatment with prostaglandin F receptor antagonists was investigated (Yu et al., 2008). The cells were exposed to hydrogen peroxide ($H_2O_2$) for 1 hour. The effects of prostaglandin analogues and benzalkonium chloride, which is the most widely used preservative in commercially available eye drops, on trabecular meshwork were investigated by preincubation of nonstressed or hydrogen peroxide ($H_2O_2$)-treated cells with 1:100 diluted commercial solutions of bimatoprost, travoprost, and latanoprost or their corresponding BAC concentrations. Pretreatment with BAC further increased the typical glaucomatous trabecular meshwork changes, which were characterized by cell loss, increased accumulation of extracellular matrix and cellular senescence in vitro. These effects were reduced by preincubation with prostaglandin analogues in hydrogen peroxide ($H_2O_2$)-treated and non-stressed cells. There was no reduction in the presence of prostaglandin F receptor antagonists in hydrogen peroxide ($H_2O_2$)-treated cells. These data suggest that oxidative stress-induced trabecular meshwork changes can be minimized by the use of prostaglandin analogues and prevention of oxidative stress exposure to the trabecular meshwork may help to reduce the progression of primary open angle glaucoma.

A refined monosodium luminal, Galavit, has antioxidant and antiinflammatory effects in human (Butorov et al., 2005) and glaucomatous mice (Jiang et al., 2006). The immunohistochemical distribution of glutathione, glutamine synthetase, and glutamate was examined in normal C57BL/6 mice (negative control), glaucomatous DBA2J mice (positive control), and glaucomatous DBA/2J mice treated with Galavit (Gionfriddo et al., 2009). Serial sections were immunogold stained for glutamate, glutamine synthetase and total glutathione, followed by image analysis for staining patterns and density. Focal decreases in glutamate immunostaining were common in the inner nuclear layer of glaucomatous DBA/2J retinas, but not in C57BL/6 or Galavit-treated glaucomatous DBA/2J retinas. Decreases in glutathione and glutamine synthetase immunostaining were found in glaucomatous DBA/2J retinal regions where neuronal glutamate immunostaining was reduced. Retinas from Galavit-treated glaucomatous DBA/2J had no significant decreases in inner nuclear layer levels of glutamate, glutathione, or glutamine synthetase. The data suggest that the antioxidant Galavit may prove to be effective in delaying or preventing retinal dysfunction and damage in at least some types of glaucoma.

## 7. Conclusions

Oxidative and nitrative processes have an important role in the pathogenesis of glaucomatous neurodegeneration (figure 5).

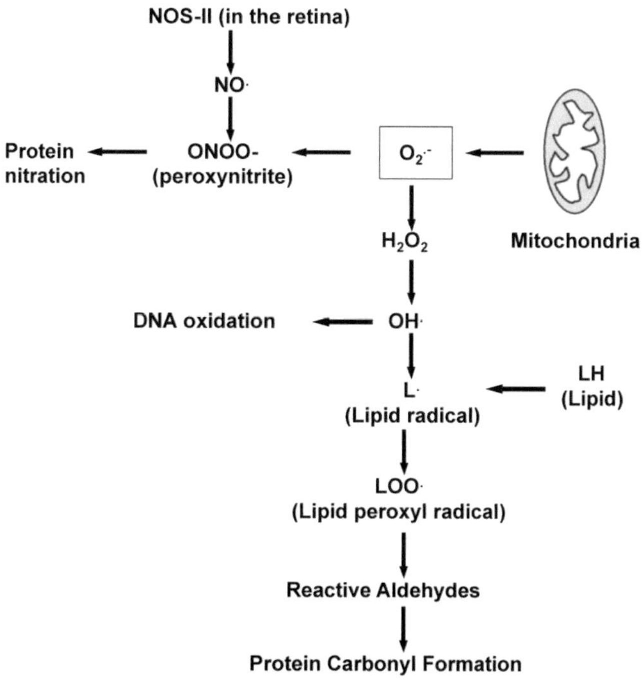


Fig. 5. Scheme of retinal oxidative damage

Despite all documentation of experimental data there is still limited understanding to whether free radical generation is a primary or a secondary event in glaucomatous neurodegeneration. As discussed herein, oxidative damage in the cellular components of the trabecular meshwork could directly affect the regulation of the extracellular matrix structure and lead to an alteration in the flow of the aqueous humor. Perturbation of the eye's outflow will thus cause an elevation in intraocular pressure, leading to clinical onset of glaucoma. In such set of circumstances, oxidative stress can be considered as a secondary event in the pathogenesis of glaucoma. Retinal oxidative injury occurring in models of elevated intraocular pressure or in normal tension glaucoma could also directly damage the retinal ganglion cell layer, leading to glaucomatous optic neuropathy. Continued trials of therapeutic interventions to reduce *in vivo* oxidative stress seem relevant in patients with the disease. Probably, an effective mode of protective therapy would be to start the therapeutic interventions at an early stage of the disease and target specific sites of reactive species generation. It is desirable that future studies and clinical trails will further advance our understanding on mechanisms of neuronal degeneration in glaucoma and help in the design of more effective therapies.

## 8. Acknowledgement

This work was supported by a grant from Akdeniz University Research Foundation (No.: 2007.01.0103.018).

## 9. References

Albrecht J., Sonnewald U., Waagepetersen H. S., & Schousboe A. (2007) Glutamine in the central nervous system:function and dysfunction. *Front Biosci.* 1, 12, (Jan 2007), 332-43.

Alderton W. K., Cooper C. E., & Knowles R. G. (2001). Nitric oxide synthases: structure, function and inhibition. *Biochem J.* 357(Pt 3), (Aug 2001), 593-615.

Andrews R. M., Griffiths P. G., Johnson M. A. & Turnbull D. M. (1999). Histochemical localisation of mitochondrial enzyme activity in human optic nerve and retina. *Br J Ophthalmol.* 83, 2, (Feb 1999), 231-5.

Aslan M., Freeman B. A. (2007). Redox-dependent impairment of vascular function in sickle cell disease. *Free Radic Biol Med.* 43, 11, (Dec2007), 1469-83.

Aslan M., Ryan T. M., Townes T. M., Coward L., Kirk M. C., Barnes S., Alexander C. B., Rosenfeld S. S., & Freeman BA. (2003) .Nitric oxide-dependent generation of reactive species in sickle cell disease. Actin tyrosine induces defective cytoskeletal polymerization. *J Biol Chem.* 278, 6, ( Feb 2003), 4194-204.

Aslan M., Yücel I., Akar Y., Yücel G., Ciftçioğlu M. A., & Sanlioglu S. (2006) Nitrotyrosine formation and apoptosis in rat models of ocular injury. *Free Radic Res.* 40, 2, (Feb 2006), 147-53.

Aslan M., Yucel I., Ciftcioglu A., Savaş B., Akar Y., Yucel G., & Sanlioglu S.(2007) Corneal protein nitration in experimental uveitis. *Exp Biol Med (Maywood).*232, 10, (Nov 2007), 1308-13.

Asregadoo, E. R. (1979). Blood levels of thiamine and ascorbic acid in chronic open-angle glaucoma. *Ann Ophthalmol.* 11, 7, (Jul 1979), 1095-1100.

Babior B. M., Lambeth J. D., & Nauseef W. (2002). The neutrophil NADPH oxidase. *Arch Biochem Biophys.* 397, 2, (Jan 2002), 342-4.

Babizhayev M. A, Bunin AYa. (1989). Lipid peroxidation in open-angle glaucoma. *Acta Ophthalmol (Copenh)*. 67, 4, (Aug 1989), 371-7.
Beckman J. S., Beckman T. W., Chen J., Marshall P. A., & Freeman B. A. (1990). Apparent hydroxyl radical production by peroxynitrite: implications for endothelial injury from nitric oxide and superoxide. *Proc Natl Acad Sci U S A*. 87, 4,(Feb 1990), 1620-4.
Becquet F., Courtois Y., & Goureau O. (1997). Nitric oxide in the eye: multifaceted roles and diverse outcomes. *Surv Ophthalmol*. 42, 1, (Jul-Aug 1997), 71-82.
Bergamini C. M., Gambetti S., Dondi A., & Cervellati C. Oxygen, reactive oxygen species and tissue damage. *Curr Pharm Des*. 10, 14, (2004),1611-26.
Bierhaus A., Hofmann M. A., Ziegler R., & Nawroth P. P. (1998) AGEs and their interaction with AGE-receptors in vascular disease and diabetes mellitus. I. The AGE concept. *Cardiovasc Res*. 37 ,3, (Mar 1998), 586-600
Blair I. A. (2008). DNA adducts with lipid peroxidation products. *J Biol Chem*.283, 23, (Jun 2008), 15545-9.
Brownlee M., Cerami A., & Vlassara H. (1988). Advanced glycosylation end products in tissue and the biochemical basis of diabetic complications. *N Engl J Med*. 318, 20, (May 1988), 1315-21.
Butorov I. V., Nikolenko, I. A., & Butorov S. I. (2005). Efficacy of galavit in patients with duodenal ulcer. *Klin Med (Mosk)*. 83, 8, (2005), 72-5.
Caprioli J., Ishii Y., & Kwong J. M. Retinal ganglion cell protection with geranylgeranylacetone, a heat shock protein inducer, in a rat glaucoma model. *Trans Am Ophthalmol Soc*. 101, (2003), 39-50; discussion 50-1.
Caprioli J., Kitano S., & Morgan J. E. (1996). Hyperthermia and hypoxia increase tolerance of retinal ganglion cells to anoxia and excitotoxicity. *Invest Ophthalmol Vis Sci*. 37, 12,(Nov 1996), 2376-81.
Cassina A. M., Hodara R., Souza J. M., Thomson L., Castro L., Ischiropoulos H., Freeman B. A., Radi R. (2000). Cytochrome c nitration by peroxynitrite. *J Biol Chem*. 275, 28, (Jul 2000), 21409-15.
Chakravarthy U., Stitt A. W., McNally J., Bailie J. R., Hoey E. M., & Duprex P. (1995). Nitric oxide synthase activity and expression in retinal capillary endothelial cells and pericytes. *Curr Eye Res*. 14, 4, (Apr 1995), 285-94.
Chance B., Sies H., & Boveris A. (1979). Hydroperoxide metabolism in mammalian organs *Physiol Rev*. 59, 3, (Jul 1979), 527-605.
Chen F., Castranova V., Shi X., & Demers L. M.(1999). New insights into the role of nuclear factor-kappaB, a ubiquitous transcription factor in the initiation of diseases. *Clin Chem*. 45, 1, (Jan 1999), 7-17.
Choi J. H., Ryu Y. W., & Seo J. H. (2005). Biotechnological production and applications of coenzyme Q10. *Appl Microbiol Biotechnol*.68, 1, (Jul 2005), 9-15.
Choi J., Kim K. H., Jeong J., Cho H. S., Lee C. H., & Kook M. S. Circadian fluctuation of mean ocular perfusion pressure is a consistent risk factor for normal-tension glaucoma. *Invest Ophthalmol Vis Sci*. 48, 1, (Jan 2007), 104-11
Chung H. S., Haris A., Kristinsson J. K., Ciulla T. A., Kagemann C., & Ritch R. (1999). Ginkgo biloba extract increases ocular blood flow velocity. *J Ocul Pharmacol Ther*. 15, 3, (Jun 1999), 233-40.
Collins A. R., Horváthová E. (2001). Oxidative DNA damage, antioxidants and DNA repair: applications of the comet assay. *Biochem Soc Trans*. 29, 2, (May 2001), 337-41.

Cort A., Ozturk N., Akpinar D., Unal M., Yucel G., Ciftcioglu A., Yargicoglu P., Aslan M. (2010) Suppressive effect of astaxanthin on retinal injury induced by elevated intraocular pressure. *Regul Toxicol Pharmacol.* 58, 1, (Oct 2010), 121-30.

Costarides A. P., Riley M. V. & Gren K. (1991). Roles of catalase and the glutathione redox cycle in the regulation of anterior-chamber hydrogen peroxide. *Ophthalmic Res.* 23, 5, (1991), 284-94.

Daff S. (2010). NO synthase: structures and mechanisms. *Nitric Oxide.* 23, (Aug 2010), 1-11.

Danshina P. V., Schmalhausen E. V., Avetisyan A. V., & Muronetz V. I. (2001). Mildly oxidized glyceraldehyde-3-phosphate dehydrogenase as a possible regulator of glycolysis. *IUBMB Life.* 51, 5, (May 2001), 309-14.

De La Paz M. A., Epstein D. L. (1996). Effect of age on superoxide dismutase activity of human trabecular meshwork. *Invest. Ophthalmol. Vis. Sci.* 37, (1996), 1849–1853.

Dickinson D. A., Iles K. E., Watanabe N., Iwamoto T., Zhang H., Krzywanski D. M., & Forman H. J. (2002). 4-hydroxynonenal induces glutamate cysteine ligase through JNK in HBE1 cells. *Free Radic. Biol. Med.* 33, 7, (Oct 2002), 974.

Dickinson D. A., Levonen A. L., Moellering D. R., Arnold E. K., Zhang H., Darley-Usmar V. M., & Forman H. J. (2004). Human glutamate cysteine ligase gene regulation through the electrophile response element. *Free Radic. Biol. Med.* 37, 8, (Oct 2004), 1152–1159.

Dizdaroglu M. (1992). Oxidative damage to DNA in mammalian chromatin. *Mutat. Res.* 275, 3-6, (Sep 1992), 331–342.

Esterbauer H., Schaur R. J., & Zollner H. (1991). Chemistry and biochemistry of 4-hydroxynonenal, malonaldehyde and related aldehydes. *Free Radic. Biol. Med.* 11, 1, (1991), 81-128.

Fantone J. C., Ward P. A. (1982). Role of oxygen-derived free radicals and metabolites in leukocyte-dependent inflammatory reactions. *Am. J. Pathol.* 107,(1982), 395–418.

Fechtner R. D., Weinreb R. N. (1994). Mechanisms of optic nerve damage in primary open angle glaucoma. Surv. Ophthalmol. 39, 1, (Jul-Aug 1994), 23-42.

Feilchenfeld Z., Yucel Y. H., & Gupta N. (2008). Oxidative injury to blood vessels and glia of the pre-laminar optic nerve head in human glaucoma. *Exp. Eye Res.* 87, 5, (Nov 2008), 409-414.

Filipowicz W., Bhattacharyya S. N., & Sonenberg N. (2008). Mechanisms of post-transcriptional regulation by microRNAs: are theanswers in sight? *Nat Rev Genet* 9, 5, (Nov 2008), 102-14.

Freeman B. A., Crapo J. D. (1982). Biology of disease: free radicals and tissue injury. *Lab. Invest.* 47, 5, (Nov 1982), 412–426.

Fridovich I. (1986). Superoxide dismutases. *Adv. Enzymol. Relat. Areas Mol. Biol.* 58,(1986), 61–97.

Fu M. X., Wells-Knecht K. J., Blackledge J. A., Lyons T. J., Thorpe S. R. & Baynes J. W. (1994). Glycation, glycoxidation, and cross-linking of collagen by glucose. Kinetics, mechanisms, and inhibition of late stages of the Maillard reaction. *Diabetes* 43, 5, (May 1994), 676–683.

Gartaganis S. P., Patsoukis N. E., Nikolopoulos D. K., & Georgiou C. D. (2007) Evidence for oxidative stress in lens epithelial cells in pseudoexfoliation syndrome. *Eye* 21, 11, (Nov 2007), 1406–1411.

Gherghel D., Griffiths H. R., Hilton E. J., Cunliffe I. A., & Hosking S. L. (2005). Systemic reduction in glutathione levels occurs in patients with primary open-angle glaucoma. *Invest. Ophthalmol. Vis. Sci.* 46, 3, (Mar 2005), 877–883.

Gionfriddo J. R., Freeman K. S., Groth A., Scofield V. L., Alyahya K., & Madl J. E. (2009). Alpha-Luminol prevents decreases in glutamate, glutathione, and glutamine synthetase in the retinas of glaucomatous DBA/2J mice. Vet Ophthalmol.;12, 5, (Sep-Oct 2009), 325-32.

Gottanka J., Johnson D. H., Martus P., & Lütjen-Drecoll E. (1997). Severity of optic nevre damage in eyes with POAG is correlated with changes in the trabecular meshwork. *J. Glaucoma* 6, 2, (Apr 1997), 123–133.

Harada T., Harada C., Nakamura K., Quah H. M., Okumura A., Namekata K., Saeki T., Aihara M., Yoshida H., Mitani A., & Tanaka K. (2007). The potential role of glutamate transporters in the pathogenesis of normal tension glaucoma. *J. Clin. Invest.* 117, (2007), 1763–1770.

Heneka M. T., Loschmann P. A., Gleichmann M., Weller M., Schulz J. B.,Wullner U., & Klockgether T. (1998). Induction of nitric oxide synthase and nitric oxidemediated apoptosis in neuronal PC12 cells after stimulation with tumor necrosis factor-alpha/lipopolysaccharide. J. Neurochem. 71, 1, (Jul 1998), 88–94.

Henry T. D., Archer S. L., Nelson D., Weir E. K., & From A. H. (1990). Enhanced chemiluminescence as a measure of oxygen-derived free radical generation during ischemia and reperfusion. Circ. Res. 67, 6, (Dec 1990), 1453–1461.

Hogg N., Kalyanaraman B., Joseph J., Struck A., & Parthasarathy S. (1993). Inhibition of low-density lipoprotein oxidation by nitric oxide. Potential role in atherogenesis. *FEBS Lett.* 334, 2, (Nov 1993), 170–174.

Hortelano S., Alvarez A. M., & Boscá L. (1999). .Nitric oxide induces tyrosine nitration and release of cytochrome c preceding an increase of mitochondrial transmembrane potential in macrophages. *FASEB J.* 13, 15, (Dec 1999), 2311–2317.

Hu J., Van Eldik L. J. (1996). S100 beta induces apoptotic cell death in cultured astrocytes via a nitric oxide-dependent pathway. *Biochim. Biophys. Acta.*1313, (19969, 239–245.

Izzotti A. (2003). DNA damage and alterations of gene expression in chronic-degenerative diseases. *Acta. Biochim. Pol.* 50, 3, (Oct 2003), 145–154.

Jiang Y., Scofield V. L., Yan M., Qiang W., Liu N., Reid A. J., Lynn W. S., & Wong P. K.(2006). Retrovirus-induced oxidative stress with neuroimmunodegeneration is suppressed by antioxidant treatment with a refined monosodium alpha-luminol (Galavit). *J Virol.* 80, 9, (May 2006), 4557-69.

Jun C. D., Oh C. D., Kwak H. J., Pae H. O., Yoo J. C., Choi B. M., Chun J. S., Park R. K., & Chung H. T. (1999) Overexpression of protein kinase C isoforms protects RAW 264.7 macrophages fromnitric oxide-induced apoptosis: involvement of c-Jun N-terminal kinase/stress-activated protein kinase, p38 kinase, and CPP-32 protease pathways. *J. Immunol.* 162, (1999), 3395–3401.

Kalmar B., & Greensmith L. (2009) Induction of heat shock proteins for protection against oxidative stress. *Adv Drug Deliv Rev.* 61, 4, (Apr 2009), 310-8.

Kanner J., German J. B. & Kinsella J. E. (1987). Initiation of lipid peroxidation in biological systems. Crit. Rev. Food Sci. Nutr. 25, 4, (1987), 317-364.

Kim Y. M., Bombeck C. A. & Billiar T. R. (1999). Nitric oxide as a bifunctional regulator of apoptosis. *Circ. Res.* 84, 3, (Feb 1999), 253–256.

Ko M. L., Peng P. H., Ma M. C., Ritch R., & Chen C. F. (2005). Dynamic changes in reactive oxygen species and antioxidant levels in retinas in experimental glaucoma. *Free Radic. Biol. Med.* 39, 3, (Aug 2005), 365–373.

Koliakos G. G., Konstas A. G., Schlötzer-Schrehardt U., Hollo G., Katsimbris I. E., Georgiadis N. & Ritch R. (2003). 8-Isoprostaglandin F2a and ascorbic acid concentration in the aqueous humour of patients with exfoliation syndrome. *Br. J. Ophthalmol.* 87, 3, (Mar 2003), 353–356.

Kruman I., Bruce-Keller A. J., Bredesen D., Waeg G., & Mattson M. P. (1997). Evidence that 4-hydroxynonenal mediates oxidative stress-induced neuronal apoptosis. *J. Neurosci.* 17, (1997), 5089–5100.

Lancaster Jr. J. R. (1997). A tutorial on the diffusibility and reactivity of free nitric oxide. *Nitric Oxide* 1, 1, (Feb 1997), 18–30.

Lapolla A., Traldi P., & Fedele D. (2005). Importance of measuring products of nonenzymatic glycation of proteins. *Clin. Biochem.* 38, 2, (Feb 2005), 103–115.

Lin L. (2006). RAGE on the toll road? *Cell. Mol. Immunol.* 3, 5, (Oct 2006), 351-358.

Lindquist S., Craig E. A.(1988). The heat-shock proteins. *Annu. Rev. Genet.* 22, (1988), 631–677.

Linser P. J., Sorrentino M., & Moscona A. (1984). Cellular compartmentalization of carbonic anhydrase-C and glutamine synthetase in developing and mature mouse neural retina. Brain Res. 315, 1, (Mar 1984), 65–71.

Liu B., Neufeld A. H. (2000). Expression of nitric oxide synthase-2 (NOS-2) in reactive astrocytes of the human glaucomatous optic nerve head. *Glia* 30, (2000), 178–186.

Loschen G., Azzi A., Richter C., & Flohe L. (1974). Superoxide radicals as precursors of mitochondrial hydrogen peroxide. *FEBS Lett.* 42, (1974), 68–72.

Luna C., Li G., Liton P. B., Qiu J., Epstein D. L., Challa P., & Gonzalez P. (2009a). Resveratrol prevents the expression of glaucoma markers induced by chronic oxidative stress in trabecular meshwork cells. *Food Chem Toxicol.* 47, 1, (Jan 2009), 198-204.

Luna C., Li G., Qiu J., Epstein D. L. & Gonzalez, P. (2009b). Role of miR-29b on the regulation of the extracellular matrix in human trabecular meshwork cells under chronic oxidative stress. *Mol Vis.* 15, (Nov 2009), 2488-97.

Luo C., Yang X., Kain A. D., Powell D. W., Kuehn M. H., & Tezel G.(2010). Glaucomatous tissue stress and the regulation of immune response through glial Toll-like receptor signaling. *Invest Ophthalmol Vis Sci.* 51, 11, (Nov 2010), 5697-707.

MacPherson, J. C., Comhair S. A., Erzurum S. C., Klein D. F., Lipscomb M. F., Kavuru M. S., Samoszuk M. K. & Hazen SL. (2001). Eosinophils are a major source of nitric oxide-derived oxidants in severe asthma: characterization of pathways available to eosinophils for generating reactive nitrogen species. *J. Immunol.* 166, 9, (May 2001), 5763–5772.

Malone P. E., Hernandez M. R. (2007). 4-Hydroxynonenal, a product of oxidative stress, leads to an antioxidant response in optic nerve head astrocytes. *Exp. Eye Res.* 84, (2007), 444–454.

Mannervik B., Alin P., Guthenberg C. Jensson H., Tahir M. K., Warholm M., & Jornvall H. (1985). Identification of three classes of cytosolic glutathione transferase common to several mammalian species: correlation between structural data and enzymatic properties. *Proc. Natl. Acad. Sci. U. S. A.* 82, 21, (Nov 1985), 7202–7206.

Marnett L. J., Riggins J. N., & West J. D. (2003). Endogenous generation of reactive oxidants and electrophiles and their reactions with DNA and protein. *J. Clin. Invest* 111, 5, (Mar 2003), 583–593.

May J. M. (1999). Is ascorbic acid an antioxidant for the plasma membrane? *Faseb J.* 13, 9, (Jun 1999), 995–1006.

Moreno, M. C., Campanelli J., Sande P., Sanez D. A., Keller Sarmiento M. I. & Rosenstein R. E. (2004). Retinal oxidative stress induced by high intraocular pressure. *Free Radic. Biol. Med.* 37, 6, (Sep 2004), 803–812.

Morrow J. D. (2000). The isoprostanes: their quantification as an index of oxidant stres status in vivo. *Drug. Metab. Rev.* 32, 3-4, (Aug-Nov 2000), 377–385.

Mozaffarieh M., Grieshaber M. C., Orgül S. & (2008a). Flammer J. The potential value of natural antioxidative treatment in glaucoma. Surv Ophthalmol. 53, 5, (Sep-Oct 2008), 479-505.

Mozaffarieh M., Grieshaber M. C., & Flammer J. (2008b). Oxygen and blood flow: players in the pathogenesis of glaucoma. Mol. Vis. 14, (Jan 2008), 224–233.

Neufeld A. H., Sawada A., & Becker B. (1999). Inhibition of nitric-oxide synthase 2 by aminoguanidine provides neuroprotection of retinal ganglion cells in a rat model of chronic glaucoma. *Proc. Natl. Acad. Sci. U. S. A.* 96, 17, (Aug 1999), 9944–9948.

Nikjoo H., O'Neill P., Terrissol M., Goodhead D. T. (1994). Modelling of radiationinduced DNA damage: the early physical and chemical event. *Int. J. Radiat. Biol.* 66, 5, (Nov 1994), 453–457.

Olsen KW., Moras, D. & Rossmann M. G. (1975). Sequence variability and structure of D-glyceraldehyde-3-phosphate dehydrogenase. *J. Biol. Chem.* 250, 24, (Dec 1975), 9313–9321.

Park C. S., Pardhasaradhi K., Gianotti C., Villegas E. & Krishna G. (1994). Human retina expresses both constitutive and inducible isoforms of nitric oxide synthase mRNA. *Biochem. Biophys. Res. Commun.* 205, 1, (Nov 1994), 85–91.

Peng H. B., Libby P., & Liao J. K. (1995). Induction and stabilization of I kappa B alpha by nitric oxide mediates inhibition of NF-kappa B. *J. Biol. Chem.* 270, (1995), 14214–14219.

Perez M. T., Larsson B., Alm P., Andersson K. E., & Ehinger B. (1995). Localisation of neuronal nitric oxide synthase-immunoreactivity in rat and rabbit retinas. *Exp. Brain Res.* 104, (1995), 207–217.

Poli G., Leonarduzzi G., Biasi F. & Chiarpotto E. (2004). Oxidative stress and cell signalling. *Curr. Med. Chem.* 11, 9, (May 2004), 1163–1182.

Poli G., Schaur J. (2000). 4-Hydroxynonenal in the pathomechanisms of oxidative stress. *IUBMB Life* 50, 4-5, (Oct-Nov 2000), 315–321.

Pollack M., Yang I. Y., Kim H. Y., Blair I. A. & Moriya M. (2006). Translesion DNA Synthesis across the heptanone–etheno-2'-deoxycytidine adduct in cells. *Chem. Res. Toxicol.* 19, (2006), 1074–1079.

Pratico D. (1999). F(2)-isoprostanes: sensitive and specific non-invasive indices of lipid peroxidation in vivo. *Atherosclerosis.* 147, 1, (Nov 1999), 1-10.

Pun P. B., Lu J. & Moochhala S. (2009). Involvement of ROS in BBB dysfunction. Free *Radic. Res.* 43, 4, (Apr 2009), 348-364.

Quaranta L., Bettelli S., Uva M. G., Semeraro F., Turano R. & Gandolfo E. (2003). Effect of Ginkgo biloba extract on preexisting visual field damage in normal tension glaucoma. *Ophthalmology.* 110, 2, (Feb 2003), 359-62; discussion 362-4.

Radi R., Denicola A. & Freeman B. A. (1999). Peroxynitrite reactions with carbon dioxidebicarbonate. Methods Enzymol. 301,(1999), 353–367.

Ransohoff R. M., Perry V. H. (2009). Microglial physiology: unique stimuli, specialized responses. *Annu. Rev. Immunol.* 27, (2009), 119-145.

Reed J. C. (2000). Mechanisms of apoptosis. *Am. J. Pathol.* 157, 5, (Nov 2000),1415–1430.

Reznick A. Z., Packer L. (1994). Oxidative damage to proteins: spectrophotometric method for carbonyl assay. *Methods Enzymol.* 233, (1994), 357-363.

Rhone M., Basu A. (2008). Phytochemicals and age-related eye diseases. *Nutr Rev.* 66, 8, (Aug 2008), 465-72.

Richer S. P., Rose R. C. (1998). Water soluble antioxidants in mammalian aqueous humor: interaction with UV B and hydrogen peroxide. *Vis. Res* 38, 19, (Oct 1998), 2881–2888.

Riley M. V. (1990). Physiologic neutralization mechanisms and the response of the corneal endothelium to hydrogen peroxide. *Clao J.* 16, 1, (Jan-Mar 1990), 16–21.

Ritch R. (2000). Potential role for Ginkgo biloba extract in the treatment of glaucoma. *Med Hypotheses* 54, 2, (Feb 2000), (221-35).

Ritch R., Schlotzer-Schrehardt U. (2001). Exfoliation syndrome. *Surv. Ophthalmol.* 45, 4, (Jan-Feb 2001), 265–315.

Ritch R., Schlotzer-Schrehardt U. & Konstas A. G. (2003). Why is glaucoma associated with exfoliation syndrome? *Prog. Retin. Eye Res.* 22, 3, (May 2003), 253–275.

Roberts R. L., Green J., & Lewis B. (2009) Lutein and zeaxanthin in eye and skin health. *Clin Dermatol.* 27, 2, (Mar-Apr 2009), 195-201.

Rodriguez C., Mayo J. C., Sainz R. M., Antolín I., Herrera F., Martín V. & Reiter R. J. (2004). Regulation of antioxidant enzymes: a significant role for melatonin. *J Pineal Res.* 36, 1, (Jan 2004), 1-9

Rubbo H., Darley-Usmar V., & Freeman B. A. (1996). Nitric oxide regulation of tissue free radical injury. *Chem. Res. Toxicol.* 9, 5, (Jul-Aug 1996), 809–820.

Sa´enz D. A., Turjanski A. G. & Sacca G. B. (2002) Physiological concentrations of melatonin inhibit the nitridergic pathway in the Syrian hamster retina. *J Pineal Res* 33, 1, (Aug 2002), 31-6.

Saccà S. C., Izzotti A., Rossi P. & Traverso C. (2007). Glaucomatous outflow pathway and oxidative stress. *Exp. Eye Res.* 84, (2007), 389–399.

Sacca S. C., Pascotto A., Camicione P., Capris P. & Izzotti A. (2005). Oxidative DNA damage in the human trabecular meshwork: clinical correlation in patients with primary open-angle glaucoma. *Arch. Ophthalmol.* 123, 4, (Apr 2005), 458–463.

Saeki K., Kobayashi N., Inazawa Y., Zhang H., Nishitoh H., Ichijo H., Saeki K., Isemura M. & You A. (2002). Oxidation-triggered c-Jun N-terminal kinase (JNK) and p38 mitogen-activated protein (MAP) kinase pathways for apoptosis in human leukaemic cells stimulated by epigallocatechin-3-gallate (EGCG): a distinct pathway from those of chemically induced and receptor-mediated apoptosis. *Biochem. J.* 368 (Pt3), (Dec 2002), 705–720.

Salmon J. F. (2008). *Glaucoma.* Riordan-Eva P., Whitcher J. P., Asbury T. (Eds.),. *Vaughan & Asbury's General Ophthalmology* 17th ed. Chapter 11. McGraw-Hill, New York, pp. 212–222.

Sarih M., Souvannavong V. & Adam A. (1993). Nitric oxide synthase induces macrophage death by apoptosis. Biochem. *Biophys. Res. Commun.* 191, 2, (Mar 1993), 503–508.

Schmalhausen E. V., Nagradova N. K., Boschi-Muller S., Branlant G. & Muronetz V. I. (1999). Mildly oxidized GAPDH: the coupling of the dehydrogenase and acyl phosphatase activities. *FEBS Lett.* 452, (1999), 219–222.

Schwartz M. (2003). Macrophages and microglia in central nervous system injury: are they helpful or harmful? *J. Cereb. Blood Flow Metab.* 23, 4, (Apr 2003), 385-394.

Schwartz M., Kipnis J. (2002). Autoimmunity on alert: naturally occurring regulatory CD4(+)CD25(+) T cells as part of the evolutionary compromise between a 'need' and a 'risk'. *Trends Immunol.* 23, 11,(Nov 2002), 530-534.

Shacter E. (2000). Protein oxidative damage. *Methods Enzymol.* 319, (2000), 428–436.

Shareef S., Sawada A. & Neufeld A. H. (1999). Isoforms of nitric oxide synthase in the optic nerves of rat eyes with chronic moderately elevated intraocular pressure. *Invest. Ophthalmol. Vis. Sci.* 40, (1999), 2884–2891.

Shigenaga M. K., Aboujaoude E. N., Chen Q. & Ames B. N. (1994). Assays of oxidative DNA damage biomarkers 8-oxo-2'-deoxyguanosine and 8-oxoguanine in nuclear DNA and biological fluids by high-performance liquid chromatography with electrochemical detection. *Methods Enzymol.* 234, (1994), 16–33.

Spiteller G. (2002). Do changes in the cell membrane structure induce the generation of lipid peroxidation products which serve as first signalling molecules in cell to cell communication? *Prostaglandins Leukot. Essent. Fat. Acids* 67, 2-3, (Aug-Sep 2002), 151–162..

Spiteller G. (2006). Peroxyl radicals: inductors of neurodegenerative and other inflammatory diseases. Their origin and how they transform cholesterol, phospholipids, plasmalogens, polyunsaturated fatty acids, sugars, and proteins into deleterious products. *Free Radic. Biol. Med.* 41, 3, (Aug 2006), 362–387.

Stadtman E. R., Berlett B. S. (1997). Reactive oxygen-mediated protein oxidation in aging and disease. *Chem. Res. Toxicol.* 10, (1997), 485–494.

Stadtman E. R., Oliver C. N. (1991). Metal-catalyzed oxidation of proteins. Physiological consequences. *J. Biol. Chem.* 266, 4, (Feb 1991), 2005–2008.

Stefani G., Slack F. J. (2008). Small non-coding RNAs in animal development. *Nat Rev Mol Cell Biol.* 9, 3, (Mar 2008), 219-30.

Takahashi N., Iwasaka T. & Sugiura T. (1989). Effect of coenzyme Q10 on hemodynamic response to ocular timolol. *J Cardiovasc Pharmacol* 14, 3, (Sep 1989), 462-8.

Tezel G., Yang X., Luo C., Kain A. D., Powell D. W., Kuehn M. H. & Kaplan H. J. (2010). Oxidative stress and the regulation of complement activation in human glaucoma. *Invest Ophthalmol Vis Sci.* 51, 10, (Oct 2010), 5071-82.

Tezel G. (2010). The immune response in glaucoma: A perspective on the roles of oxidative stres *Exp Eye Res.* 2010 Aug 13. [Epub ahead of print]

Tezel G., Luo C. & Yang X. (2007). Accelerated aging in glaucoma: immunohistochemical assessment of advanced glycation end products in the human retina and optic nerve head. *Invest. Ophthalmol. Vis. Sci.* 48,3, (Mar 2007), 1201-1211.

Tezel G., Yang X. & Cai J. (2005). Proteomic identification of oxidatively modified retinal proteins in a chronic pressure-induced rat model of glaucoma. *Invest. Ophthalmol. Vis. Sci.* 46, 9, (Sep 2005), 3177-3187.

Tomasetti M., Alleva R. & Borghi B. (2001). In vivo supplementation with coenzyme Q10 enhances the recovery of human lymphocytes from oxidative DNA damage. *FASEB J* 15, 8, (Jun 2001), 1425-7.

Tripathi R. C., Chan W. F., Li J. & Tripathi B. J. (1994). Trabecular cells express the TGF-beta 2 gene and secrete the cytokine. *Exp. Eye Res.* 58, 5, (May 1994), 523–528..

Vasan S., Foiles P. & Founds H. (2003). Therapeutic potential of breakers of advanced glycation end product-protein crosslinks. *Arch. Biochem. Biophys.* 419, 1, (Nov 2003), 89–96.

Wallace D. C. (19999. Mitochondrial diseases in man and mouse. *Science* 283, (1999), 1482–1488.

Wu L., Fan, J. & Belasco J. G. (2006). MicroRNAs direct rapid deadenylation of mRNA. *Proc Natl Acad Sci USA.* 103, 11, (Mar 2006), 4034-9.

Xu H., Chen M. & Forrester J. V. (2009). Para-inflammation in the aging retina. *Prog. Retin. Eye Res.* 28, 5, (Sep 2009), 348-368.

Xu X., Ichida J. M., Allison J. D., Boyd J. D., Bonds A. B. & Casagrande V. A. (2001) A comparison of koniocellular, magnocellular and parvocellular receptive field properties in the lateral geniculate nucleus of the owl monkey (Aotus trivirgatus). *J Physiol.* 531, Pt 1, (Feb 2001), 203-18.

Yagci R., Gürel A., Ersöz I., Keskin U. C., Hepşen I. F., Duman S. & Yigitoğlu R. (2006). Oxidative stress and protein oxidation in pseudoexfoliation syndrome. *Curr. Eye Res.* 31,12, (Dec 2006), 1029–1032.

Yan D. B., Coloma F. M., Metheetrairut A., Trope G. E., Heathcote J. G. & Ethier C. R. (1994). Deformation of the lamina cribrosa by elevated intraocular pressure. *Br. J. Ophthalmol.* 78 , 8, (Aug 1994), 643–648.

Yeo H. C., Helbock H. J., Chyu D. W. & Ames B. N. (1994). Assay of malondialdehyde in biological fluids by gas chromatography-mass spectrometry. *Anal. Biochem.* 220, 2, (Aug 1994), 391–396.

Yu A. L., Fuchshofer R., Kampik A. & Welge-Lüssen U. (2008). Effects of oxidative stress in trabecular meshwork cells are reduced by prostaglandin analogues. *Invest Ophthalmol Vis Sci.* 49, 11, (Nov 2008), 4872-80.

Yucel I., Akar Y., Yucel G., Ciftcioglu M. A., Keles N. & Aslan M. (2005). Effect of hypercholesterolemia on inducible nitric oxide synthase expression in a rat model of elevated intraocular pressure. *Vis. Res.* 45, 9, (Apr 2005),1107–1114.

Yucel I., Yucel G., Akar Y., Demir N., Gurbuz N. & Aslan M. (2006). Transmission electron microscopy and autofluorescence findings in the cornea of diabetic rats treated with aminoguanidine. *Can. J. Ophthalmol.* 41, 1, (Feb 2006), 60–66.

Yücel Y. H., Zhang Q., Weinreb R. N., Kaufman P. L. & Gupta N. (2001) Atrophy of relay neurons in magno- and parvocellular layers in the lateral geniculate nucleus in experimental glaucoma. *Invest Ophthalmol Vis Sci.* 42, 13, (Dec 2001), 3216-22.

Yun A. J., Murphy C. G., Polansky J. R., Newsome D. A. & Alvarado J. A.(1989). Proteins secreted by human trabecular cells. Glucocorticoid and other effects. *Invest. Ophthalmol. Vis. Sci.* 30, 9, (Sep 1989), 2012–2022.

Zanon-Moreno V., Garcia-Medina J. J., Gallego-Pinazo R., Vinuesa-Silva I., Moreno-Nadal M. A. & Pinazo-Duran M. D. (2009). Antioxidant status modifications by topical administration of dorzolamide in primary open-angle glaucoma. *Eur J Ophthalmol.* 19, 4, (Jul-Aug 2009), 565-71.

Zhou L., Li Y., Yue B. Y. (1999). Oxidative stress affects cytoskeletal structure and cellmatrix interactions in cells from an ocular tissue: the trabecular meshwork. *J. Cell. Physiol.* 180, 2, (Aug 1999), 182–189.

Zoric L., Miric D., Milenkovic S., Jovanovic P., & Trajkovic G. (2006). Pseudoexfoliation syndrome and its antioxidative protection deficiency as risk factors for agerelated cataract. *Eur. J. Ophthalmol.* 16 ,2, ( Mar-Apr 2006), 268–273.

# 6

# Excitotoxic Injury to Retinal Ganglion Cells

William A. Hare, Cun-Jian Dong and Larry Wheeler
*Allergan, Inc.*
*USA*

## 1. Introduction

In the retina, as in other parts of the central nervous system, excitatory synaptic transmission is mediated by glutamate. Excitatory synaptic transmission begins typically with a depolarization of the presynaptic (axon) terminal membrane resulting in an influx of calcium ions from the extracellular space into the presynaptic terminal. This influx of calcium ions triggers release of glutamate from the presynaptic terminal into the synaptic cleft. Glutamate then diffuses across the synaptic cleft and binds to ion channels of the post-synaptic membrane (neuronal dendrite). These glutamate-gated channels allow sodium and calcium ions to flow from the extracellular space into the post-synaptic dendritic compartment, thereby depolarizing or "exciting" the post-synaptic neuronal membrane. In order to preserve both the temporal properties and local specificity of synaptic transmission, glutamate must be cleared rapidly from the extracellular space by transporters located in neurons as well as glial cells.

It has been shown that excessive levels of excitatory activity can result in *excitotoxic* neuronal injury that is mediated ultimately by elevation of intracellular sodium and calcium concentration. Excitotoxic neuronal injury can be triggered by a wide range of primary insults and associated mechanisms that vary with location within the neuronal membrane compartment. In retinal ganglion cells (RGCs), somato-dendritic membrane is specialized for receiving synaptic inputs and integrating those conductance changes while axonal membrane is specialized for transmission of action potentials and synaptic communication. RGC dendritic membrane thus has a high density of glutamate-gated channels (Aizenman et al., 1988; Massey & Miller, 1990; Diamond & Copenhagen, 1993) while the axonal membrane has a high density of voltage-gated sodium channels (Pellegrino & Ritchie, 1984; Craner et al., 2003). RGC axons are not known to express glutamatergic channels but voltage-gated sodium channels are also expressed in somato-dendritic membrane (Wollner et al., 1988; Kaneda & Kaneko, 1991). Excessive activation of either glutamate-gated channels or voltage-gated sodium channels can result in excitotoxic injury to RGCs. Although other membrane conductances may, under some circumstances, drive excitotoxic RGC injury, this chapter will focus on mechanisms for RGC injury resulting from glutamate-gated channels and voltage-gated sodium channels.

## 2. Glutamatergic excitotoxicity

There are two general classes of glutamate-gated ion channel in the CNS: the NMDA-type and the non-NMDA type (Choi, 1988; Schoepfer et al., 1994). For both classes, glutamate is the normal endogenous ligand for channel activation but they may be distinguished by their selectivity for molecules that can bind to and activate the channel. NMDA-type channels are activated selectively by N-methyl-D-aspartate while non-NMDA channels are activated selectively by either kainate or α-amino-3-hydroxy-5-methyl-4-isoxazole-proprionic acid (AMPA). Both sub-types are permeable to sodium and calcium ions and neurons may be injured by excessive activity of either subtype. However, due to the relatively high calcium permeability of NMDA-type channels, neurons are particularly sensitive to injury resulting from overactivity of this channel subtype (Rothman & Olney, 1987). RGCs are known to express NMDA-type channels and glutamatergic excitotoxicity, mediated by NMDA channels , has been shown to be an important mechanism for RGC injury in a wide range of animal models for both acute and chronic disease including retinal ischemia (Lam et al., 1997; Lagreze et al., 1998), and glaucoma (Gu et al., 2000; WoldeMussie et al., 2002; Schuettauf et al., 2002; Hare et al., 2004a, 2004b).

Some key features of NMDA channel function are summarized in Figure 1. Under "resting" conditions, the trans-membrane potential is highly negative and the channel conductance gate is closed (A). At this high negative "resting" membrane potential, a magnesium ion is bound to a site within the channel conductance pore. When glutamate (or NMDA) binds to its receptor site, the channel opens but cannot conduct sodium or calcium ions due to block of the channel pore by magnesium (B). Unbinding of magnesium from its site within the pore requires depolarization of the neuronal membrane. That is, the probability of magnesium binding decreases with decreasing membrane polarization (C). The NMDA channel thus acts as a coincidence detector or, in the parlance of digital logic, an "AND" gate. In other words, the NMDA channel requires the simultaneous activity of non-NMDA channel synaptic input (or some other depolarizing event) in order to be "active", regardless of whether or not the channel has been "opened" by glutamate binding.

Any insult or condition that leads either to an increase in extracellular levels of glutamate or to an increase in the effect of glutamate at the post-synaptic membrane may trigger excitiotoxic neuronal injury. Ischemic insult provides one example for excitotoxic neuronal injury. Under conditions of metabolic insufficiency, cellular energy failure will be associated with loss of function in energy-dependent membrane transporters. Failure of the sodium/potassium exchanger results in loss of the transmembrane sodium gradient and depolarization of the "resting" membrane potential. Membrane dopolarization, in turn, increases the release of glutamate from presynaptic terminals and also decreases the voltage-dependent magnesium block of NMDA channel pores in the post-synaptic membrane. The resulting increase in glutamate-gated influx of sodium and calcium ions further depolarizes the cell membrane and also leads directly to cell injury through activation of calcium-dependent mechanisms as well as loss of function in membrane transporters that rely on the trans-membrane sodium gradient.

### 2.1 Glutamatergic excitotoxicity in RGCs

Glutamatergic neuronal excitotoxicity, originally described in the retina (Lucas & Newhouse, 1957), results from excessive activity of glutamate-gated ion channels and consequent increase in the intracellular levels of both sodium and calcium ions. RGCs are known to express both NMDA and non-NMDA type glutamataergic channels and are sensitive to injury from exposure to exogenously applied NMDA (Siliprandi et al., 1992;

Pellegrini & Lipton, 1993; Pang et al., 1999; Luo et al., 2001). In addition, systemic treatment with selective NMDA antagonists has shown that NMDA-type glutamatergic membrane channels make a significant contribution to RGC injury in rat (Gu et al., 2000; WoldeMussie et al., 2002) and monkey (Hare et al., 2004a, 2004b) models of experimental glaucoma.

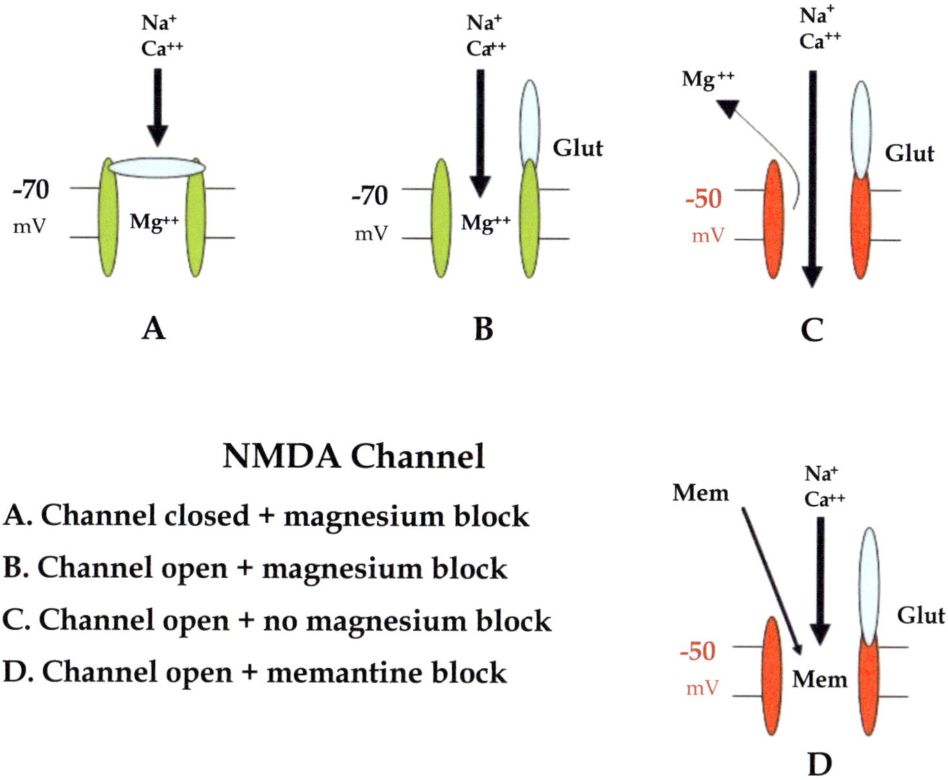


Fig. 1. Function of the NMDA-type glutamate-gated channel. Channel opening (B) requires binding of both glutamate (Glut) and glycine (not shown). See also (Choi, 1988)

Acute glutamatergic excitotoxic responses can be observed in electrophysiological recordings from single RGCs in a dark-adapted, perfused, ex-vivo rabbit retina preparation as illustrated in Figure 2. For these experiments, simultaneous recordings of the electroretinogram (ERG) and single-unit RGC responses were made. The retinal sample, beginning at the inferior margin of the optic disk as shown in panel A, was mounted RGC (vitreal) side up in the perfusion chamber as shown in panel B. The transretinal potential (ERG) was recorded as the voltage between the bath electrode and the sub-retinal electrode. The spiking activity of a single RGC was recorded using a tungsten microelectrode and the bath electrode as reference. Dim stimuli (delay = 400 msec, duration = 10 msec) were generated using a blue-green LED (λpeak = 504 nM). RGCs were classified as either "ON" or "OFF" subtype based on the response to a dim stimulus of one second duration. ON RGCs respond to this stimulus with a burst of action potentials at the stimulus onset while OFF RGCs are inhibited by the stimulus and respond with a burst of action potentials at stimulus offset (not shown).

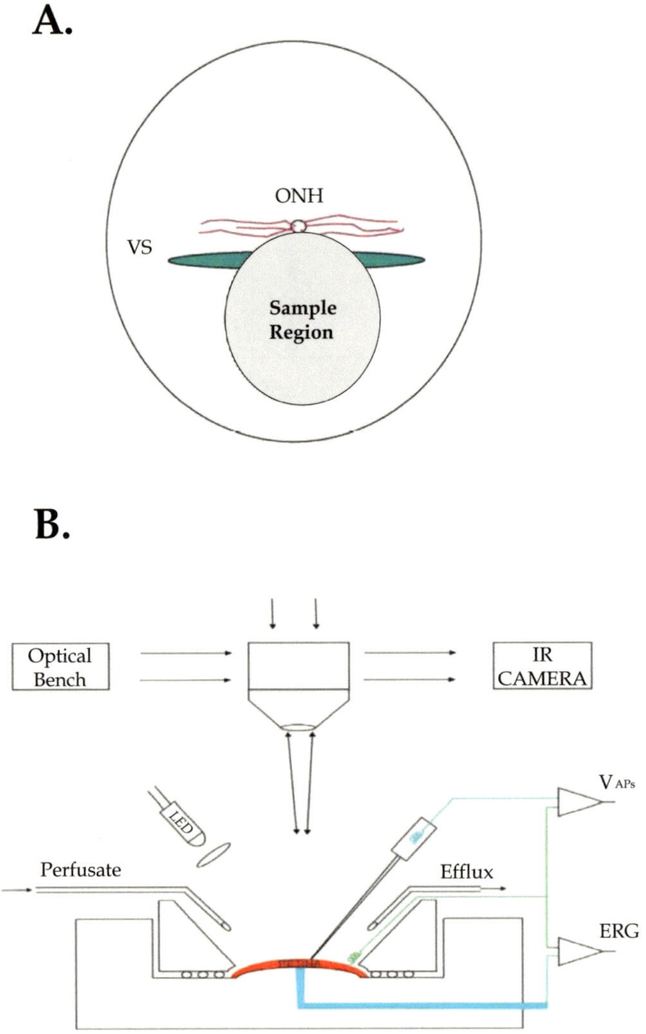


Fig. 2. Ex-vivo dark-adapted perfused rabbit retina preparation for simultaneous recording of the ERG and single-unit RGC activity. RGCs were classified as either "ON" or "OFF" subtype

Figure 3A shows the ERG (top trace) and single-unit RGC (bottom trace) responses to a dim flash delivered at 400 msec (vertical line). Note that the dim flash is below the ERG a-wave threshold and elicits a purely b-wave response. This OFF RGC exhibits a tonic level of spiking activity and responds to the dim flash with a burst of spikes at a latency of approximately 100 msec. At 2 minutes following continuous bath application of 200 μM NMDA (panel B), there is an obvious increase in the tonic level of RGC spiking activity, a reduction in spike amplitude, and no significant effect on the ERG. After 6 minutes of NMDA exposure (panel C), the RGC spike generation mechanism has failed. At 2 minutes following the switch to perfusion with 200 μM NMDA in combination with 10 μM memantine (a selective NMDA channel blocker), the RGC spike generation mechanism has begun to recover. The RGC has recovered to CONTROL levels of tonic spike frequency and amplitude by 4 minutes following addition of memantine. Clearly, application of exogenous NMDA results in an increase in tonic RGC spiking activity with a consequent rundown of the trans-membrane sodium gradient and loss of spike generation. Addition of memantine is able to completely reverse the effects of continuously applied NMDA and restore normal levels of tonic spike activity including responses to light stimuli.

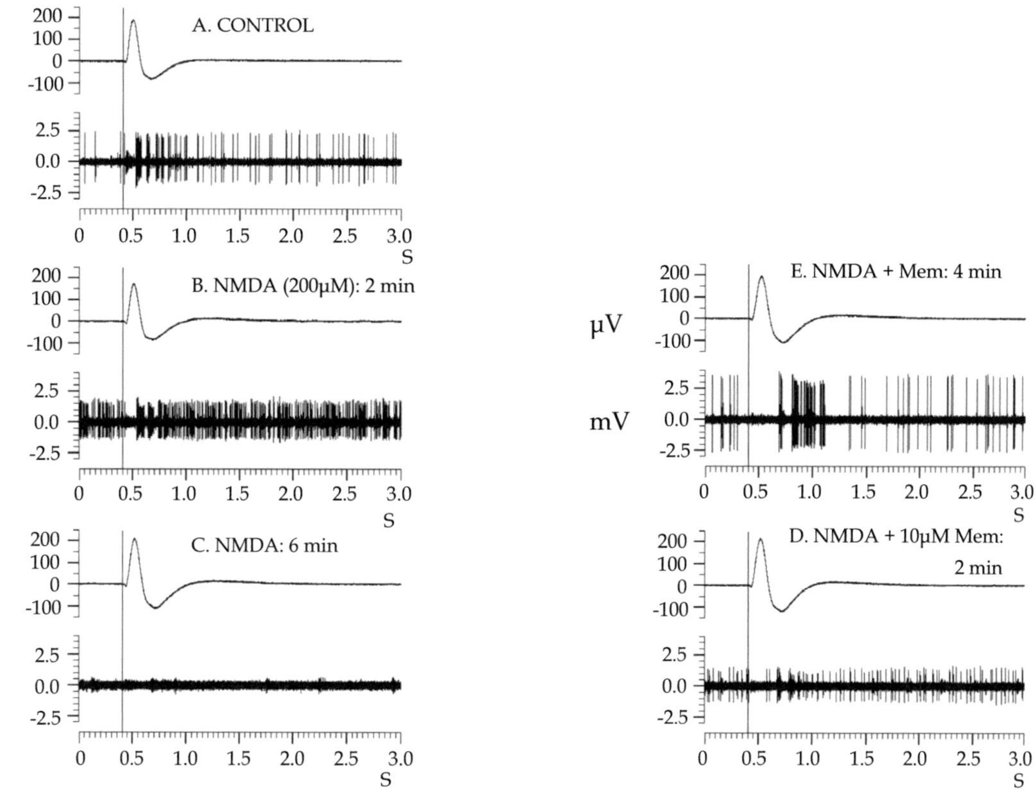


Fig. 3. Exogenous application of NMDA results in excitotoxicity in an OFF RGC that is reversed by co-application of memantine, an uncompetitive NMDA open-channel blocker. In all panels: top trace = ERG, bottom trace = single-unit RGC spikes. 10 msec duration stimulus flash onset at 400 msec (vertical line). ERG = microvolts. RGC = millivolts. (From Hare & Wheeler 2009)

Memantine is an "open channel blocker" of the NMDA channel pore (Pelligrini et al., 1992; Chen & Lipton, 1997). In order for memantine to access its binding site within the pore, the channel must be in the open configuration following binding of glutamate (or NMDA) and magnesium must unbind from its site within the pore (see Figure 1). These properties of memantine binding make it more effective to block very high (pathological) levels of NMDA receptor activity while having a lesser effect on lower (normal) levels of activity. Figure 4 summarizes results which show that application of NMDA to a different OFF RGC has a similar effect to increase tonic RGC spiking frequency and to reduce spike amplitude. In this case, NMDA-induced excitotoxic RGC activity was reversed completely by co-application of 30 μM AP5 (2-amino-5-phosphonovaleric acid). Unlike memantine, AP5 competes with glutamate (or NMDA) for its binding site on the NMDA receptor to block channel opening.

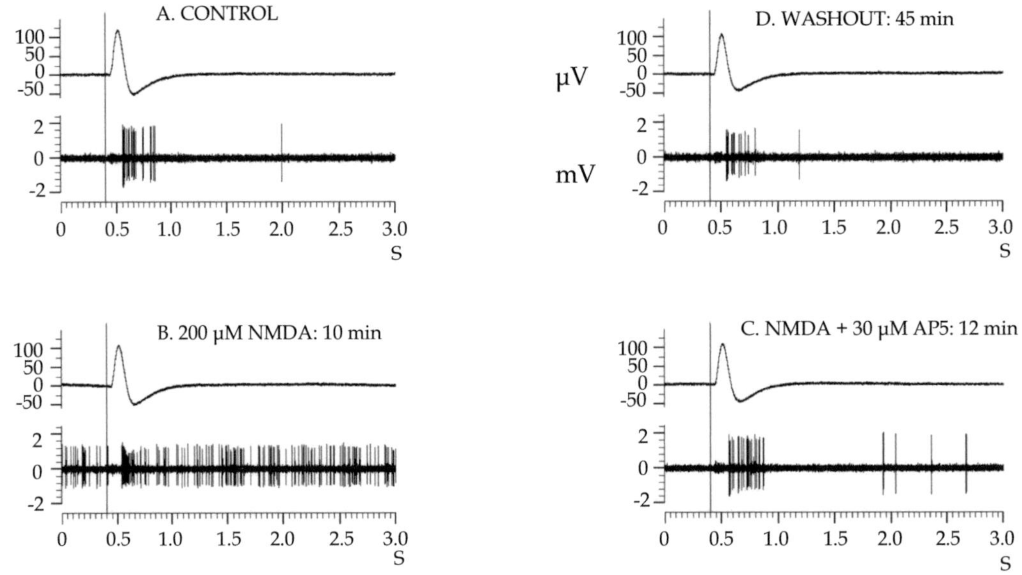


Fig. 4. NMDA-induced excitotoxicity in an OFF RGC is completely reversed by co-application of AP5, a competitive NMDA receptor antagonist. (From Hare & Wheeler, 2009)

Exogenous application of NMDA mimics the pathological condition where excessive release of glutamate into the extracellular space results in excitotoxic activity of NMDA receptors. Increased release of glutamate into the extracellular space has been reported in various models for experimental insults to CNS tissue including retina (Louzada-Junior et al., 1992; Neal et al., 1994; Kowluru et al., 2001; Nucci et al., 2005). RGCs are much less sensitive to exogenously applied glutamate since CNS tissue expresses high levels of glutamate transporters that, under normal conditions, provide for very tight regulation of extracellular glutamate levels. These transporters work to prevent exogenously applied glutamate from reaching increased levels at the post-synaptic membrane receptors. RGCs are much more sensitive to exogenously applied NMDA since it is not transported by these intrinsic glutamate buffer mechanisms. Under pathological conditions, failure of these glutamate transporters would be expected to contribute to elevations in extracellular glutamate that could drive excitotoxic RGC injury. For this reason, a different series of experiments used exogenous application of TBOA (DL-threo-β-benzyloxyaspartic acid) to block selectively retinal glutamate transporters (Izumi et al., 2002). Figure 5 shows that application of 50 μM TBOA was associated with a rapid increase in tonic spiking of this OFF RGC and reduction of spike amplitude (panel B) followed by complete block of RGC spike generation (panel C). As was seen for reversal of NMDA-induced excitotoxicity, co-application of memantine produced a rapid recovery of both spike amplitude and tonic spike frequency toward control levels (panel D). Memantine washout in the presence of continuous application of TBOA was associated with the reappearance of excitotoxic RGC spiking activity (panel E).

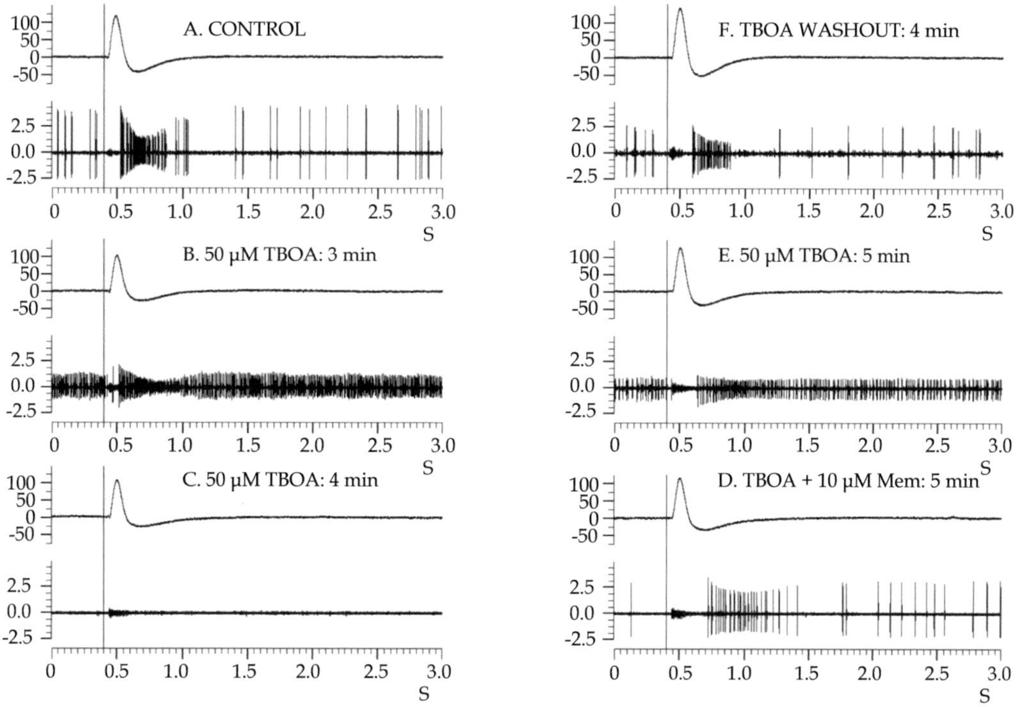


Fig. 5. For this OFF RGC, block of retinal glutamate transporters with TBOA results in excitotoxic activity that can be reversed by co-application of memantine. (From Hare & Wheeler, 2009)

Membrane depolarization resulting from cellular energy failure or other causes is thought to play an important role in excitotoxic neuronal injury. Membrane depolarization is associated with decreased binding of magnesium at its blocking site within the NMDA channel pore (see Fig. 1). For this reason, when RGCs become chronically depolarized, excitotoxic levels of NMDA channel activity can occur even in the presence of otherwise "normal" levels of extrtacellular glutamate (Zeevalk & Nicklas, 1992). The loss of voltage-dependent magnesium block can be experimentally approximated by perfusion with magnesium-free solution. The results for the ON RGC summarized in Figure 6 show that the switch to zero magnesium solution was followed by an increased rate of spiking activity and reduction of spike amplitude (panel C). This excitotoxic response is similar to that seen following perfusion with either NMDA (see Fig. 3) or TBOA (see4 Fig. 5) and was also reversed by co-application of memantine (panel D). However, the decrease in spike amplitude (spike generation failure) seen in zero magnesium typically developed more slowly than spike generation loss resulting from either NMDA or TBOA.

### 2.2 Regulation of NMDA receptor function in RGCs

We have seen how the level of NMDA receptor activity in RGCs depends upon the amount of glutamate released from pre-synaptic neurons, the removal of glutamate from the extracellular space by glutamate transporters, and the degree of voltage-dependent magnesium block set by the RGC membrane potential. It has also been shown recently that activation of alpha-2 adrenergic receptors reduces NMDA-induced responses in RGCs. This

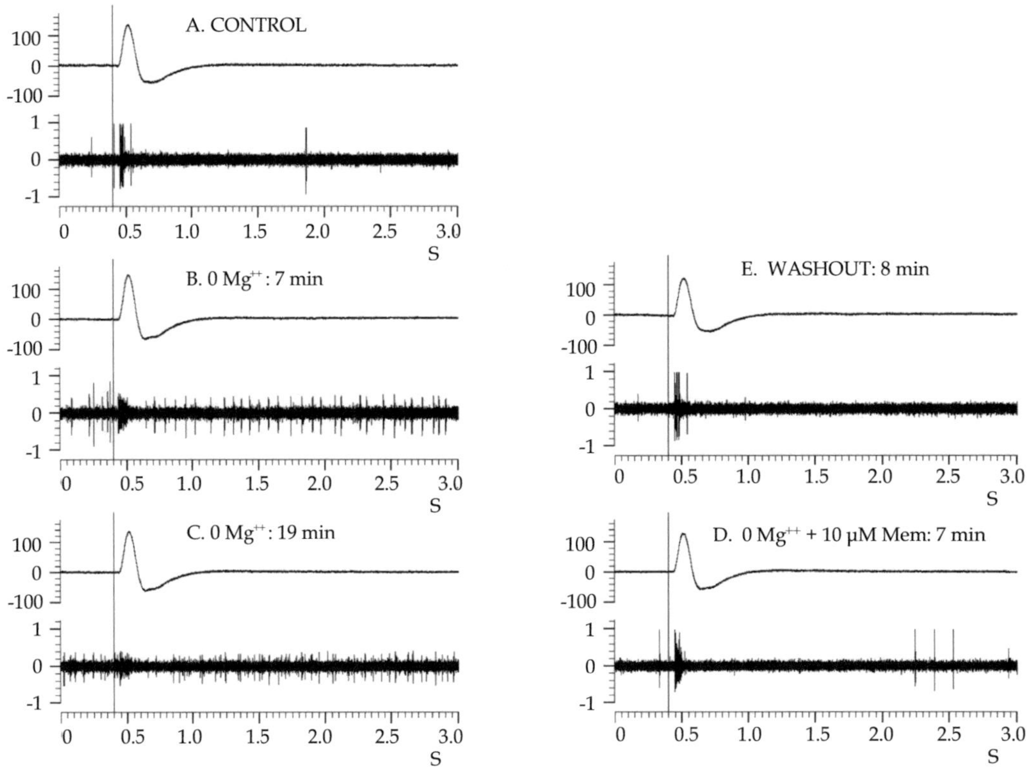


Fig. 6. Perfusion with zero magnesium results, for this ON RGC, in excitotocic activity that resembles that seen following application of either NMDA or TBOA and is also reversed by co-application of memantine. (From Hare & Wheeler, 2009)

finding results from studies using simultaneous recordings of the membrane current and cytoplasmic calcium concentration changes induced by application of NMDA. For these experiments, whole-cell current recordings were made from RGCs in a flat-mounted, perfused, ex-vivo rat retina preparation as illustrated schematically in Figure 7. For these recordings, the RGC membrane is voltage-clamped at -70 mV, close to the normal "resting" level. The recording pipette contained the calcium indicator Fluo-4 which was passively loaded into the RGC cytoplasm through diffusion. Activation of NMDA receptors was effected using local delivery of NMDA. RGC membrane current was measured using conventional voltage-clamp methods while cytoplasmic calcium measures were acquired with a spinning disk confocal fluorescence imaging system.

Results from one experiment are summarized in Figure 8 where the top panel traces represent recordings of RGC membrane current responses to local NMDA application (heavy black horizontal bar) and the bottom panel traces represent changes in cytoplasmic calcium concentration to the same NMDA applications. Note that under control conditions (red traces), NMDA induces an inward current representing an influx of sodium and calcium cations while this inward calcium flux produces an increase in cytoplasmic calcium. Continuous bath application of 10 µM memantine is associated with a severe reduction in NMDA-induced membrane current and cytoplasmic calcium signal (green traces). This effect of memantine is rapidly reversed following washout (blue traces).

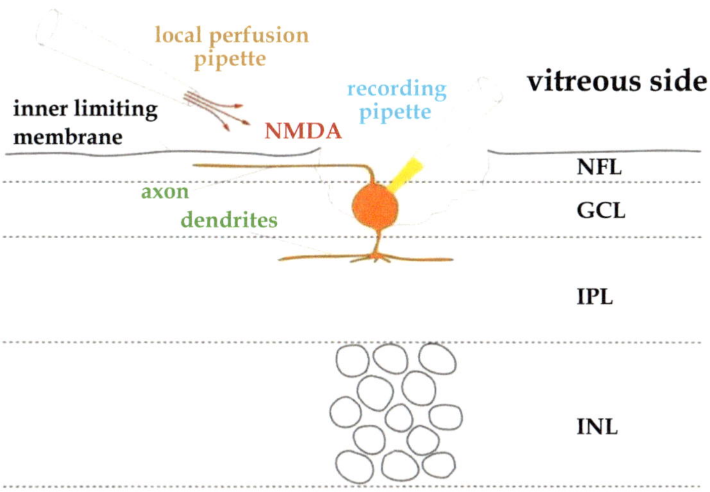


Fig. 7. Simultaneous measures of membrane current and cytoplasmic calcium level in a single RGC in the flat-mounted, perfused, ex-vivo rat retina. NFL (nerve fiber layer), GCL (ganglion cell layer), IPL (inner plexiform layer), INL (inner nuclear layer)

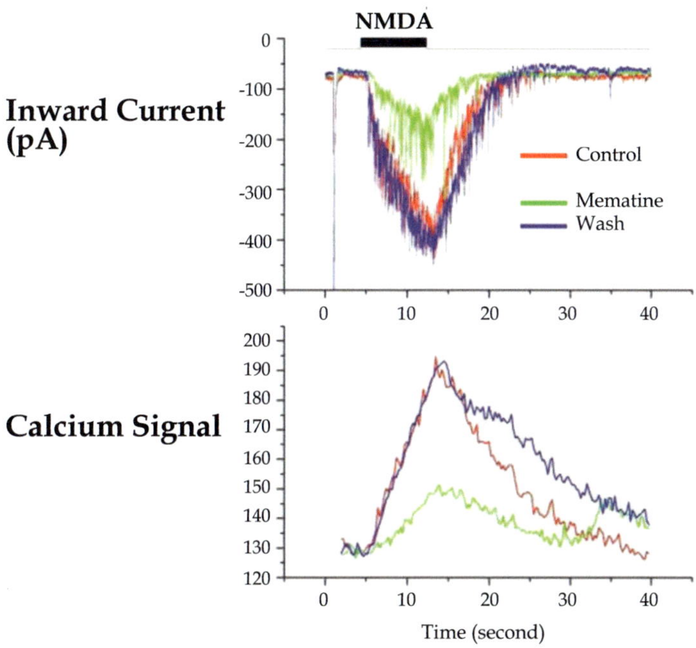


Fig. 8. NMDA-induced membrane current (upper panel) and cytoplasmic calcium signal (lower panel) in a single RGC are reduced by bath application of memantine

Recordings from a different RGC are summarized in Figure 9. The traces in panel A show that bath application of 3 μM brimonidine, a selective alpha-2 adrenergic receptor agonist, is associated with a reduction of both the NMDA-induced current and calcium signals by approximately 40% and 50%, respectively. The summary results plotted in panel C show that this effect of brimonidine to reduce NMDA-induced current and calcium signals is blocked by co-application of 15 μM atipamezole (a selective alpha-2 receptor antagonist) or by intracellular loading (via the patch pipette) of GDPβS, a G-protein inhibitor. These findings are consistent with the notion that alpha-2 receptor activation, through Gαi - mediated coupling, leads to inhibition of adenyl cylase and a consequent decline in cytoplasmic levels of cyclic AMP. In other experiments, intracellular application of Sp-cAMPS, a hydrolysis-resistant analog of cAMP, was also shown to block the effect of brimonidine to decrease NMDA-induced current and calcium signals (data not shown). Further confirmation that activation of alpha-2 receptors leads to a down regulation of NMDA receptor activity by reducing intracellular levels of cAMP is provided by results summarized in Figure 10. Intracellular application of either rolipram, a selective PDE4 inhibitor, or forskolin, an activator of adenyl cyclase, resulted in a block of the brimonidine effect.

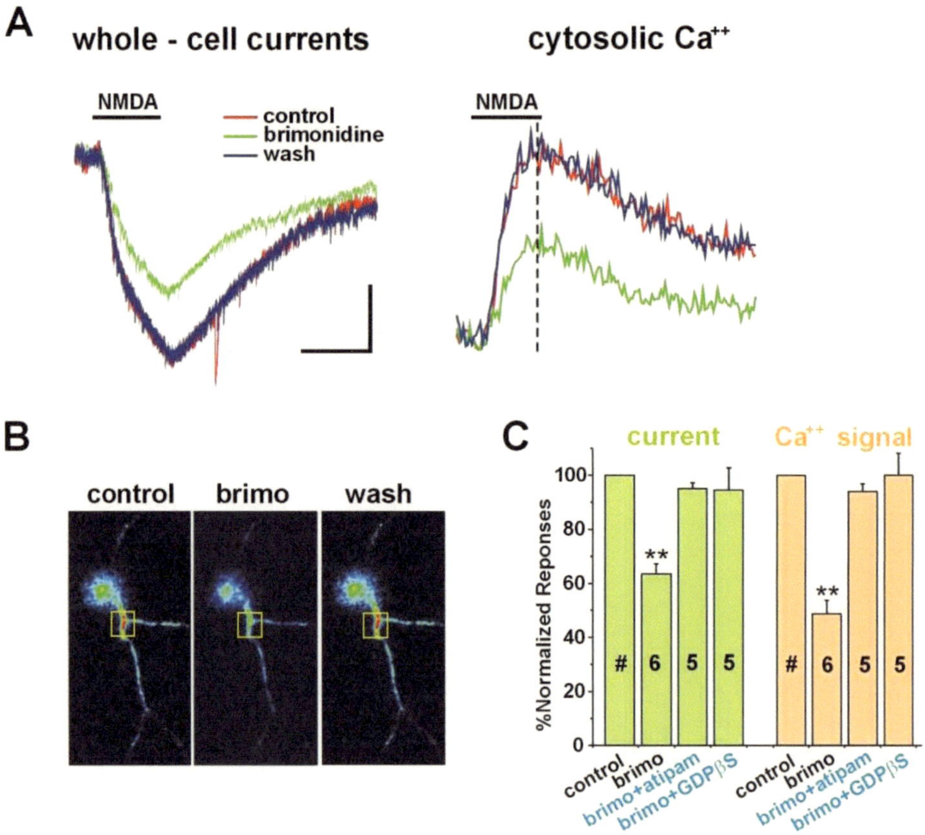


Fig. 9. Bath application of brimonidine reduces the magnitude of NMDA-induced current and calcium responses in RGCs. This effect is blocked by either an alpha-2 receptor antagonist (atipamezole; bath application) or G protein inhibitor (GDPβS; intracellular application). The yellow windows in panel B indicate RGC region used for calcium measures. (From Dong et al., 2008)

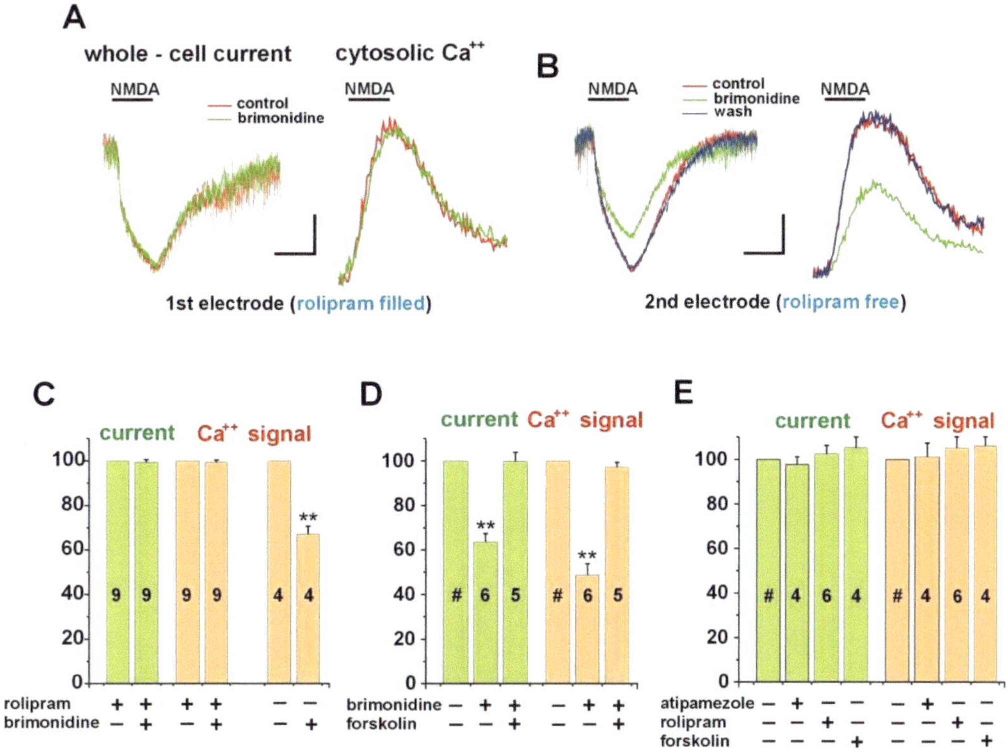


Fig. 10. Intracellular application of either rolipram (PDE4 inhibitor) or forskolin (adenyl cyclase activator) results in block of the brimonidine effect on NMDA-induced current or calcium responses in RGCs. (From Dong et al., 2008)

Results from recordings of NMDA-induced RGC responses in an ex-vivo rat retina thus show that NMDA channel function and, by extension, intracellular calcium concentration are regulated by apha-2 adrenergic receptors through Gαi-coupled inhibition of adenyl cyclase. Brimonidine treatment has been shown to prevent damage in a wide range of animal models for RGC injury including experimental glaucoma (WoldeMussie et al., 2001; Kim et al., 2007), acute retinal ischemia (Donello et al., 2001; Lafuente et al., 2002; Lai et al., 2002), optic nerve mechanical injury (Yoles et al., 1999; Ma et al., 2009), and NMDA-induced retinal excitotoxicity (Metoki et al., 2005; Dong et al., 2008); all models in which NMDA receptors have been shown to play a significant role in driving RGC injury. Two of these, a rat model for experimental glaucoma and a rabbit model for intravitreal injection of NMDA, were used to demonstrate that the protective effects of brimonidine treatment result from alpha-2 receptor mediated inhibition of adenyl cyclase activity.

Figure 11 shows that, for the rat glaucoma model used in this study, laser photocoagulation of the perilimbal vessels and episceral veins was followed, on average, by an increase in intraocular pressure (IOP) from a control level of approximately 15 mm Hg to approximately 30 mm Hg. RGC survival was quantified, at approximately 2 weeks following IOP elevation, by flat-mounting the retina and counting RGCs at 24 locations in the central and peripheral retina (panel A). RGCs were labeled using retrograde transport of rhodamine-conjugated dextran delivered directly to the retrobulbar optic nerve (panel B).

Untreated (control) glaucoma eyes lost, on average, approximately 30 % of their RGCs (panel C). Continuous dosing, using subcutaneous osmotic pumps, with either memantine (3 mg/kg/day) or brimonidine (0.18 mg/kg/day) resulted in a reduction of RGC loss to less than 10%. This protective effect of brimonidine was blocked by co-administration of either the selective PDE4 inhibitor, rolipram (0.6 mg/kg/day), or the selective alpha-2 receptor antagonist, atipamezole (0.9 mg/kg/day). None of these systemically delivered test agents had any significant effect on IOP in the laser treated eye (panel E).

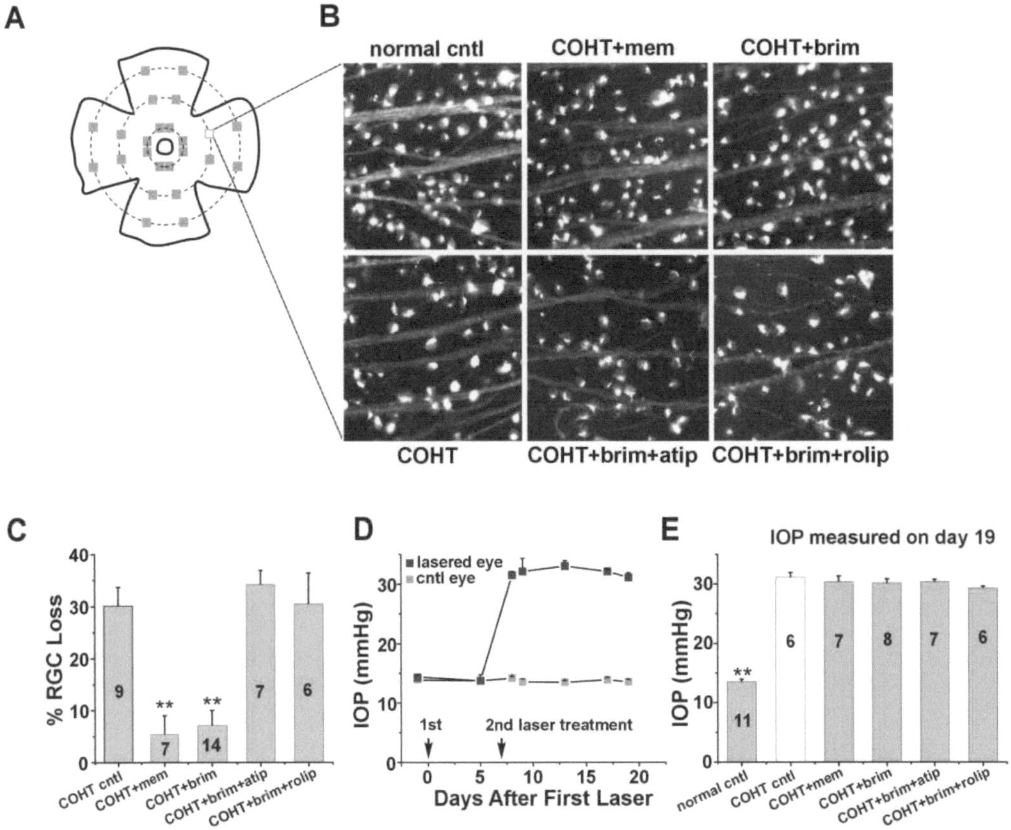


Fig. 11. Treatment with either memantine or brimonidine is associated with a reduction in the level of RGC loss in a rat model of experimental glaucoma. The protective effect of brimonidine treatment is blocked by co-administration of either an alpha-2 receptor antagonist (atipamezole) or an inhibitor of PDE4 (rolipram). (From Dong et al., 2008)

Intravitreal injection of NMDA is known to be toxic to RGCs and provides a model of RGC injury that has, as its primary insult, the overactivity of NMDA receptors. As shown in Figure 12, RGC injury following injection of NMDA into the rabbit eye was quantified by counting DAPI-labeled cells in the RGC layer. RGC layer cells (RGCs & displaced amacrine cells) were counted in a 5x5 sampling array whose superior row included the visual streak (region of highest RGC density; panelA). Intravitreal injection of 50 μL saline solution containing 3.6 micromoles of NMDA resulted in the loss, at two weeks following NMDA injection, of approximately 40 % of DAPI-labeled cells in the RGC layer (panel D). Co-injection of two different NMDA channel blockers, either MK-801 (0.12 micromoles) or memantine ( 0.36 micromoles), reduced loss to either approximately 0% or approximately 10%, respectively. Co-injection of brimonidine (3.6 nanomoles) also reduced NMDA-induced RGC loss to approximately 20% and this protection was blocked by co-injection of the combination of either brimonidine + atipamezole (24.0 nanomoles) or brimonidine + rolipram (12-120 nanomoles). While total RGC counts are plotted in panel D, averaged counts for each of the 25 sample regions from a representative animal are plotted in panel C for each treatment group.

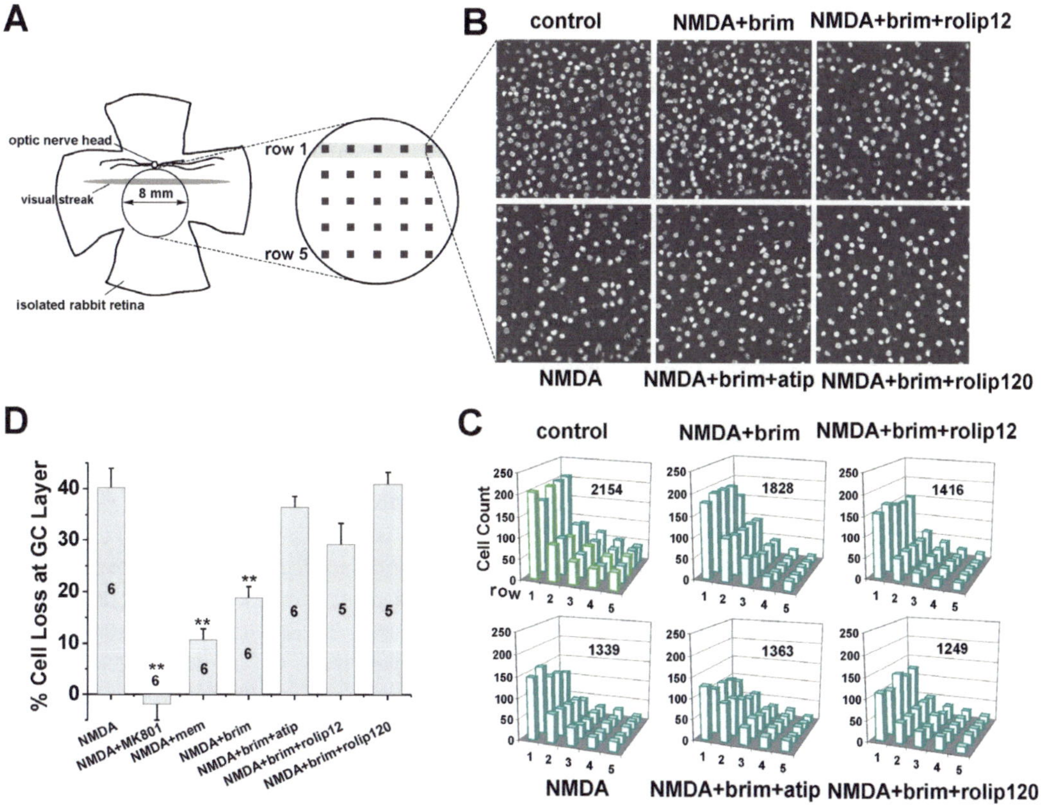


Fig. 12. Intravitreal injection of NMDA results in excitotoxic RGC loss that can be prevented or reduced with co-injection of either an NMDA channel blocker (MK-801 or memantine) or an alpha-2 receptor agonist (brimonidine). The protective effect of brimonidine is, in turn, blocked by co-injection of brimonidine in combination with a selective alpha-2 receptor antagonist (atipamezole) or by co-injection of brimonidine in combination with a PDE4 inhibitor (rolipram). (From Dong et al., 2008)

These results show clearly that RGC injury in both the rat model for experimental glaucoma and the rabbit model for NMDA-induced excitotoxicity is driven predominantly by overactivity in NMDA-type glutamate-gated channels. Treatment with either MK-801 or memantine reduces RGC injury by blocking directly the conductance pore of the NMDA channels, thereby reducing NMDA-induced increases in sodium and calcium ions. Brimonidine treatment reduces NMDA channel activity indirectly through a mechanism that includes alpha-2 receptor activation, inhibition of adenyl cyclase, and decreased levels of intracellular cAMP. Pharmacological agents that act to block brimonidine-elicited decreases in cytoplasmic cAMP also block brimonidine's action to decrease NMDA-induced currents and calcium signals in RGCs. These same agents block the protective effects of brimonidine treatment in animal models of RGC injury known to be driven predominantly by overactivity in NMDA channels.

## 3. Excitotoxicity and voltage-gated sodium channels

Visual signals are transmitted from the retina to more central visual pathways via the RGC axons. Signal transmission is coded as a temporal pattern of "spikes" or "action potentials"; each spike consisting of a regenerative depolarizing (inward) membrane current that typically travels from its generation site at the RGC soma (axon hillock) to the axon terminal in the brainstem. Axon spikes reflect the activity of voltage-gated sodium channels. At high negative resting potentials (inside negative trans-membrane voltage), these sodium channels are closed. Decreasing the membrane voltage (depolarization = decreased inside negative) activates the channels and allows sodium ions to flow down their electrochemical gradient from the extracellular space into the axonal cytoplasm. This influx of sodium ions represents an inward current that spreads passively to depolarize and activate sodium channels in the immediately neighboring (resting) axonal membrane. In this manner, local inward current, generated by voltage-gated sodium channels, propagates along the axon in a regenerative fashion and transmits a wave of membrane depolarization to the axon terminal. Good temporal bandwidth for information transfer requires that these individual spike events be of very short duration. For this reason, following activation by membrane depolarization, voltage-gated sodium channels typically inactivate rapidly in a time-dependent fashion in order to move axonal membrane voltage back toward the resting level. That is, sodium channels are activated by membrane depolarization but rapidly inactivate, even in the presence of continued membrane depolarization. This property of the sodium channels is responsible for the fact that spikes are able to travel only in one direction: away from immediately active membrane and toward membrane that is "at rest". Membrane depolarization not only activates sodium channels but also inactivates them and the channels remain inactivated until membrane potential is returned toward the resting level.

Action potential generation is thus dependent upon both the sodium gradient as well as membrane voltage. The resting transmembrane sodium gradient (intracellular concentration = low, extracellular concentration = high) is generated by energy-dependent pumps that move sodium from the cytoplasm to the extracellular space. The same pumps contribute to both the electrical and chemical transmembrane gradient for sodium ions. The transmembrane sodium gradient provides an electrochemical energy source that is used by a wide range of membrane transporters including the sodium/calcium exchanger (SCE). The SCE uses energy available from sodium ions moving down their electrochemical gradient to transport calcium ions from the cytoplasm to the extracellular space; against both the electrical (inside negative) and chemical (calcium inside is low) gradient for calcium ions. Calcium is an important regulator of many intracellular signaling pathways and its cytoplasmic concentration is very tightly regulated at levels typically lower than a resting level of 200 nM (Connor & Tseng, 1988; Kirischuk et al., 1992). Even small prolonged elevations above this level can result in irreversible injury to RGCs. Any condition resulting in a loss of the electrochemical gradient for sodium ions will also be associated with, among other things, depolarization of the axonal membrane and increases in the cytoplasmic concentration of calcium ions.

Although the mechanisms for glaucomatous RGC injury are not known, evidence suggests that a primary insult to RGC axons at or near the optic nerve head may be a significant contributor to glaucomatous vision loss (Quigley et al., 1981; Johansson, 1986). It has been proposed that IOP can generate mechanical forces at or near the lamina cribrosa resulting in direct injury to RGC axons. These same IOP-induced stresses will compromise local vascular perfusion of the tissue resulting indirectly in ischemic insult of RGC axons (Burgoyne & Downs, 2008). Mechanisms for ischemic injury to RGC axons have been explored using an isolated perfused rat optic nerve preparation in combination with methods for induction of experimental ischemia. For these studies, optic nerves were isolated (from eye to chiasm) from adult rats and mounted in a perfusion chamber between two suction electrodes as shown in Figure 13. Nerves were maintained at 37$^0$ C and perfused with bicarbonate buffered ringer saturated with 95% $O_2$ and 5% $CO_2$. At one end of the nerve, a constant voltage pulse of 50 µsec duration was used to drive depolarizing current through the tissue to bath ground. This current, if strong enough to reach threshold depolarization for axonal membrane sodium channels, initiates in each axon a spike that travels to the opposite end where it can be measured as a voltage. Since each axon can generate only a single spike in response to the brief stimulus pulse, the resulting composite voltage signal represents the temporal sum of all such single spikes generated in all activated axons. This composite response is therefore referred to as the compound action potential (CAP).

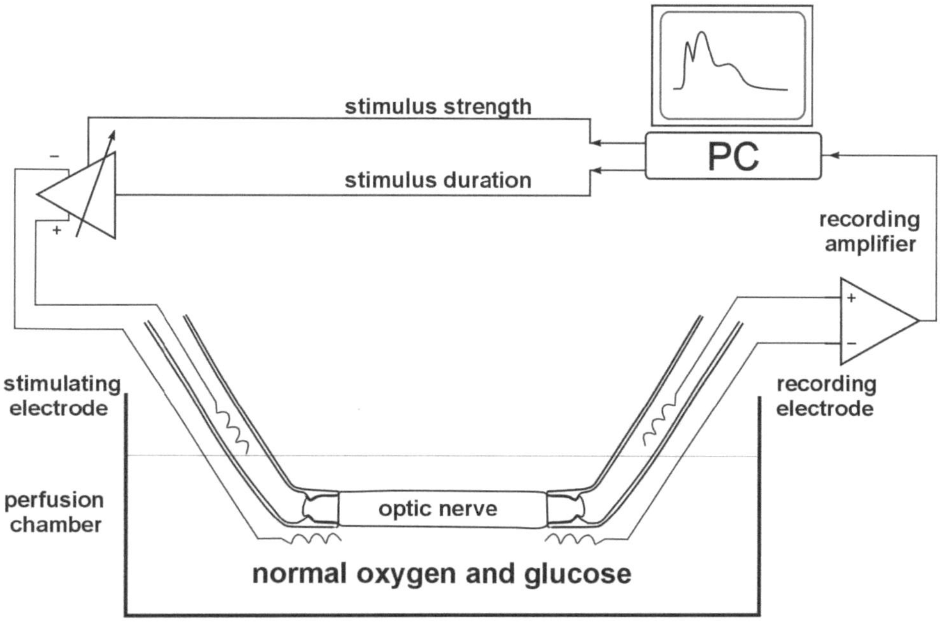


Fig. 13. Recording of the compound action potential (CAP) from the isolated rat optic nerve. (From Dong & Hare 2005)

The two panels in Figure 14 illustrate how the CAP varies with stimulus intensity. The family of traces in panel A shows how the CAP response increases in magnitude with increasing stimulus voltage. That is, increasing stimulus intensity is associated with an increasing number of activated axons. The CAP waveform also clearly represents three functionally distinct axonal populations having different conduction velocities. Although, for these short conduction lengths, there is considerable temporal overlap of the three spike populations, it can be seen that the fastest spikes (large neurons, large axons) have the lowest stimulus voltage activation threshold while the slowest spikes (small RGCs, small axons) have the highest threshold. Due to the temporal overlap of spikes from the three different groups of axons, integrated CAP response area was measured instead of peak amplitude as indicated in panel B. Panel B also shows that CAP amplitude (area) saturated at a stimulus intensity of approximately 150 volts which was used for all subsequent experiments since this intensity is expected to activate all functional axons.

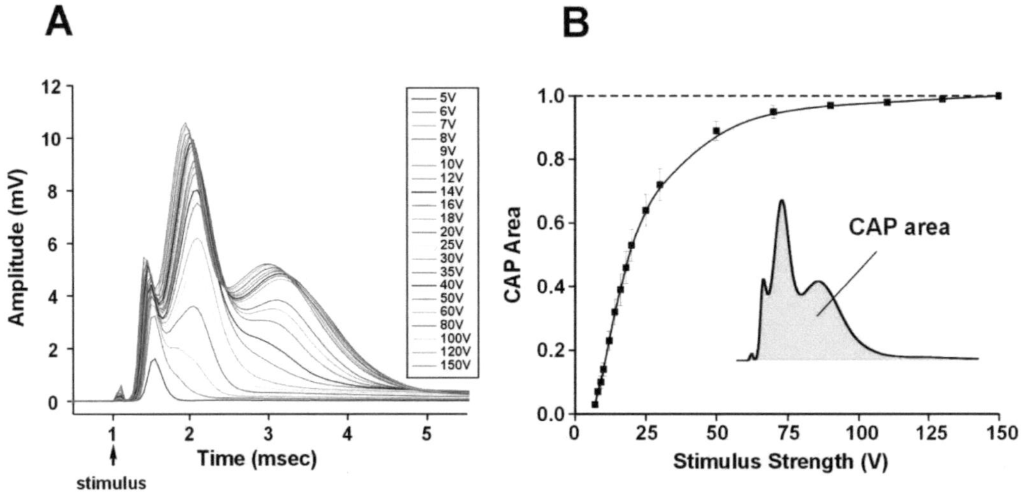


Fig. 14. CAP response as a function of stimulus intensity (voltage). Response amplitude is measured as the area of the CAP response. (From Dong & Hare, 2005)

Experimental ischemia was induced by switching to a perfusion medium which was saturated with nitrogen instead of oxygen and from which glucose was omitted (oxygen-glucose deprivation; OGD). Figure 15 shows that, following the switch to OGD, CAP amplitude declined rapidly and was almost completely blocked after 60 minutes of OGD. The switch back to control saline was associated with a partial recovery of the CAP response. This recovery was typically stable by 20 minutes following OGD washout. Responses obtained prior to OGD (1), at the end of 60 minutes OGD (2), and at 60 minutes following switch back to control saline (3), are illustrated in panel B. The inset in panel A also shows how CAP amplitude following recovery from OGD is dependent upon the duration of OGD. A standard OGD duration of 60 minutes was used for the experiments described here.

Experimental ischemia (OGD) of 60 minutes duration is associated with approximately a 70% irreversible loss of axonal function resulting from a failure of the membrane machinery responsible for spike generation and propagation. This injury results, in turn, from loss of the transmembrane sodium gradient and the subsequent elevation of intracellular calcium. According to this model, axonal energy failure leads to loss of energy-dependent sodium extrusion with consequent loss of the trans-membrane sodium gradient and resting membrane potential. Under these conditions, axonal sodium gradient and membrane voltage are further reduced due to influx of sodium ions through voltage-gated sodium channels. Although most membrane sodium channels are inactivated by membrane depolarization, a subset of these channels remains open and contributes to loss of the sodium gradient (Stys et al., 1993; Hammarstrom & Gage, 2002). Since intracellular calcium is normally regulated at very low intracellular levels by the action of a calcium extrusion mechanism (sodium/calcium exchanger), the loss of the membrane sodium gradient results in elevation of intracellular calcium and activation of calcium-dependent mechanisms for axonal injury (Stys et al., 1992; Garthwaite et al., 1999).

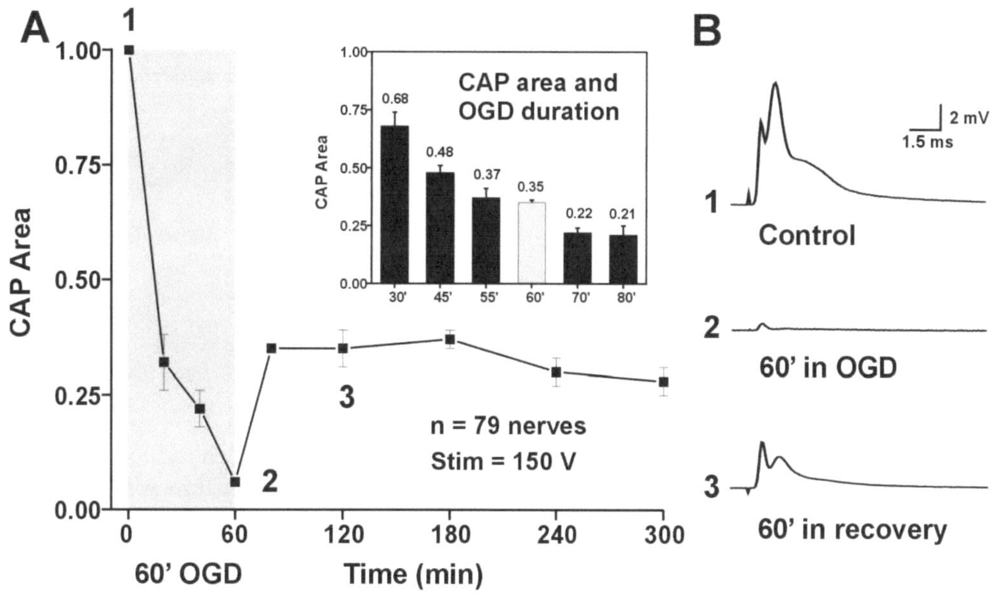


Fig. 15. OGD of 60 minutes duration is associated with irreversible loss of function in isolated rat optic nerve. (From Dong & Hare, 2005)

The dependence of OGD-induced axonal injury on the influx of sodium ions through non-inactivating voltage-gated sodium channels is illustrated by results summarized in Figure 16. Results from the control experiments of Figure 15 are re-plotted as the filled black squares in panel A. Nerves exposed to bath application of 1 mM lidocaine (open squares), a sodium channel blocker, for 20 minutes prior to OGD as well as during the 60 minute exposure to OGD, recovered a greater level of function (CAP area) than untreated nerves. Inspection of panel A shows that pre-treatment with lidocaine is associated with complete block of the CAP by the onset of OGD. At the end of OGD, lidocaine must wash out before any protective effect can be measured. These results show clearly that OGD-induced axonal injury is mediated, at least in part, by sodium influx via voltage-gated sodium channels. This was further tested in experiments where the nerves were perfused with sodium-free medium for 20 minutes prior to and during OGD as summarized in Figure 17. The open squares plotted in panel A show that removal of sodium ions from the extracellular space reduces axonal functional loss associated with OGD; supporting the notion that injury depends significantly on the net flux of sodium ions from the extracellular space to the axonal cytoplasm.

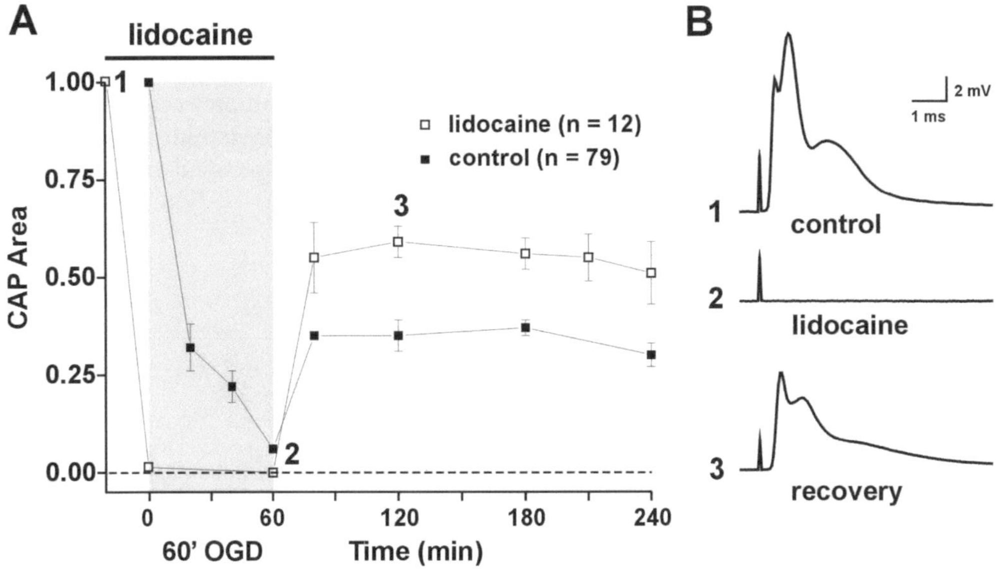


Fig. 16. Blockade of voltage-gated sodium channels with bath application of 1 mM lidocaine (for 20 minutes preceding OGD and during OGD) reduces OGD-induced axonal injury. (From Dong & Hare, 2005)

Removal of calcium from the perfusion medium is also associated with a reduction of OGD-induced axonal injury. Figure 18 shows that perfusion with zero-calcium medium for 20 minutes before as well as during OGD resulted in a reduction of OGD-induced axonal injury. Results from experiments using either a sodium channel blocker (lidocaine; Figure 16), zero sodium medium (Figure 17), or zero calcium medium (Figure 18) are summarized for comparison in Figure 19. Prevention of sodium overload is clearly associated with reduced OGD-induced axonal injury. The fact that perfusion with zero calcium medium, in the presence of normal extracellular sodium levels and functioning voltage-gated sodium channels, is able to reduce axonal injury suggests that increased intracellular calcium is the major driver of injury and that intracellular sodium overload leads to injury, in large part, by reducing extrusion of axonal calcium by the sodium/calcium exchanger. In fact, if the sodium gradient and membrane potential are decreased sufficiently, the exchanger can run in reverse mode to actually transport calcium into the cell and further accelerate increases in intracellular calcium.

These experiments show how intracellular sodium overload, by reducing calcium extrusion via the sodium/calcium exchanger, leads to injury of RGC axons indirectly through the elevation of intracellular calcium. Of course, sodium overload may also contribute to axonal injury resulting from loss of function in other sodium-dependent membrane transporters that, in addition to the sodium/calcium exchanger, are also necessary for axonal function/survival. For this model of acute experimental ischemic insult axonal injury is driven predominantly by failure of membrane calcium transport. Voltage gated sodium channels are also found in somato-dendritic RGC membrane where the sodium/calcium

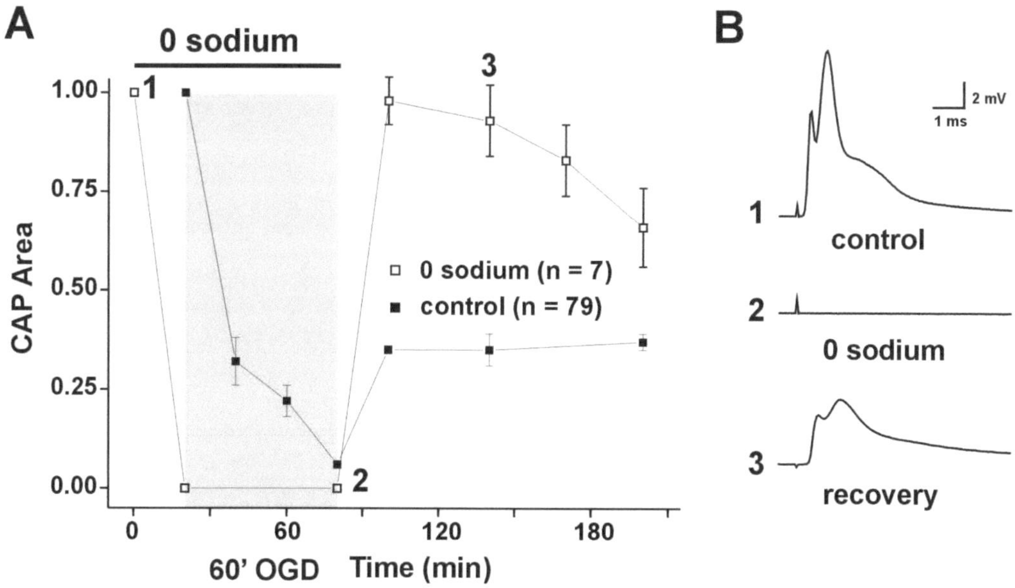


Fig. 17. Removal of sodium ions from the extracellular space (perfusion with zero sodium medium), both prior to and during OGD, reduces OGD-induced axonal injury. For zero sodium medium, sodium chloride was replaced with lithium chloride and sodium bicarbonate was replaced with choline bicarbonate. (From Dong & Hare, 2005)

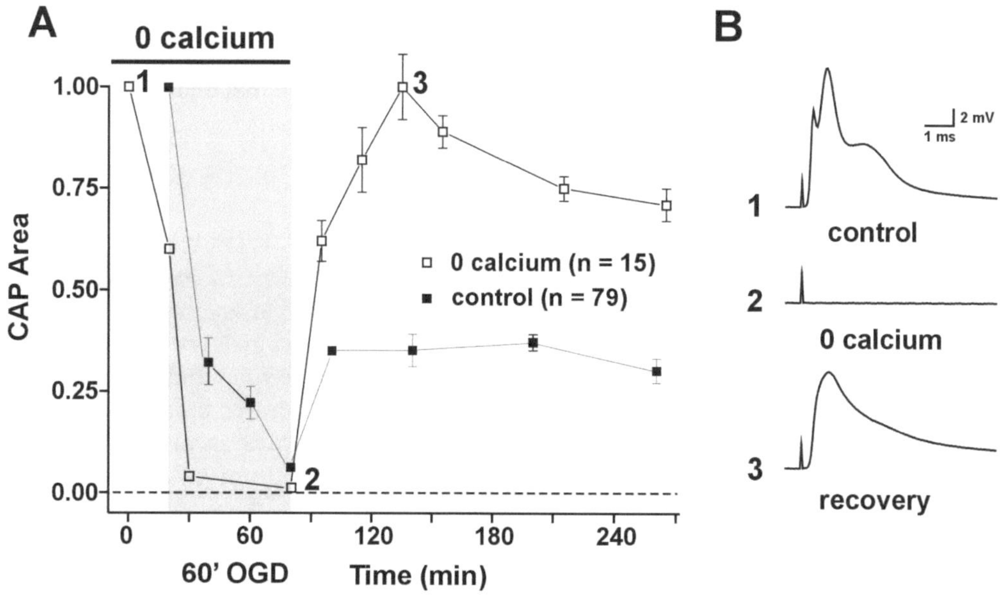


Fig. 18. Perfusion with zero-calcium medium is associated with a reduction of OGD-induced axonal injury. Calcium was omitted from the medium and replaced with 5 mM EGTA (calcium buffer). (From Dong & Hare, 2005)

exchanger is also an important mechanism for regulation of intracellular calcium at low levels. However, models of injury to the somato-dendritic compartment are complicated by the fact that glutamate-gated channels and voltage-gated calcium channels provide additional sources for entry of sodium and calcium ions that also contribute to RGC injury.

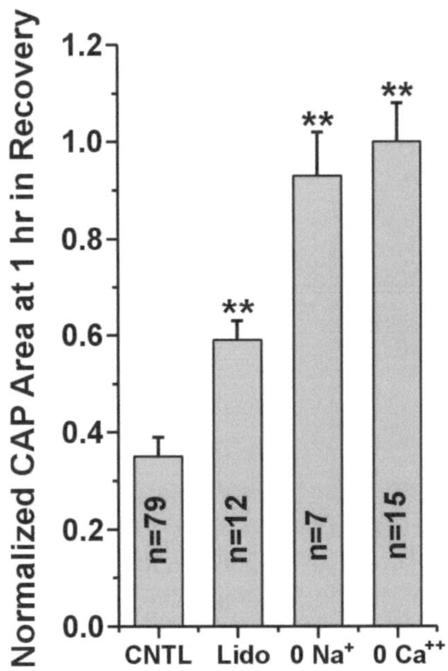


Fig. 19. Summary of results for experiments showing that blockade of sodium channels (Lido), perfusion with zero-sodium medium (0 $Na^+$), or perfusion with zero-calcium medium (0 $Ca^{++}$) is associated with a reduction in OGD-induced axonal injury. (From Dong & Hare, 2005)

## 4. Conclusion

Although the precise mechanism for glaucomatous injury to RGCs is not known, glutamate-gated ion channels and voltage-gated sodium channels are known to contribute to RGC injury resulting from a wide range of insults in both in-vitro and animal models including experimental glaucoma. Under "normal" conditions, these channels participate in the transmission of excitatory signals between neurons in the retina and central visual pathways. Under pathological conditions, overactivity of these same channels may result in elevation of intracellular sodium concentration, loss of the electrochemical transmembrane gradient for sodium ions, decreased calcium extrusion via the sodium/calcium exchanger, elevation of intracellular calcium, and activation of calcium dependent intracellular mechanisms for RGC injury.

## 5. Acknowledgement

The authors acknowledge the participation of Yuanxing Guo and Peter Agey in much of the work presented in this chapter.

## 6. References

Aizenman, E., Frosch, MP. & Lipton, SA. (1988) Responses mediated by excitatory amino acid receptors in solitary retinal ganglion cells, *Journal of Physiology* Vol.(396):75-91.

Burgoyne, CF. & Downs, JC. (2008) Premise and prediction-how optic nerve head biomechanics underlies the susceptibility and clinical behavior of the aged optic nerve head, *Journal of Glaucoma* Vol. (17):318-328.

Chen, HS., Pellegrini, JW.,Aggarwal, SK., Lei, SZ., Warach, S., Jensen, FE. & Lipton, SA. (1992) Open-channel block of N-methyl-D-aspartate (NMDA) responses by memantine: therapeutic advantage against NMDA receptor-mediated neurotoxicity, *Journal of Neuroscience* Vol.(12):4427-4436.

Chen, HS. & Lipton, SA. (1997) Mechanism of memantine block of NMDA-activated channels in rat retinal ganglion cells: uncompetitive antagonism, *Journal of Physiology* Vol.(499):27-46.

Choi, DW. (1988) Glutamate neurotoxicity and diseases of the nervous system, *Neuron* Vol.(1):623-634.

Connor, JA. & Tseng, HY. (1988) Measurement of intracellular $Ca^{++}$ in cerebellar purkinje neurons in culture: Resting distribution and response to glutamate, *Brain Research Bulletin* Vol.(21):353-361.

Craner, MJ., Lo, AC., Black, JA. & Waxman, SG. (2003) Abnormal sodium channel distribution in optic nerve axons in a model of inflammatory demyelination, *Brain* Vol.(126):1552-1561.

Diamond, JS. & Copenhagen, DR. (1993) The contribution of NMDA and non-NMDA receptors to the light-evoked input-output chacteristics of retinal ganglion cells, *Neuron* Vol.(11):725-738.

Donello, JE., Padillo, EU., Webster, ML., Wheeler, LA. & Gil, DW. (2001) alpha(2)-adrenergic agonists inhibit vitreal glutamate and aspartate accumulation and preserve retinal function after transient ischemia, *Journal of Pharmacology and Experimental Therapeutics* Vol.(296):216-223.

Dong, CJ. & Hare, WA. (2005) Contribution to ischemic injury of rat optic nerves by intracellular sodium overload, *Documenta Ophthalmologica* Vol.(110):15-23.

Dong, CJ., Guo, Y., Agey, P., Wheeler, L. & Hare, WA. (2008) Alpha2 adrenergic modulation of NMDA receptor function as a major mechanism of RGC protection in experimental glaucoma and retinal excitotoxicity, *Investigative Ophthalmology & Visual Science* Vol.(49):4515-4522.

Garthwaite, G., Brown, G., Batchelor, AM., Goodwin, DA. & Garthwaite, J. (1999) Mechanisms of ischemic damage to central white matter axons: A quantitative histological analysis using rat optic nerve, *Neuroscience* Vol.(94):1219-1230.

Gu, Z., Yamamoto, T., Kawase, C., Matsubara, M., Kawase, K., Sawada, A. & Kitazawa, Y. (2000) Neuroprotective effect of N-methyl-D-aspartate receptor antagonists in an experimental glaucoma model in the rat, *Nippon Ganka Gakkai Zasshi* Vol.(104):11-16.

Hammarstrom, AKM. & Gage, PW. (2002) Hypoxia and persistent sodium current, *European Biophysical Journal* Vol.(31):323-330.

Hare, WA., WoldeMussie, E., Lai, RK., Ton, H., Ruiz, G., Chun, T. & Wheeler, L. (2004a) Efficacy and safety of memantine treatment for reduction of changes associated with experimental glaucoma in monkey, I: Functional measures, *Investigative Ophthalmology & Visual Science* Vol.(45):2625-2639.

Hare, WA., WoldeMussie, E., Weinreb, R., Ton, H., Ruiz, G., Wijono, M., Feldmann, B., Zangwill, L. & Wheeler, L. (2004b) Efficacy and safety of memantine treatment for reduction of changes associated with experimental glaucoma in monkey, II: Structural measures, *Investigative Ophthalmology & Visual Science* Vol.(45):2640-2651.

Hare, WA. & Wheeler, L. (2009) Experimental glutamatergic excitotoxicity in rabbit retinal ganglion cells: Block by memantine, *Investigative Ophthalmology & Visual Science* Vol.(50):2940-2948.

Izumi, Y., Shimamoto, K., Benz, AM., Hammerman, SB., Olney, JW. & Zorumski, CF. (2002) Glutamate transporters and retinal excitotoxicity, *Glia* Vol.(39):58-68.

Johansson, JO. (1986) Retrograde axoplasmic transport in rat optic nerve in vivo. What causes blockage at increased intraocular pressure?, *Experimental Eye Research* Vol.(43):653-660.

Kaneda, M. & Kaneko, A. (1991) Voltage-gated sodium currents in isolated retinal ganglion cells of the cat: relation between the inactivation kinetics and the cell type, *Neuroscience Research* Vol.(11):261-275.

Kim, HS., Chang, YI., Kim, JH. & Park, CK. (2007) Alteration of retinal intrinsic survival signal and effect of alpha2-adrenergic receptor agonist in the retina of the chronic ocular hypertension rat, *Visual Neuroscience* Vol.(24):127-139.

Kirischuk, S., Pronchuk, N. & Verkhratsky, A. (1992) Measurements of intracellular calcium in sensory neurons of adult and old rats, *Neuroscience* Vol.(50):947-951.

Kowluru, RA., Engerman, RL., Case, GL. & Kern, TS. (2001) Retinal glutamate in diabetes and effect of antioxidants, *Neurochem. Int.* Vol.(38):385-390.

Lafuente, MP., Villegas-Perez, MP, Mayor, S., Aguilera, ME., Miralles de Imperial, J. & Vidal-Sanz, M. (2002) Neuroprotective effects of brimonidine against transient ischemia-induced retinal ganglion cell death: a dose response in vivo study, *Experimental Eye Research* Vol.(74):181-189.

Lagreze, WA., Knorle, R., Bach, M. & Feuerstein, TJ. (1998) Memantine is neuroprotective in a rat model of pressure-induced ischemia, *Investigative Ophthalmology & Visual Science* Vol.(39):1063-1066.

Lai, RK., Chun, T., Hasson, D., Lee, S., Mehrbod, F. & Wheeler, L. (2002) Alpha-2 adrenoceptor agonist protects retinal function after acute retinal ischemic injury in the rat, *Visual Neuroscience* Vol.(19):175-185.

Lam, TT., Siew, E., Chu, R. & Tso, MO. (1997) Ameliorative effect of MK-801 on retinal ischemia, *Journal of Ocular Pharmacology and Therapeutics* Vol.(13):129-137.

Louzada-Junior, P., Dias, JJ., Santos, WF., Lachat, JJ., Bradford, HF. & Coutinho-Netto, J. (1992) Glutamate release in experimental ischemia of the retina: an approach using microdialysis, *Journal of Neurochemistry* Vol.(59):358-363.

Lucas, DR. & Newhouse, JP. (1957) The toxic effect of sodium L-glutamate on the inner layers of the retina, *A.M.A. Archives of Ophthalmology* Vol.(58):193-201.

Luo, X., Heidinger, V., Picaud, S., Lambrou, G., Dreyfus, H., Sahel, J. & Hicks, D. (2001) Selective excitotoxic degeneration of adult pig retinal ganglion cells in vitro, *Investigative Ophthalmology & Visual Science* Vol.(42):1096-1106.

Ma, K., Xu, L., Zhang, H., Zhang, S., Pu, M. & Jonas, JB. (2009) Effect of brimonidine on retinal ganglion cell survival in an optic nerve crush model, *American Journal of Ophthalmology* Vol.(147):326-331.

Massey, SC. & Miller, RF. (1990) N-methyl-D-aspartate receptors of *ganglion* cells in rabbit retina, *Journal of Neurophysiology* Vol.(63):16-30.

Metoki, T., Ohguro, H., Ohguro, I., Mamiya, K., Ito, T. & Nakazawa, M. (2005) Study of effects of antiglaucoma eye drops on N-methyl-D-aspartate-induced retinal damage, *Japanese Journal of Ophthalmology* Vol.(49):453-461.

Neal, MJ., Cunningham, JR., Hutson, PH. & Hogg, J. (1994) Effects of ischemia on neurotransmitter release from the isolated retina, *Journal of Neurochemistry* Vol.(62):1025-1033.

Nucci, C., Tartaglione, R., Rombola, L., Morrone, LA., Fazzi, E. & Bagetta, G. (2005) Neurochemical evidence to implicate elevated glutamate in the mechanisms of high intraocular pressure (IOP)-induced retinal ganglion cell death in rat, *Neurotoxicology* Vol.(26):935-941.

Pang, IH., Wexler, EM., Nawy, S., DeSantis, L. & Kapin, MA. (1999) Protection by eliprodil against excitotoxicity in cultured rat retinal ganglion cells, *Investigative Ophthalmology & Visual Science* Vol.(40):1170-1176.

Pellegrini, JW. & Lipton, SA. (1993) Delayed administration of memantine prevents N-methyl-D-aspartate receptor-mediated neurotoxicity, *ANN. Neurology* Vol.(33):403-407.

Pellegrino, RG. & Ritchie, JM. (1984) Sodium channels in the axolemma of normal and degenerating rabbit optic nerve, *Proceedings of the Royal Society (London)* Vol.(222):155-160.

Quigley, HA., Addicks, EM., Green, WR. & Maumenee, AE. (1981) Optic nerve damage in glaucoma II. The site of injury and susceptibility to damage, *Archives of Ophthalmology* Vol.(99):635-649.

Rothman, SM. & Olney, JW. (1987) Excitotoxicity and the NMDA receptor, *Trends In Neurosciences* Vol.(10):299-302.

Schoepfer, R., Monyer, H., Sommer, B., Wisden, W., Sprengel, R., Kuner, T., Lomeli, H., Herb, A, Kohler, M. & Burnashev, N. (1994) Molecular biology of glutamate receptors, *Progress in Neurobiology* Vol.(42):353-357.

Shuettauf, F., Quinto, K., Naskar, R. & Zurakowski, D. (2002) Effects of anti-glaucoma medications on ganglion cell survival: the DBA/2J mouse model, *Vision Research* Vol.(42):2333-2337.

Siliprandi, R., Canella, R., Carmignoto, G., Schiavo, N., Zanellato, A., Zanoni, R. & Vantini, G. (1992) N-methyl-D-aspartate-induced neurotoxicity in the adult rat retina, *Visual Neuroscience* Vol.(8):567-573.

Stys, PK., Waxman, SG. & Ransom, BR. (1992) Ionic mechanisms of anoxic injury in mammalian CNS white matter: Role of $Na^+$ channels and $Na^+$-$Ca^{+2}$ exchanger, *The Journal of Neuroscience* Vol.(12):430-439.

Stys, PK., Sontheimer, H., Ransom, BR. & Waxman, SG. (1993) Noninactivating tetrodotoxin-sensitive $Na^+$ conductance in rat optic nerve axons, *Proceedings of the National Academy of Science* Vol.(90):6976-6980.

Wolde Mussie, E., Ruiz, G., Wijono, M. & Wheeler, L. (2001) Neuroprotection of retinal ganglion cells by brimonidine in rats with laser-induced chronic ocular hypertension, *Investigative Ophthalmology & Visual Science* Vol.(42):2849-2855.

Wolde Mussie, E., Yoles, E., Schwartz, M., Ruiz, G. & Wheeler, L. (2002) Neuroprotective effect of memantine in different retinal injury models in rats, *Journal of Glaucoma* Vol.(11):474-480.

Wollner, DA., Scheinman, R. & Catterall, W. (1988) Sodium channel expression and assembly during development of retinal ganglion cells, *Neuron* Vol.(8):727-737.

Yoles, E., Wheeler, L. & Schwartz, M. (1999) Alpha2-adrenoceptor agonists are neuroprotective in a rat model of optic nerve degeneration, *Investigative Ophthalmology & Visual Science* Vol.(40):65-73.

Zeevalk, GD. & Nicklas, WJ. (1992) Evidence that the loss of the voltage-dependent $Mg^{2+}$ block at the N-methyl-D-aspartate receptor underlies receptor activation during inhibition of neuronal metabolism, *Journal of Neurochemistry* Vol.(59):1211-1220.

# 7

# Neuroprotection in Glaucoma

Brett H. Mueller II[1], Dorota L. Stankowska[2] and Raghu R. Krishnamoorthy[2]
[1]*Department of Pharmacology and Neuroscience*
[2]*Department of Cell Biology and Anatomy,*
*North Texas Eye Research Institute*
*University of North Texas Health Science Center; Texas*
*USA*

## 1. Introduction

Glaucoma is an age related heterogeneous group of diseases affecting 70 million people worldwide that is commonly associated with elevated intraocular pressure due to impairment of the outflow pathway of the trabecular meshwork, and characterized by pathological changes in optic nerve head, and lamina cribosa, leading to visual field defects and eventual blindness due to apoptosis of retinal ganglion cells (RGCs) (Clark and Yorio, 2003; Fraser and Wormald, 1999; and Lipton, 2003). The predominant risk factor for patients that suffer from glaucoma is elevation of intraocular pressure (IOP) (Fatma, et al. 2008). Elevated IOP imposes strain on the unmyelinated portion of axons of the RGCs, at the optic nerve head where they take a 90 degree turn to traverse to their final destination at the lateral geniculate nucleus in the thalamus of the brain, or to the superior colliculus in lower vertebrate animals (Quigley 1981). This strain on the axons of the RGCs at the optic nerve head is thought to be the initiating primary insult that damages the axons of the RGCs, inhibiting retrograde transport of neurotrophic factors produced in the brain, and eventually leading to cell death of RGCs (Quigley 1981). This primary insult is hypothesized to initiate a release of noxious secondary factors including glutamate, endothelin, and tumor necrosis-factor-α from injured RGCs and proliferating astrocytes going through reactive gliosis (Clark and Yorio 2003; Prasanna et al., 2010; Tezel and Wax, 2000; Tezel et al., 2001; Tezel and Wax 2004; Nakazawa et al. 2006). These secondary factors are also hypothesized to be associated with RGC death. Other mechanisms include ischemia/hypoxia at the optic nerve head, which could trigger release of glutamate, endothelin-1 (ET-1) and TNF-α from astrocytes, which could contribute to neurodegeneration.
Currently used treatment modalities for glaucoma are agents targeted at lowering IOP and preventing the primary insult contributing to RGC apoptosis. If the main cause of RGC death is axotomy due to pressure induced trauma to axons at the optic nerve head, then a reduction of IOP should protect the remainder of RGCs and halt the progression of this disease process. Although IOP in glaucoma patients is often held within "normal" ranges, the disease process and RGC death can still progress. Additionally, patients with IOP measurements of 6-10 mmHg (normal being 10-20 mmHg) can still develop glaucoma (normal tension glaucoma), thus suggesting that elevation of IOP is not the only predisposing factor for patients that suffer from glaucoma, and suggests that there may be

secondary causes of RGC apoptosis during the progression of this heterogeneous disease process (Bahrami 2006). However, what remains unclear are the secondary factors contributing to the continual apoptotic cell death of the RGCs after the hypothesized initial insult to axons, causing optic nerve damage at the lamina cribosa. Commonly proposed secondary factors that appear to be implicated in this self-perpetuating model of RGC death include free radical formation, glutamate excitotoxicity, and trophic factor withdrawal. Agents that can block these noxious agents need to be studied for their potential role as neuroprotective agents that can protect injured and uninjured RGCs, enhance viability and functionality after exposure to both primary and secondary causes of RGC death during this disease process. These neuroprotectants can be administered as adjunct therapies to IOP lowering agents with a view to provide better therapeutic options aimed at treating both the major risk factor (IOP elevation) as well as secondary pathological process (RGC death) of glaucoma.

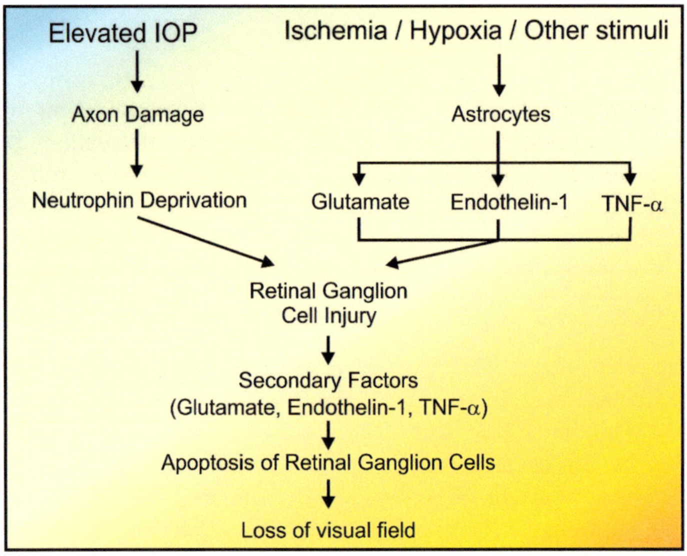


Fig. 1. Mechanisms underlying neurodegeneration in glaucoma. Elevated intraocular pressure (IOP) is a well known risk factor contributing to axon loss and retinal ganglion cell death. Other factors including ischemia/hypoxia and lesser known glaucomatous stimuli have been hypothesized to contribute to release of other mediators including glutamate, endothelin-1 and TNF-α from astrocytes which produce degenerative effects on RGCs. Damage to RGCs could unleash secondary factors which contribute to apoptosis of RGCs and subsequent loss of visual field

Much of the studies conducted in the area of neuroprotection to treat glaucoma has been conducted in animal models where IOP is chronically elevated for a few weeks to months in order to monitor RGC survival when different neurotrophic agents are administered. IOP is artificially elevated in these animal models using several experimental approaches: hypertonic saline injections of the episcleral vessels in the eye causing venous congestion (Morrison et al. 1997), by injection of hypertonic saline into the limbal plexus causing sclerosis of trabecular meshwork (Johnson et al. 2009), through laser-induced damage to the trabecular meshwork causing impairment of aqueous humour outflow (Levkovitch-Verbin et al. 2002), or by trabecular meshwork obstruction by injecting polystyrene beads (Sappington et al. 2010). Researchers also use DBA/2J mice carrying inherent genetic mutation in the glycoprotein nmb-like protein (Gpnmb) and tyrosinase-related protein 1b (Tyrp 1b) genes which causes iris atrophy late in the lifespan of these mice (John et al. 1998). This atrophy causes sloughing off of the iris pigment which clogs the meshwork and leads to elevation of IOP and RGC loss (Anderson et al. 2002). Some studies also use a more acute *in vivo* model of RGC death called optic nerve crush, in which the axons protruding from the posterior pole of the eye are physically crushed using forceps (Heacock and Agranoff, 1976; Benowitz et al., 1981). This acute *in vivo* model causes considerable RGC death after 1-2 weeks following the crush; therefore, this experimental paradigm enables researchers to quickly screen a variety of agents for neuroprotective properties (Danesh-Meyer 2011). The optic nerve crush is a traumatic optic neuropathy model producing damage to optic nerve axons, however it has provided insight into the neuroprotective ability of various test compounds administered intravitreally (Danesh-Meyer 2011). In addition, the optic nerve crush model has also been useful to study other systemic factors conferring neuroprotection. For instance, it was found that a T-cell-mediated immune response directed against self-antigens residing in the site of damage can be beneficial for the injured optic nerve or spinal cord (Schwartz 2004).

Drugs for neuroprotection to treat glaucoma have to reach the axons and somas of the RGCs. It would be ideal to administer these neuroprotectants as eyedrops; however, the eye possesses key barriers that would impede pharmaceutical agents from penetrating to the back of the eye. The most notable barriers include the precorneal tear clearance and the selective corneal epithelial barrier (Ghate and Edelhauser 2008). The traditional means available to administer pharmaceutical agents to the posterior segment of the eye include: intravenous or oral (which has poor bioavailability with increasing risks of systemic side effects), intravitreal injections (which has excellent bioavailability but carries the inherent risk of ocular infections), or periocular injections (Ghate and Edelhauser 2008). More recent drug delivery systems that could serve to administer neuroprotectants to the posterior pole of the eye include nanoparticles and viral vectors which hold much promise to prolong effective treatment to the retina and optic nerve. Nanoparticles can administer a prolonged stead flow of neuroprotective compounds to the back of the eye for a long period of time (Diebold and Calonge 2010). Additionally, both nanoparticles and viral vectors could be used to administer gene therapies in order to up-regulate potent protective genes, and down-regulate neurodegenerative genes. Specifically, gene therapy through viral vectors has gained some momentum in recent years especially after treatment of patients suffering from Leber's congenital amaurosis, using adeno-associated viral vector encoding RPE65, showed promising results of safety and efficacy (Bainbridge et al. 2008).

A number of studies have been conducted over the past 30 years to identify neuroprotective molecules to protect the neurons in central nervous system (CNS) from acute (stroke) and chronic neurological diseases (e.g. Alzheimer, Parkinson, and glaucomatous optic neuropathy), with numerous encouraging preclinical neuroprotective outcomes, however most clinical studies done to demonstrate neuroprotection in humans failed to show efficacy. Only three neuroprotective drugs have been demonstrated to improve outcomes in human clinical trails: riluzole for amytrophic lateral sclerosis, memantine for moderate to severe Alzheimer disease (Bensimon et al. 1994, Lacomblez et al. 1996, Reisberg et al. 2003) and brimonidine for low pressure glaucoma (Krupin et al. 2011). Memantine and riluzole have failed to have a dramatic impact on the progression of these neurological diseases

(Danesh-Meyer and Levin 2009). From the perspective of clinical trails aimed at developing neuroprotective therapies in glaucoma, the memantine trial was disappointing and failed to demonstrate efficacy in two large multicenter clinical trails at sites worldwide (Allegran 2008). Brimonidine ($\alpha 2$ adrenergic agonist) was another drug given to a small group of patients suffering from ischemic optic neuropathy, where the treated and untreated groups did not show any statistical significant difference in visual field tests (Wilhelm 2006). However, a recent promising study of brimonidine treatment in patients suffering from low-pressure glaucoma, suggests that patients treated with brimonidine are less likely to have worsening of visual fields compared to patients treated with timolol (Krupin et al., 2011). Further studies are required to determine the long term neuroprotective and clinical efficacy of brimonidine in glaucoma patients.

A review article written by Levin and Danesh Meyer (2010) go on to describe the disparity between pre-clinical neuroprotective data and clinical trails. They emphasize lack of appropriate animal models for each neurological disease, appropriate dose of the neuroprotective compounds, timing of the neuroprotective agent administration, poor pre-clinical study designs, premature initiation of clinical trails, problems in execution of neuroprotection clinical trails, and choice of clinical end points. Some or all of these factors may result in the disparity that is observed between pre-clinical experimental results, and clinical trials.

The difficulty in finding an appropriate animal model for neurological diseases is that for most neurological diseases, it is unclear why and how certain specific subpopulations of neurons die. For example in glaucoma, increasing levels of IOP is the major risk factor for patients suffering from glaucoma. In fact, when an individual's IOP reaches 21 mm Hg or higher (normal values being close to 16 mm Hg), IOP lowering agents are administered as a preventative measure so that patients do not develop glaucoma. However, the Baltimore Eye Survey published in 1991 demonstrated that more than half of all the glaucomatous eyes tested in this prospective cohort had IOPs under 21mmHg, whether they were being treated with IOP lowering agents or not (Sommer et al. 1991). Yet, the only animal models used to mimic the disease of glaucoma are those that artificially elevate IOP. Therefore, there is a paucity of animal models that accurately mimic the disease process of primary open angle glaucoma.

Other impediments in the discovery of neuroprotective compounds in clinical trails from promising pre-clinical data is trying to identify the correct therapeutic dose for these neurological diseases in humans (Danesh-Meyer and Levin 2009). Knowing how much of a drug reaches its therapeutic target in the retina is a challenge. Also, most pre-clinical studies looking at the neuroprotective compounds often administer these compounds before the glaucomatous insult (Danesh-Meyer and Levin 2009). This never happens in clinical practice, as most patients enrolled in these neuroprotective clinical trials have advanced disease pathology. Lastly, many investigators carrying out pre-clinical animal studies looking at neuroprotection often are not blinded to the animal getting the therapeutic agent (Danesh-Meyer and Levin 2009). This could inadvertently bias the researcher that is trying to demonstrate neuroprotective efficacy in an animal model. If researchers can adopt a set standard of rules that more closely mimics the rules applied to patients going through clinical trials, perhaps fewer drugs will show promising pre-clinical data (Bebarta 2003). However, those drugs which show pre-clinical efficacy in animal models with standardized protocols could be more closely investigated in order to discover a more effective neuroprotective compound in humans that can treat glaucoma. Moreover, interventions in different steps of the neurodegenerative pathways could have an additive effect to bolster neuroprotective effects.

The failure of the memantine clinical trial for treating glaucoma has generated skepticism over the discovery of neuroprotective agents to treat glaucoma. Memantine is a drug that blocks the toxic effects of glutamate excitoxicity by antagonizing N-methyl-D-aspartate (NMDA) receptors (Chen et al. 1992 and Parsons et al. 1993). Glutamate excitotoxicity and its effects on RGCs are not without controversy. Studies have demonstrated that glutamate excitotoxicity has toxic effects on primary hippocampal neurons but not on primary RGCs. A thorough investigation by Ullian et al. (2004) which showed that primary RGCs cultured in the presence of 500 μM glutamate for 1 hour did not cause apoptosis of these cells. However, hippocampal neurons treated with glutamate for 1 hour produced almost 100% death of these cultured cells. While this is one report of inability of glutamate to kill RGCs, it does demonstrate that perhaps there may be different levels of susceptibility to the same noxious stimuli between different types of neurons in the CNS. If excitotoxicity does not occur in RGCs, then there is less likelihood of memantine to work as a neuroprotective compound in patients suffering from glaucoma. It is not completely clear how RGCs are dying in the disease process of glaucoma. Without fully understanding the mechanisms of cell death in neurodegenerative diseases, it is difficult to develop strategies for neuroprotection. Perhaps, the lack of a comprehensive understanding of the pathways leading to degeneration in the CNS is a stumbling block in the development of a neuroprotective compound in humans.

As mentioned earlier, most of the molecular studies done on neurons have been performed on cortical neurons, not RGCs. Additionally, researchers have identified up to 22 different morphological distinct RGC subtypes in a mouse retina (Sun et al., 2002; Badea and Nathans, 2004, Kong et al., 2005, Coombs et al., 2006; Völgyi et al, 2009). Even though it is assumed that all these RGCs behave in a similar fashion, it is unclear if each subtype of RGCs has its own set of distinct rules for survival and functionality. Besides, it is not known if some of these subtypes of RGCs are the ones that are consistently dying in glaucoma. This adds even more complexity to the research that is being conducted in neuroprotection. Lastly, an emerging area of research being conducted is the investigation of neuronal cell death in the lateral geniculate nucleus (LGN) in glaucoma (Gupta et al., 2006). The LGN is a subcortical structure that receives the axons of the RGCs, and relays that information to the visual cortex. The LGN has been demonstrated to show apoptotic changes after intravitreal NMDA injections (Shimazawa et al., 2007; Suemori et al., 2006; Ito et al., 2008). Additionally, it is one of the hypothesized reasons for why nearly 50% RGC loss is needed to cause visual field loss, and why the initial loss of RGCs does not cause any noticeable defect in visual function (Quigley et al. 1989). Perhaps there is a need to also look at the neuroprotective capabilities of various compounds in the retina and the brain. This is another emerging area of interest that is poised to draw a lot of attention in the coming years, and will probably help to unveil some of the key mechanisms underlying apoptosis of RGCs in the disease process of glaucoma.

Many neuroprotective agents targeting various proposed pathological mechanisms associated with RGC death in glaucoma have been tested. These include calcium channel blockers, trophic factors, and anti-apoptotic factors (Danesh-Meyer 2011). Other neuroprotective strategies include, blocking the toxic effects of TNF-α and endothelin, and providing immunomodulation (Frank et al. 2009, Krishnamoorthy et al. 2008, Nakazawa et al. 2006, Schober et al. 2008, Schwartz, 2004). Other studies have demonstrated that mesenchymal stem/stromal cell transplantation can also provide robust neuroprotective effects in rat models of glaucoma (Bull et al. 2009 and Johnson et al. 2010). This chapter focuses on those therapies which have demonstrated pre-clinical neuroprotective effects against excitotoxicity, blocking pathological influxes of calcium, and neurotrophin withdrawal. Additionally, a section will discuss emerging neuroprotectants including endothelin antagonists, TNF antagonists and sigma-1 receptor agonists as potential therapeutic targets in treating RGC degeneration.

## 2. Neurotrophins and their role in neuroprotection

This section will discuss the role of neurotrophins in promoting neuroprotection under conditions of neurotrophin deprivation observed in several models of glaucomatous optic neuropathy. The various types of neurotrophins and their receptors as well as their downstream signaling pathways will be briefly described. Results obtained after different strategies for neurotrophin delivery in animal models of glaucoma will be discussed.

### 2.1 Neurotrophins their function and structure

Neurotrophins (NTs) are a family of proteins that promote survival (Hempstead BL, 2006), development and function (Reichardt LF, 2006) of neurons and maintenance of the nervous system. They could be considered as the growth factors of the nervous system and are secreted primarily by the target tissue innervated by neurons. Typically, during development, only those neurons that make synaptic contact with target cells releasing neurotrophins survive, while others neurons that unable to gather trophic support are eliminated *via* apoptosis. The term trophic is widely used to point to a pro-survival action towards target cells by signaling molecules, including neurotrophins (NTs). Neurotrophins are the member of the neurotrophic factors (NTFs) family (Table 1). The NT family is composed of Nerve Growth Factor (NGF), brain-derived neurotrophic factor (BDNF), Neurotrophin-3 (NT-3) and Neurotrophin-4/5 (NT-4/5). Other related class of proteins include several neurotrophic factors which provide trophic support to RGCs.

| Neurotrophic factor group | Neurotrophic factor member | Main receptors |
|---|---|---|
| Neurotrophins | Nerve Growth Factor (NGF) | TrkA, p75 |
| | Brain Derived Neurotrophic Factor (BDNF) | TrkB, p75 |
| | Neurotrophin-3 (NT3) | TrkC, TrkA, TrkB, p75 |
| | Neurotrophin-4/5 (NT4/5) | TrkB,TrkA, TrkC, p75 |
| Other NTFs | Ciliary Neurotrophic Factor (CNTF), Leukemia Inhibitory Factor (LIF), Transforming Growth Factor $\beta$ 1-3 (TGF$\beta$1 -3 ), Transforming Growth Factor $\alpha$(TGF$\alpha$), Glial Cell Line-Derived Neurotrophic Factor (GDNF), Neurturin (NTN), Persephin (PSP), Artemin (ARTN), Fibroblast Growth Factor (FGF), Neuritin -1, Insulin-like Growth Factors 1-2 (IGF-1, IGF-2), Stem Cell Factor (SCF), Platelet-Derived Growth Factor (PDGF), Erythropoietin (Epo) | |

Table 1. Neurotrophic factor groups, members and main receptors

In addition to synthesis of neurotrophins in the brain, all of them are locally produced in the retina. NGF's (Liu et al 2010) and NT-3's (Seki et al, 2004) mRNA were found in the retina. BDNF and NT4/5 are expressed by RGCs (Vecino et al., 2002, Spalding et al., 2004) and by Muller cells in the retina (Seki et al., 2005). Other sources of neurotrophins in the eye include the lamina cribrosa cells and optic nerve head astrocytes which were found to express both NTs and Trk receptors (Lambert et al., 2001). BDNF is synthesized primarily in the brain and together with its receptor TrkB is taken up by RGC axon terminals and transported retrogradely to the somas of RGCs. Table 2 shows chromosomal localization of NT receptors.

| Receptor | chromosome | Reference |
|---|---|---|
| p75 | 17q21-q22 | (Huebner et al., 1986) |
| TrkA | 1q21-q22 | (Weier et al., 1995) |
| TrkB | 9q22.1 | (Nakagawara et al., 1995) |
| TrkC | 15q25 | (Valent et al., 1997) |

Table 2. Chromosomal localizations of neurotrophin receptor genes. The BDNF protein is coded by the bdnf gene. In humans, this gene is located on chromosome 11p13 (Maisonpierre et al., 1991) and codes for a 247 aa protein. NT-3 gene *nt-3* is located on human chromosome 12p13 (Maisonpierre et al., 1991) codes for a 257 aa protein. Human *nt-4/5* gene encodes the NT-4/5 protein comprising of 210 aa and is localized to chromosome 19 band q13.3 (BERKemeier et al., 1992). NGF (299 aa protein) is coded by a gene located on chromosome 1p13.1 (www.kegg.com)

All neutrophins are synthesized as large precursors and they have analogous biochemical characteristics (Sariola et al., 1994; Barbacid 1995). They contain nerve growth factor family signature ([GSRE]-C-[KRL]-G-[LIVT]-[DE]-x(3)-[YW]-x-S-x-C). BDNF, NT-3 and NT-4/5 have been found to be structurally and functionally related to NGF (Lo DC, 1992). NGF is a protein of about 120 residues. It contains six cysteines which are involved in intra-chain disulphide bonds. Representation of the structure of NGF is shown on Figure 2. All neutrophins in modified mature forms are secreted and act as dimers

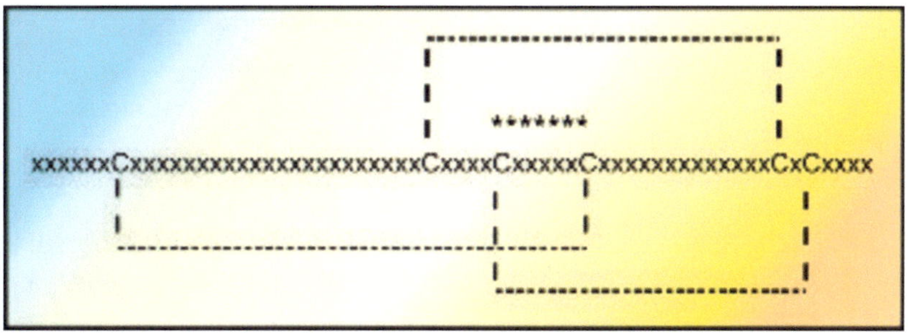


Fig. 2. Schematic representation of the structure of NGF. The signature pattern for the NGF family contains the middle region which includes two of the six cysteines involved in formation of disulfide bonds. (Stucture taken from http://www.expasy.org/prosite/PDOC 00221). Where: 'C': conserved cysteine involved in a disulfide bond, '*' position of the pattern

**2.2 Neutrophin receptors TrkA, TrkB, TrkC and p75. Signaling through NT receptors**

The neurotrophins in general are able to bind to two types of receptors. The high-affinity binding occurs *via* Tropomyosin Receptor Kinase (TrkA, TrkB or TrkC) and low affinity

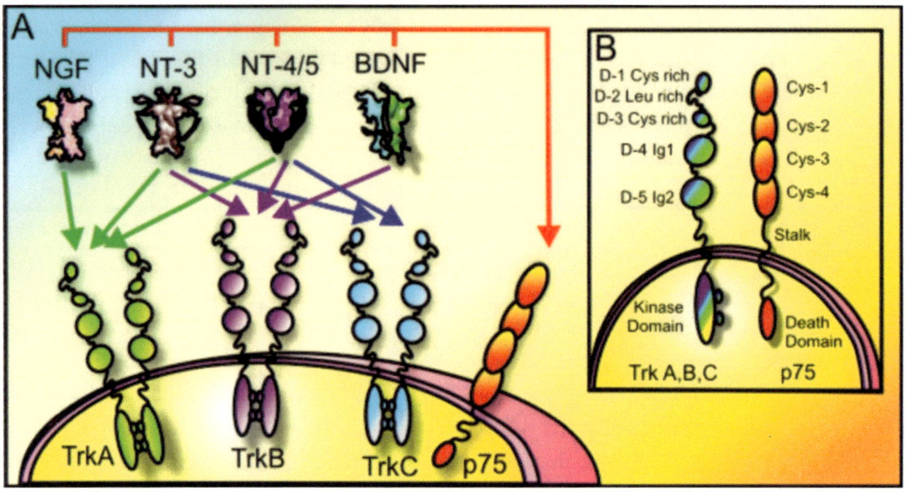


Fig. 3. A) Preferred receptors for neurotrophins are shown by color coding: Green for TrkA, purple for TrkB and Blue for TrkC. All Neutrophins bind to p75 (Red arrow). B) Schematic representation of the Trk and p75 receptors showing individual domains

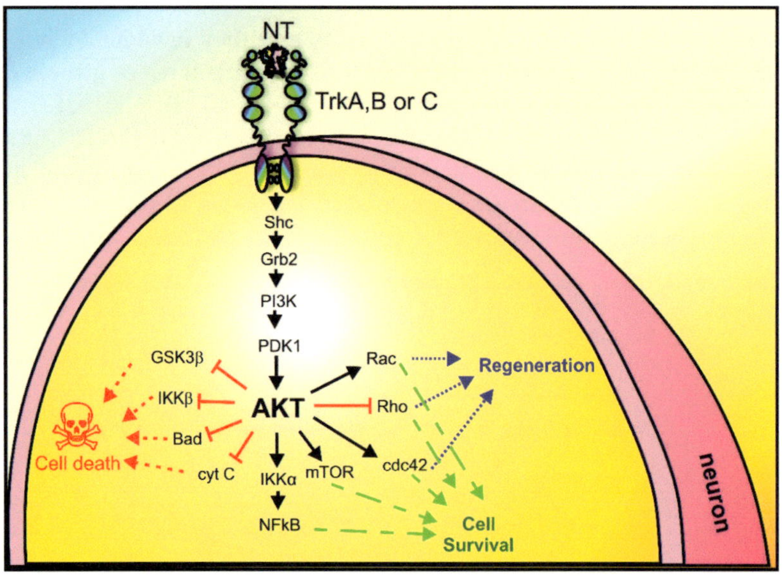


Fig. 4. AKT survival pathway activated by neurotrophins. Binding of neurotrophins to Trk receptors activates signal transduction pathway leading to activation of AKT which has an effect on several effectors. By inhibiting GSK3β, IKKβ, Bad and cytochrome C release, AKT prevents cell death. On the other hand cell survival responses are also activated by AKT through NFκB, mTor, Rac and cdc42 mediated mechanisms

binding through common neurotrophin receptor p75 (p75NTR know also as LNGFR). Receptor p75 has no tyrosine kinase domain (Greene and Kaplan, 1995; Chao and Hempstead, 1995). Preferentially, NGF binds to TrkA, BDNF and NT-4/5 bind to TrkB and NT-3 binds to TrkC (Figure 3). However, NT-3 and NT-4/5 have the ability to also bind to all the Trk receptors with different affinities. All NTs bind to the p75 receptor, which is a member of tumor necrosis factor superfamily (Figure 3).

Binding of neurotrophin to Trk type receptor induces dimerization and transphosphorylation (MacPhee et al, 1999) followed by activation of signaling cascades leading in general to pro-survival cellular responses (Figure 5). However, specific cell responses to NT-dependent Trk activation, depend upon the cell context and the balance of associated adaptors and kinase proteins. A common feature of neurotrophin signaling through Trk has been activation of MAP kinases (Marshall, 1995). Trk dependent antiapoptotic and growth pathways are mediated by cytoplasmic adaptors proteins Shc (SHC), fibroblast growth factor receptor substrate 2 ( FRS-2) and others effectors including phosphatidyl inositol 3-kinase (PI3-K) and phospholipase C gamma (PLCγ1) (Chao, 2003; Huang and Reichardt, 2003). PI3-kinase activates the RAC serine/threonine-protein kinase (AKT) pathway that supports cell survival and protein synthesis. Binding of NT to Trk receptors induces the PI3-K→AKT→mTOR pathways evoking pro-survival and/or pro-growth cellular responses. Trk receptors are receptor tyrosine kinases which activate the prototypical Ras→Raf→MEK→ERK1/2 growth promoting pathway and PLCγ1 supports activation of the PKC pathway. Trk dimers promotes also phosphorylation of ankyrin-rich membrane spanning protein (ARMS) causes formation of CrkL-C3G complex, resulting in Rap1-dependent sustained ERK activation leading to pro-survival events (Arevalo et al, 2004).

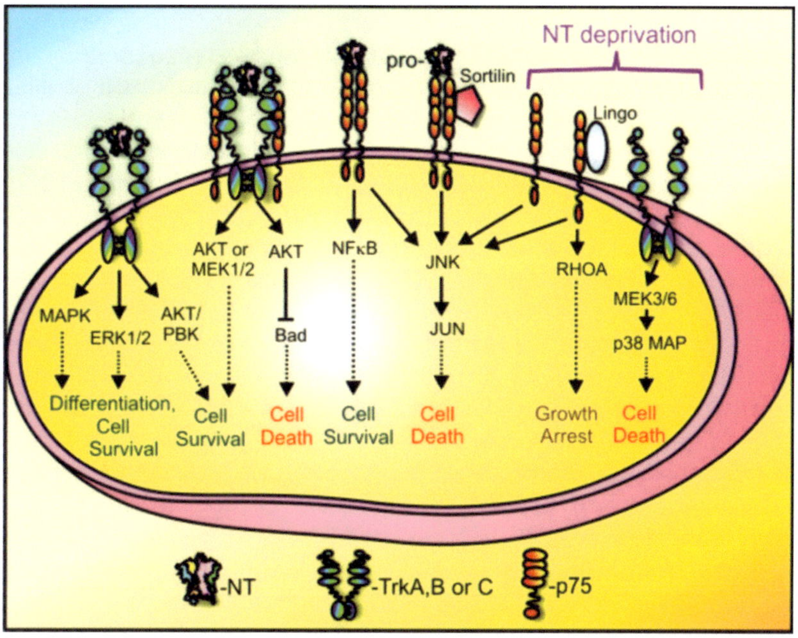


Fig. 5. A simplified summary of the NT signaling pathways. NTs binding to Trk receptors activate primarily a cell survival response. p75 receptors have predominantly cell death and growth arrest promoting effects

Trk receptors have different isoforms, some of which are deficient in the catalytic tyrosine kinase intracellular domain and their role is so far unknown (Barbacid 1995). Trk receptors may switch from pro-survival to pro-apoptotic action in the absence of its specific ligands (Calissano et al. 2010). During conditions of NT deprivation Trk signaling leads to cell death. The same effect can be caused by an over-production of TrkA which may induce a switch from an ERK→CREB pro-survival pathway to a MEK3/6→p38MAP pro-apoptotic cascade (Figure 5). It has been demonstrated that during NTs deprivation, the pro-apoptotic protein Bad is associated with Bcl-2/Bcl-xl at the mitochondrial membrane and inhibits Bcl-2/Bcl-xl, promoting cell death (Lodish et al., 2000).

A well established function of the p75 receptor is to promote cell death. When p75 receptor does not interact with Trk it promotes pro-apoptotic signal cascades. Signaling mediated through receptor p75 and its partner leucine rich repeat and Ig domain containing 1 (LINGO-1) is coupled to the mitochondrial apoptotic pathway (Nykjaer, 2005). Recently two binding partner proteins namely, ankyrin repeat - rich membrane spanning protein (ARMS) and Fas apoptosis inhibitory molecule (FAIM) were found to interact with p75 as well as Trk and modulate their signaling pathways thereby promoting survival (Chang et al, 2004, Sole et al, 2004). Moreover, when p75 interacts with pro-neutrophins bound to Vsp10p-domain receptor Sortilin, forming a ternary complex, it causes a pro-apoptotic response through TNF-α (Chikar et al 2008 and Nykjaer et al, 2004). p75 receptor can also positively regulate Trk receptor mediated pro-survival events by forming complex with Trk receptor facilitating its binding to NTs (Huang and Reichardt, 2003). p75 is able to promote neuronal survival *via* nuclear factor kappa B (NFκB) signaling (Hamanoue et al, 1999). The simplified signaling pathways regulating neuronal pro-survival or death depending on receptor, receptor-ligand or receptor-receptor-ligand interaction are presented in Figure 5.

### 2.3 Theory of neurotrophin deprivation and its relevance to glaucoma

During embryonic development, RGCs elongate neurites towards their targets within the brain. These targets actively secrete NTs in particular BDNF. When there is an insufficient supply of NTs to developing RGCs they undergo apoptosis (Meyer-Franke et all, 1995). In adult retinas, similar processes could take place. When a stable complex of NT and its Trk receptor is formed it is taken up by endocytosis and transported retrogradely up the axon to cell body (Ibáñez, 2007). Retrograde and orthograde axonal transport can be blocked by elevated intraocular pressure (elevated IOP) (Johansson, 1988). During conditions of elevated IOP, retrograde transport of NTs and Trk complexes is blocked and their accumulation occurs at the optic nerve head. This phenomenon is believe to be a main cause of neurotrophic deprivation in RGCs (Quigley et al., 2000, Pease et al., 2000) and may lead to neurodegenerative changes seen in glaucoma. Johnson et al. (2000) showed that a gradual depletion of BDNF and NT-4/5 occurs in the proximal optic nerve and in the superior region of the retina, as a possible response to elevated IOP. It is known that the survival of adult RGCs is maintained by transported as well as locally produced NTs (Raju et al., 1994). The blockage of retrograde transport of NTs causes gradual depletion of NTs in the retina. It seems that NTs trafficked from the brain can help in RGC survival in cases of injury, where the efficacy of local neurotrophins is not sufficient.. During glaucoma, in the situation of injury to RGCs, decreased local production of NTs in the retina as well as additional obstruction to retrograde transport could have significant implications in disease progression. The obstruction of retrograde transport precipitated by posterior displacement of the lamina cribrosa due to elevated IOP is the main hypothesis underlying glaucomatous optic neuropathy (Quigley et al., 2000, Pease et al., 2000). Figure 6 shows the mechanisms involved in the blockage of retrograde transport of growth factors due to ischemia or increased IOP.

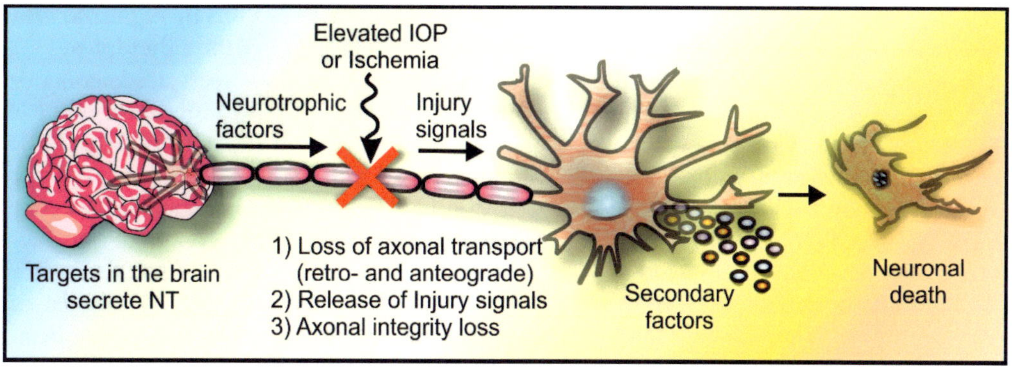


Fig. 6. Schematic representation of blockade of transport of neutrophic factors

While there is acceptance that neurotrophin deprivation leads to glaucoma, several studies found transiently elevated levels of NTs (BDNF and NT3) in the retina after injury. In acute optic nerve injury like optic nerve crush, there was an initial short term increase in retinal BDNF and TrkB levels (Hirsch et al., 2000) followed by a a decrease in TrkB receptors below normal level which had a correlation to apoptosis of RGCs (Chen and Weber, 2004). One plausible explanation for the short term increase in retinal BDNF and TrkB levels might be endogenous synthesis of NTs in response to the cessation of axonal transport. There was a loss of BDNF and NT-4/5 from the superior retina which coincided with evidence of axonal degeneration during elevated IOP in rats (Johnson et al., 2000). However, neurotrophin deprivation by itself could not be the only explanation for RGC death during glaucoma. As discussed earlier, NTs are locally produced in the retina (Ugolini, 1995, Seki, 2005). It is possible that in case of retrograde transport blockade, NTs expressed in situ should serve as proper compensation to the brain derived NTs. However, there is no clear agreement about the relative contribution of brain and locally derived NTs towards neuronal survival, as well as various effects of NTs on somal and axonal compartments (Quigley et al., 2000, Kimpinski et al., 1997 and Kuruvilla et al., 2000).

### 2.4 Promoting RGC survival in experimental models of neurotrophin deprivation

Exogenous NTs administration can decrease RGC loss during axonal injury; however, so far this strategy resulted only in temporary effects (Clarke et al., 1998, Di Polo et al., 1998, Isenmann et al., 1998, Bahr, 2000). This could be due to a deficit in Trk receptors in injured RGCs (Chen and Weber, 2004). Coassin et al. (2008) demonstrated that during elevated IOP retinal NGF expression was upregulated and it correlated with RGC death, mainly as the ratio of TrkA to p75 was shifted toward pro-apoptotic p75. Rudzinski et al. (2004) suggested that RGC apoptosis during elevated IOP was not only due to neurotrophic factor deprivation, but also dysfunction of NT receptors and their signaling pathways. It is clear that mere administration of NTs would not be efficacious as a neuroprotective strategy, suggesting that a concurrent regulation of receptor expression would be necessary for optimal neuroprotection.

#### 2.4.1 Pure protein delivery

Sawai et al (1996) investigated the effect of brain- derived neurotrophic factor (BDNF), neurotrophin NT-4/5, or NT-3 on retinal ganglion cell (RGC) axons regeneration in the retinas of rats after optic nerve transection. The authors found that intravitreal injections of BDNF as well as NT4/5 were able to increase the branch median lengths by eightfold which could have implications for RGCs regrowth into their CNS targets in future therapies.

In many experimental studies, axotomy or severe nerve crush has been used as a nerve injury model. Administration of BDNF after optic nerve injury in a cat model resulted in a 55% increase in ganglion cell survival 1 week after nerve crush and 79% by the second week. Combined introduction of BDNF to the eye as well as the visual cortex increased these values further by 17%. Based on the results it was concluded that combined treatments of the eye and brain targets presented more effective approaches against nerve injury and RGC survival (Weber et al., 2010). Administration of 200 µg/mL NGF eye drops has been shown to be neuroprotective for RGC in rat eyes by inhibiting apoptosis of RGCs in animals with glaucoma. More significantly, the authors tested the same eye drops on three human glaucoma patients for three months. Patients were evaluated for changes in pattern electroretinography, visual field and visual evoked potential assays. The NGF topical administration caused improvements in inner retinal function, however no placebo controls were included in this study (Lambiase et al, 2009). In another study Colafrancesco et al. (2011) produced elevated IOP by hypertonic saline intravitreal injections into rat eyes to investigate the role of NGF on damaged RGCs and axons. Pressure elevation transiently caused an increase in NGF in the retina, followed by a drastic drop below normal levels leading to RGC apoptosis. This study showed that non-invasive, topic delivery of NGF as eye drops protected RGCs from degeneration and death. It is however unclear how NGF could penetrate the eye and reach higher order brain structures to produce therapeutic effects.

#### 2.4.2 Gene therapy

Gene therapy has emerged as a promising avenue for the treatment of ocular disorders after the successful phase I clinical trial for Leber's Congenital Amaurosis using AAV-mediated gene delivery of the RPE65 gene (Bainbridge et al. 2008). Gene therapy as a delivery method to the retina using viral vectors has also been successful in several animal models of eye diseases including retinal degeneration, inherited retina degeneration, retinitis pigmentosa or canine childhood blindness (Martin et al., 2003). Using an experimental rat glaucoma model, it was shown that AAV mediated administration of BDNF to the RGCs significantly increased RGC survival (up to 52%) after 4 weeks of IOP elevation (Martin et al, 2003). In another study, Cheng et al. (2002) overexpressed TrkB receptor using AAV vector and combined this therapy with exogenous intraocular injections of pure BDNF, and found an increase in RGC survival. Their results indicated that TrkB-induced RGC rescue was caused by activation of the MEK →MAPK but not the PI-3K→AKT pathway. In another approach to protect RGCs, Di Polo et al. (1998) targeted BDNF to the Muller cells and found a 4.5-fold increase in surviving RGCs, 16 days post-injury in an optic nerve axotomy model in rats.

#### 2.4.3 Intravitreal transplantation

Intraocular transplantation of progenitor or stem cells is a rapidly growing research field. Despite the fact that transplantation is a very attractive approach, many barriers to clinical efficacy remain such as an acute immune response and rejection of the transplants. To overcome these difficulties subsequent multiple immunosuppressive therapies either alone or in combination with exogenous erythropoietin or chondroitinase ABC treatment have been used in parallel. There is a question of ethical issues connected to stem cell therapy. Transplantation of progenitor or stem cells is an emerging approach for treating neurodegenerative conditions of the CNS, and in particular the retina. It has been suggested that the neuroprotective effects of transplanted cells occur *via* the production and secretion of NTFs (Bull et al., 2008). So far, many different cell types including bone marrow mesenchymal stem cells (Inoue et al., 2007), embryonic stem (ES) cells (Banin et al., 2006) and neuronal stem cells (Grozdanic et al.,2006) have been used for the treatment of retinal degeneration and were found to integrate into the retina and differentiate into mature cell types. Transplantation of photoreceptor precursors to rhodopsin-deficient mice retinas resulted in incorporation and differentiation of progenitors to fully functional photoreceptors (MacLaren et al., 2006 and Bartsch et al., 2008). Similar strategies could be used for RGCs, but the mechanism could be more complicated. In the rat model of raised IOP by laser treatment, oligodendrocyte precursor cells (OPCs) were intravitreally transplanted to the retina. Transplanted OPCs survived up to 12 weeks post surgery and were found to localize in proximity to the RGCs. The transplanted cells increased survival rate of injured RGCs by up to 60% (Bull et al., 2009). Use of MSCs derived from bone marrow of patients is therapeutically very attractive because it allows autologous transplantation and has less ethical issues. This strategy was successfully used in an elevated IOP rat model by Yu et al. (2006) which resulted in significant RGC neuroprotection.

### 2.4.4 Neuroprotection *via* NT receptors and/or their downstream signaling modifications

Increasing NT concentrations was not always sufficient for neuronal survival and/or regeneration and the effects of administration of NTs were usually only transient. In some cases intraocular injections of NTs promoted neuronal survival; however, they also produced axonal dystrophy (Pernet et al., 2006). As previously discussed, there needs to be a balance between NTs and their receptors (Trk and p75), which depending on the cellular context can trigger contrary biological effects (anti- or pro- survival). Since there were difficulties with long-term stable administration of NTs in animal models of glaucoma and retinopathy, the selective agonists of Trk receptors or antagonists of p75 or their downstream pathway components have been studied as anti-glaucoma treatments. Combinations of growth factors and antagonist of protein forming complexes with Trk receptors can promote a sustained and efficacious rescue of ganglion cells. For instance, in the rat experimental model of laser derived ocular hypertension, an antagonist of LINGO-1, which was known to form a complex with TrkB receptor, produced its inhibition and long term protection of RGCs. This study showed that combined treatment of RGC by intravitreal injections of BDNF and LINGO-1-Fc provided long lasting neuroprotection after elevated IOP. This treatment was responsible for stable activation of the TrkB receptor (Fu et al., 2009).

Therapeutic use of NGF has been able to only partially rescue RGCs from apoptosis and failed because the action depends on the receptor (TrkA or p75). This was supported by the finding that the TrkA receptor agonist (peptidomimetic D3) was effective in the treatment of experimental glaucoma caused by elevated IOP and decreased RGCs loss by 25% (She et al., 2007). However the best results were obtained by a combination of a TrkA receptor agonist together with a pressure lowering drug (betaxolol) in which 90% reduction of RGCs loss was observed (Shi et al., 2007). The synergistic effect of a combination of NGF and peptidomimetic TrkA agonist, along with a peptidomimetic p75 antagonist prevented RGC cells loss following optic nerve transection (Lebrun-Julien et al., 2009). p75 increased production of neurotoxic proteins TNF-α and α(2)-macroglobulin. p75 was found to be expressed by the majority of glia and Muller cells and TrkA was found mainly in RGCs (Lebrun-Julien et al., 2009). In another study, wild type NGF failed to protect RGCs in tested models of glaucoma and nerve axotomy. NGF-C, a NGF selective agonist of TrkA, which does not bind to p75, was found to increase neuronal survival by 17% two weeks following axotomy and by 13% in a ocular hypertension glaucoma model. Other approaches used an anti-NGF monoclonal antibody (mAb NGF30) blocking NGF binding to p75 without changes in NGF-TrkA interaction. This treatment caused a doubling of RGC survival post-axotomy and a 15% increase in RGC survival in an ocular hypotension model. Moreover, authors tested p75 receptor antagonists (THX-B and LM-24) in ON axotomy and ocular hypotension and found 37% and 21% RGC survival in the two experimental models. Antagonists of p75 inhibit TNF-α and α(2)-macroglobulin expression and were found to be neuroprotective in ON axotomy and ocular hypertension (Bai et al, 2010). Other approaches have employed Trk B agonists to produce neuroprotective effects. Unfortunately, many TrkB agonists were not able to fully mimic neuroprotective functions of BDNF on TrkB receptors. To discover small molecules having similar potency as BDNF, the authors developed a cell-based apoptotic assay and identified a potent TrkB agonist, deoxygedunin. Deoxygeduin was able to activate only TrkB, in a BDNF-independent manner evoking antiapoptotic cell pathways (ERK1/2 and AKT activation). When intravenously injected into mice (5mg/kg), deoxygeduin penetrated the blood brain barrier and strongly mimicked BDNF, in terms of its neuroprotective ability (Jang et al., 2010).

There are many complications in developing and testing new active ligands with greater specificity for pro-survival NTF receptors. Due to those difficulties, there were strategies developed to avoid receptor *per se* and activate downstream pro-survival pathways. There is still an incomplete understanding of the complexity of NT receptors signaling pathways, in particular to differentiate between target-mediated and cell body-mediated neurotrophin signaling. Zhou et al. (2005) hypothesized that stable activation of pro-survival ERK1/2 kinase, which is a downstream effector of Trk receptors, inhibits RGC death. Since MEK1 is a direct upstream activator of ERK1/2, increase in MEK1 should activate ERK1/2 expression. The authors found significant RGC protection in the AAV-MEK1 mice, with up to 60% greater survival compared to control mice after the $5^{th}$ week of treatment (Zhou et al., 2005). Another study evaluated the neuroprotective effect of modification of downstream NTs effectors. A NK-4 cyanine dye produced neurotrophic effects and promoted neurite-outgrowth and cell proliferation of PC12 cells. Action of NK-4 was dependent on activation of PI3K-AKT but occurred independently of Trk. NK-4 additionally induced phosphorylation of AKT kinase. The authors showed increased cell count indicative of enhanced survival in the treated group versus control (Ohta et al., 2011).

Another key target for neuroprotection of RGCs is Rho kinase which is a member of the serine-threonine family of protein kinases activated by the small G protein Rho. Rho kinase inhibition has been shown to be beneficial for IOP regulation in patients and also enhances RGC survival and axon regeneration (Rao and Epstein, 2007). An attempt to modify downstream signaling of NT receptors was to stably inactivate Rho GTPase, which was shown previously to be a downstream effector of p75 /LINGO-1/Nogo-R complex which formation leads to cell death (Nykjaer et al., 2005). It is also known that neurotrophin (NGF, BDNF or NT-3) binding abolished RhoA activation. Inactivation of Rho proteins mimicked the effect of neurotrophins by increasing the rate of neurite elongation. (Yamashita et al., 2005). Bertrand et al. (2007) used multiple intraocular injections of membrane permeable C3-like Rho antagonists and found that sustained Rho inactivation acts as a pro-survival mechanism following optic nerve injury showing a 1.5 fold increase in RGCs survival. Co-receptor of p75 - NogoR can activate Rho kinase in a p75 dependent manner. In neurons, Rho has been shown to play a role in the regulation of apoptosis. The Rho antagonist C3–05 (to suppress Rho activation) was tested in the rodent model of acute nerve injury. In mice and rats treated with Rho-C3–05 the extent of cell death was significantly reduced by ~50% post- injury. The correlation between Rho kinase and p75 receptor was based on co-localization of active Rho with p75 after injury. Rho inactivation after injury inhibited apoptosis by preventing the synthesis of pro-apoptotic p75 receptor (Wang et al., 2002). The Rho antagonist C3-07 was successfully used in another study resulting in survival of RGCs by 1.5 fold after optic nerve lesion (Bertrand et al., 2007).

#### 2.4.4.1 Other neuroprotective approaches

Shi et al. (2008) studied α-2-macroglobulin (α2-M) inhibitors for their neuroprotective abilities. It was found that α-2M act as a sink for NTs and therefore inhibits their bioavailability during glaucoma. The authors elevated IOP in rats by cauterization and by the Morrison's model to test their hypothesis that neutrophic deficit is due to neutralization of neutrophins by α-2M. They proved that blocking α-2M, using specific inhibiting antibodies against α-2M was protective for RGCs even without lowering IOP (29% protection). Together with normalization of IOP the neutralization effect were even more pronounced (35% protection) (Shi et al., 2008).

Erythropoietin (Epo) is a glycoprotein hormone, synthesized in the kidney secreted by interstitial cells of the adrenal cortex in response to tissue hypoxia. Epo is a neurotrophic factor that could be developed as a new drug for neurological disorders. Epo posses a specific Epo/Epo-receptor system in the CNS and cerebrospinal fluid (Buemi et al., 2002). Zhong et al. (2007) studied the neuroprotective effects of intraperitoneal administration of erythropoietin(Epo) in the DBA/2J mouse model of glaucoma. Treatment with Epo at doses of 3000, 6000, and 12,000 U/kg body weight per week promoted RGC survival in DBA/2J glaucomatous mice without affecting IOP. These results suggested that Epo may be used as a potential therapeutic neuroprotectant in glaucoma. Since Epo does not cross the blood-brain barrier (BBB) there is a tendency to recombine its structure that way that it will became permeable to BBB. Boado et al. (2010) developed new drug (HIRMAb(IgG)-EPO fusion protein) enabling Epo to cross the BBB.

### 2.4.5 Potential methods for NTs delivery

Topical eye drops, intraocular injections and systemically-administered compounds have been the conventional systems for delivering drugs to glaucomatous eye. However, these methods have many limitations and disadvantages. First, there is a factor of patient compliance, efficacy, side effects and absorption of the chemical. Several methods were discovered recently to improve long-term delivery of the drug, control dosage and reduce side effects. The goal might be achieved by different strategies such a slow-release biodegradable microspheres devices commonly made of poly-DL-lactic-co-glycolic acid (PLGA). PLGA spheres can be filled with chosen NT or receptor agonist which when intraocularly injected will result in slow, sustained drug release (Ward et al., 2007). Devices can be filled with not only NTs or receptor agonist/antagonist. It could be also fortified with chemical compounds which have the ability to activate pro-survival or inhibit pro-apoptotic pathways, downstream to NTs. It is also possible to deliver viral constructs or siRNAs to the retina: however, genetic manipulation of human cells always represents a potential biohazard issue. The other new method for sustained delivery of glaucoma medication involves incorporation of the drug into a punctal plug. This method is already used for patients suffering from dry eye syndrome. Another approach is usage of solid lipid nanoparticles loaded with neuroprotective drugs. Researchers have reported promising results from experiments using laboratory-created nanoparticles to deliver a glaucoma medication (Li et al., 2011). Investigations into this approach for treating glaucoma were in very early stages. This approach can also be used for NTs delivery. Animal experiments using nanoparticles demonstrated that they can actively migrate through the vitreous and neurosensory retinal layers, reaching the retinal pigment epithelium and choroid. This capability has proved to be useful particularly in treatment of retinal degeneration diseases. Nanotechnology can be used in ophthalmology to treat retinal degenerative disease with gene therapy, prosthetics, and regenerative nanomedicine (Zarbin et al., 2010). Another emerging technology for drug delivery to the eye is encapsulated cell technology (ECT). ECT has also been developed to treat diseases of the central nervous system and the eye (Tao et al., 2002). ECT could be applied to neurodegeneration treatment in glaucomatous eyes. This device can serve as a source of neurotrophic factors produced by encapsulated cells in the eye. Such an approach was already successfully used to delivery CNTF in a dog model of retinitis pigmentosa.

## 3. Calcium channel blockers

Calcium channel blockers (CCBs) have a therapeutic potential in treating glaucomatous optic neuropathy. However, their therapeutic potential as neuroprotectants has not yet been fully realized to treat glaucoma or other chronic neurodegenerative diseases. This section will discuss the importance of neuronal calcium signaling under normal physiological conditions. Secondly this section will then discuss the proposed hypothesis of calcium dysregulation in playing a key role in apoptosis, and the proposed mechanism of ischemia-reperfusion that has been demonstrated to occur in some cases of glaucoma. Lastly, this section will then discuss CCBs as neuroprotective pharmaceutical agents, retinal vessel dilators, and IOP lowering agents.

Under physiological conditions, calcium is an important neuronal intracellular signaling molecule found at very low cytoplasmic concentrations (100 nM) under normal non-excited states (1-2 mM extracellularly). This low intracellular calcium concentration allows a strong inward electrochemical gradient, and facilitates the ability for calcium to be used as a quick communicator to activate and suppress a number of different genes and signaling pathways that are critical for neuronal survival, long term potentiation, and synaptic plasticity. Interestingly, it seems that not all calcium influx is considered equal. Different subset of neuronal signaling pathways can be activated depending on which channel is used to mediate calcium conduction inside neurons.

RGCs are the output neurons of the retina that conveys all the visual information obtained from the retina to the brain. Different synaptic inputs are received on the dendrites of RGCs from bipolar cells and amacrine cells. The normal flow of electrical potentials through the retina is initiated at the back of the retina starting from the photoreceptor cells. The electrical information then travels from photoreceptor cells to bipolar cells, and finally to RGCs.

Glutamate is the main excitatory neurotransmitter that is released from photoreceptor cells and biopolar cells. Typically horizontal cells and amacrine cells modulate the electrical signal at the outer and inner plexiform layers respectively. Figure 7 shows various layers of the retina(A) and a representative retina flat mount (B).

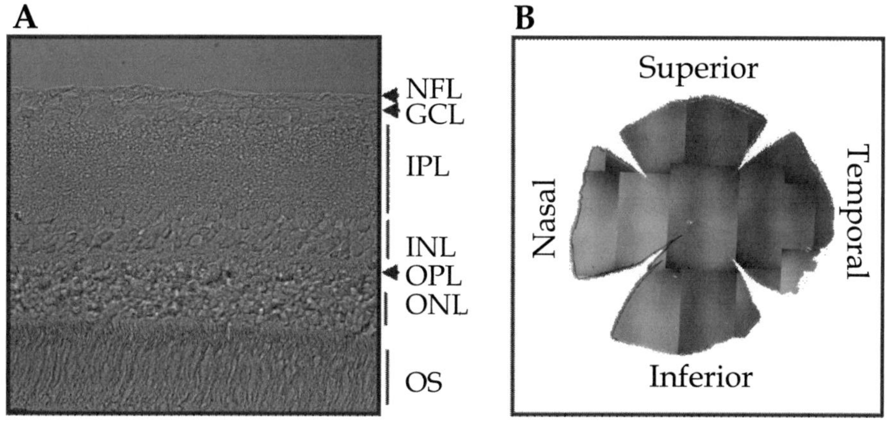


Fig. 7. A. Organization of the retinal layers. Confocal microscopic image of a rat retina section. The different layers of the retina are indicated in the picture: Nerve fiber layer (NFL), Ganglion cell layer (GCL), Inner plexiform layer (IPL), Inner nuclear layer (INL), Outer plexiform layer (OPL), Outer nuclear layer (ONL) and Outer Segment (OS). B. Representative flat mount showing different areas of the retina including superior, inferior, nasal and temporal

Once glutamate is released from the axonal terminals of bipolar cells, it will migrate through the synaptic cleft to interact with glutamate receptors found on the dendrites of RGCs. Glutamate receptors are divided into two main classes: ionotropic and metabotropic. The ionotropic glutamate receptors are further divided into NMDA and non-NMDA subtypes. The non-NMDA receptors are also known as AMPAr and Kainate receptors. NMDA receptors are known for their ability to be highly permeable to $Ca^{2+}$ ion influx once they are activated. Typically NMDA receptors need both glutamate and glycine to be activated. However, NMDA receptors are subject to a $Mg^{2+}$ blockade preventing calcium ion influx when the membrane potential is at rest (-90 to -70 mV). This $Mg^{2+}$ can only be removed from the NMDA receptor complex once the membrane potential of the dendrites reaches between -20 and -30 mV. (Mayer et al., 1984; Ozawa et al., 1998) The $Mg^{2+}$ blockade is typically relieved by raising the membrane potential through the activation of non-NMDA receptors. The stimulation of these ionotropic receptors causes excitatory postsynaptic currents that then go to further activate voltage gated calcium channels (VGCCs). VGCCs are divided into two major classes of $Ca^{2+}$ channels based upon the membrane potential that opens them. There are low-voltage activated (LVA) and high-voltage activated (HVA) channels. These channels can be further divided into T-type which is the LVA and L-, N-, P/Q, and R-type which are all HVA. Of the VGCCs, L-type is the one that is associated with calcium-mediated neuronal injury because of the prolong calcium influx that occurs when this channel is activated (Mark et al., 2001). Additionally, prolonged stimulation of VGCCs and NMDA channels has been shown in cortical neurons to suppress mitochondrial movement in the dendrites (Li et al., 2004).

Under normal physiological conditions, calcium signaling inside neurons mediates a number of second messenger pathways. For example, when calcium influx occurs through neuronal L-type VGCCs that are encoded by the CaV1.2 and CaV1.3 pore-forming subunits, the channel has the ability to activate CREB, MEF, and NFAT that can lead to the expression of genes like *c-fos* and *bdnf* (Graef et al., 1999; Mao et al., 1999; Sheng et al., 1990; Morgan and Curran, 1986; Murphy et al., 1991; Zafra et al., 1990). Similarly, NMDA receptors expressing NR2A-containing glutamate receptors have demonstrated to promote long term potentiation through Ras-GRF2 and ERK MAP kinase activation (Flammer et al., 1994). It is evident that calcium signaling through ionotropic glutamate receptors and VGCCs are essential and needed for neuronal survival and functionality. However, one caveat in all of these studies is that the data has not been replicated in primary RGCs. So though, it can be assumed that RGCs are an excitatory neuron and probably do behave in a similar fashion to cortical excitatory neurons, there is not much information to determine if cell survival and long term potentiation pathways are also activated in RGCs when NMDA and L-type VGCCs are activated.

In chronic neurological disease processes, it is plausible that the beneficial effects that occur from neuronal calcium signaling are suppressed, and an overload of calcium causes activation of the apoptotic cascade. For example, normal stimulation of intrasynaptic NMDA receptors under physiological conditions causes activation of many pro-survival pathways which lead to phosphorylation of cAMP response element-binding protein (CREB) through activation of calmodulin-dependent protein (CaM) kinase pathway and Ras-extracellular signal-regulated kinase 1/2 (ERK1/2) pathway (Hardingham et al., 2001; Wu et al., 2001; and Hardingham et al., 2001b). However, extrasynaptic NMDA stimulation suppresses CREB activation through the inactivation of Ras-ERK1/2 pathway (Hardingham et al., 2002; Hardingham et al., 2002b; and Ivanov et al. 2006). These opposing pathways are activated through similar receptors in different neuronal locations and demonstrate the importance of compartmentalization of calcium signaling in the neuron. When the same ionotropic calcium channel is stimulated, the location of that channel dictates the secondary pro-survival/pro-apoptotic pathways that are stimulated. It is clear from all these studies that basal calcium signaling is beneficial for the neuron, but overstimulation of these extrasynaptic NMDA receptors is detrimental for neuronal survival causing stimulation of apoptotic enzymes including calcineurin and calpain.

Calcineurin is a calmodulin-dependent serine-threonine phosphatase that activates Bad through dephosphorylation. This dephosphorylation causes BAD to dissociated from the inhibiting protein 14-3-3 and cause it to move into the mitochondrial outer membrane. Once Bad is on the outer mitochondrial members, it will bind to anti-apoptotic Bcl-2 or Bcl-XL and promote release of cytochrome c. (Wang et al., 1999; Heckman et al., 2006) Calcineurin activation and cytochrome c release has been linked with RGC death after optic nerve crush. (Huang et al., 2005) Lastly, RGC death has been shown to be attenuated in experimental models of optic nerve crush after treatment with a calcineurin inhibitor, FK506 (Huang et al., 2005).

Calpain is a $Ca^{2+}$-dependent cysteine protease that is implicated in many neurodegenerative diseases such as Alzheimer's disease, Parkinson's disease and Huntington's disease (Nixon, 2003; Goll et al., 2003) Calpain activates calcineurin and transforms it into its constitutively activated form. Calpain activation has been detected in rat experimental glaucoma, (Huang et al., 2010) while its inactivation has demonstrated protection against excitotoxic neuronal cell death *in vitro* and *in vivo* (Wu et al., 2004).

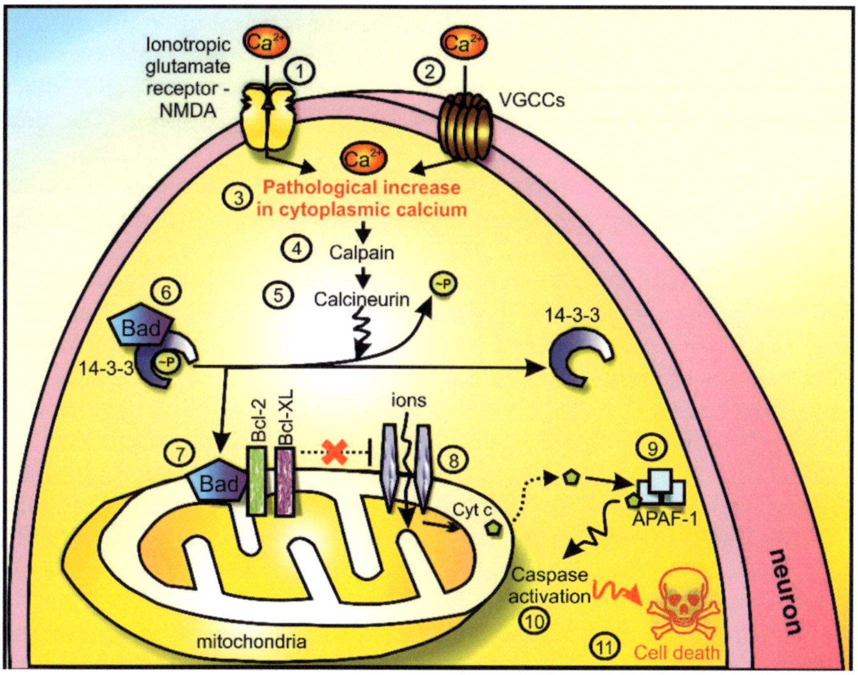


Fig. 8. Calcium-induced apoptotic changes in neurons. Intracellular calcium in increased through the sequential actions of NMDA and voltage-dependent calcium channels. Elevated $Ca^{2+}$ activates a number of factors including calpain and calcineurin which have downstream effects on substrates. Calcineurin activation promotes dephosphorylation of Bad which in turn initiates mitochondrial dysfunction by its interaction with Bcl2 or Bcl-XL. The disruption of mitochondria releases cytochrome c which activates the apoptotic cascade

Calcium channel blockers (CCBs) are pharmaceutical agents geared at halting calcium influx across cellular membranes and decreasing intracellular calcium levels. These agents are widely used clinically to control patients suffering from benign essential hypertension, angina pectoris, cardiac arrhythmias (like atrial fibrillation and paroxysmal supraventricular tachycardia), and pulmonary hypertension. CCBs have been studied to treat many of the chronic neurological diseases afflicting individuals worldwide. CCBs could in theory act as neuroprotectants to help preserve neuronal viability, especially by halting the upstream activation of calcium sensitive apoptotic proteins (calcineurin and calpain) and can prevent permanent damage from the late stage activation of apoptosis (Loetscher et al., 2001). Many of the theories implicated in RGC death in glaucoma involve some form of calcium dysregulation. So if an appropriate CCB can be identified to treat RGCs vulnerable to apoptosis, then this pharmaceutical agent could halt the activation of many apoptotic pathways early on in the activation of the cell-death pathway. Additionally, CCBs have therapeutic potential in decreasing IOP and increasing retinal blood flow. Therefore, it is possible that a CCB treatment could act as a "silver bullet glaucoma therapy" by decreasing IOP, increasing retinal blood, and protecting RGCs by maintaining calcium homeostasis by acting as a neuroprotectant. The rest of this section will highlight CCBs as a pharmaceutical treatment to treat glaucoma as a neuroprotectant, retinal vessel vasodilator, and IOP reducing molecule.

The use of CCBs to treat glaucoma as a neuroprotectant is based upon the assumption that two fundamental molecular hypothesizes implicated in RGC death in glaucoma are correct. These two hypothesizes are that glutamate excitotoxicity exist, and that calcium dysregulation occurs and activates apoptotic enzymes in glaucoma. The debate over glutamate excitotoxicity as a pathological correlate to RGC death in glaucoma is addressed in the glutamate excitotoxicity portion of this chapter. There does appear to be evidence, as mentioned above, that calcium dysregulation does occur prior to RGC death. Drugs that are geared at blocking calcium ion influx mainly target two classes of ion channels, NMDA receptors and L-type VGCCs. The section on excitotoxicity will touch upon treatments that have shown neuroprotective potential through the blockade of NMDA receptors.

Of the drugs that have been developed and used to treat human pathological conditions, there are three classes of drugs geared at blocking L-type VGCCs. These three main classes are the phenylalkylamine (PAA), or verapamil-like CCBs, the benzothiazepine (BTZ), or diltiazem-like CCBs, and the dihydropyridine (DHP), or nifedipine-like CCBs (Araie and Mayana, 2010). In animal studies, intraperitoneal injections of nifedipine showed neuroprotection and improved b-wave amplitude when rats received retinal ischemic damage (Crosson et al., 1990) Lomerizine is another L-type and T-type CCB that has demonstrated to have neuroprotective effects on ischemic retinal neurons in both *in vitro* and *in vivo* (Toriu et al., 2000). In primary RGC cultures exposed to hypoxic conditions (5% normal partical pressure), iganidipine, nimodipine, and lomerizine demonstrated robust RGC protection (Yamada et al., 2006; Chen et al., 2007).

Another pharmaceutical agent that has demonstrated neuroprotection to RGCs by blocking calcium currents is betaxolol, a β1-adrenoceptor antagonists (Araie and Mayana, 2010). This molecule has demonstrated to have binding affinity to L-type VGCCs and NMDA, and has been shown to decrease calcium influx through the cellular plasma membrane. (Melena et al., 1999; Bessho et al., 1991; Hester et al., 1994; Hoste and Sis, 1998; Setoguchi et al., 1995; Dong et al., 2006; Nagata et al., 2008) Considering the potential that blocking L-type VGCCs has demonstrated as being a neuroprotectant as described above, their may be therapeutic potential for treating patients afflicted with glaucoma with betaxolol as well. Betaxolol may act as an IOP lowering agent and as a neuroprotectant by blocking pathological influxes of calcium through L-type VGCCs. (Hirooka et al., 2000) Topical application of betaxolol has also been reported to induce expression of BDNF in the rat retina. (Wood et al., 2001). In vivo experiments also demonstrated protection through the attenuation of retinal damage to rabbits and rats subjected to ischemic insult (Wood et al., 2001; Wood et al., 2003; Osborne et al., 1999; Osborne et al., 2004; Cheon et al., 2002) or to rat eyes injected with NMDA or kainic acid (Osborne et al., 1999; Cheon et al., 2006). However given betaxolol's L-type VGCC blocking effect, when this drug was tested next to timolol in a large comparative human clinical trial, there was no difference in disease progression between those patients taking either timolol or betaxolol (Watson et al., 2001; Araie et al., 2003). Lastly, in another human clinical trial, the conversion rate from ocular hypertension to glaucoma between betaxolol and placebo was not attenuated between the two treatment groups (Kamal et al., 2003).

The predominant theory of what precipitates the cascade of RGC death in glaucoma is the mechanical compression theory highlighted above. However, another theory of retinal ischemia reperfusion has been put forth to account for RGC loss as a consequence of insufficient retinal blood flow (Flammer, 1994). The retina receives its blood supply from the central retinal artery which is a branch from the ophthalmic artery (Olver, 1998). Insufficient blood flow to the retina is able to produce glaucomatous-like visual field defects, and researchers have speculated that patients suffering from normal tension glaucoma could be developing glaucomatous optic neuropathy because of a vasospastic syndrome (Flammer et al., 1987; Broadway and Drance 1998). Research studies have actually demonstrated that patients suffering from glaucoma are more prone to suffer from vasospastic episodes (Gasser and Flammer, 1991; Rojanapongpun and Drance, 1993; O'Brien 1998). In fact, in some glaucoma patients, improvements are seen in retinal circulation and visual field defects when patients are treated with CCBs (Flammer and Guthauser, 1987; Guthauser et al., 1988).

As mentioned above, CCBs have the ability to block intracellular calcium influx, which can lead to relaxation of vascular smooth muscle and enable enhanced blood flow to perfuse certain organs. There are numerous studies that have been conducted in looking at the effects of nifedipine, nicardipine, verapamil, nimodipine, nilvadipine, and lomerizine on ocular blood flow and their abilities to counteract retinal vasospasm. In a prospective clinical trial, Kitazawa et al. (1989) treated 25 patients suffering from normal tension glaucoma with oral nifedipine for 6 months and was able to demonstrate improved visual fields. However, another study performed by Harris et al. (1997) showed that 6-month treatment with oral nifedipine in 21 patients failed to demonstrated significant difference in visual field and spatal contrast sensitivity. Another prospective study performed on patients with open angle glaucoma showed that a 3 month treatment with nifedipine had no affect on improving visual fields compared with the control group (Rainer et al., 2001). In contrast, nimodipine has demonstrated in multiple prospective clinical trials to improve visual function in normal tension glaucoma patients (Bose et al., 1995; Piltz et al., 1998; Boehm et al., 2003; Luksch et al., 2005) How some of these CCBs demonstrated improvement in visual function in patients suffering from glaucoma is unknown, but perhaps it could have been through both a vasodilator affect, and a direct neuroprotective effect on the RGCs.

A final therapeutic target for CCBs is their ability to lower IOP when given topically. The mechanism of action of CCBs in lowering IOP is still controversial. L-type VGCCs have been shown to exist on both human and bovine trabecular meshwork (TM) cells (Steinhausen et al., 2000; Wiederholt et al., 2000; Thieme et al., 2005). Ciliary epithelial cells also have DHP-sensitive, VGCCs (Farahbakhsh et al., 1994). CCBs act by decreasing in-flow through its effects on ciliary epithelial cells, or improve outflow through its effects on the TM cells. Out of all the therapies used to treat glaucoma, CCBs have the capability to lower IOP while also increasing retinal blood flow and protecting RGCs from pathological influxes of cytoplasmic calcium.

Though there is a lot of evidence correlating pathological influx of cytoplasmic calcium with RGC death, the fact of the matter is that there are probably many pathological pathways acting in concert with one another to elicit RGC apoptosis (Qu et al., 2010). For example, astrocytes and retinal glial cells can fail to take up glutamate from the excess glutamate that is being released from damaged RGCs in glaucoma (Adachi et al., 1998; Danbolt, 2001) Therefore, excitoxicity then can cause pathological influx of calcium ions through overactivation of NMDA receptors and VGCCs. This elevation of calcium ions can not only cause activation of calcium specific apoptotic enzymes, but also generate large amounts of free radicals which can in-turn cause oxidative stress (Tezel, 2006). So therefore, it is not only important to investigate potential therapeutic targets that are geared at protecting RGCs from cell death caused by glaucomatous optic neuropathy insults, but it is just as important to understand basic cellular and molecular mechanisms underlying neuronal cell death in glaucoma.

## 4. Glutamate excitotoxicity

Excitotoxicity is a process by which excitatory amino acids such as glutamic acid (glutamate) and aspartic acid produce overstimulation of their receptors leading to neurotoxicity and/or neurodegeneration. Glutamate is a major excitatory neurotransmitter both in the brain and in the retina. The excitatory neurotransmitters in the brain include glutamate and aspartate, while the inhibitory neurotransmitters include GABA, glycine and taurine. In the retina, glutamate is the primary neurotransmitter that is involved in the visual transduction pathway. Glutamate is an $\alpha$-amino acid containing a second carboxylic acid (-COOH) group attached to the $\gamma$-carbon atom. In the CNS, glutamate does not cross the blood brain barrier, hence in neurons, glutamate is made from $\alpha$-ketoglutarate, an intermediate of the TCA cycle. Another source of glutamate is the conversion of glutamine obtained from glial cells to glutamate within neurons. This cycle is described in Figure 9.

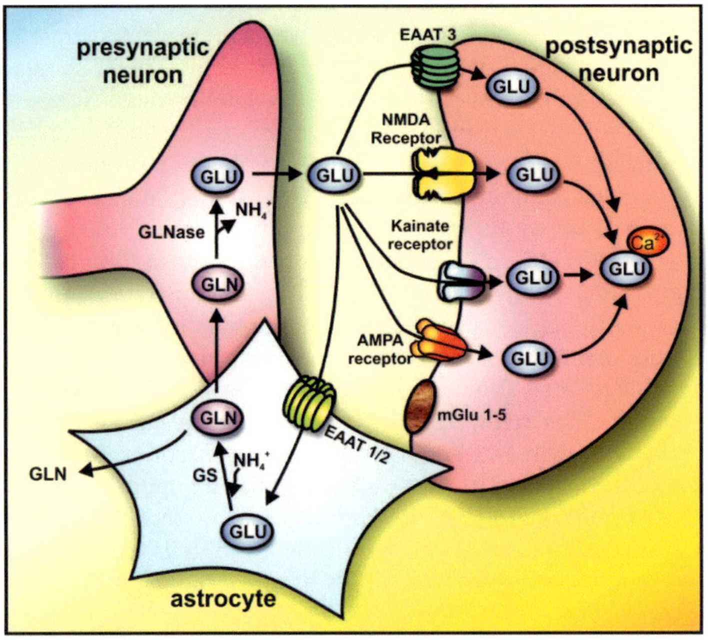


Fig. 9. The Glutamate-Glutamine cycling between neurons and glia. Glutamate (GLU) is taken up by glial cells and converted to glutamine (GLN) by the enzyme glutamine synthase (GS). Glutamine is transported by the action of excitatory amino acid transporters (EAATs) back to the neurons where it is converted back to glutamate by the enzyme glutaminase (GLNase)

Glutamate is generated by the enzyme, glutaminase, in the endoplasmic reticulum, packaged in the golgi apparatus into membrane-bound vesicles and transported down the axon by anterograde axonal transport on microtubules to the synaptic junctions. The membranes of the vesicles merge with the synaptic membrane and glutamate is released by exocytosis into the synaptic space. Upon release into the synapse, glutamate binds to glutamate receptors in the post-synaptic membranes. There are two principal classes of glutamate receptors: ionotropic and metabotropic receptors. Ionotropic receptors are ligand-gated ion channels which produce an influx of calcium and sodium ions upon binding to glutamate and similar agonists. Metabotropic receptors are G-protein coupled receptors which couple ligand binding to intracellular signal transduction mechanisms mediated by a variety of second messengers including cAMP and intracellular calcium. Excitotoxicity is mediated by ionotropic receptors which can be characterized into various subtypes according to the type of the selective agonist including, N-methyl D-aspartate (NMDA), α-amino-3-hydroxy-5-methyl-4-isoxazolepropionate (AMPA) and kainate. These agonists are not naturally occurring, but have a structural resemblance to glutamate. Glutamate binds to and activates all three classes of receptors namely, NMDA, AMPA and kainate receptors. NMDA receptor activation is important for synaptic plasticity which plays a key role in memory and learning. However, overstimulation of NMDA receptors contributes to elevation of intracellular calcium leading to neuronal injury.

The NMDA receptor has a tetrameric structures composed of two subunits of NR1 and NR2 subunits (Figure 10). There are four subtypes of NR2 subunits called NR2A, NR2B, NR2C and NR2D. Other related subunits including NR3 and NR4 have inhibitory effect on receptor activity. Activation of the NMDA receptor requires binding of two molecules of glutamate and two molecules of glycine which acts as a co-agonist. The AMPA receptor (AMPAr) also functions as a tetramer comprised of four different types of subunits including GluR1 to GluR4. Most AMPA receptors have a structure comprising of a combination of a dimer of GluR2 with a dimer of either GluR1, GluR3 or GluR4 (Figure 10). Each subunit of the AMPA receptor has a binding site for glutamate. Binding of glutamate to AMPA receptors causes an opening of the ion channel leading to an influx of sodium ions. AMPA and kainate receptors play an important role in facilitating rapid excitatory neurotransmission by rapid conduction of $Na^+$ ions. AMPA receptors in the retina are also permeable to $Ca^{2+}$ ions. Electrical stimulation of a presynaptic neuron causes glutamate release which activate AMPA receptors in the post-synaptic neuron. Activation of AMPAr causes depolarization of the post-synaptic neuron. However glutamate binding to NMDA receptors in weakly depolarized postsynaptic neurons is not sufficient to trigger activation of the receptors. NMDA receptors possess a high conductance $Ca^{2+}$ channels which in normal resting state have a magnesium block that prevents activation of the channel. However, high frequency activation of the AMPAr (due to arrival of a train of nerve impulses) causes a release of the magnesium block of the NMDA receptors producing an influx of calcium ions. AMPArs have a dual role in neuroprotection depending upon their spatiotemporal pattern of expression. Increased expression of GluR1 in neurons has been demonstrated to facilitate dendrite outgrowth and synaptogenesis, while increased expression of GluR2 preserves existing dendritic arbors (Prithiviraj et al., 2008). This dynamic receptor moves into and out of the plasma membrane, and when the AMPAr complex is comprised of both the GluR1 and GluR2 subunits, it is correlated with synaptogenesis and long term potentiation (LTP) (Malinow and Malenka, 2002).

Under pathological conditions, when neurons are under stress, AMPAr is also implicated in cell death by excitotoxicity through the increase permeability of AMPAr to calcium ions by the endocytosis of GluR2 (Beattie et al., 2010). During elevation of IOP in a rodent model, GluR2 expression in the dying RGCs demonstrated a decreased level of expression, implying that this decrease level of GluR2 expression made the RGCs more susceptible to calcium overload through the increased permeability of calcium through the AMPArs. Typically AMPArs are impervious to calcium ion influx when GluR2 is associated with the AMPAr complex on the plasma membrane. So how can increased AMPAr expression be implicated both as a neuroprotective, neurotrophic physiological cellular process, and also associated with increased neuronal excitotoxicity when neurons are under pathological stress? The answer appears to be in the ability to maintain GluR2 expression in the AMPAr complex in order to impede calcium ion influx through AMPAr on the plasma membrane while maintaining the beneficial role that AMPAr (GluR1/GluR2) plays in promoting dendritic outgrowth and promoting LTP (Gainey et al., 2009). Kainate receptors also have a tetrameric structure comprising of a combination of GluR5, GluR6 and GluR7 subunits. The role of kainite receptors is not as well understood as the NMDA and AMPA receptors (Figure 10).

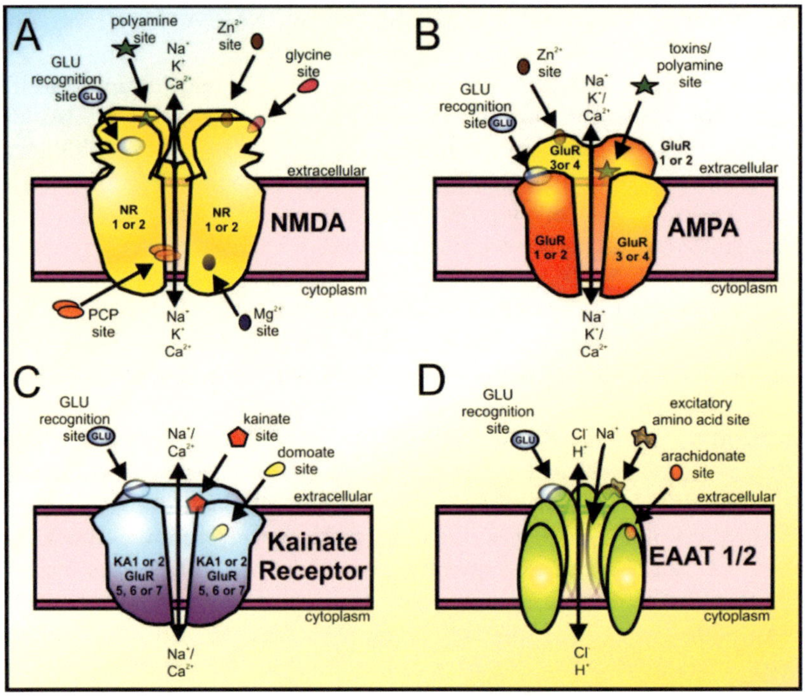


Fig. 10. Classes of glutamate receptors and transporters. Glutamate acts by binding to three main classes of receptors including NMDA (A), AMPA (B) and Kainate receptors (C) which are ligand-gated ion channels. All the glutamate receptors are permeable to sodium, and calcium ions. NMDA receptor is a tetramer comprising of two subunits of NR1 and NR2. AMPA receptor contains four different types of subunits called GluR 1 to GluR4. Kainate receptors are also tetrameric in structure and their subunits are named KA1 and KA2 and GluR5 to GluR7. EAAT is a excitatory glutamate transporter which is a high affinity sodium dependent membrane-bound carrier protein having a ion channel-like structure

While glutamate is the primary neurotransmitter in the vertical pathway of the retina (from photoreceptor to bipolar cells to ganglion cells), abnormal increase in glutamate has been thought contribute to retinal injury. One of the earliest observations describing glutamate excitotoxicity was made by Hayashi in 1954 who observed seizure activities in brain after administration of glutamate to neonatal mice. Subsequently, Lucas and Newhouse (1957) reported that postnatal mice fed with monosodium glutamate show loss of inner retinal neurons. These observations were the basis of "glutamate excitotoxicity" hypothesis in glaucoma. Excitotoxicity has also been shown to occur in clinical conditions including traumatic brain injury, stoke, epilepsy, and also in various neurodegenerative diseases including Huntington disease, amyotrophic lateral sclerosis, AIDS dementia. Elevation of intracellular calcium is thought to be the primary mechanism leading to excitotoxicity by glutamate. The intracellular calcium levels are maintained at low levels (typically 100 nM in most cell types), while extracellular calcium concentrations are much higher (1 to 2 mM). NMDA receptors activation cause calcium influx into cells which produces membrane depolarization and this activates voltage-dependent calcium channels. Opening of these channels amplifies the calcium response, thereby exacerbating calcium overload in the cells. Calcium levels homeostasis maintained by a variety of calcium pumps and antiporters in the plasma membrane, endoplasmic reticulum and mitochondria. $Ca^{2+}$-ATPases use energy inherent in ATP hydrolysis to pump calcium ions across the plasma membrane by active transport. These pumps have high affinity but low capacity, pumping out one $Ca^{2+}$ ion for each molecule of ATP hydrolyzed. Sodium calcium exchangers act as antiporters use the sodium gradient across the plasma membrane to exchange calcium ions for sodium ions. However under conditions of ischemia, due to poor energy (ATP) production, the sodium gradients across cell membranes are decreased thereby affect the ability antiporters to extrude $Ca^{2+}$ ions (Figure 11). All these factors contribute to elevation of cytosolic calcium. Increase in cytosolic calcium activates a variety of signaling molecules that influence the fate of cell survival. For example calcium binds to calmodulin and activate CaM kinase II which phosphorylates a variety of substrates, various enzymes and transcription factors. Calcium activates calpains which degrades essential cellular proteins. Calcium also activates endonucleases and promotes cleavage of genomic DNA.

One of the key targets of elevated intracellular calcium is the mitochondria, which undergoes changes that could lead to opening of the permeability transition pore (Nickells, 2004). The mitochondrial calcium antiporter is a low affinity high capacity calcium transporter that pumps calcium ions into the mitochondria upon elevation of cytoplasmic calcium. $Ca^{2+}$ build up in the mitochondria produces mitochondrial swelling by dissipating the voltage gradient between the outer and inner mitochondrial membrane. The inner mitochondrial membrane is flexible and thrown into multiple folds called cristae, and is therefore able to withstand the increase in volume. However the outer mitochondria membrane is unable to accommodate the increase in volume and ruptures, leading to release of cytochrome c from the mitochondria. The released cytochrome c forms a complex with apoptotic protein activating factor-1 (APAF-1) and caspase 9 to form the apoptosome which in turns activates the caspases which cleave a variety of structural and regulatory protein thereby leading to apoptotic death of cells.

Excitatory amino acid transporters (EAATs): After glutamate is released into the synaptic cleft, it is not degraded since there are no extracellular enzymes for its degradation. Glutamatergic transmission is terminated by rapid uptake of glutamate by a variety of specific glutamate transporters which are called excitatory amino acid transporters (EAATs) (Beretta et al., 2003). There are several classes of EAATs including EAAT1 (GLAST), EAAT2 (GLT), EAAT3 (EAAC), EAAT4 and EAAT5 (expressed mainly in the retina) each of which is encoded by distinct genes (Beretta et al., 2003). EAAT1 expression has been observed mainly in astrocytes throughout the CNS. EAAT1 is a plasma membrane bound protein and rarely detected in the cytoplasm. EAAT2 is also a plasma membrane protein expressed in astrocytes in various cerebral areas. EAAT3 is a major excitatory amino acid transporter in the neurons and highly expressed in hippocampus, cerebellum, and basal ganglia. EAAT4 expressed has been observed both in the cytoplasm and plasma membrane. EAAT4 is

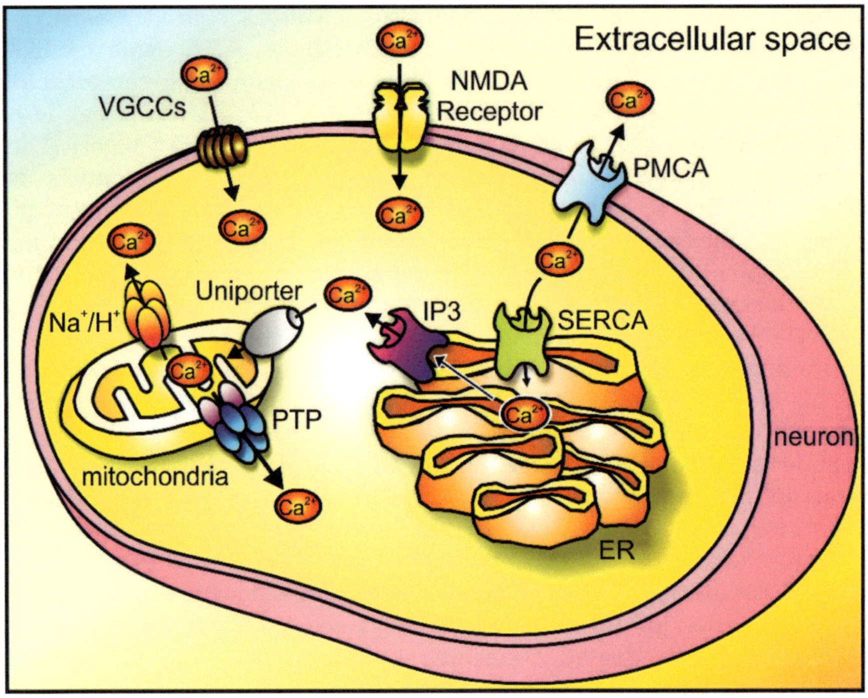


Fig. 11. Calcium homeostasis in cells. Intracellular calcium is elevated mainly by ionotropic receptors (for example, glutamate receptors), which in turn could activate voltage-sensitive calcium channels and store-operated channels. Elevated intracellular $Ca^{2+}$ can produce a variety of cellular changes by binding to calmodulin and activating various signaling pathways or can be sequestered into the endoplasmic reticulum or mitochondria. Sarcoplasmic reticulum $Ca^{2+}$-ATPase (SERCA) pumps promote uptake of $Ca^{2+}$ into the endoplasmic reticulum. On the other hand, activation of inositol-1,4,5-trisphosphate ($IP_3$) receptors in the endoplasmic reticulum or sarcoplasmic reticulum promote release of $Ca^{2+}$ from these intracellular stores . The resting calcium is maintained at 100 nM by both uptake into the ER and $Ca^{2+}$ release from cells by the action of plasma-membrane $Ca^{2+}$-ATPase (PMCA). The mitochondria has a uniporter that takes up $Ca^{2+}$ from the cytosol, however it can release it by reversal of the uniporter. Other mechanisms contributing to release of $Ca^{2+}$ from the mitochondria include $Na^+/H^+$-dependent $Ca^{2+}$ exchange, or opening of the permeability transition pore (PTP). $Ca^{2+}$ efflux from cells occurs mainly by the PMCA, which binds calmodulin and has a high affinity for $Ca^{2+}$

localized in the plasma membrane mainly in Purkinje cells. Expression of EAATs is decreased by conditions of transient global ischemia. Treatment with different cytokines including tumor necrosis factor-α (TNF-α), interferon-γ and interleukin-1β have been shown to inhibit glutamate uptake. TNF-α appears mediate this effect by decreasing GLAST and GLT expression in astrocytes. TNF-α levels have been shown to be elevated in glaucoma primarily in glial cells (Nakagawa et al., 2006; Tezel, 2008) and this could be one factor that contributing to glutamate elevation during glaucomatous insults. These observations are significant in the light of recent studies which suggest that glial activation is an early and key event in glaucoma disease progression (Nickells, 2007).

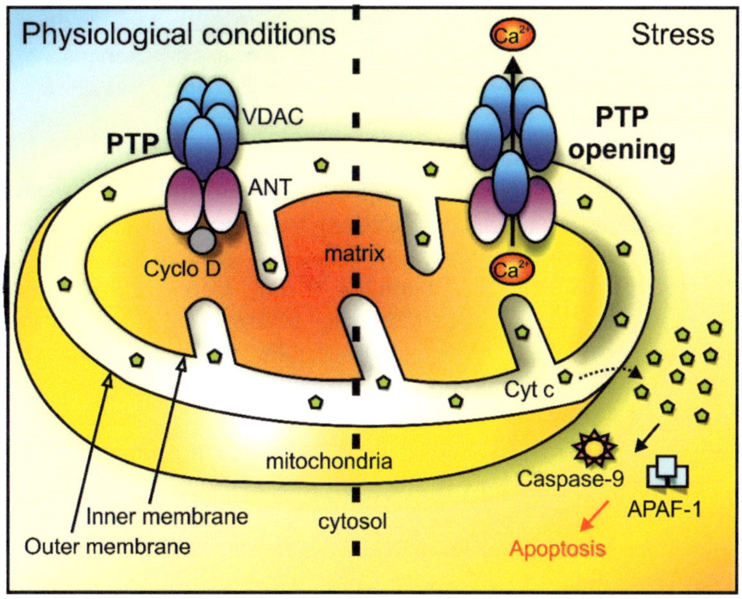


Fig. 12. $Ca^{2+}$ and Mitochondrial Permeability Transition Pore. One of the consequences of elevation of intracellular calcium is the opening of permeability transition pore, which is a conductance pore comprising of a complex of adenine nucleotide translocator (ANT) (in the inner mitochondrial membrane) and voltage-dependent anion channel (in the outer membrane). Under conditions of cellular stress, the complex forms an open pore at the junction of the outer and inner mitochondrial membrane. Opening of the opens dissipates the ionic gradient across the mitochondrial membrane, produces mitochondrial swelling and release of $Ca^{2+}$ from the mitochondria. Cytochrome c (Cyt c) is another factor that is released from the mitochondria due to opening of the PTP and rupture of the outer mitochondrial membrane. The released cytochrome c forms a complex with procaspase 9 and apoptotic protein activating factor-1 (APAF-1) to activate the caspase cascade and promote apoptosis

### 4.1 Glutamate elevation in glaucoma

Excitotoxicity due to elevation of glutamate concentrations is an attractive hypothesis to account for retinal ganglion cell death in glaucoma. However, there is no consistent evidence for increased glutamate in animal models of glaucoma. Dreyer et al (1996) found a 2-fold increase in glutamate levels in human glaucoma patients compared to control subjects. The study also found 6-8 fold higher levels of vitreal glutamate in monkeys with experimentally-induced ocular hypertension. Another study found 5-fold higher levels of glutamate in dogs with primary glaucoma, compared with normal dogs. However two subsequent studies carried out in primates found no significant increase in vitreal glutamate in IOP elevated monkey eyes, compared to those in control eyes (Carter-Dawson et al., 2002; Wamsley et al., 2005). It is possible that the confounding factors such as increased activity of EAATs in glial cells that could be masking the increased glutamate concentrations that may occur in a narrow time window following ocular hypertension. Another significant omission in many of these studies is assessment of glutamate levels in the retina, since glial cells in the retina including Muller cells and astrocytes could be paracrine sources of glutamate that contribute to excitotoxiciy. A more detailed analysis of various retinal sources of glutamate is necessary for a comprehensive assessment of glutamate elevation in glaucoma.

### 4.2 Excitotoxic cell death of retinal ganglion cells

Excitotoxicity is a recurring theme in the pathogenesis of retinal ganglion cell death, however the detailed cellular and biochemical mechanisms have eluded understanding for the past five decades. There are several unanswered questions about the relevance of excitotoxicity in glaucoma. The basic premise of elevation of glutamate needs further evaluation in both animal models of ocular hypertension and in human patients. If an increase in glutamate concentrations does occur in glaucoma, it is unclear if it is secondary to ischemia/hypoxia at the optic nerve head. Treatment with MK801 an NMDA glutamate receptor antagonist prevented apoptotic cell death of RGCs in ischemic rat retina after 12 h after insult (Ju et al., 2008). If an increase in glutamate occurs independent of ischemia, the underlying mechanisms for glutamate efflux from glial cells are not yet clear. The major line of evidence for excitotoxic cell death of retinal ganglion cells was from animal studies in which injection of nanomolar amounts of NMDA produce a loss of inner retinal neurons, particularly the retinal ganglion cells and inner plexiform layers. For instance, studies (Silliprandi et al., 1992) have shown that a single intravitreal injection of 20 nmole of NMDA resulted in 70% loss of cells with a soma diameter of greater than 8 microns in the ganglion cell layer, which were presumed to be retinal ganglion cells. Similar observations were made by Manabe and Lipton (2002) who demonstrated 80% retinal ganglion cell death after intravitreal injection of 20 nmole of NMDA in rats. Treatment with MK801, an uncompetitive NMDA antagonist was shown to block NMDA-mediated loss of retinal ganglion cells. A more detailed analysis of retinal ganglion cell death by excitotoxicity emerged from in vitro studies using primary cultures of retinal ganglion cells. Using chick retinal cells, Ferreira et al. demonstrated that under sodium-free conditions (to block activation of VGCC), calcium entry through NMDA receptors was sufficient to produce cell death. Hahn et al. (1988) showed that the extracellular $Ca^{2+}$ concentration, plays a key role in glutamate-induced cell death in retinal ganglion cells. Under these conditions, both $Mg^{2+}$ and the amino acid antagonist MK-801 [(+)-5-methyl-10,11-dihydro-5H-dibenzo-(alpha,gamma)-cyclohepten-5, 10-imine maleate], blockers of N-methyl-D-aspartate receptor-coupled ion channels, completely blocked cell death induced by glutamate. The study suggests that $Ca^{2+}$ entry through N-methyl-D-aspartate-activated channels is responsible for retinal ganglion cell death. Another NMDA antagonist, eliprodil (1 μM) was also found be very effective in protecting cultured retinal ganglion cells from NMDA-mediated cell death (Pang et al., 1999). Activation of p38 MAP kinase appears to mediate some of the neurotoxic effects of NMDA since treatment with SB203580 (a specific inhibitor of p38 MAP kinase) is effective in protecting against NMDA-mediated cell death (Manabe and Lipton, 2003). Most of the studies that demonstrate an acute effect of NMDA in producing neurodegeneration in the inner retina, may have limited relevance to primary open angle glaucoma which is a chronic neurodegenerative disease, in which clinical manifestation occurs over a period of several years. Perhaps, it would be worthwhile to study the involvement of metabotropic glutamate receptors in neurodegeneration in glaucoma. One study reported changes in several metabotropic glutamate receptors, particularly mGluR2 which was increased nearly 10-fold after ocular hypertension in DBA/2J mice (Dyka et al., 2004). Additional studies are needed to analyze the significance of changes in metabotropic glutamate receptors in glaucoma and their role in neurodegeneration.

Despite numerous observations about excitotoxic cell death of retinal ganglion cells and loss of inner plexiform layer, one study reported no effect of NMDA on retinal ganglion cells (Ullian et al., 2004). The study found that NMDA treatment killed mainly the amacrine cells, while retinal ganglion cells were unaffected. This study was unable to reproduce the NMDA-mediated cell death of cultured primary retinal ganglion cells that was observed in many of the previous studies. There are many possibilities for this apparent discrepancy between various research findings about excitotoxicity in retinal ganglion cells. RGCs are highly dependent on trophic factor-mediated signaling for their cell survival. Many of the earlier studies employed NMDA treatment in cell culture conditions that did not have the optimum levels of neurotrophins and trophic factors which could account for differences in the findings. Depending upon the concentration of neurotrophins in the culture medium of retinal ganglion cells, there could be variation in viability of the cells, which could account for variations in the data for excitotoxicity. For instance BDNF has been shown to inhibit the activation of Bim, a pro-apoptotic factor that is important for promoting apoptosis of trophic-factor deprived RGCs. Thus the experimental conditions of primary culture could greatly influence the outcome of experiments when excitotoxicity of NMDA is assessed in primary cultures of retinal ganglion cells. The localization of NMDA receptors is another factor contributing to susceptibility to excitotoxicity. Chen and Diamond (2002) report that NMDA receptors are localized predominantly in the extrasynaptic region suggesting that NMDA receptors are less likely to be overactivated by synaptic events. It is unclear how this distribution of receptors would contribute to excitotoxicity of retinal ganglion cells.

Cell culture experiments with glutamate are often problematic due to poor solubility of L-glutamic acid and high concentrations of glutamate tend to generate artifacts due to acidification of the cell culture medium. Some investigators use monosodium glutamate to circumvent this problem, but it is unclear if this has different binding properties to glutamate receptors. It would be interesting to analyze glutamate levels in a chronic animal model of ocular hypertension and determine if NMDA antagonist would be effective as neuroprotective agents in these experimental models of glaucoma.

Since NMDA receptor activity, is important for synaptic plasticity and normal neuron physiology, many NMDA antagonist that block all NMDA activity have undesirable side effects. In contrast, studies by Stuart Lipton's group demonstrated that memantine, an adamantane derivative, preferentially blocks excessive NMDA receptor activity without disrupting normal activity (Lipton, 2004). Memantine acts as an open-channel blocker by preferential binding when there is overstimulation of the receptor and does not appreciably bind to the receptor channel and interfere with normal channel activity and neurotransmission. Memantine was found to be well tolerated in patients and has been approved by FDA for treatment of dementia in Alzheimer's disease patients. Studies with the uncompetitive NMDA antagonist, memantine, met with a degree of success in ocular hypertensive rats. However phase III clinical trials with memantine were largely unsuccessful and patients showed no improvement in visual field. This study raises several issues about the contribution of NMDA receptor activation in neurodegeneration in glaucoma patients. The involvement of glutamate excitotoxicity in retinal ganglion cell death needs further investigation and further studies are necessary to understand its relevance to neurodegeneration in glaucoma.

## 5. Alpha-2-adrenergic agonists

Alpha-2 adrenergic agonists including clonidine and brimonidine have been known to reduce intraocular pressure, however clonidine produces a number of undesirable cardiovascular side effects. Brimonidine has a structure similar to clonidine, and is effective loweing IOP both in normotensive and ocular hypertensive primates (Burke and Potter, 1986). The mechanism underlying its ocular hypotensive effects are possibly related to reducing aqueous humor formation, since alpha-2-adrenergic receptors have been shown to be expressed in the iris and ciliary body. In recent years, studies have shown that in addition to lowering IOP, brimonidine has neuroprotective effects in animal models of glaucoma (Wheeler et al., 2003; Ahmed et al., 2001). For instance, in a rat model of elevated IOP, brimonidine administration initiated 10 days after IOP elevation prevented any further loss of ganglion cells. In vehicle- or timolol-treated rats, ganglion cell loss continued to occur (Woldmussie et al., 2001). In another glaucoma model, seven days after inducing transient ischaemia, there was loss of approximately half of the RGC population. Topical pre-treatment with 0.1% or 0.5% brimonidine attenuated ischaemia-induced RGC death. Brimonidine appers to preserve RGC survival and protect against a variety of glaucomatous insults. For instance, Lee et al. (2010) showed that brimonidine increased survival of rat RGCs in the presence of glutamate neurotoxicity, oxidative stress, and hypoxia.

## 6. Other emerging targets for neuroprotection

### 6.1 Endothelins

Endothelin-1 (ET-1) is a potent vasoactive peptide (Yanagisawa et al., 1988), has gained attention for its neurodegenerative role in glaucoma (Yorio et al., 2002). However the precise mechanisms underlying ET-1 mediated neurodegeneration are not completely understood. ET-1 levels are elevated in the aqueous humor of primary open angle glaucoma patients (Noske et al., 1997; Tezel et al., 1997) and in animal models of glaucoma (Kallberg et al., 2002; Thanos and Naskar 2004; and Prasanna et al., 2005). The clinical relevance of these findings is not completely clear but it appears plausible that ET-1 in aqueous humor could be secreted in response to an increase in IOP. There is considerable evidence to suggest that ET-1 could produce optic nerve damage similar to that seen in glaucoma. For instance, continuous peribulbar administration of ET-1 in primates produces optic nerve damage, similar to that seen in glaucoma (Orgul et al., 1996; Cioffi and Sullivan, 1999). Lau et al. (2005) have shown that a single ET-1 injection into rat eyes promoted loss of retinal ganglion cells, accompanied by increased GFAP labeling in the Muller cells end feet and astrocytic cell layer in retina and optic nerve. Chauhan et al. (2004) demonstrated that chronic administration of low doses ET-1 that do not appreciably alter blood flow in the retrobulbar region of the optic nerve, also results in a progressive loss of retinal ganglion cells and their axons without changes in optic disc morphology.

Since all known actions of ET-1 occur through binding to its receptors, it is important to understand which receptors may be mediating its damaging effects in glaucomatous optic neuropathy. Endothelin-1 acts mainly through two classes of receptors, the ETA and ETB receptors (Rubanyi and Polokoff, 1994). Both ETA and ETB belong to the rhodopsin superfamily of G-protein coupled receptors. Recently studies suggest that the endothelin B (ETB) receptor may be involved in mediating ET-1's neurodegenerative effects. For instance, Wang et al. (2006) showed increased immunohistochemical staining for ETB receptors in human glaucomatous optic nerves as compared with age-matched controls Rogers et al. (1997) demonstrated an increase in ETB expression in glial cells in the optic nerve, after optic nerve transection. ET-1 acts through its receptors to promote proliferation and activation of optic nerve head astrocytes, which are key steps in the progression of glaucoma (Prasanna et al., 2002). Yang et al. (2007) showed that ETB mRNA expression in the retina increased in a rodent elevated IOP model of glaucoma, from as early as 1 day and persisted up to 8 weeks of IOP elevation. It therefore appears that endothelin receptor activation could be an early event in the etiology of glaucoma. Krishnamoorthy et al. (2008) showed that ETB receptor expression is increased in RGCs after intravitreal injection of ET-1 and this was accompanied by apoptosis of RGCs. ET-1 mediated apoptosis was attenuated in ETB receptor-deficient rats (Krishnamoorthy et al., 2008). Recent studies from Simon John's lab showed that blocking endothelin receptors using bosentan (antagonist for both ETA and ETB receptors) is neuroprotective in a mouse ocular hypertension model of glaucoma (Howell et al., 2011). It is becoming increasingly evident from several corroborative observations that the endothelin system may play a pivotal role in neurodegeneration in glaucoma. Together these studies suggest the possibility of using endothelin antagonists as potential neuroprotective agents for glaucoma treatment.

### 6.2 Sigma-1 receptor

Sigma-1 receptors have emerged as a promising new neuroprotective candidate to protect RGCs from many of the noxious factors that are associated with the disease process of glaucoma (Dun et al., 2007). Sigma-1 receptors are a 26 kD transmembrane protein found on the endoplasmic reticulum (ER) that translocate from the ER to interact with ionotropic channels located on the plasma membrane (Hayahsi and Su 2007). This molecular signaling pathway enables the ubiquitously expressed sigma-1 receptor to associate and regulate many ligand gated ion channels that are found on the plasma membrane of many different cell types throughout the body (Hayashi and Su 2007; Zhang and Cuevas 2002). Sigma-1 receptors have been shown to be expressed in the retina, with the predominating level of expression in the retinal ganglion cell layer (Liu et al., 2010). There are several factors that contribute to neuroprotective ability of sigma receptors. Sigma-1 receptor's ability to bind and associate with L-type voltage gated calcium channels, regulate neuronal intracellular calcium concentrations when exposed to ischemic conditions, prevent glutamate excitotoxicity of RGCs when exposed to sigma-1 agonist (+)-pentazocine are some of the key mechanisms underlying sigma-1's neuroprotective effects (Tchedre et al., 2008; Katnik at al., 2006; Dun et al., 2007). Other pathways affected by sigma-1 receptor include attenuation of intrinsic death signal of glutamate-exposed retinal cell lines, which is a likely candidate to maintain the viability, and homeostatic intracellular calcium regulation of RGCs when they are exposed to a number of noxious stimuli that cause RGC apoptosis (Tchedre and Yorio 2008). Lastly, sigma-1 receptor stimulation has also demonstrated *in vivo* protection against retinal degeneration in a diabetic retinopathy animal model (Smith et al., 2008). More pre-clinical research needs to be preformed to demonstrate the neuroprotective efficacy of sigma receptors in glaucomatous animal models.

### 6.3 Tumor necrosis factor-α

Another molecule that has emerged as a key contributor to glaucoma progression is the cytokine, tumor necrosis factor-α (TNF-α) (Tezel, 2008). In the anterior chamber of the eye,

TNF-α could have beneficial effects by promoting outflow through conventional and uveoscleral pathways (Husain et al., 2008). However, TNF-α appears to produce damaging effects in the posterior segment of the eye. Several publications point to the involvement of TNF-α in glaucomatous neurodegeneration. Yang et al. (2007) showed an increase in TNF-α receptor 1A expression in an ocular hypertension model of glaucoma in rodents. Increased labeling for TNF-α and its receptor was observed in glaucomatous eyes compared to controls (Tezel et al., 2001). In the same study, double immunofluorescence suggested TNF-α labeling mainly in glial cells, while TNF-α receptors were found mainly on RGCs. In a mouse model of ocular hypertension, Nakazawa et al. (2008) found increased concentrations of TNF-α in the retina, which was followed by microglial activation and loss of RGCs. The authors found that RGC loss was greatly attenuated in TNF-receptor 2-deficient mice, suggesting that TNF-α acts through TNF receptor-2 to produce neurodegeneration in glaucoma (Nakazawa et al., 2006). TNF-α promotes ET-1 release from ciliary non-pigmented ciliary epithelial cells (Prasanna et al., 1998) as well as retinal pigmented epithelium (Narayan et al., 2003), suggesting that some of TNF-α's effects could be due to the downstream effects of endothelins. The role of TNF-α in glaucomatous degeneration is an evolving area of research with important implications for further research.

### 6.4 CD44

CD44 is a transmembrane glycoprotein which acts as a receptor for hyaluronic acid. Recent work by several groups suggests that soluble CD44 is significantly increased in aqueous humor of primary open angle glaucoma patients (Choi et al., 2005; Budak et al., 2009; Mokbel et al., 2010). The 32kDa ectodomain fragment of soluble CD44 was found have toxic effects both in the trabecular meshwork and ganglion cells *in vitro*. The cyotoxicity of CD44 was blocked by administration of anti-CD44 antibody in vitro (Choi et al., 2005). CD44 was also found to be increased in other models of neurodegeneration such as RDS mice which is characterized by inherited retinal degeneration (Krishnamoorthy et al., 2000). More work is needed in this developing area of research to fully understand the contribution of CD44 to glaucomatous pathophysiology.

## 7. Concluding remarks

While the present treatment modalities for glaucoma are effective in terms of lowering intraocular pressure and slowing down neurodegeneration, there are issues with long term application of medications particularly their side effects due to prolonged use. Besides, neurodegenerative effects continue to occur in some patients despite lowering IOP. It is clear that there are numerous targets that could be exploited for developing a neuroprotective agent to reduce axon loss and apoptosis of RGCs. However, it would be imperative to develop stringent measures to assess the efficacy and potency of various test compounds in animal models of glaucoma. After careful analysis using a battery of tests and cellular and molecular assays for neuroprotection, an efficacious candidate drug could make significant progress in clinical trials, so that there would be a good chance for success with neuroprotection in humans. This would involve a concerted effort among basic scientists, clinicians and pharmacologists and should result in the development of the first generation of neuroprotective treatments for glaucoma.

## 8. Acknowledgements

The authors thank Dr. Thomas Yorio for critically reading the manuscript and providing several useful comments and suggestions.

## 9. References

Adachi,K.,Kashii,S.,Masai,H.,Ueda,M.,Morizane,C.,Kaneda,K.,Kume,T.,Akaike,A., Honda,Y. (1998).Mechanism of the pathogenesis of glutamate neurotoxicity in retinal ischemia. *Graefes Arch. Clin. Exp. Ophthalmol.* Vol. 236, pp. 766-774.

Allergan Inc, Press Releases on Memantine Trials, Fourth Quarter Operating Results, Jan 30 2008 http://www.allergan.com/newsroom/index.htm

Anderson, M.G., Smith, R.S., Hawes, N.L., Zabaleta, A., Chang, B., Wiggs, J.L. & John SW. (2002). Mutations in genes encoding melanosomal proteins cause pigmentary glaucoma in DBA/2J mice. *Nat Genet.* 30: 81-5.

Araie, M., and Mayama, C. (2010) Use of calcium channel blockers for glaucoma, Progress in Retinal and Eye Research, 2010, 1-18

Araie, M., Azuma, I., Kitazawa, Y., 2003. Influence of topical betaxolol and timolol on visual field in Japanese open-angle glaucoma patients. Jpn. J. Ophthalmol. Vol. 47, pp. 199-207.

Arévalo, J.C., Yano, H., Teng, K.K. & Chao, M.V. (2004 ). A unique pathway for sustained neurotrophin signaling through an ankyrin-rich membrane-spanning protein. *EMBO J.* 23:2358-68.

Badea T.C., and Nathans J. (2004). Quantitative analysis of neuronal morphologies in the mouse retina visualized by using a genetically directed reporter. J Comp Neurol 480:. 331–351

Bähr, M. (2000). Live or let die - retinal ganglion cell death and survival during development and in the lesioned adult CNS. *Trends Neurosci.* 23:483-90.

Bahrami H. (2006) Causal models in primary open angle glaucoma. *Ophthalmic Epidemiol.* 4:291-298.

Bai, Y., Dergham, P., Nedev, H., Xu, J., Galan, A., Rivera, J.C., ZhiHua, S., Mehta, H.M., Woo, S.B., Sarunic, M.V., Neet, K.E. & Saragovi, H.U. (2010). Chronic and acute models of retinal neurodegeneration TrkA activity are neuroprotective whereas p75NTR activity is neurotoxic through a paracrine mechanism. *J Biol Chem.* 285:39392-39400

Bainbridge, J.W., Smith, A.J., Barker, S.S., Robbie, S., Henderson, R., Balaggan, K., Viswanathan, A., Holder, G.E., Stockman, A., Tyler, N., Petersen-Jones, S., Bhattacharya, S.S., Thrasher,A.J., Fitzke, F.W., Carter, B.J., Rubin, G.S., Moore, A.T. & Ali, R.R. (2008) Effect of gene therapy on visual function in Leber's congenital amaurosis. *N Engl J Med* 358:2231–2239.

Banin, E., Obolensky, A., Idelson, M., Hemo, I., Reinhardtz, E., Pikarsky, E., Ben-Hur, T. & Reubinoff, B. (2006). Retinal incorporation and differentiation of neural precursors derived from human embryonic stem cells. *Stem Cells.* 24:246-57.

Barbacid, M. (1995). Neurotrophic factors and their receptors. *Curr Opin Cell Biol.* 7(2):148-55.

Bartsch, U., Oriyakhel, W., Kenna, P.F., Linke, S., Richard, G., Petrowitz, B., Humphries, P., Farrar, G.J. & Ader, M. (2008). Retinal cells integrate into the outer nuclear layer and differentiate into mature photoreceptors after subretinal transplantation into adult mice. *Exp Eye Res.* 86(4):691-700

Beattie, M.S., Ferguson, A.R. & Bresnahan, J.C. (2010) AMPA-receptor trafficking and injury-induced cell death. *Eur J Neurosci.* 32:290-297.

Bebarta, V., Luyten, D. & Heard K. (2003) Emergency medicine animal research: does use of randomization and blinding affect the results?, *Acad Emerg Med.* 10: 684–687

Benowitz, L.I., Shashoua, V.E. & Yoon, M.G. (1981) Specific changes in rapidly transported protein during regeneration of the goldfish optic nerve. *J Neurosci.* 1: 300-7.

Bensimon, G., Lacomblez, L. & Meininger, V. (1994) A controlled trial of riluzole in amyotrophic lateral sclerosis: ALS/Riluzole Study Group, N Engl J Med 330: 585-591.

Beretta, S., Begni, B. & Ferrarese C (2003) Pharmacological manipulation of glutamate transport *Drug News Perspect.* 16:435-445.

Berkemeier, L.R., Ozçelik, T., Francke, U. &Rosenthal, A. (1992). Human chromosome 19 contains the neurotrophin-5 gene locus and three related genes that may encode novel acidic neurotrophins. *Somat Cell Mol Genet.* 18:233-245.

Bertrand, J., Di Polo, A. & McKerracher, L. (2007). Enhanced survival and regeneration of axotomized retinal neurons by repeated delivery of cell-permeable C3-like Rho antagonists. *Neurobiol Dis.* 25(1):65-72

Bessho, H., Suzuki, J., and Tobe, A., (1991). Vascular effects of betaxolol, a cardioselective b-adrenoceptor antagonist, in isolated rat arteries. Jpn. J. Pharmacol. 55: 351-358.

Boado, RJ., Hui, EK., Lu, JZ., Pardridge, WM. (2010). Drug targeting of erythropoietin across the primate blood-brain barrier with an IgG molecular Trojan horse. *J Pharmacol Exp Ther.* 333:961-969.

Boehm, A.G., Breidenbach, K.A., Pillunat, L.E., Bernd, A.S., Mueller, M.F., Koeller, A.U., (2003). Visual function and perfusion of the optic nerve head after application of centrally acting calcium-channel blockers. *Graefes Arch. Clin. Exp. Ophthalmol.* 241: 34-38.

Bose, S., Piltz, J.R., Breton, M.E., (1995). Nimodipine, a centrally active calcium antagonist, exerts a beneficial effect on contrast sensitivity in patients with normal-tension glaucoma and in control subjects. *Ophthalmology* 102: 1236-1241.

Broadway, D.C., Drance, S.M., 1998. Glaucoma and vasospasm. *Br. J. Ophthalmol.* Vol 82 pp. 862–870.

Budak YU, Akdogan M, Huysal K. Aqueous humor level of sCD44 in patients with degenerative myopia and primary open-angle glaucoma. (2009)BMC Res Notes. 2:224.

Buemi, M., Cavallaro, E., Floccari, F., Sturiale, A., Aloisi, C., Trimarchi, M., Grasso, G., Corica, F., Frisina, N. (2002). Erythropoietin and the brain: from neurodevelopment to neuroprotection. *Clin Sci (Lond).* 103:275-82.

Bull N.D., Irvine K.A., Franklin R.J.M, Martin K.R. (2009) Transplanted oligodendrocyte precursor cells reduce neurodegeneration in a model of glaucoma. *Invest Ophthalmol Vis Sci.* 50:4244–4253.

Calissano, P., Amadoro, G., Matrone, C., Ciafrè, S., Marolda, R., Corsetti, V., Ciotti, MT., Mercanti, D., Di Luzio, A., Severini, C., Provenzano, C., Canu, N. (2010). Does the term 'trophic' actually mean anti-amyloidogenic? The case of NGF. *Cell Death Differ.* 17:1126-1133.

Carter-Dawson, L., Crawford, M.L., Harwerth, R.S. & Smith, E.L. 3rd., Feldman, R., Shen, F.F., Mitchell, C.K. & Whitetree, A. (2002) Vitreal glutamate concentrations in monkey with experimental glaucoma. *Invest. Ophthalmol. Vis. Sci.* 43: 2633-2637

Chang, MS., Arevalo, JC., Chao, MV. (2004). Ternary complex with Trk, p75, and an ankyrin-rich membrane spanning protein. *J Neurosci Res.* 78:186-92

Chao, MV. & Hempstead, BL (1995). p75 and Trk: a two-receptor system. *Trends Neurosci.* 18:321-326

Chao, MV. (2003). Neurotrophins and their receptors: a convergence point for many signalling pathways. *Nat Rev Neurosci.* 4:299-309.

Chauhan, B.C., LaVatte, T.L., Jollimore, C.A., Yu, P.K., Reitsamer, H.A., Kelly, M.E.M., Yu, D-Yi., Tremblay, F. & Archibald, MA. (2004) Model of endothelin-1-induced chronic optic neuropathy in rat. *Invest. Ophthalmol. Vis. Sci.* 45: 144-152.

Chen H-SV, Pellegrini JW, Aggarwal SW, Lei SZ, Warach S, Jensen FE and Lipton SA. (1992). Open-channel block of N-methyl-d-aspartate (NMDA) responses by memantine: therapeutic advantage against NMDA receptor-mediated neurotoxicity. *J Neurosci* 12: 4427-4436.

Chen, H. & Weber, AJ. (2004). Brain-derived neurotrophic factor reduces TrkB protein and mRNA in the normal retina and following optic nerve crush in adult rats. *Brain Res.* 1011:99-106.

Chen, S. & Diamond, J.S. (2002) Synaptically released glutamate activates extrasynaptic NMDA receptors on cells in the ganglion cell layer of rat retina. J. Neurosci. 22: 2165-2173.

Chen, Y.N., Yamada, H., Mao, W., Uchida, S., Matsuyama, S., Aihara, M., and Araie, M.(2007). Hypoxia-induced retinal ganglion cell death and the neuroprotective effects of beta-adrenergic antagonists. Brain Res. 1148: 28-37.

Cheng, L., Sapieha, P., Kittlerova, P., Hauswirth, WW., Di Polo, A. (2002). TrkB gene transfer protects retinal ganglion cells from axotomy-induced death in vivo. *J Neurosci.* 22:3977-86

Cheon, E.W., Kim, Y.H., Cho, Y.Y., Kim, H.J., Kang, S.S., Cho, G.J., Yoo, J.M., Song, J.K., Choi, W.S., 2002. Betaxolol, a b1-adrenoceptor antagonist, protects a transient ischemic injury of the retina. Exp. Eye Res. 75: 591-601.

Cheon, E.W., Park, C.H., Kim, Y.S., Cho, C.H., Chung, Y.C., Kwon, J.G., Yoo, J.M., Choi, W.S., Cho, G.J., 2006. Protective effects of betaxolol in eyes with kainic acid-induced neuronal death. Brain Res. 1069: 75-85.

Chikar, JA., Colesa, DJ., Swiderski, DL., Di Polo, A., Raphael, Y., Pfingst, BE. (2008). Over-expression of BDNF by adenovirus with concurrent electrical stimulation improves cochlear implant thresholds and survival of auditory neurons. *Hear Res.* 245:24-34.

Choi J, Miller AM, Nolan MJ, Yue BY, Thotz ST, Clark AF, Agarwal N, Knepper PA. (2005) Soluble CD44 is cytotoxic to trabecular meshwork and retinal ganglion cells in vitro. Invest Ophthalmol Vis Sci. 46:214-222.

Cioffi, G.A. & Sullivan, P. (1999) The effect of chronic ischemia on the primate optic nerve. *Eur. J. Ophthalmol.* 9: S34-S36

Clark, A.F. & Yorio, T. *Ophthalmic Drug Discovery. Nature Review Drug Discovery.* 2: 448-459

Clarke, PG., Posada, A., Primi, MP., Castagné, V. (1998). Neuronal death in the central nervous system during development. *Biomed Pharmacother.* 52:356-62.

Coassin, M., Lambiase, A., Sposato, V., Micera, A., Bonini, S., Aloe, L. (2008). Retinal p75 and bax overexpression is associated with retinal ganglion cells apoptosis in a rat model of glaucoma. *Graefes Arch Clin Exp Ophthalmol.* 246:1743-1749.

Colafrancesco, V., Parisi, V., Sposato, V., Ross,i S., Russo, MA., Coassin, M., Lambiase, A., Aloe, L. (2011). Ocular application of nerve growth factor protects degenerating retinal ganglion cells in a rat model of glaucoma. *J Glaucoma.* 20:100-108

Coombs J, Van Der List D, Wang G-Y, Chalupa LM. (2006). Morphological properties of mouse retinal ganglion cells. *Neuroscience* 140: 123–136.

Crosson, C.E., Willis, J.A., Potter, D.E. (1990). Effect of the calcium antagonist, nifedipine, on ischemic retinal dysfunction. J. Ocul. Pharmacol. 6: 293-299.

Danbolt, N.C.,2001.Glutamate uptake.*Prog.Neurobiol.* 65: 1-105.

Danesh-Meyer H.V. &Levin L. A. (2009) Neuroprotection: Extrapolating from Neurologic Diseases to the Eye. American Journal of Ophthalmology 148: 186-191.

Danesh-Meyer, H.V. (2011). Neuroprotection in glaucoma: recent and future directions. *Current Opinion in Ophthalmology* 22: 78-86

Di Polo, A., Aigner, LJ., Dunn RJ., Bray, GM., Aguayo, AJ. (1998). Prolonged delivery of brain-derived neurotrophic factor by adenovirus-infected Müller cells temporarily rescues injured retinal ganglion cells. *Proc Natl Acad Sci U S A.* 95:3978-3983.

Diebold, Y. & Calonge, M. (2010)Applications of nanoparticles in ophthalmology. Progress in Retinal and Eye Research: 29: 596-609

Dong, Y., Ishikawa, H., Wu, Y., Shimizu, K., Goseki, T., Yoshitomi, T. (2006). Effect and mechanism of betaxolol and timolol on vascular relaxation in isolated rabbit ciliary artery. Jpn. J. Ophthalmol. 50:504-508.

Dryer, E.B., Zurakowski, D., Schumer, R.A., Podos, S.M, & Lipton, S.A. (1996) Elevated glutamate levels in the vitreous body of humans and monkeys with glaucoma. *Arch. Ophthalmol.* 114: 299-305.

Dun Y, Thangaraju M, Prasad P, Ganapathy V, Smith SB. (2007) Prevention of excitotoxicity in primary retinal ganglion cells by (+)-pentazocine, a sigma receptor-1 specific ligand. *Invest Ophthamol Vis Sci.* Vol. 48:4785-4794.

Dyka, F.M., May, C.A. & Enz, R. (2004) Metabotropic glutamate receptors are differentially regulated under elevated intraocular pressure. *J. Neurochem.* 90: 190-202.

Farahbakhsh, N.A., Cilluffo, M.C., Chronis, C., Fain, G.L., (1994). Dihydropyridinesensitive Ca2þ currents in rabbit ciliary body epithelial cells. *Exp. Eye Res.* 58:197-205.

Fatma, N., Kubo, E., Sen, M., Agarwal, N., Thoreson, W.B., Camras, C.B. & Singh, D.P. (2008)Peroxiredoxin 6 delivery attenuates TNF-alpha-and glutamate-induced retinal ganglion cell death by limiting ROS levels and maintaining $Ca^{2+}$ homeostasis. *Brain Res.*1233:63-78.

Ferreira, I.L., Duarte, C.B. & Carvalho, A.P. (1996) $Ca^{2+}$ influx through glutamate receptor-associated channels in retina cells correlates with neuronal cell death. *Eur J Pharmacol.* 302(1-3):153-62.

Flammer J.(1994) The vascular concept of glaucoma. *Surv Ophthalmol.* Vol. 38 (May 1994) Suppl:S3-6. Review.

Flammer, J., Guthauser, U., (1987). Behandlung chorioidaler Vasospasmen mit Kalziumantagonisten. *Klin. Monatsbl. Augenheilkd.* 190:299–300.

Flammer, J., Guthauser, U., Mahler, F., 1987a. Do ocular vasospasms help cause low-tension glaucoma? *Doc. Opthalmol. Proc. Ser.* 49: 397–399.

Frank T., Schlachetzki J.C., Göricke B., Meuer K., Rohde G., Dietz G.P., Bähr M., Schneider A., Weishaupt J.H. (2009) Both systemic and local application of granulocyte-colony stimulating factor (G-CSF) is neuroprotective after retinal ganglion cell axotomy. *BMC Neurosci.* 10: 49-59.

Fraser S., Wormald R. Ophhthalmology (eds yanoff, M. & duker, J. S.). . 1999,12:1.1-12:1.6.

Fu, Q.L., Li, X., Yip, H.K., Shao, Z., Wu, W., Mi, S., So, K.F. (2009). Combined effect of brain-derived neurotrophic factor and LINGO-1 fusion protein on long-term survival of retinal ganglion cells in chronic glaucoma. *Neuroscience.* 162:375-82

Gainey, M.A., Hurvitz-Wolff, J.R., Lambo, M.E. & Turrigiano GG. (2009) Synaptic scaling requires the GluR2 subunit of the AMPA receptor. *Journal of Neuroscience.* 29:6479-6489.

Gasser, P., and Flammer, J. (1991). Blood-cell velocity in the nailfold capillaries of patients with normal-tension and high-tension glaucoma. *Am. J. Ophthalmol.* 111:585–588.

Ghate, D. and Edelhauser, H.F. (2008) Barriers to Glaucoma Drug Delivery. *J Glaucoma* 17:147-156

Goll DE, Thompson VF, Li H, Wei W, Cong J. (2003) The calpain system. *Physiol Rev.* Vol. 83: 731-801. Review

Graef IA, Mermelstein PG, Stankunas K, Neilson JR, Deisseroth K, Tsien RW, Crabtree GR. (1999) L-type calcium channels and GSK-3 regulate the activity of NF-ATc4 in hippocampal neurons. *Nature.* 401: 703-708.

Greene, L.A. & Kaplan, D.R. (1995). Early events in neurotrophin signalling via Trk and p75 receptors. *Curr Opin Neurobiol.* 5:579-87.

Grozdanic, S.D., Ast, A.M., Lazic, T., Kwon, Y.H., Kardon, R.H., Sonea, I.M., Sakaguchi, D.S. (2006). Morphological integration and functional assessment of transplanted neural progenitor cells in healthy and acute ischemic rat eyes. *Exp Eye Res.* 82:597-607.

Gupta N., Ang L.C., Noel de T.L., Bidaisee L., Yu¨ cel Y.H.(2006) Human glaucoma and neural degeneration in intracranial optic nerve, lateral geniculate nucleus, and visual cortex. *Br J Ophthalmol.* 90: 674–678.

Guthauser, U., Flammer, J., Mahler, F. (1988). The relationship between digital and ocular vasospasm. *Graefes Arch. Clin. Exp.Ophthalmol.* 226: 224–226.

Hahn, J.S., Aizenman, E. & Lipton, S.A. (1988) Central mammalian neurons normally resistant to glutamate toxicity are made sensitive by elevated extracellular $Ca^{2+}$: toxicity is blocked by the N-methyl-D-aspartate antagonist MK-801. *Proc. Natl. Acad. Sci.* 85:6556-60.

Hamanoue, M., Middleton, G., Wyatt, S., Jaffray, E., Hay R.T., Davies, AM. (1999) p75-mediated NF-kappaB activation enhances the survival response of developing sensory neurons to nerve growth factor. *Mol Cell Neurosci.* 14:28-40

Hardingham, G. E. & Bading, H. (2002b) Coupling of extrasynaptic NMDA receptors to a CREB shut-off pathway is developmentally regulated. *Biochim. Biophys. Acta* 1600: 148–153.

Hardingham, G. E., Arnold, F. J. & Bading, H. (2001a) Nuclear calcium signaling controls CREB-mediated gene expression triggered by synaptic activity. *Nature Neurosci.* 4, 261–267.

Hardingham, G. E., Arnold, F. J. & Bading, H. (2001b)A calcium microdomain near NMDA receptors: on switch for ERK-dependent synapse-to-nucleus communication. *Nature Neurosci.* 4: 565–566.

Hardingham, G. E., Fukunaga, Y. & Bading, H. Extrasynaptic NMDARs oppose synaptic NMDARs by triggering CREB shut-off and cell death pathways. *Nature Neurosci.* 5, 405–414 (2002a).

Harris, A., Evans, D.W., Cantor, L.B., Martin, B. (1997). Hemodynamic and visual function effects of oral nifedipine in patients with normal-tension glaucoma. *Am. J. Ophthalmol.* 124:296-302.

Hayashi T, Su T.P.(2007) Sigma-1 receptor chaperones at the ER-mitochondrion interface regulate $Ca^{2+}$ signaling and cell survival. *Cell.* 131:596-610.

Heacock, A.M. & Agranoff, B.W. (1976) Enhanced labeling of a retinal protein during regeneration of optic nerve in goldfish. *Proc Natl Acad Sci USA.* 73: 828-832.

Hekman, M., Albert, S., Galmiche, A., Rennefahrt, U.E., Fueller, J., Fischer, A., Puehringer, D., Wiese S. & Rapp, U.R. (2006) Reversible membrane interaction of BAD requires two C-terminal lipid binding domains in conjunction with 14-3-3 protein binding, *J. Biol. Chem.* 281:17321–17336.

Hempstead, B.L. (2006). Dissecting the diverse actions of pro- and mature neurotrophins. *Curr Alzheimer Res* 3 (1): 19–24.

Hester R.K., Chen Z., Becker E.J., McLaughlin M., DeSantis L. (1994) The direct vascular relaxing action of betaxolol, carteolol and timolol in porcine long posterior ciliary artery. *Surv Ophthalmol.* 38: Suppl:S125-34.

Hirooka, K., Kelly, M.E., Baldridge, W.H., Barnes, S. (2000). Suppressive actions of betaxolol on ionic currents in retinal ganglion cells may explain its neuroprotective effects. Exp. Eye Res. 70: 611-621.

Hirsch, S., Labes, M., Bähr, M. (2000). Changes in BDNF and neurotrophin receptor expression in degenerating and regenerating rat retinal ganglion cells. *Restor Neurol Neurosci.*,17:125-134

Hoste, A.M., Sys, S.U. (1998). $Ca^{2+}$ channel-blocking activity of propranolol and betaxolol in isolated bovine retinal microartery. J. Cardiovasc. Pharmacol. 32: 390-396.

Howell, G.R., Macalinao, D.G., Sousa G.L., Walden, M., Soto, I., Kneeland, S.C., Barbay, J.M., King, B.L., Marchant, J.K., Hibbs, M., Stevens, B., Barres, B.A., Clark, A.F., Libby, R.T. & John, S.W. (2011) Molecular clustering identifies complement and endothelin induction as early events in a mouse model of glaucoma. *J Clin Invest.* doi: 10.1172/JCI44646.
http://www.kegg.com/dbget-bin/www_bget?hsa:4803

Huang W., Fileta J., Rawe I., Qu J., Grosskreutz C.L. (2010) Calpain activation in experimental glaucoma. *Invest Ophthalmol Vis Sci.* 51: 3049-3054.

Huang, W., Fileta, J.B., Dobberfuhl, A., Filippopolous, T., Guo, Y., Kwon G. & Grosskreutz, C.L. (2005) Calcineurin cleavage is triggered by elevated intraocular pressure, and calcineurin inhibition blocks retinal ganglion cell death in experimental glaucoma, *Proc. Natl. Acad. Sci. U.S.A.* 102: 12242–12247.

Huebner, K., Isobe, M., Chao, M., Bothwell, M., Ross, AH., Finan, J., Hoxie, JA., Sehgal, A., Buck, CR., Lanahan, A (1986). The nerve growth factor receptor gene is at human chromosome region 17q12-17q22, distal to the chromosome 17 breakpoint in acute leukemias. *Proc Natl Acad Sci U S A.* 83(5):1403-7.

Husain, S., Yates, P.W., Crosson, C.E. (2008). Latanoprost-induced changes in rat intraocular pressure: direct or indirect? J *Ocul Pharmacol Ther.* 24:367-72.

Ibáñez, C.F. (2007). Message in a bottle: long-range retrograde signaling in the nervous system. *Trends Cell Biol.* 17(11):519-28

Inoue, Y., Iriyama, A., Ueno, S., Takahashi, H., Kondo, M., Tamaki, Y., Araie, M., Yanagi, Y. (2007). Subretinal transplantation of bone marrow mesenchymal stem cells delays retinal degeneration in the RCS rat model of retinal degeneration. *Exp Eye Res.* 85:234-241.

Isenmann, S., Klöcker, N., Gravel, C., Bähr ,M. (1998). Short communication: protection of axotomized retinal ganglion cells by adenovirally delivered BDNF in vivo. *Eur J Neurosci.* 10:2751-6

Ito Y, Shimazawa M, Inokuchi Y, Fukumitsu H, Furukawa S, Araie M, Hara H.(2008) Degenerative alterations in the visual pathway after NMDA-induced retinal damage in mice. *Brain Res* 1212: 89–101.

Ivanov A., Pellegrino C., Rama S., Dumalska I., Salyha Y., Ben-Ari Y., Medina I. (2006) Opposing role of synaptic and extrasynaptic NMDA receptors in regulation of the extracellular signal-regulated kinases (ERK) activity in cultured rat hippocampal neurons. J Physiol. 572(Pt 3):789-98.

Jang, S.W., Liu, X., Chan, C.B., France, S.A., Sayeed, I., Tang, W., Lin, X., Xiao, G., Andero, R., Chang, Q., Ressler, K.J., Ye, K. (2010). Deoxygedunin, a natural product with potent neurotrophic activity in mice. *PLoS One.* 5(7):e11528.

Johansson, J.O. (1988). Inhibition and recovery of retrograde axoplasmic transport in rat optic nerve during and after elevated IOP in vivo. *Exp Eye Res*, 46 (2): 223-7

John, S.W., Smith, R.S., Savinova, O.V., Hawes, N.L,., Chang, B., Turnbull, D., Davisson, M., Roderick, T.H. & Heckenlively, J.R. (1998) Essential iris atrophy, pigment dispersion, and glaucoma in DBA/2J mice. *Invest Ophthalmol Vis Sci,* 39(6):951-962

Johnson T.V., Bull N.D., Hunt D.P., Marina N., Tomarev S.I., Martin K.R. (2010) Neuroprotective effects of intravitreal mesenchymal stem cell transplantation in experimental glaucoma. *Invest Ophthalmol Vis Sci* , 51(4): 2051–2059.

Johnson, E.C., Guo, Y., Cepurna, W.O. and Morrison, J.C. (2009) Neurotrophin roles in retinal ganglion cells survival: lessons from rat glaucoma models. *Exp Eye Res* 88(4):808-815.

Johnson, E.C., Deppmeier, L.M., Wentzien, S.K., Hsu, I., Morrison, J.C. (2000). Chronology of optic nerve head and retinal responses to elevated intraocular pressure. *Invest Ophthalmol Vis Sci.* 41(2):431-42.

Ju W.K., Lindsey J.D., Angert M., Patel A., Weinreb R.N. (2008) Glutamate receptor activation triggers OPA1 release and induces apoptotic cell death in ischemic rat retina. Mol Vis.,14: 2629-2638.

Kallberg, M.E.., Brooks, D.E.., Garcia-Sanchez, G.A.., Komaromy, A.M.., Szabo, N.J., and Tian, L. (2002). Endothelin-1 levels in aqueous humor of dogs with glaucoma. *J. Glaucoma* 11(2): 105-109.

Kamal, D., Garway-Heath, D., Ruben, S., O'Sullivan, F., Bunce, C., Viswanathan, A., Franks, W., Hitchings, R., (2003). Results of the betaxolol versus placebo treatment trial in ocular hypertension. Graefes Arch. Clin. Exp. Ophthalmol. 241(3), 196-203.

Katnik C., Guerrero W.R., Pennypacker K.R., Herrera Y., Cuevas J. (2006) Sigma-1 receptor activation prevents intracellular calcium dysregulation in cortical neurons during in vitro ischemia. *J Pharmacol Exp Ther*, 319( 3): 1355-1365.

Kimpinski, K., Campenot, R.B., Mearow, K. (1997). Effects of the neurotrophins nerve growth factor, neurotrophin-3, and brain-derived neurotrophic factor (BDNF) on neurite growth from adult sensory neurons in compartmented cultures. *J Neurobiol.* 33(4):395-410

Kitazawa, Y., Shirai, H., Go, F.J., (1989). The effect of Ca2þ-antagonist on visual field in low-tension glaucoma. *Graefes Arch. Clin. Exp. Ophthalmol.* 227(5),408-412.

Kong J-H, Fish D.R., Rockhill R.L., Masland R.H. (2005). Diversity of ganglion cells in the mouse retina: unsupervised morphological classification and its limits. *J Comp Neurol* Vol. 489(3): 293–310.

Krishnamoorthy, R., Agarwal, N., Chaitin, M.H. (2000) Upregulation of CD44 expression in the retina during the rds degeneration. Brain Res Mol Brain Res. 77(1):125-30.

Krishnamoorthy, R.R., Rao, V.R., Dauphin, R., Prasanna, G., Johnson, C., Yorio, T. (2008) Role of the ETB receptor in retinal ganglion cell death in glaucoma. Can J Physiol Pharmacol , 86 (6), 380-393.

Krupin, T, Liebmann, J.M, Greenfield, D.S, Ritch, R., Gardiner, S. Low-Pressure Glaucoma Study Group. (2011) A randomized trial of brimonidine versus timolol in preserving visual function: results from the Low-Pressure Glaucoma Treatment Study. Am J Ophthalmol. 151(4):671-81.

Kuruvilla, R., Ye, H., Ginty, DD. (2000). Spatially and functionally distinct roles of the PI3-K effector pathway during NGF signaling in sympathetic neurons. *Neuron.* 27(3):499-512.

Lacomblez, L., Bensimon, G., Leigh, P.N., Guillet, P., Powe, L., Durrleman, S., Delumeau, J.C. & Meininger, V. (1996) A confirmatory dose-ranging study of riluzole in ALS: ALS/Riluzole Study Group-II, Neurology ,47(6 Suppl 4):S242-50.

Lambert, W., Agarwal, R., Howe, W., Clark, AF., Wordinger, RJ. (2001). Neurotrophin and neurotrophin receptor expression by cells of the human lamina cribrosa. *Invest Ophthalmol Vis Sci.* 42(10):2315-2323.

Lambiase, A., Aloe, L., Centofanti, M., Parisi, V., Mantelli, F., Colafrancesco, V., Manni, GL., Bucci, MG., Bonini, S., Levi-Montalcini, R. (2009). Experimental and clinical evidence of neuroprotection by nerve growth factor eye drops: Implications for glaucoma. *Proc Natl Acad Sci U S A.* 106(32):13469–13474

Lau, J., Dang, M., Hockmann, K. & Ball AK (2005) Effects of acute delivery of endothelin-1 on retinal ganglion cell loss in the rat. *Exp. Eye Res.* 82(1):132-145.

Lebrun-Julien, F., Morquette, B., Douillette, A., Saragovi, HU., Di Polo, A. (2009). Inhibition of p75(NTR) in glia potentiates TrkA-mediated survival of injured retinal ganglion cells. *Mol Cell Neurosci.* 40(4):410-20

Levin, L.A. & Danesh-Meyer, H.V. (2010) Lost in translation: bumps in the road between bench and bedside. *JAMA* 303(15): 1533-1534.

Levkovitch-Verbin, H., Quigley, H.A., Martin, K.R., Valenta, D., Baumrind. L.A. & Pease, M.E. (2002) Translimbal laser photocoagulation to the trabecular meshwork as a model of glaucoma in rats. *Invest Ophthalmol Vis Sci.* 43(2): 402-10.

Lewin, G.R. & Barde, Y.A. (1996). Physiology of the neurotrophins. *Annu Rev Neurosci.* 19:289-317.

Li, R., Jiang, S., Liu, D., Bi, X., Wang, F., Zhang, Q., Xu, Q. (2011). A potential new therapeutic system for glaucoma: solid lipid nanoparticles containing methazolamide. *J Microencapsul.* 28(2):134-41

Li, Z., Okamoto, K., Hayashi, Y., Sheng, M. (2004) The Immportance of Dendritic Mitochondria in the Morphogenesis and Plasticity of Spines and Synapses. *Cell,* 119(6), 873-887.

Lipton, S.A. (2003) Possible role for memantine in protecting retinal ganglion cells from glaucomatous damage. *Surv Ophthalmol.* 48,Suppl 1:S38-46.

Lipton, S.A. (2004) Failures and successes of NMDA receptor antagonists: Molecular basis for the use of open channel blockers like memantine in the treatment of acute and chronic neurologic insults. NeuroRx 1(1): 101-110.

Liu LL, Wang L., Zhong Y. M., Yang X.L. (2010) Expression of sigma receptor 1 mRNA and protein in rat retina. *Neuroscience*. 167(4), 1151-1159.

Liu, X., Wang, D., Liu ,Y., Luo, Y., Ma, W., Xiao, W., Yu, Q. (2010). Neuronal-driven angiogenesis: role of NGF in retinal neovascularization in an oxygen-induced retinopathy model. *Invest Ophthalmol Vis Sci.*,51(7):3749-57

Lodish, H, BERK., A, Zipursky, S. L, Matsudaira, P, Baltimore, D, Darnell, J E. (1999). Molecular Cell Biology. 4th ed. New York: *W H Freeman & Co,*. Section 23.8

Loetscher, H., Niederhauser, O., Kemp, J., Gill, R., (2001). Is caspase-3 inhibition a valid therapeutic strategy in cerebral ischemia? *Drug Discov. Today* 6(13): 671-680.

Luksch, A., Rainer, G., Koyuncu, D., Ehrlich, P., Maca, T., Gschwandtner, M.E., Vass, C., Schmetterer, L., (2005). Effect of nimodipine on ocular blood flow and colour contrast sensitivity in patients with normal tension glaucoma. *Br. J. Ophthalmol.* 89(1), 21-25.

MacLaren, R.E., Pearson, R.A., MacNeil, A., Douglas, R.H., Salt, T.E., Akimoto, M., Swaroop, A., Sowden, JC., Ali RR. (2006). Retinal repair by transplantation of photoreceptor precursors. *Nature*. 444(7116):203-207.

MacPhee, I. & Barker, P.A. (1999). Extended ceramide exposure activates the trkA receptor by increasing receptor homodimer formation. *J Neurochem*. 72(4):1423-1430.

Maisonpierre, P.C., Le Beau, M.M., Espinosa, R 3rd., Ip NY., Belluscio, L., de la Monte SM., Squinto, S., Furth, ME., Yancopoulos, GD. (1991). Human and rat brain-derived neurotrophic factor and neurotrophin-3: gene structures, distributions, and chromosomal localizations. *Genomics* 10 (3): 558–568.

Malinow, R. & Malenka, R.C. AMPA receptor trafficking and synaptic plasticity. (2002) *Annu Rev Neuroscience.*, 25:103-126.

Manabe S. & Lipton S.A. (2003) Divergent NMDA signals leading to proapoptotic and antiapoptotic pathways in the rat retina. Invest. Ophthalmol. Vis. Sci. 44(1):385-392.

Mao Z, Bonni A, Xia F, Nadal-Vicens M, Greenberg ME.(1999) Neuronal activity-dependent cell survival mediated by transcription factor MEF2. *Science*. 286(5440), 785-790.

Mark, L.P., Prost, R.W., Ulmer, J.L., Smith, M.M., Daniels, D.L., Strottmann, J.M., Brown, W.D. & Hacein-Bey L (2001) Pictorial review of glutamate excitotoxicity: Fundamental concepts for neuroimaging. *Am. J. Neuroradiol.* 22(10): 1813-1824.

Marshall, C. (1995) Specificity of receptor tyrosine kinase signalling: transient versus sustained extracellular signal-regulated kinase activation. *Cell* 80(2): 179–185

Martin, K.R., Quigley, H.A., Zack, D.J., Levkovitch-Verbin, H., Kielczewski, J., Valenta, D., Baumrind, L., Pease, M.E., Klein, R.L., Hauswirth, W.W. (2003). Gene therapy with brain-derived neurotrophic factor as a protection: retinal ganglion cells in a rat glaucoma model. *Invest Ophthalmol Vis Sci.* 44(10):4357-65

Mayer M. L., Westbrook G. L., and Guthrie P. B. (1984) Voltage-dependent block by $Mg^{2+}$ of NMDA responses in spinal cord neurones. *Nature* 309(5965):261-3..

Melena, J., Wood, J.P.M., Osborne, N.N., (1999). Betaxolol, a β1-adrenoceptor antagonist, has an affinity for L-type Ca2þ channels. *Eur. J. Pharmacol.* 378(3), 317-322.

Meyer-Franke, A., Kaplan, M.R., Pfrieger, F.W., Barres, B.A. (1995). Characterization of the signaling interactions that promote the survival and growth of developing retinal ganglion cells in culture. *Neuron*, 15(4): 805–819

Mokbel T.H., Ghanem A.A., Kishk H, Arafa L.F., El-Baiomy A.A. (2010) Erythropoietin and soluble CD44 levels in patients with primary open-angle glaucoma. Clin Experiment Ophthalmol. 38(6):560-655.

Morgan J.I, Curran T. (1986). Role of ion flux in the control of c-fos expression. *Nature.* 322(6079): 552-555.

Morrison, J.C., Moore, C.G., Deppmeier, L.M., Gold, B.G., Meshul, C.K. and Johnson, E.C. (1997) A rat model of chronic pressure-induced optic nerve damage. *Exp Eye Res.* 64: 85–96.

Murphy, T.H., Worley, P.F., Baraban, J.M. (1991) L-type voltage-sensitive calcium channels mediate synaptic activation of immediate early genes. *Neuron.* 7 (4), 625-35.

Nagata, T., Ueno, S., Morita, H., Kubota, T., Toyohira, Y., Tsutsui, M., Tawara, A., Yanagihara, N., (2008). Direct inhibition of N-methyl-D-aspartate (NMDA)-receptor function by antiglaucomatous b-antagonists. J. Pharmacol. Sci. 106(3), 423-434.

Nakagawara, A., Liu, XG., Ikegaki, N., White, PS., Yamashiro, DJ., Nycum LM., Biegel JA., Brodeur GM. (1995). Cloning and chromosomal localization of the human TRK-B tyrosine kinase receptor gene (NTRK2). *Genomics.* 25(2):538-46.

Nakazawa T., Nakazawa C., Matsubara A., Noda K., Hisatomi T., She H., Michaud N, Hafezi-Moghadam A, Miller JW, Benowitz LI. (2006) Tumor necrosis factor-alpha mediates oligodendrocyte death and delayed retinal ganglion cell loss in a mouse model of glaucoma. J Neurosci. 26(49), 12633–12641.

Nakazawa, T., Nakazawa, C., Matsubara, A., Noda, K., Hisatomi ,T., She, H., Michaud, N., Hafezi-Moghadam A., Miller JW., Benowitz LI. (2006). Tumor necrosis factor-alpha mediates oligodendrocyte death and delayed retinal ganglion cell loss in a mouse model of glaucoma. *J Neurosci.* 26(49):12633-12641.

Nakazawa, T., Nakazawa, C., Matsubara, A., Noda, K., Hisatomi, T., She, H., Michaud, N., Hafezi-Moghadam, A., Miller, J.W. & Benowitz LI (2006) Tumor necrosis factor-alpha mediates oligodendrocyte death and delayed retinal ganglion cell loss in a mouse model of glaucoma. *J. Neurosci.* 26(49): 12633-12641.

Narayan, S., Prasanna, G., Krishnamoorthy, RR., Zhang, X., Yorio, T. (2003). Endothelin-1 synthesis and secretion in human retinal pigment epithelial cells (ARPE-19) :differential regulation by cholinergics and TNF-alpha. *Invest Ophthalmol Vis Sci.*44(11):4885-4894.

Nickells, R.W. (2004) The molecular biology of retinal ganglion cell death: caveats and controversies. *Brain Res. Bull.* 62(6): 439-446.

Nickells, R.W. (2007) From ocular hypertension to ganglion cell death: a theoretical sequence of events leading to glaucoma. *Canadian J. Ophthalmol.* 42(2):278-287.

Nixon, R.A. (2003) The calpains in aging and aging-related diseases, *Ageing Res. Rev.* 2(4) , 407–418.

Noske, W., Hensen, J.., and Wiederholt, M. (1997). Endothelin-like immunoreactivity in aqueous humor of primary open angle glaucoma and cataract patients. *Grafes Arch. Clin. Exp. Ophthamol.* 235(9): 551-552.

Nykjaer, A., Lee, R., Teng, KK., Jansen, P., Madsen, P., Nielsen, MS., Jacobsen, C., Kliemannel, M., Schwarz, E., Willnow, TE., Hempstead, BL., Petersen, CM. (2004). Sortilin is essential for proNGF-induced neuronal cell death. *Nature.* 26,427(6977):843-8

Nykjaer, A., Willnow, TE., Petersen, CM. (2005). p75NTR-live or let die. *Curr Opin Neurobiol.* 15(1):49-57

O'Brien, C., (1998) Vasospasm and glaucoma. *Br. J. Ophthalmol.* 82, 855–856.

Ohta, H., Arai, S., Akita, K., Ohta, T., Fukuda, S. (2011). Neurotrophic effects of a cyanine dye via the PI3K-Akt pathway: attenuation of motor discoordination and neurodegeneration in an ataxic animal model. *PLoS One.* 6(2):e17137.

Olver, J.M., (1998). Angioarchitecture of the human optic nerve. In: Bisantis, C., Carella, G. (Eds.), Vascular System of the Optic Nerve. Innovation-News-Communication, Rome, pp. 29–44.

Orgul, S., Cioffi, G.A., Bacon, D.R. & Van Buskirk, E.M. (1996) An endothelin-1 induced model of chronic optic nerve ischemia in rhesus monkeys. *J. Glaucoma* 5: 135-138.

Osborne, N.N., Casson, R.J., Wood, J.P., Chidlow, G., Graham, M., Melena, J., (2004). Retinal ischemia: mechanisms of damage and potential therapeutic strategies. Prog. Retin. Eye Res. 23, 91-147.

Osborne, N.N., DeSantis, L., Bae, L.H., Ugarte, M., Wood, J.P.M., Nash, M.S., Chidlow, G., (1999). Topically applied betaxolol attenuates NMDA-induced toxicity to ganglion cells and the effects of ischaemia to the retina. Exp. Eye Res. 69, 331-342.

Ozawa S., Kamiya H., and Tsuzuki K. (1998) Glutamate receptors in the mammalian central nervous system. *Prog. Neurobiol.* 54, 581–618.

Pang I.H., Wexler E.M., Nawy S., DeSantis L., Kapin M.A. (1999) Protection by eliprodil against excitotoxicity in cultured rat retinal ganglion cells. Invest. Ophthalmol. Vis. Sci. 40:1170-1176.

Parsons C.G., Gruner R., Rozental J., Millar J. and Lodge D. (1993). Patch clamp studies on the kinetics and selectivity of N-methyl-d-aspartate receptor antagonism by memantine (1-amino-3,5-dimethyladamantane). *Neuropharmacology* 32(12), 1337-1350.

Pease, M.E., McKinnon, S.J., Quigley, H.A., Kerrigan-Baumrind, L.A., Zack, D.J. (2000). Obstructed axonal transport of BDNF and its receptor TrkB in experimental glaucoma. *Invest Ophthalmol Vis Sci*, 41: 764–774

Pernet, V., Di Polo, A. (2006). Synergistic action of brain-derived neurotrophic factor and lens injury promotes retinal ganglion cell survival, but leads to optic nerve dystrophy in vivo. *Brain.* 129(Pt 4):1014-26

Piltz, J.R., Bose, S., Lanchoney, D., (1998). The effect of nimodipine, a centrally active calcium antagonist, on visual function and macular blood flow in patients with normal-tension glaucoma and control subjects. *J. Glaucoma* 7, 336-342.

Prasanna, G., Dibas, A., Tao, W., White, K., Yorio, T. (1998). Regulation of endothelin-1 in human non-pigmented ciliary epithelial cells by tumor necrosis factor-alpha. *Exp Eye Res.* 66: 9-18.

Prasanna, G., Hulet, C., Desai, D., Krishnamoorthy, R.R., Narayan, S., Brun, A.M., Suburo, A.M. & Yorio T. (2005) Effect of elevated intraocular pressure on endothelin-1 in a rat model of glaucoma. *Pharmacol Res.* 51: 41-50.

Prasanna, G., Krishnamoorthy, R., Clark, AF., Wordinger, RJ., Yorio, T.(2002) . Human optic nerve head astrocytes as a target for endothelin-1. *Invest Ophthalmol Vis Sci.* 43: 2704-13.

Prasanna, G., Krishnamoorthy, R., Yorio, T. (2010) Endothelin, astrocytes and glaucoma. *Experimental Eye Research.* doi:10.1016/j.exer.2010.09.006

Prithviraj, R., Kelly, K.M., Espinoza-Lewis, R., Hexom, T., Clark, A.B.& Inglis, F.M. (2008) Differential regulation of dendrite complexity by AMPA receptor subunits GluR1 and GluR2 in motor neurons. *Dev Neurobiol.* 1:247-264.

Qu J, Wang D, Grosskreutz C.L. (2010) Mechanisms of retinal ganglion cell injury and defense in glaucoma. *Exp Eye Res*. 91(1), 48-53.

Quigley H.A., Dunkelberger G.R., Green W.R. (1989) Retinal ganglion cell atrophy correlated with automated perimetry in human eyes with glaucoma. *Am J Ophthalmol* 107, 453–464.

Quigley, H.A., Addicks, E.M., Green, W.R, & Maumenee, A.E. (1981) Optic nerve damage in human glaucoma. II. the site of injury and susceptibility to damage. *Arch Ophthalmol*. 99:635-649.

Quigley, H.A., McKinnon, S.J., Zack, D.J., Pease, M.E., Kerrigan-Baumrind, L.A., Kerrigan, D.F., Mitchell, R.S. (2000). Retrograde axonal transport of BDNF in retinal ganglion cells is blocked by acute IOP elevation in rats. *Invest Ophthalmol Vis Sci*. 41(11):3460-6

Rainer, G, Kiss, B., Dallinger, S., Findl, O., Georgopoulos, M., Vass, C., Menapace, R., Polak K., Eichler, H.G., Wolzt, M., Schmetterer, L.(2001) A double masked placebo controlled study on the effect of nifedipine on optic nerve blood flow and visual field function in patients with open angle glaucoma. *Br J Clin Pharmacol*. 52:210-212.

Raju, T.R., Rao, M.S., Nagaraja, T.N., Meti, B.L., Schulz, M. (1994). Retinal ganglion cell survival and neurite regeneration in vitro after cell death period are dependent upon target derived trophic factor and retinal glial factor(s). *Brain Res*. 21,664(1-2):247-51.

Rao, V.P., Epstein, D.L. (2007) Rho GTPase/Rho kinase inhibition as a novel target for the treatment of glaucoma. *BioDrugs*. 21:167-77.

Reichardt, L.F ( 2006). Neurotrophin-regulated signalling pathways. *Philos. Trans. R. Soc. Lond., B, Biol. Sci*. 361 (1473): 1545–64.

Reisberg, B., Doody, R., Stoffler, A., Schmitt, F., Ferris, S. & Mobius, H.J. (2003) Memantine in moderate-to-severe Alzheimer's disease, *N Engl J Med* 348:1333-1341

Rogers, S.D., Demaster E., Catton, M., Ghilardi, J.R., Levin, L.A., Maggio, J.E. & Mantyh, P.W. (1997) Expression of endothelin-B receptors by glia in vivo is increased after CNS injury in rats, rabbits and humans. *Exp. Neurol*. 145: 180-195.

Rojanapongpun, P., Drance, S.M. (1993) The response of blood flow velocity in the ophthalmic artery and blood flow of the finger to warm and cold stimuli in glaucomatous patients. *Graefes Arch. Clin. Exp. Ophthalmol*. 231:375–377.

Rubanyi, G.M. & Polokoff, M.A. (1994) Endothelins: molecular biology, biochemistry, pharmacology and pathophysiology. *Pharmacol. Rev*. 46: 325-415.

Rudzinski, M., Wong, T.P., Saragovi, H.U. (2004). Changes in retinal expression of neurotrophins and neurotrophin receptors induced by ocular hypertension. *J Neurobiol*. 15,58(3):341-54.

Sappington, R.M., Carlson, B.J., Crish, S.D. & Calkins, D.J. (2010). The microbead occlusion model: a paradigm for induced ocular hypertension in rats and mice. *Invest Ophthalmol Vis Sci*. 51:207-216

Sariola, H., Sainio, K., Arumäe, U., Saarma, (1994). M. Neurotrophins and ciliary neurotrophic factor: their biology and pathology. Ann Med. 26(5):355-63.

Sawai, H., Clarke, D.B., Kittlerova, P., Bray, G.M., Aguayo, A.J. (1996). Brain-derived neurotrophic factor and neurotrophin-4/5 stimulate growth of axonal branches from regenerating retinal ganglion cells. *J Neurosci*. 15,16(12):3887-94.

Schober M.S., Chidlow G, Wood J.P, Casson R.J. (2008) Bioenergetic-based neuroprotection and glaucoma. *Clin Experimental Ophthalmol* 36:377–385.

Schwartz M. (2004) Optic nerve crush: protection and regeneration. Brain Res Bull. 15,62(6):467-71.

Seki, M., Fukuchi, T., Tanaka, T., Nawa, H., Takei, N., Abe, H. (2004) Quantitative analyses of mRNA and protein levels of neurotrophin-3 in the rat retina during postnatal development and aging. *Jpn J Ophthalmol.*,48(5):460-4.

Seki, M., Tanaka, T., Sakai, Y., Fukuchi, T., Abe, H., Nawa, H., Takei ,N. (2005). Müller Cells as a source of brain-derived neurotrophic factor in the retina: noradrenaline upregulates brain-derived neurotrophic factor levels in cultured rat Müller cells. *Neurochem Res.* 30(9):1163-70.

Setoguchi, M., Ohya, Y., Abe, I., Fujishima, M. (1995) Inhibitory action of betaxolol, a b1-selective adrenoceptor antagonist, on voltage-dependent calcium channels in guinea-pig artery and vein. Br. J. Pharmacol. 115:198-202.

Sheng, M., McFadden, G., Greenberg, M.E.(1990) Membrane depolarization and calcium induce c-fos transcription via phosphorylation of transcription factor CREB. *Neuron.* 4. 571-582

Shi, Z., Birman, E., Saragovi, HU. (2007). Neurotrophic rationale in glaucoma: a TrkA agonist, but not NGF or a p75 antagonist, protects retinal ganglion cells in vivo. *Dev Neurobiol.* 67(7):884-94. Erratum in: *Dev Neurobiol.* 2007 Sep 15,67(11):1547-8.

Shi, Z., Rudzinski, M., Meerovitch, K., Lebrun-Julien, F., Birman, E., Di Polo, A., Saragovi, HU. (2008). Alpha2-macroglobulin is a mediator of retinal ganglion cell death in glaucoma. *J Biol Chem.* 24,283(43):29156-65

Shimazawa, M., Inokuchi, Y., Ito, Y., Murata, H., Aihara, M., Miura, M., Araie, M., Hara, H. (2007) Involvement of ER stress in retinal cell death. *Mol Vis.* Vol. 13:578–587.

Siliprandi R., Canella R., Carmignoto G., Schiavo N., Zanellato A., Zanoni R.,Vantini G. (1992) N-methyl-D-aspartate-induced neurotoxicity in the adult rat retina. Vis. Neurosci. 8(6):567-573.

Smith SB, Duplantier J, Dun Y, Mysona B, Roon P, Marin PM, Ganapathy V. (2008). In vivo protection against retinal neurodegeneration by sigma receptor 1 ligand (+) pentazocine. *Invest Ophthamol Vis Sci.* 49:4154-4161.

Sole, C., Dolcet, X., Segura, M.F., Gutierrez, H., Diaz-Meco, M.T., Gozzelino, R., Sanchis, D., Bayascas, JR., Gallego, C., Moscat, J., Davies, AM., Comella, JX. (2004). The death receptor antagonist FAIM promotes neurite outgrowth by a mechanism that depends on ERK and NF-kapp B signaling. *J Cell Biol.* 8,167(3):479-92

Sommer, A., Tielsch, J.M., Katz, J., Quigley, H.A., Gottsch, J.D., Javitt J. and Singh K. (1991) Relationship between intraocular pressure and primary open angle glaucoma among white and black Americans. The Baltimore Eye Survey. Arch Ophthalmol 109:1090-5

Spalding, K.L., Rush, R.A., Harvey, A.R. (2004). Target-derived and locally derived neurotrophins support retinal ganglion cell survival in the neonatal rat retina. *J Neurobiol.* 5,60(3):319-27.

Steinhausen, K., Stumpff, F., Strauss, O., Thieme, H., Wiederholt, M., (2000). Influence of muscarinic agonists and tyrosine kinase inhibitors on L-type Ca(2þ) channels in human and bovine trabecular meshwork cells. *Exp. Eye Res.* 70:285-293.

Suemori S, Shimazawa M, Kawase K, Satoh M, Nagase H, Yamamoto T, Hara H.(2006) Metallothionein, an endogenous antioxidant, protects against retinal neuron damage in mice. *Invest Ophthalmol Vis Sci.* 47 (3975–3982)

Sun W, Li X, He S. (2002). Large-scale morphological survey of mouse retinal ganglion cells. *J Comp Neurol* 451:(115–126)

Tao, W., Wen, R., Goddard, MD., Sherman, SD., O'Rourke, PJ., Stabila, PF., Bell, WJ., Dean, BJ., Kauper, KA., Budz, VA., Tsiaras, WG., Acland, GM ., Pearce-Kelling, S., Laties, AM., Aguirre GD (2002). Encapsulated cell-based delivery of CNTF reduces photoreceptor degeneration in animal models of retinitis pigmentosa. Invest Ophthalmol Vis Sci. 43:3292-3298

Tchedre, K.T., Huang, R.Q., Dibas, A., Krishnamoorthy, R.R., Dillon, G.H., Yorio, T. (2008) Sigma-1 receptor regulation of voltage gated calcium channels involves a direct interaction. *Invest Ophthamol Vis Sci.* 49:4993-5002.

Tchedre, K.T., Yorio, T.(2008) Sigma-1 receptors protect RGC-5 cells from apoptosis by regulating intracellular calcium, bax levels, and caspase-3 activation. *Invest Ophthamol Vis Sci.* 49:2577-2588

Tezel, G. & Wax, M.B. (2000) Increased production of tumor necrosis factor-alpha by glial cells exposed to simulated ischemia or elevated hydrostatic pressure induces apoptosis in cocultured retinal ganglion cells. *J Neurosci.* 20:8693–8700.

Tezel, G. & Wax, M.B. (2004) The immune system and glaucoma. *Curr Opin Ophthalmol.* 15:80–84.

Tezel, G.(2008) TNF-alpha signaling in glaucomatous neurodegeneration. *Prog Brain Res.* 173:409-21.

Tezel, G., Li, L.Y., Patil, R.V., Wax, M.B.(2001). TNF-alpha and TNF-alpha receptor-1 in the retina of normal and glaucomatous eyes. *Invest Ophthalmol Vis Sci.*42:1787-94.

Tezel,G. (2006) Oxidative stress in glaucomatous neurodegeneration: mechanisms and consequences.Prog.Retin.EyeRes. 25:490-513.

Tezel., G.., Kass, M.A.., Kolker, A.E.., Becker B, Wax MB. (1997). Plasma and aqueous endothelin levels in primary open angle glaucoma. *J. Glaucoma* 6: 83-89.

Thanos, S. & Naskar, R. (2004). Correlation between retinal ganglion cell death and chronically developing inherited glaucoma in a new rat mutant. *Exp. Eye Res.* 79:119-29

Thieme, H., Steinhausen, K., Ottlecz, A., Lambrou, G.N., Strauss, O., Wiederholt, M., Rosenthal, R. (2005) Effects of unoprostone and endothelin 1 on L-type channel currents in human trabecular meshwork cells. *Ophthalmic Res.* 37:293-300.

Toriu, N., Akaike, A., Yasuyoshi, H., Zhang, S., Kashii, S., Honda, Y., Shimazawa, M., Hara, H.(2000) Lomerizine, a $Ca^{2+}$ channel blocker, reduces glutamate-induced neurotoxicity and ischemia/reperfusion damage in rat retina. *Exp Eye Res.* 70:475-84.

Ugolini, G., Cremisi, F., Maffei, L. (1995). TrkA, TrkB and p75 mRNA expression is developmentally regulated in the rat retina. *Brain Res.* 15,704(1):121-4.

Ullian, E.M., Barkis, W.B., Chen, S., Diamond, J.S. &, Barres, B.A. (2004) Invulnerability of retinal ganglion cells to NMDA excitotoxicity. *Mol Cell Neurosci.* 26:544-57.

Valent, A., Danglot, G., Bernheim, A. (1997). Mapping of the tyrosine kinase receptors trkA (NTRK1), trkB (NTRK2) and trkC(NTRK3) to human chromosomes 1q22, 9q22 and 15q25 by fluorescence in situ hybridization. *Eur J Hum Genet.* 5(2):102-4.

Vecino, E., García-Crespo, D., García, M., Martinez-Millán, L., Sharma, SC., Carrascal, E. (2002). Rat retinal ganglion cells co-express brain derived neurotrophic factor (BDNF)and its receptor TrkB. *Vision Res.* 42(2):151-7. Erratum in: *Vision Res.* 2010 21,50(9):926.

Völgyi, B., Chheda, S., Bloomfield, S.A.,(2009) Tracer coupling patterns of the ganglion cell subtypes in the mouse retina. *J Comp Neurol.* 512:664-87.

Wamsley, S., Gabelt, B.T., Dahl, D.B., Case, G,L., Sherwood, R.W., May, C.A., Hernandez, M.R. and Kaufman PL.(2005) Vitreous glutamate concentration and axon loss in monkeys with experimental glaucoma. *Arch Ophthalmol.* 123:64-70.

Wang, H.G., Pathan, I.M., Ethell, S., Krajewski, Y., Yamaguchi, F., Shibasaki, F., McKeon, F., Bobo, T., Franke, T.F. & Reed J.C. (1999) $Ca^{2+}$-induced apoptosis through calcineurin dephosphorylation of BAD, *Science* 284:339–343.

Wang, K.C., Kim, J.A., Sivasankaran, R., Segal, R., He Z. (2002). P75 interacts with the Nogo receptor as a co-receptor for Nogo, MAG and OMgp. *Nature.* 7,420(6911):74-8.

Wang, L., Fortune, B., Cull, G., Dong, J & Cioffi GA (2006) Endothelin B receptor in human glaucoma and experimentally induced optic nerve damage. *Arch. Ophthalmol.* 124:717-24

Ward, M.S., Khoobehi, A., Lavik, E.B., Langer, R., Young, M.J. (2007). Neuroprotection of retinal ganglion cells in DBA/2J mice with GDNF-loaded biodegradable microspheres. *J Pharm Sci.* 96(3):558-68.

Watson, P.G., Barnett, M.F., Parker, V., Haybittle, J., (2001) A 7 year prospective comparative study of three topical beta blockers in the management of primary open angle glaucoma. Br. J. Ophthalmol. 85:962-968.

Weber, A.J., Viswanáthan, S., Ramanathan, C., Harman, C.D. (2010). Combined application of BDNF to the eye and brain enhances ganglion cell survival and function in the cat after optic nerve injury. *Invest Ophthalmol Vis Sci.* 51(1):327–334

Weier, H.U., Rhein, A.P., Shadravan, F., Collins, C., Polikoff, D. (1995). Rapid physical mapping of the human trk protooncogene (NTRK1) to human chromosome 1q21-q22 by P1 clone selection, fluorescence in situ hybridization (FISH), and computer-assisted microscopy. *Genomics.* 20,26(2):390-3.

Wiederholt, M., Thieme, H., Stumpff, F., (2000). The regulation of trabecular meshwork and ciliary muscle contractility. *Prog. Retin. Eye Res.* 19:271-295.

Wilhelm, B, Lüdtke, H, Wilhelm, H, BRAION Study Group. Efficacy and tolerability of 0.2% brimonidine tartrate for the treatment of acute non-arteritic anterior ischemic optic neuropathy (NAION): a 3-month, double-masked, randomised, placebo-controlled trial. Graefes Arch Clin Exp Ophthalmol. 2006

Wood, J.P.M., Desantis, L., Chao, H.-M., Osborne, N.N. (2001) Topically applied betaxolol attenuates ischaemia-induced effects to the rat retina and stimulates BDNF mRNA. Exp. Eye Res. 72:79-86.

Wood, J.P.M., Schmidt, K.-G., Melena, J., Chidlow, G., Allmeier, H., Osborne, N.N. (2003) The b-adrenoceptor antagonists metipranolol and timolol are retinal neuroprotectants: comparison with betaxolol. Exp. Eye Res. 76:505-516.

Wu, H.Y., Tomizawa, K., Oda, Y., Wei, F.Y., Lu, Y.F., Matsushita, M., Li, S.T., Moriwaki, A., Matsui, H. (2004) Critical role of calpain-mediated cleavage of calcineurin in excitotoxic neurodegeneration. *J Biol Chem.* 279:4929-40.

Wu, G. Y., Deisseroth, K. & Tsien, R. W. (2001) Activitydependent CREB phosphorylation: convergence of a fast, sensitive calmodulin kinase pathway and a slow, less sensitive mitogen-activated protein kinase pathway. *Proc. Natl Acad. Sci. USA* 98:2808–2813.

Yamada, H., Chen, Y.N., Aihara, M., Araie, M. (2006) Neuroprotective effect of calcium channel blocker against retinal ganglion cell damage under hypoxia. Brain Res. 1071:75-80.

Yamagishi, S., Fujitani, M., Hata, K., Kitajo, K., Mimura, F., Abe, H., Yamashita, T. (2005). Wallerian degeneration involves Rho/Rho-kinase signaling. *J Biol Chem.* 27,280(21):20384-8.

Yanagisawa, M, Kurihara, H, Kimura, S, Tomobe, Y, Kobayashi, M, Mitsui, Y, Yazaki, Y, Goto, K, Masaki, T. (1988) A novel potent vasoconstrictor peptide produced by vascular endothelial cells. Nature. 332(6163):411-5.

Yang, Z., Quigley, H.A., Pease, M.E., Yang, Y., Qian J., Valenta, D. & Zack, D.J. (2007) Changes in gene expression in experimental glaucoma and optic nerve transection: the equilibrium between protective and detrimental mechanisms. *Invest. Ophthalmol. Vis. Sci.* 48:5539-5548.

Yorio, T., Krishnamoorthy, R. & Prasanna, G. (2002) Endothelin: Is it a contributor to glaucoma pathophysiology? *J Glaucoma.* 11:259-70.

Yu, S., Tanabe, T., Dezawa, M., Ishikawa, H., Yoshimura, N. (2006). Effects of bone marrow stromal cell injection in an experimental glaucoma model. *Biochem Biophys Res Commun.* 16,344(4):1071-9.

Zafra, F., Hengerer, B., Leibrock, J., Thoenen, H., Lindholm, D.(1990) Activity dependent regulation of BDNF and NGF mRNAs in the rat hippocampus is mediated by non NMDA glutamate receptors. *EMBO J.* 9:3545-50.

Zarbin, M.A., Montemagno, C., Leary, J.F., Ritch, R. (2010). Nanotechnology in ophthalmology. *Can J Ophthalmol.* 45(5):457-76

Zhang, H, Cuevas, J.(2002) Sigma receptors inhibit high-voltage-activated calcium channels in rat sympathetic and parasympathetic neurons. *J Neurophysiol.* 87:2867-2879.

Zhong, L., Bradley, J., Schubert, W., Ahmed, E., Adamis, AP., Shima, DT., Robinson, GS., Ng YS. (2007). Erythropoietin promotes survival of retinal ganglion cells in DBA/2J glaucoma mice. *Invest Ophthalmol Vis Sci.* 48(3):1212-8.

Zhou, Y., Pernet, V., Hauswirth, WW., Di Polo, A. (2005). Activation of the extracellular signal-regulated kinase 1/2 pathway by AAV gene transfer protects retinal ganglion cells in glaucoma. *Mol Ther.* 12(3):402-12.

# 8

# Neural Mechanisms Underlying Brimonidine's Protection of Retinal Ganglion Cells in Experimental Glaucoma

Cun-Jian Dong, William A. Hare and Larry Wheeler
*Department of Biological Sciences, Allergan Inc*
*The United States of America*

## 1. Introduction

Glaucoma is a neurodegenerative disease characterized by a progressive loss of retinal ganglion cells (RGCs), the output neurons of the retina. Elevated intraocular pressure (IOP) has long been recognized as a major risk factor for human glaucoma (Kass et al., 1980; Quigley et al., 1994; Tsai & Kanner, 2005). Indeed, in animal models of glaucoma, ranging from rodents (Johnson & Tomarev, 2010) to primates (Gaasterland & Kupfer, 1974; Hare et al., 2004), elevated IOP produced either biophysically (Gaasterland & Kupfer, 1974; WoldeMussie et al., 2001) or genetically (Anderson et al., 2001; Ju et al., 2009) can lead to RGC degeneration similar to that found in human glaucoma (Quigley, 2005).

A common and effective treatment for glaucoma is the use of IOP lowering topical drugs that act at a variety of cellular targets, such as the α2 and β adrenergic receptors (Tsai & Kanner, 2005). However, in many patients, the disease continues to progress despite successful IOP reduction with topical drugs (Heijl et al., 2002; Vasudevan et al., 2011).

Brimonidine, a selective α2 receptor agonist, is the active ingredient in one class of topical IOP lowering drugs, such as Alphagan® and Alphagn-P®. Brimonidine has been shown to protect RGCs in experimental glaucoma (WoldeMussie et al., 2001; Dong et al., 2008), retinal ischemia (Donello et al., 2001; Lai et al., 2002), optic nerve injury (Yoles et a., 1999), and retinal excitotoxicity (Dong et al., 2008). In experimental glaucoma, brimonidine's neuroprotective effect appears to be independent of its IOP lowering action (Dong et al., 2008; Hernandez et al., 2008). More recently, in a randomized, double-masked, multicenter clinical trial, brimonidine has been shown to be more effective in slowing disease progression (visual field loss), compared with timolol (a β blocker), despite the fact that the mean treated IOP was similar in both treatment groups at all time points (Krupin 2011). These clinical data suggest that brimonidine may have a *direct* RGC protective effect that is independent of its IOP lowering action in human low-pressure glaucoma, similar to that found in experimental glaucoma (Dong et al., 2008; Hernandez et al., 2008).

In this chapter, we will summarize the results of our recent studies on the mechanisms that underlie brimonidine's protection of RGCs in experimental glaucoma and retinal excitotoxicity. We will first describe the properties of RGCs and the *ex vivo* and *in vivo* models used in our studies on the mechanisms of RGC injury and protection. Then we will discuss neuronal $Ca^{++}$ signaling in health and disease, as well as the properties of the $\alpha2$ receptor and its intracellular signaling pathways responsible for brimonidine mediated neuroprotection. A particular emphasis will be placed on the role of the $\alpha2$ receptor in modulation of retinal $Ca^{++}$ signaling pre- and postsynaptic to RGCs. Finally, we will briefly discuss other beneficial effects of brimonidine in retinal disease models reported in the literature.

## 2. Properties of RGCs

The vertebrate retina is a part of the central nervous system (CNS) and RGCs are a type of CNS projection neuron (Dowling, 1987; Rodieck, 1973). Unlike all other types of retinal neurons that receive their synaptic inputs and send the outputs within the retina, RGCs receive synaptic input at the inner plexiform layer (IPL) of the retina, but transmit their output at locations far away from the retina via long axons (a major component of the optic nerve). Also unlike the majority of the retinal neurons, such as photoreceptors, bipolar cells, and horizontal cells, that use only graded potentials to transmit the visual signal, RGCs are the only retinal neurons that use *exclusively* action potentials (nerve spikes) to transmit signals to their postsynaptic neurons at higher brain centers, such as lateral geniculate nucleus and superior colliculus (Dowling, 1987; Ito et al., 2008; Rodieck & Watanabe, 1993).

While these unique functional and structural properties of RGCs are required for long-range signaling as projection neurons, they also cause significantly elevated metabolic demand due to increased energy (ATP) usage to prevent intracellular ionic imbalance resulting from the high frequency spiking activity and for long-range bidirectional axonal transport. This elevated metabolic demand likely makes RGCs more susceptible to various stresses under pathophysiological conditions, such as intracellular $Ca^{++}$ dysregulation (Dong et al., 2008), metabolic challenge caused by elevated IOP (Baltan et al., 2010) or vascular abnormality (Moore et al., 2008), and axonal ionic imbalance such as $Na^{+}$ overload (Dong & Hare, 2005; Waxman et al., 1994).

## 3. *Ex vivo* and *in vivo* models used in determination of the mechanisms of RGC injury and $\alpha2$ protection

In order to determine the mechanisms that underlie high IOP induced RGC degeneration in experimental glaucoma and protection by brimonidine, we used two *ex vivo* models: live rat retinal slice (Dong et al., 2007) and the isolated, flat-mount rat and rabbit retina (Dong et al., 2008) and two *in vivo* models: a rat chronic ocular hypertensive glaucoma model (WoldeMussie et al., 2001; Dong et al., 2008) and a rabbit retinal excitotoxicity model (Dong et al., 2008). We use the *ex vivo* models to study intracellular signaling pathways of the $\alpha2$ receptor and its interactions with the voltage- and transmitter-gated $Ca^{++}$ channels, namely the L-type $Ca^{++}$ channel and the NMDA receptor. We use *in vivo* models to test our hypotheses based on our findings from the *ex vivo* models. Rodent ocular hypertensive models of various kinds have been widely used in glaucoma research (Johnson & Tomarev, 2010). However, the other three models, namely the retinal slice, *in situ* RGCs in the isolated retina, and the rabbit retinal excitotoxicity model, are not commonly used. We therefore will briefly describe their unique features and utility in glaucoma research.

### 3.1 Live retinal slice

Both the retinal slice and isolated flat-mount retina are *ex vivo* preparations that retain rather well natural intercellular neural connections/interactions and have neuronal gene express patterns that are very similar to those under *in vivo* conditions. And yet, they allow experimentation under more controlled conditions than possible under *in vivo* conditions. For example, the compositions of extracellular media can be controlled precisely and changed rapidly and retinal neurons can be accessed readily for electrophysiological recording and optical imaging/labeling while still maintaining connections with their neighboring neurons and other supporting cells such as glial cells. Therefore, these *ex vivo* preparations are particularly useful for studies aiming at understanding the mechanisms of eye diseases and drug action.

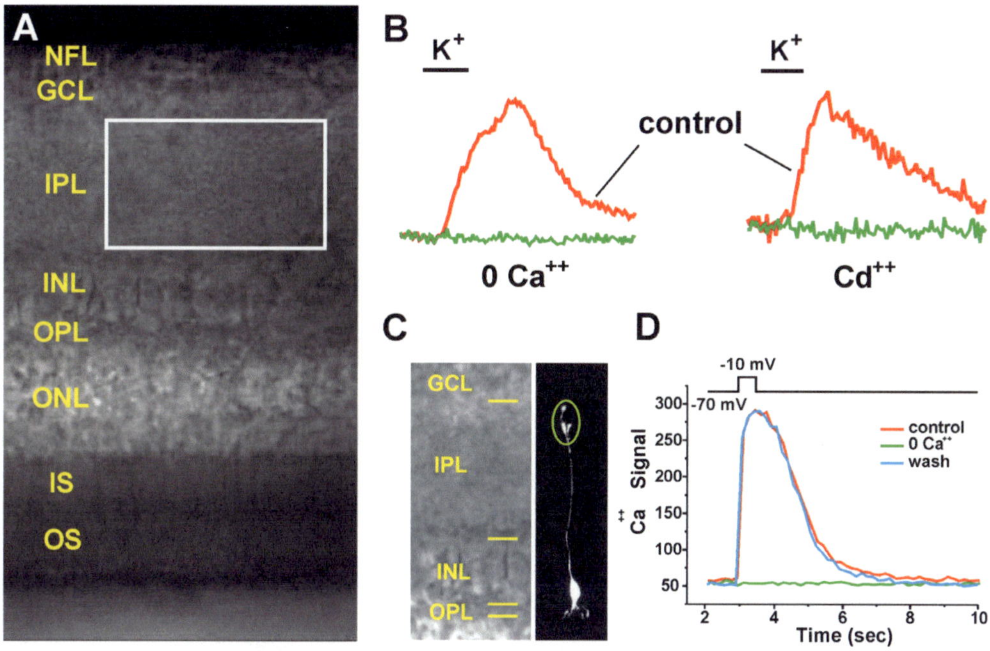


Fig. 1. The live rat retinal slice preparation. See the text for details

Intracellular $Ca^{++}$ plays a critical role in neuronal signal processing and communication, such as neurotransmitter release from presynaptic axon terminals. It is also a key signaling molecule to trigger cell apoptosis/death under pathophysiological conditions (see the next section below). Figure 1A shows an acutely cut and superfused rat retinal slice in which the major retinal layers (nerve fiber layer, NFL; ganglion cell layer, GCL; inner plexiform layer, IPL; inner nuclear layer, INL; outer plexiform layer, OPL; outer nuclear layer, ONL; photoreceptor inner segment, IS; photoreceptor outer segment, OS) are easily visible under the microscope with a water immersion objective. When retinal slices are loaded with a membrane permeable fluorescent $Ca^{++}$ dye (Fluo-4 AM), changes in cytosolic free $Ca^{++}$ under various experimental conditions can be recorded with a confocal imaging system (for technical details see Dong et al., 2007). Membrane depolarization induced by a 5-8 sec rapid perfusion of high $K^+$ Ringer solution elicited a robust $Ca^{++}$ signal (red traces in Fig. 1B) at

IPL where RGCs communicate with their presynaptic neurons, such as bipolar and amacrine cells. A representative area for the $Ca^{++}$ measurement at IPL is indicated by the white rectangle in Fig. 1A. The high $K^{+}$ induced $Ca^{++}$ signals were abolished completely after perfusing with either a $Ca^{++}$-free Ringer solution or normal Ringer solution that contained 100 μM $Cd^{++}$, a broad-spectrum $Ca^{++}$ channel blocker (green traces in Fig. 1B). This indicates that the signal is generated by $Ca^{++}$ influx through depolarization activated $Ca^{++}$ channels at IPL.

The $Ca^{++}$ influx into bipolar cell synaptic terminals (located at IPL) is likely a major contributor to the depolarization induced $Ca^{++}$ signal shown in Fig. 1B. Bipolar cells are key presynaptic partners of RGCs. Bipolar cells release glutamate (Matsui et al., 1998) as their neurotransmitter at the synaptic terminals to communicate with RGCs and amacrine cells and $Ca^{++}$ influx is needed to trigger the release. Therefore, it is not surprising that voltage-gated $Ca^{++}$ channels are highly concentrated at bipolar cell terminals for glutamate release (Pan, 2000, 2001). When these $Ca^{++}$ channels are over activated under pathophysiological conditions, such as retinal ischemia, glutamate released from bipolar terminals could be a major contributor to the significantly elevated extracellular glutamate that can cause excessive activation of the NMDA receptor on RGCs and lead to RGC dysfunction/death.

The right panel of Fig. 1C shows the confocal image of a $Ca^{++}$ dye labeled bipolar cell from a live rat retinal slice. The major parts of the cell, the dendrites, soma, axon, and synaptic terminals (indicated by the green oval), are clearly visible. The $Ca^{++}$ dye (a cell membrane-impermeable version of Fluo-4) was delivered to the bipolar cells intracellularly via a patch-clamp electrode (not shown). Membrane depolarization induced by a 0.5 sec voltage step from the holding potential of -70 mV to -10 mV through the recording electrode elicited at the bipolar cell terminals a large cytosolic free $Ca^{++}$ signal (Fig. 1D, arbitrary units) that was completely eliminated by removing $Ca^{++}$ from the Ringer solution. $Ca^{++}$ channels in the CNS, particularly those at presynaptic terminals, are important drug targets and *in situ* bipolar terminals provide an excellent *ex vivo* system for the studies on neuromodulation of presynaptic $Ca^{++}$ channel activity by brimonidine and other neuroactive drugs/drug candidates.

### 3.2 *In situ* RGCs in the isolated flat-mount retina

Because of the selective vulnerability of RGCs in glaucoma, a detailed characterization of physiological and pharmacological properties of RGCs can help to understand the mechanism of RGC injury in glaucoma and the mechanism of action of neuroprotective drugs, such as brimonidine, as well as to identify novel drug targets for the treatment of glaucoma. *In situ* RGCs in the acutely isolated, superfused retina (Fig. 2) offer a unique opportunity to study the pharmacological properties and intracellular signaling pathways of various neural active drugs and drug candidates on RGCs without significantly altering retinal synaptic connections and RGC gene expression pattern compared to RGC cell lines or even primary cultures.

Fig. 2A shows a bright field image of a piece of live isolated, superfused rabbit retina viewing from the vitreous side. The axon bundles (the main component of the nerve fiber layer) of RGCs are visible. After the inner limiting membrane and nerve fiber layer were carefully poked through and the debris were removed with a cleaning glass micropipette, somas of *in situ* RGCs were revealed and whole-cell recordings could be performed with patch-clamp electrodes (Fig. 2B). We routinely include a membrane-impermeable $Ca^{++}$ dye in the patch electrodes. Therefore, neurotransmitter agonist (such as NMDA) induced transmembrane currents and cytosolic free $Ca^{++}$ signals can be measured simultaneously. Fig. 2C shows the NMDA (applied with the co-agonist glycine) induced inward current and $Ca^{++}$ signal from an *in situ* RGC. A transient light response from that RGC is also visible immediately after the onset of the excitation light for $Ca^{++}$ imaging. After electrophysiological and optical recordings, the identity of the recorded cell can be confirmed with confocal imaging (Fig. 2D).

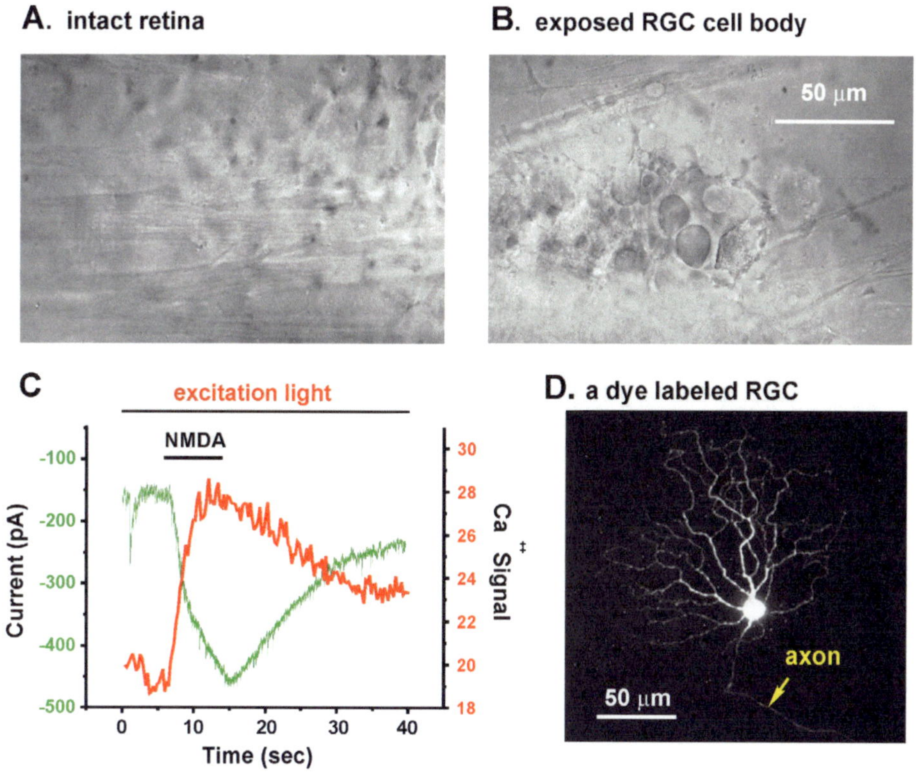


Fig. 2. *In situ* RGCs in the isolated, superfused rabbit retina. See the text for details

### 3.3 Rabbit retinal excitotoxicity model

Excessive activation of glutamate receptors, particularly the NMDA receptor, has been suggested as a key factor that contributes to high IOP induced RGC loss in experimental glaucoma, regardless how IOP is elevated and what animal species is selected (Dong et al., 2008; Hare et al., 2004; Ju et al., 2009; WoldeMussie et al., 2002).

Intravitreal injection of NMDA, a selective agonist of the NMDA sub-type of ionotropic glutamate receptor, can also induced RGC loss by directly activating the NMDA receptor on RGCs. The rat (Siliprandi et al., 1992) and mouse (Ito et al., 2008) retinal NMDA models have been used in glaucoma research to explore the mechanism of RGC injury and to evaluate efficacy of potential RGC protective drug candidates. However, relatively hard to perform intravitreal injection and lack of macular-like structure are two major disadvantages of the rodent models.

We therefore developed a rabbit retinal NMDA model (Fig. 3, see also Dong et al., 2008). The rabbit has large eyes and it's significantly easier to conduct multiple intravitreal injections in rabbit eyes with low risk of causing accidental retinal or lens damage (both of which can affect RGC survival directly or indirectly). This facilitates *in vivo* studies on the mechanisms of RGC protection by brimonidine or other novel neuroprotective agents.

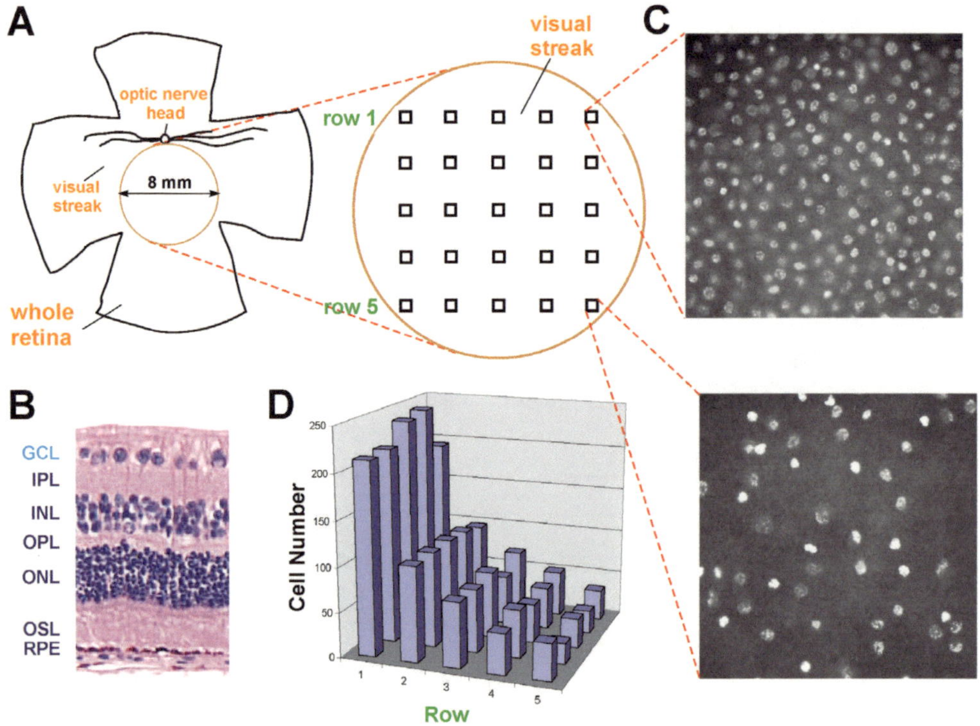


Fig. 3. The rabbit model to evaluate NMDA excitotoxicity. See the text for details

The rabbit retina also has a visual streak that is an elongated macular-like structure that has the highest density of neurons in the retina (Fig. 3C and 3D). This allows us to study the differential vulnerability of RGCs located at the center (visual streak) versus more peripheral retinal locations, which may provide an important clue as to why the central visual fields are more resistant to glaucomatous injury in human glaucoma (Dong et al., 2011). Fig. 3A shows an isolated rabbit retina. We routinely cut out a circular piece (8 mm in diameter) from the central retina using the optic nerve head as a marker to ensure that we compare the same regions of the retina between different experimental groups. We count the neurons in the ganglion cell layer at 25 locations in a 5x5 array using a computer-controlled automated microscope stage (see Dong et al., 2008 for technical details). The circular piece of the retina is aligned carefully so that the first row of 5 sites is located within the visual streak (Fig. 1A). Fig. 1B shows a representative cross section of H&E stained rabbit retina. The individual dots in Fig. 1C are nuclei of RGCs and displaced amacrine cells in the ganglion cell layer labelled with a fluorescent nuclear dye (DAPI). The density of the neurons drops rapidly from the visual streak (row 1) to more peripheral retina (rows 2 to 5). Fig. 1D shows the 3D plot of the cell density profile based on neuron density of these 25 sites.

## 4. Intracellular $Ca^{++}$ dysregulation and neurodegeneration

There is compelling evidence that intracellular $Ca^{++}$ dysregulation is a key contributor to neurodegeneration in a wide range of CNS degenerative diseases, such as Alzheimer's disease and Parkinson's disease (Bezprozvanny, 2009). In addition to age and genetically related changes in intracellular $Ca^{++}$ handling, $Ca^{++}$ overload as a result of excessive activation of voltage- and ligand-gated $Ca^{++}$ channels on the neuronal cell membrane, particularly the NMDA receptor, plays a central role in intracellular $Ca^{++}$ dysregulation (Choi, 1985; Choi et al., 1988). The NMDA receptor is a type of ionotropic glutamate receptor that is coupled to a cation channel which has a high $Ca^{++}$ permeability (MacDermott et al., 1986; Sattler & Tymianski, 2001). It is therefore sometimes called the ligand-gated $Ca^{++}$ channel. Unlike the other types of ionotropic glutamate receptors (such as AMPA and kainate receptors) that desensitize rapidly and significantly in the continuous presence of the agonist (Hestrin et al., 1990; Lukasiewicz et al., 1995), the NMDA receptor shows significantly less desensitization in the continuous presence of the agonists (MacDermott et al., 1986; Matsui et al., 1998) and is therefore particularly effective in causing intracellular $Ca^{++}$ overload when excessively activated.

Intracellular $Ca^{++}$ overload can trigger neuronal apoptosis via a number of cross-amplifying pathways, including $Ca^{++}$-activated proteases and their downstream effectors such as calpain and calpain-activated caspases (Das et al., 2005; Sharma & Rohrer, 2004), mitochondrial dysfunction and damage directly produced by $Ca^{++}$ overload (Starkov et al., 2004), and $Ca^{++}$ dependent cytosolic overproduction of free radicals (Brennan et al., 2009; Sattler et al., 1999).

### 4.1 NMDA receptor, intracellular $Ca^{++}$ dysregulation, and RGC degeneration

Intracellular $Ca^{++}$ dysregulation/overload caused by deregulated retinal glutamatergic transmission is also likely a key mechanism that causes RGC dysfunction (Hare & Wheeler, 2009) and degeneration in disease states, such as acute retinal ischemia (Lagreze et al., 1998) and experimental glaucoma (Dong et al., 2008; Harada et al., 2007; Ju et al., 2009). For example, vulnerability of RGCs in acute retinal ischemia is associated not only with NMDA receptor activity (Lagreze et al., 1998), but also with significantly elevated vitreal glutamate level (Donello et al., 2001; Lagreze et al., 1998). Brimonidine not only protects RGCs in retinal ischemia, but also significantly reduced vitreal glutamate concentration (Donello et al., 2001), suggesting that it either prevents excessive release of glutamate or enhances its uptake, or both.

## 5. The $\alpha 2$ adrenergic receptor

The $\alpha 2$ adrenergic receptor is a G-protein coupled receptor (GPCRs, Fig. 4) that can signal through both $G_{\alpha}$ and $G_{\beta\gamma}$ subunits (Delaney et al., 2007; Maze, 1991). In the CNS, the major functional role of the $\alpha 2$ receptor is modulation of neurotransmitter release (Starke, 2001). This action is through the classical *presynaptic* inhibition either by inhibiting $Ca^{++}$ channels (Boehm, 1999; Starke, 2001), activating $K^{+}$ channels (Bünemann et al., 2001), or reducing active release sites (Delaney et al., 2007). Presynaptic inhibition by the $\alpha 2$ receptor in the brain is mediated by the $G_{\beta\gamma}$ subunits (Fig. 4B, see also Delaney et al., 2007).

The $\alpha 2$ receptor is coupled to $G_{\alpha i/o}$ (i for inhibition of adenylate cyclase and o for olfactory type). When signaling through the $G_{\alpha}$ subunit, $\alpha 2$ receptor activation leads to inhibition of adenylate cyclase, resulting in a reduction of cAMP production. cAMP is an important intracellular second messenger that modulates many aspects of cellular function through interacting with various downstream effectors (Maze, 1991), such as protein kinase A. Alpha 2 receptors are known to be expressed in retinal neurons, including retinal bipolar cells (Dong et al., unpublished results) and RGCs (Kalapesi et al., 2005).

### 5.1 Suppression of NMDA receptor function by brimonidine

As shown in Fig. 2, robust NMDA induced transmembrane currents and cytosolic free $Ca^{++}$ signals can be recorded from *in situ* RGCs in the isolated, superfused retina when they are voltage-clamped close to their resting membrane potential at -70 mV. We reported (Dong et al., 2008) that pretreatment with brimonidine produced a significant suppression of both of these NMDA induced signals in RGCs (Fig. 5B and 5C). NMDA (plus glycine) was applied with a local perfusion micropipette (Fig. 5A) that was connected to a computer-controlled, multi-channel drug delivery system in a 0 $Mg^{++}$ Ringer. This allowed rapid delivery and removal of NMDA as well as effective activation of the NMDA receptor without the voltage-dependent $Mg^{++}$ block. Brimonidine and atipamezole (a selective $\alpha 2$ antagonist) were delivered using both bath (the whole-chamber) and the local perfusion systems. The $Ca^{++}$ dye and some tool compounds, such as GDP-βS, were delivered intracellularly to the RGC using the recording pipette.

The suppressive effect of brimonidine on NMDA responses is mediated by the $\alpha 2$ receptor, because this effect was completely blocked (Fig. 5C) by a highly selective $\alpha 2$ antagonist, atipamezole (Virtanen, 1989). Brimonidine's effect is direct on RGCs since it was also completely blocked (Fig. 5C) by intracellularly applied GDP-βS, a membrane impermeable GPCR inhibitor that blocks exchange of GDP for GTP on the $G_{\alpha}$ subunit of the G-protein (Fig. 4A), an obligate event required for $\alpha 2$ receptor activation. Other intracellularly delivered tool compounds that act at various sites along the $\alpha 2$ receptor signaling pathway also blocked brimonidine's effect on NMDA receptor function (see section 5.2), confirming that brimonidine's effect is direct on RGCs, not an indirect effect through other retinal cells.

### 5.2 Brimonidine suppresses NMDA receptor function through the $G_{\alpha i}$ pathway

Using tool compounds acting at different sites along the $G_{\alpha i}$ signaling pathway (Fig. 4), we have obtained compelling evidence that brimonidine's effect on NMDA receptor function is mediated almost exclusively by the $G_{\alpha i}$ pathway (Dong et al., 2008). We found that SQ22536, a selective inhibitor of adenylate cyclase (Fabbri et al., 1991), mimicked the effect of brimonidine on NMDA receptor function (Fig. 6A). On the other hand, forskolin (abbreviated as "forsk" in Fig. 6B), an activator of AC (de Souza et al., 1983), blocked the effect of brimonidine (abbreviated as "brimo" in Fig. 6B). This suggests that intracellular cAMP is an important regulator of NMDA receptor function in RGCs (Fig. 6C). A reduction of adenylate cyclase activity, produced either indirectly by brimonidine via $\alpha 2$ receptor activation (Fig. 6D) or directly by SQ222536 (Fig. 6A & 6E), can lead to the same effect: suppression of NMDA receptor function likely through a decrease in intracellular cAMP concentration. On the other hand, forskolin blocks brimonidine's effect likely through neutralizing brimonidine's effect on adenylate cyclase activity and therefore preventing significant alteration of intracellular cAMP concentration (Fig. 6B & 6F).

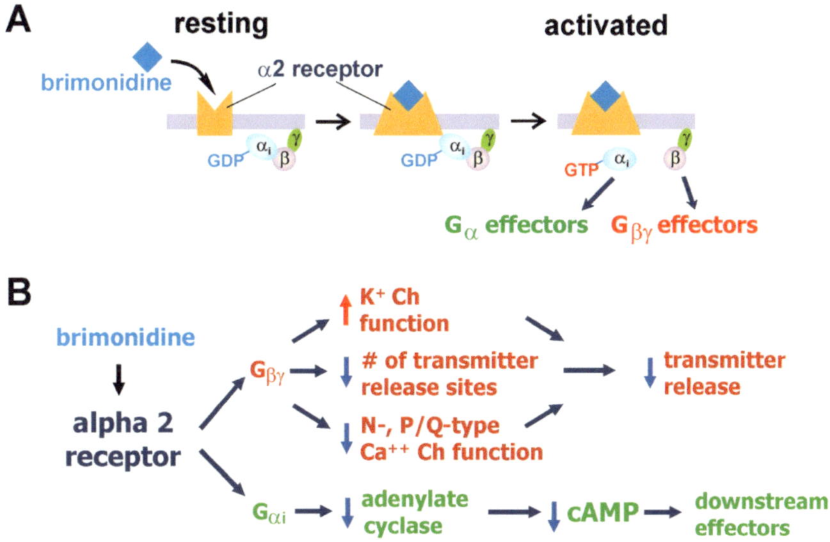


Fig. 4. Activation and intracellular signaling pathways of the α2 receptor

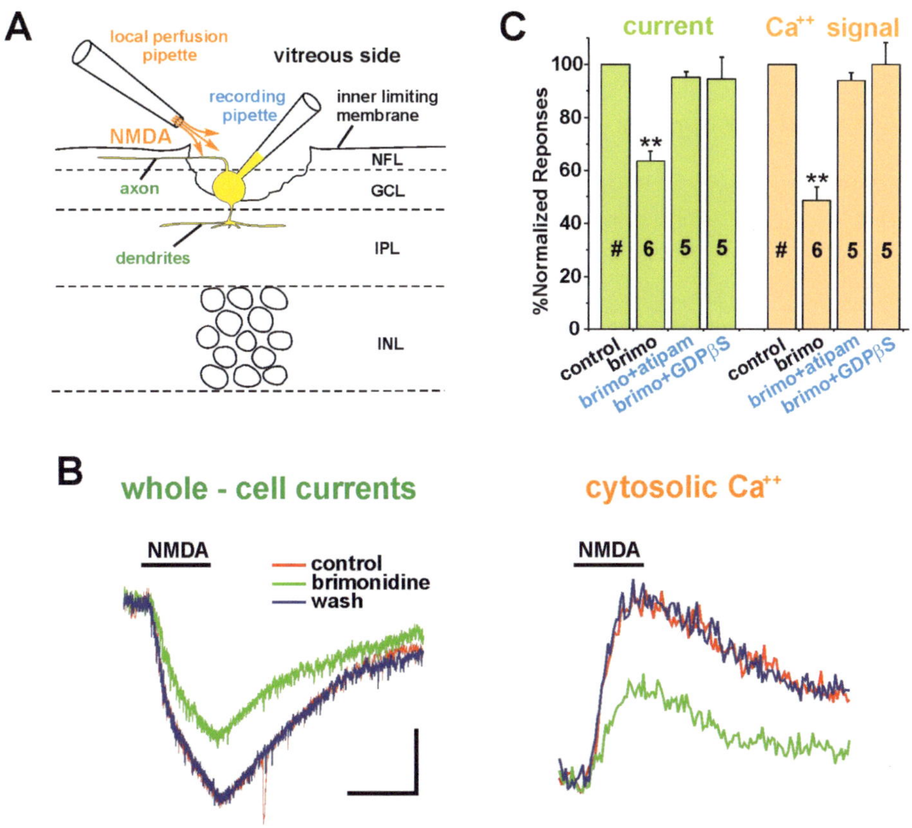


Fig. 5. Brimonidine modulation of NMDA receptor function. See the text for details

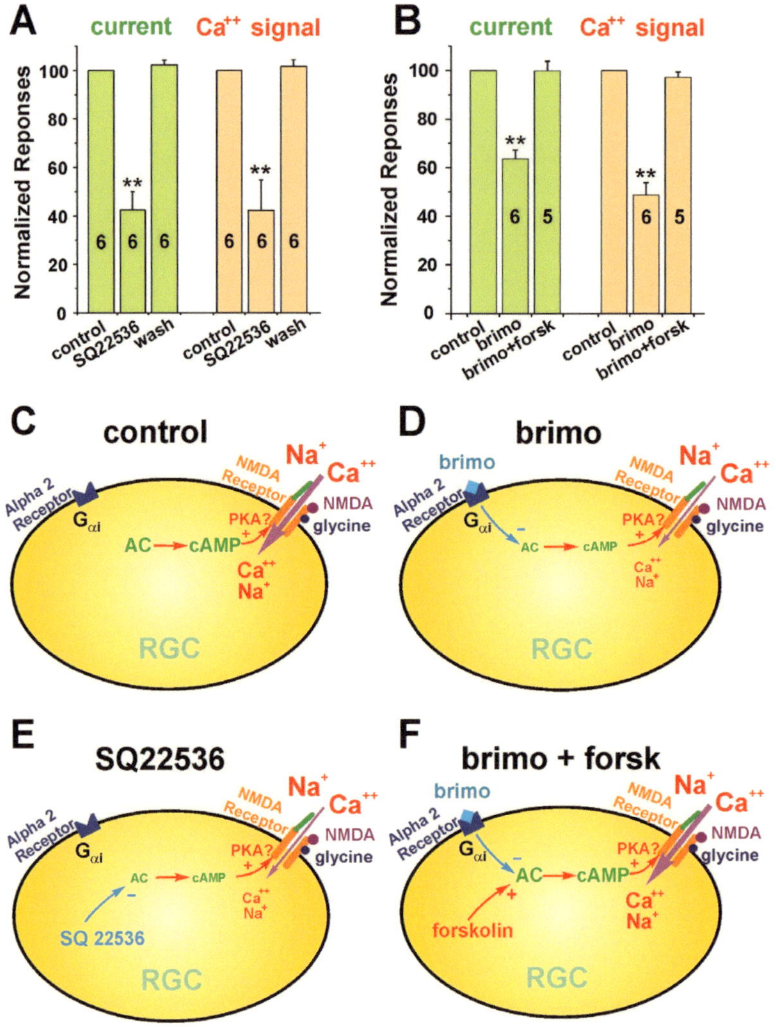


Fig. 6. Effects of an adenylate cyclase (AC) inhibitor and activator. See the text for details

Results with other tool agents provide additional support that brimonidine's effect is mediated by the $G_{\alpha i}$ pathway. To avoid potential global indirect effects of intracellularly acting tool agents on recorded RGCs, we applied those agents intracellularly through the recording pipette. Therefore, the effects are largely limited within the recorded RGCs. Intracellular application of Sp-cAMPS, a synthetic cell-permeable, hydrolysis-resistant cAMP analog, blocks *completely* brimonidine's effect on NMDA receptor function (Fig. 7A). To confirm that the lack of brimonidine's effect is indeed due to the presence of intracellular Sp-cAMPS, but not because of damage caused by patch-clamping, we recorded the same group of RGCs twice: in the presence and absence of Sp-cAMPS. After the first set of recordings were done with the electrode attached (Fig. 7A), we successfully removed the Sp-cAMPS-filled recording electrodes from 5 RGCs without causing significant damage to those cells. After waiting for a few minutes to allow the residual intracellular Sp-cAMPS to diffuse out of the RGCs and wash away, we observed a typical brimonidine-induced suppression of NMDA induced $Ca^{++}$ signal in the *same* group of RGCs (Fig. 7B, note: the $Ca^{++}$ dye delivered intracellularly by the electrode is a membrane impermeable form of Fluo-4 and therefore stayed inside the RGCs even after the electrode was removed). Thus, "clamping" intracellular cAMP level experimentally with equivalent synthetic cAMP analog is able to eliminate *completely* brimonidine's effect.

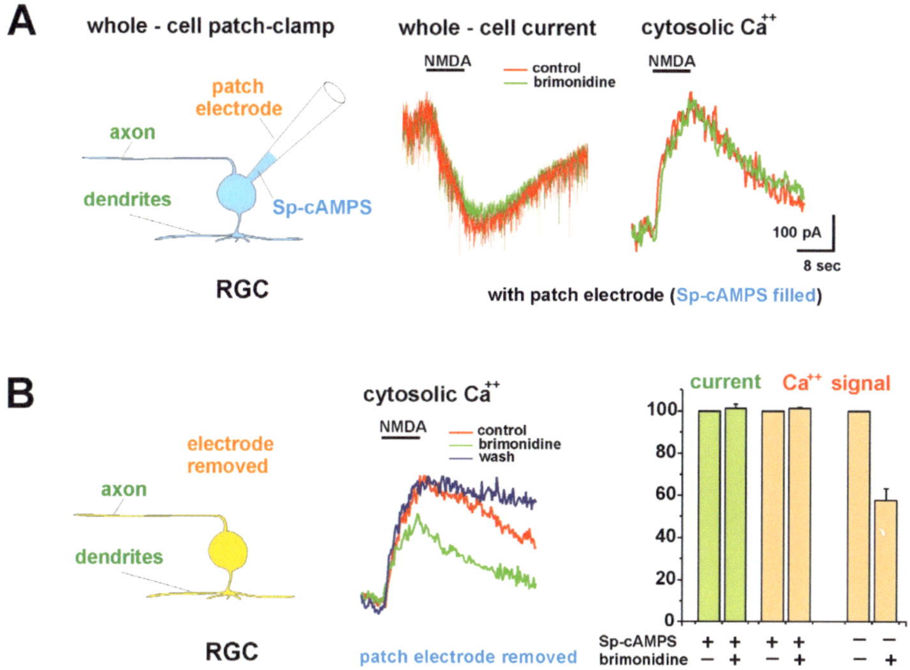


Fig. 7. Brimonidine's effect is blocked by intracellular application of a cAMP analog

In another experiment, we attempted to maintain *endogenous* intracellular cAMP level in RGCs through blocking its active degradation by phosphodiesterases (PDE). When rolipram, a type 4 PDE (a cAMP specific PDE) inhibitor (Teixeira et al., 1997), was intracellularly delivered through the recording electrode into a RGC, brimonidine's suppressive effect on the NMDA receptor mediated transmembrane current and cytosolic free $Ca^{++}$ signal was also completely blocked (Fig. 8A). In this RGC, we succeeded not only in removing the rolipram-filled electrode but also in re-recording the same RGC with a second, rolipram-free electrode. This allowed both electrical and optical recordings being repeated in the absence of the PDE inhibitor and typical brimonidine's effect on NMDA responses was observed (Fig. 8B). These results demonstrate that preserving endogenous cAMP level through blocking its active degradation by PDE is also able to *completely* eliminate brimonidine's effect, confirming that brimonidine's effect is mediated by the $G_{\alpha i}$–AC–cAMP pathway coupled to the α2 receptor.

Fig. 9 summarizes the sites of action of various tool compounds used in our studies to dissect out the intracellular signaling pathway through which brimonidine modulates NMDA receptor function. Among the tool agents, SQ22536 mimics brimonidine's effect by a direct inhibition of the adenylate cyclase. Those in red are all able to block brimonidine's effect at the different sites along the $G_{\alpha i}$ mediated signaling pathway. With these tool agents, we have demonstrated clearly that brimonidine can down modulate NMDA receptor function in RGCs and this brimonidine's effect is mediated predominantly, if not exclusively, by the $G_{\alpha i}$–AC–cAMP pathway coupled to the α2 receptor.

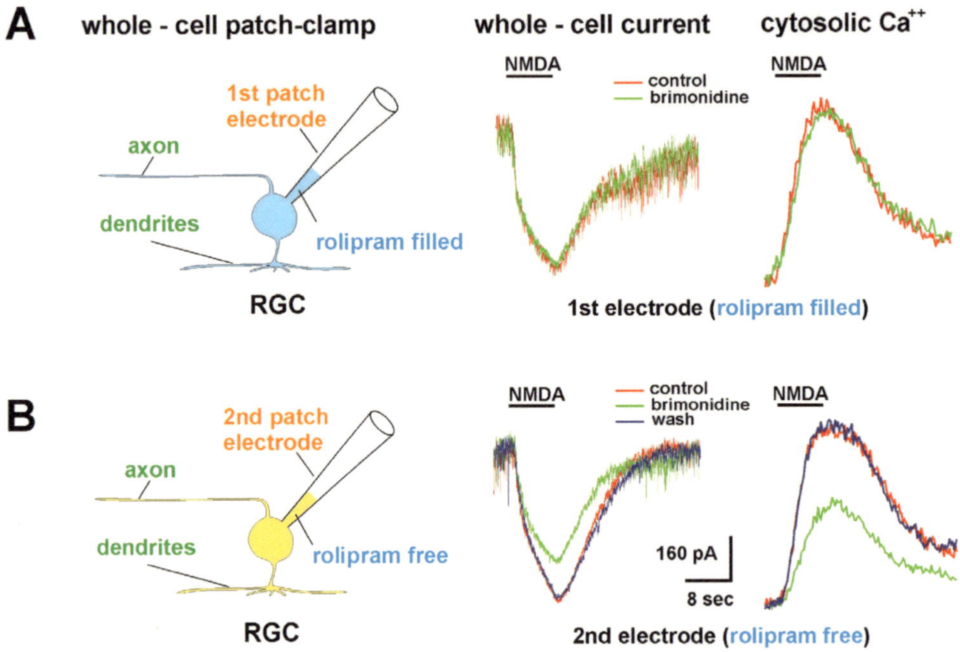


Fig. 8. Brimonidine's effect is blocked by intracellular application of a PDE-4 inhibitor

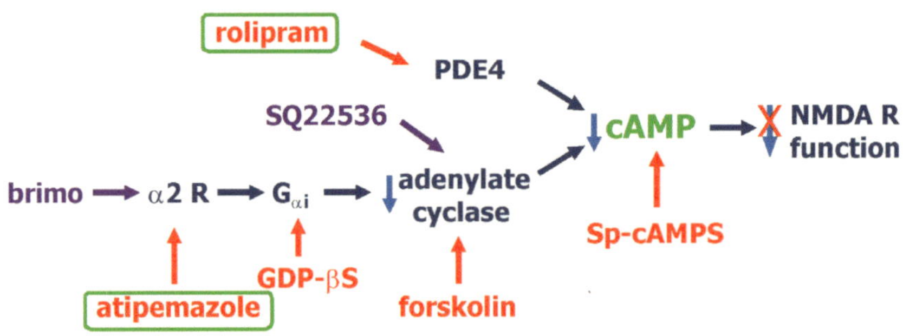


Fig. 9. The sites of action of the tool agents used along the $G_{\alpha i}$–AC–cAMP pathway

## 6. Validation in *in vivo* models

To test whether α2 receptor mediated modulation of NMDA receptor function in *in situ* RGCs contributes significantly to RGC protection by brimonidine in *in vivo* models, we evaluated in *in vivo* models two of the tool agents, atipamezole and rolipram (Fig. 9), that have a proven CNS bioavailability after systemic application. Only a minority of all tool agents that work well in *in vitro* models can be used in *in vivo* models for target validation or proof of concept due to practical reasons such as systemic toxicity, bioavailability, and unfavorable pharmacokinetics. Atipamezole and rolipram have already been successfully used in many whole animal studies for other purposes and are therefore chosen for use in our *in vivo* validation experiments.

### 6.1 Rat glaucoma model

The first *in vivo* model we tested is a rat glaucoma model. In this rat model, elevated IOP (from approximately 15 to 32 mmHg) produced by laser photocoagulation of episclearal and limbal veins leads to approximately 30% RGC loss evaluated at 3 weeks following the laser treatment (WoldeMussie et al., 2001; Dong et al., 2008). We used subcutaneous osmotic pumps to deliver brimonidine alone or in combination with atipamezole or rolipram. Memantine, an NMDA receptor channel blocker, was also used as a positive control to confirm the role of the NMDA receptor in RGC injury in this experimental glaucoma model (WoldeMussie et al, 2002).

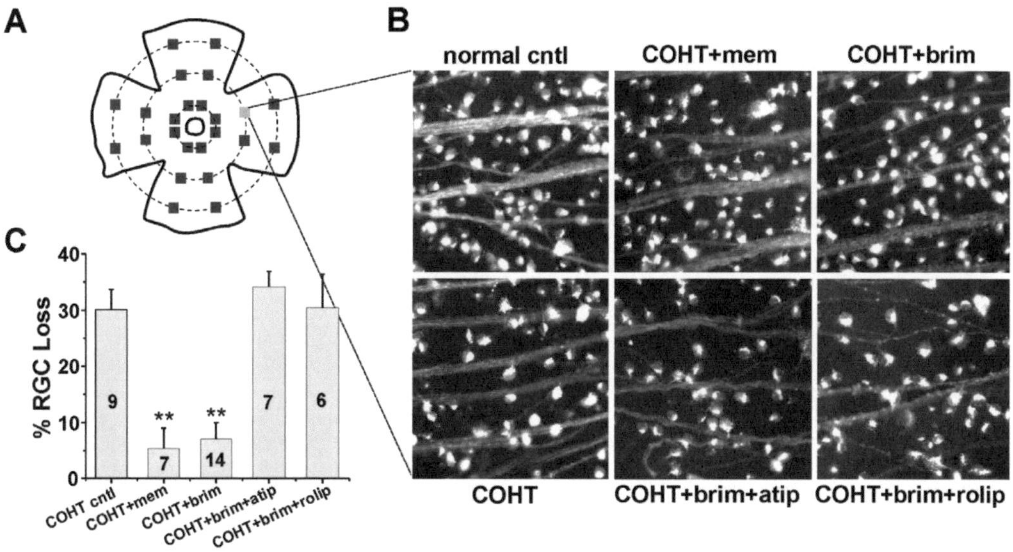


Fig. 10. Brimonidine's protection of RGCs in the rat glaucoma model is mediated by the $G_{\alpha i}$–AC–cAMP signaling pathway coupled to the α2 receptor. See the Dong et al., 2008 for technical details

We used a computer-controlled automated microscope stage and counted dextran tetramethylrhodamine retrogradely labeled RGCs at 24 sites (Fig. 10A). Fig. 10B shows representative images from an intermediate retinal location taken from a normal rat and glaucomatous rats under various treatment conditions: laser treatment alone (COHT for chronic ocular hypertension), COHT treated with memantine (COHT+mem), brimonidine (COHT+brim), brimonidine plus atipamezole (COHT+brim+atip), brimonidine plus rolipram (COHT+brim+rolip). Both memantine and brimonidine provided substantial protection of RGCs in this rat glaucoma model (Fig. 10C), consistent with the observations reported in previous studies (WoldeMussie et al., 2001, 2002). We found that brimonidine's protective effect was completely blocked by co-administration of atipamezole, verifying for the first time that brimonidine's effect is indeed mediated by the α2 receptor. Furthermore, RGC protection by brimonidine was also *completely* blocked by co-administration of rolipram, a novel finding that identifies PDE-4 as a key endogenous player contributing to brimonidine's protection of RGCs. Together these *in vivo* results suggest strongly that the $G_{\alpha i}$-AC-cAMP signaling pathway coupled to the α2 receptor, described above in *in situ* RGCs, is responsible for RGC protection by brimonidine in this rat glaucoma model.

### 6.2 Rabbit retinal NMDA model

In animal glaucoma models, ranging from mouse to monkey (including the rat model used here), NMDA receptor mediated excitotoxicity is a major contributor to RGC injury regardless whether IOP elevation is produced biophysically (Dong et al., 2008; Hare et al., 2004; WoldeMussie et al., 2002) or genetically (Ju et al., 2009). We have demonstrated that brimonidine down-modulates NMDA receptor function through the α2 receptor coupled $G_{\alpha i}$-AC-cAMP signaling pathway (see Fig. 4 and Fig. 9 above). We also showed that the same $G_{\alpha i}$ pathway is responsible for brimonidine's protection of RGCs in the rat glaucoma model (Fig. 10). Therefore, it is likely that brimonidine protects RGCs in the glaucoma models, at least in part, through attenuation of NMDA receptor mediated excitotoxicity.

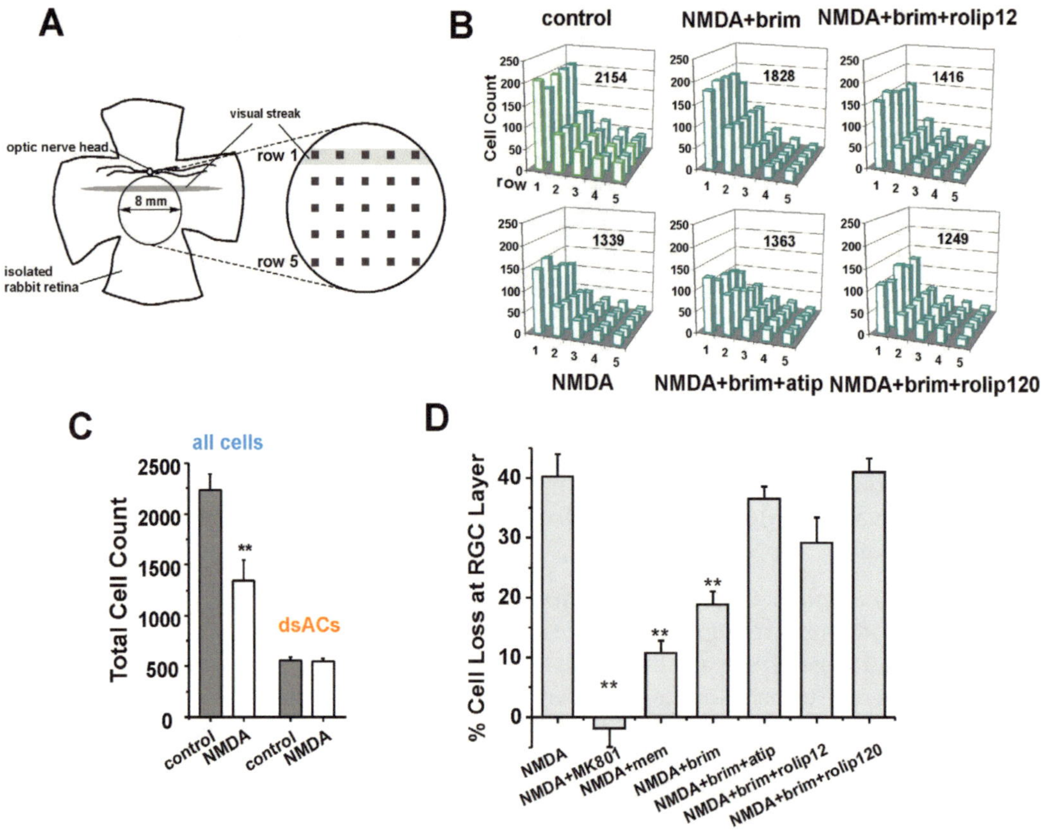


Fig. 11. Brimonidine's protection of RGCs in the rabbit retinal NMDA model is mediated by the $G_{\alpha i}$-AC-cAMP signaling pathway coupled to the α2 receptor. See the text for details

To test this *directly*, we used the rabbit retinal NMDA excitotoxicity model described in section 3 above (Fig. 3). We counted the total number of all neurons in the ganglion cell layer at 25 sites (Fig. 11A) at 2 weeks following intravitreal application of NMDA alone or in combination with other tool agents (Fig. 11D). These tool agents were applied intravitreally 3 times: 1 hour prior to NMDA injection, co-injected with NMDA, and 24 hours following NMDA injection (See Dong et al., 2008 for details). In the rabbit retinal ganglion cell layer, approximately two-thirds of the neurons are RGCs and the remaining one-third are displaced amacrine cells, predominantly displaced starburst amacrine cells (dsACs, 85% of all displace amacrine cells, Vaney, 1984; Vaney et al., 1981). These dsACs can be selectively labeled with a very low dose of DAPI (4',6-diamidino-2-phenylindole, a fluorescent nuclear dye, Vaney et al., 1981; Dong et al., 2010). We found that these dsACs are resistant to NMDA excitotoxicity: the same intravitreal dose of NMDA (3.6 μmol) that produced a substantial cell loss at ganglion cell layer had no effect on dsACs (Fig. 11C), indicating a selective vulnerability of RGCs to NMDA receptor mediated excitotoxicity.

RGC loss produced by intravitreal injection of NMDA is caused by excessive activation of NMDA receptors on RGCs since it can be completely blocked by MK801 (Fig. 11D), a potent and selective NMDA receptor channel blocker (Thompson et al., 1990). RGC loss can also be significantly attenuated by memantine (a less potent, but safer NMDA channel blocker, Fig. 11D). Pretreatment with brimonidine produced a significant protection of RGCs against NMDA excitotoxicity. This protective effect was completely blocked by co-pretreatment with the α2 receptor antagonist atipamezole (Fig. 11D), verifying that brimonidine's protection of RGCs against NMDA excitotoxicity is mediated by the α2 receptor. The PDE-4 inhibitor, rolipram, also blocked brimonidine's effect in a dose-dependent manner at 12 and 120 nmol (Fig. 11D), indicating that this effect is mediated by the $G_{\alpha i}$–AC–cAMP signaling pathway coupled to the α2 receptor (Fig. 4).

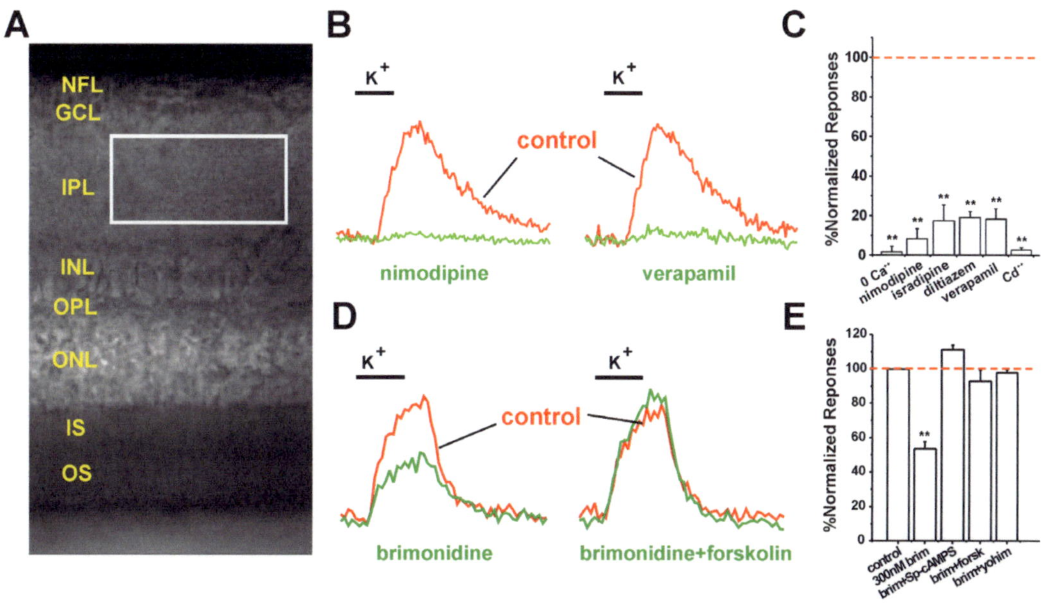


Fig. 12. Brimonidine modulation of L-type Ca++ channel function at IPL. See the text for details

We have shown with *in situ* RGCs that brimonidine modulates NMDA receptor function through the α2 receptor coupled $G_{\alpha i}$–AC–cAMP signaling pathway (Dong et al, 2008; see section 5 above). We have also shown that brimonidine protects RGCs through the same $G_{\alpha i}$–AC–cAMP signaling pathway in both experimental glaucoma and retinal NMDA excitotoxicity models (Figs. 10 and 11). Together, our *ex vivo* and *in vivo* data suggest strongly that brimonidine modulation of NMDA receptor function is a major mechanism of RGC protection in experimental glaucoma.

## 7. Modulation of retinal L-type $Ca^{++}$ channel function by brimonidine at IPL

In addition to modulation of NMDA receptor function postsynaptically in RGCs, brimonidine was also found to modulate the function of voltage-gated $Ca^{++}$ channel at IPL (Dong et al., 2007), a major retinal synaptic layer where communication between RGCs and their presynaptic partners, such as bipolar cells, takes place. In the most regions of CNS, release of neurotransmitters are mediated by voltage-gated N- and P/Q types of $Ca^{++}$ channels (Reid et al., 2003). However, in the retina the L-type $Ca^{++}$ channel plays a dominant role in transmitter release, particularly at photoreceptor and bipolar cell synaptic terminals where glutamate is released (Morgans et al., 2005; Pan, 2000, 2001; Tachibana et al., 1993).
Using several commonly used L-type $Ca^{++}$ channel blockers, we demonstrated that the depolarization (using a high K+ Ringer) induced $Ca^{++}$ signals at IPL were mediated predominantly by the L-type $Ca^{++}$ channel (Dong et al., 2010; see also Fig. 12B & 12C). We also showed that brimonidine down modulated this L-type channel mediated $Ca^{++}$ signal (Dong et al., 2007; see also Fig. 12D). Brimonidine's effect was blocked by Sp-cAMPS, forskolin, and yohimbine (a selective α2 antagonist), indicating that the effect is also mediated by the α2 receptor coupled $G_{\alpha i}$–AC–cAMP signaling pathway (Fig. 12E).
A major contributor to the depolarization induced $Ca^{++}$ signal at IPL is the presynaptic terminals of bipolar cells (Fig. 1C & 1D) where L-type $Ca^{++}$ channels are expressed in high density for glutamate release (Pan, 2000, 2001; Tachibana et al., 1993). We found at the presynaptic terminals from individual *in situ* bipolar cells (Fig. 1C) that the $Ca^{++}$ signal induced by a depolarization voltage step applied through a patch-clamp electrode (Fig. 1D) was also modulated by brimonidine (unpublished observation). Thus, together our results suggest that preventing presynaptic glutamate overrelease by brimonidine is likely an additional neural mechanism contributing to brimonidine's protection of RGCs in experimental glaucoma and acute retinal ischemia. It is also consistent with the observation that brimonidine application reduced vitreal glutamate concentration in acute retinal ischemia (Donello et al., 2001).

## 8. Other neuroprotective effects by brimonidine

In addition to preventing RGC $Ca^{++}$ overload by modulating activities of both voltage-gated (Fig. 12) and ligand-gated (Fig. 5) $Ca^{++}$ channels that are pre- and post-synaptic to RGCs, brimonidine can also up-regulate survival factors/pathways in the retina. For example, in acute retinal ischemia, brimonidine's neuroprotection is associated with up-regulation of basic fibroblast growth factor, bcl-2, bcl-xl, as well as activation of the PI3 kinase/protein kinase B (Akt) and extracellular-signal-regulated kinase (ERK) pathways (Lai et al., 2002). We believe that some of these beneficial effects of brimonidine may be related to its modulation of NMDA receptor function (Fig. 5). For example, increased expression of bcl-2 and decrease expression of Bax (a proapoptosis member in the bcl-2 family) is associated with blockage of the NMDA receptor by memantine in a mouse glaucoma model (DBA/2J, Ju et al., 2009).

In experimental glaucoma (Lambert et al., 2011) and acute retinal ischemia (López-Herrera et al., 2002), brimonidine also preserves retrograde and anterograde axonal transport in RGCs. This brimonidine's effect may be related to its action on preventing intracellular $Ca^{++}$ overload in RGCs via modulation of NMDA receptor function (Fig. 5), since a healthy soma and unimpaired mitochondrial function are required to provide energy needed for effective transport. It is well established that mitochondria dysfunction caused by NMDA receptor mediated $Ca^{++}$ overload plays a central role in neuronal cell death in disease states (Pivovarova & Andrews, 2010; Stout et al., 1998). Indeed, in experimental glaucoma, it has been shown recently that RGC injury is associated with NMDA receptor mediated mitochondrial dysfunction and can be prevented by NMDA receptor blockade with memantine (Ju et al., 2009).

## 9. Conclusion

Neuronal $Ca^{++}$ dysregulation, particularly $Ca^{++}$ overload caused by excessive activation of the NMDA receptor and voltage-gated $Ca^{++}$ channels, is an important common final pathway leading to neural dysfunction/death in a wide range of CNS neurodegenerative diseases (Bezprozvanny, 2009).

Our *ex vivo* and *in vivo* findings have provided strong evidence that functional modulation of the NMDA receptor (Fig. 4) and the L-type $Ca^{++}$ channel (Fig. 12) in the retina are two key mechanisms through which brimonidine protects RGCs in animal models of glaucoma and retinal excitotoxicity. Brimonidine also upregulates pro-survival molecules and pathways (Lai et al., 2002). These mechanisms may contribute to brimonidine's IOP-independent preservation of visual function in human glaucoma (also a CNS neurodegenerative disease) observed in a recent randomized, double-masked, multicenter clinical trial (Krupin at al., 2011).

## 10. Acknowledgement

The authors would like to thank Yuanxing Guo and Peter Agey for their important contribution to the *ex vivo* and *in vivo* experiments described in this chapter.

## 11. References

Anderson, M.G., Smith, R.S., Savinova, O.V., Hawes, N.L., Chang, B., Zabaleta, A., Wilpan, R., Heckenlively, J.R., Davisson, M., & John, S.W. (2001). Genetic modification of glaucoma associated phenotypes between AKXD-28/Ty and DBA/2J mice. *BMG Genetics.*, Vol. 2, No. 1.

Baltan, S., Inman, D.M., Danilov, C.A., Morrison, R.S., Calkins, D.J., Horner, P.J. (2010). Metabolic vulnerability disposes retinal ganglion cell axons to dysfunction in a model of glaucomatous degeneration. *J. Neurosci.*, Vol. 30, No. 16, 5644-5652.

Bezprozvanny, I. (2009). Calcium signaling and neurodegenerative diseases. *Trends. Mol. Med.*, Vol. 15, No. 3, 89-100.

Boehm, S. (1999). Presynaptic alpha2-adrenoceptors control excitatory, but not inhibitory, transmission at rat hippocampal synapses. J. Physiol., Vol. 519. Part 2, 439-449.

Brennan, A.M., Suh, S.W., Won, S.J., Narasimhan, P., Kauppinen, T.M., Lee, H., Edling, Y., Chan, P.H., & Swanson, R.A. (2009). NADPH oxidase is the primary source of superoxide induced by NMDA receptor activation. *Nat. Neurosci.*, Vol. 12, No. 7, 857-863.

Bünemann, M., Bücheler, M.M., Philipp, M., Lohse, M.J., & Hein, L. (2001). Activation and deactivation kinetics of alpha 2A- and alpha 2C-adrenergic receptor-activated G protein-activated inwardly rectifying K+ channel currents. *J. Biol. Chem.*, Vol. 276, No. 50, 47512-47517.

Choi, D.W. (1985). Glutamate neurotoxicity in cortical cell culture is calcium dependent. *Neurosci. Lett.*, Vol. 58, No. 3, 293-297.

Choi, D.W., Koh, J.Y., & Peters, S. (1988). Pharmacology of glutamate neurotoxicity in cortical cell culture: attenuation by NMDA antagonists. *J. Neurosci.*, Vol. 8, No. 1, 185-196.

Das, A., Sribnick, E.A., Wingrave, J.M., Del Re, A.M., Woodward, J.J., Appel, S.H., Banik, N.L., Ray, S.K. (2005). Calpain activation in apoptosis of ventral spinal cord 4.1 (VSC4.1) motoneurons exposed to glutamate: calpain inhibition provides functional neuroprotection. *J. Neurosci. Res.*, Vol. 81, No. 4, 551-562.

Delaney, A.J, Crane. J.W., & Sah, P. (2007). Noradrenaline modulates transmission at a central synapse by a presynaptic mechanism. *Neuron*, Vol. 56, No. 5, 880-892.

de Souza, N.J., Dohadwalla, A.N., & Reden, J. (1983). Forskolin: a labdane diterpenoid with antihypertensive, positive inotropic, platelet aggregation inhibitory, and adenylate cyclase activating properties. *Med. Res. Rev.*, Vol. 3, No. 2, 201-219.

Donello JE, Padillo EU, Webster ML, Wheeler LA, Gil DW. (2001). Alpha(2)-Adrenoceptor agonists inhibit vitreal glutamate and aspartate accumulation and preserve retinal function after transient ischemia. *J. Pharmacol. Exp. Ther.*, Vol. 296, No. 1, 216-223.

Dong, C-J., Guo, Y., Wheeler, L., & Hare, W.A. (2007). α2 Adrenergic Receptor-Mediated Modulation of Cytosolic $Ca^{++}$ Signals at the Inner Plexiform Layer of the Rat Retina. *Invest. Ophthalmol. Vis. Sci.*, Vol. 48, No. 3, 1410-1415.

Dong, C-J., Guo, Y., Agey, P., Wheeler, L., & Hare, W.A. (2008). α2 Adrenergic Modulation of NMDA Receptor Function as a Major Mechanism of RGC Protection in Experimental Glaucoma and Retinal Excitotoxicity. *Invest. Ophthalmol. Vis. Sci.*, Vol. 49, No. 10, 4515-4522.

Dong, C-J., Guo, Y., Agey, P., Wheeler, L., & Hare, W.A. (2010). Nimodipine enhancement of α2 adrenergic modulation of NMDA receptor via a mechanism independent of Ca2+ channel blocking. *Invest. Ophthalmol. Vis. Sci.*, Vol. 51, No. 10, 4174-4180.

Dong, C-J., & Hare, W.A. (2005). Contribution to ischemic injury of rat optic nerves by intracellular sodium overload. *Doc. Ophthalmol.*, Vol. 110, No. 1, 15-23.

Dong, C-J., Guo, Y., Agey, P., & Hare, W.A. (2011). *In vivo* Location-dependent Differential Vulnerability of Rabbit RGCs to Excitotoxicity. ARVO Annual Meeting, Fort Lauderdale, FL, USA, May 2011.

Dowling, J.E. (1987). *The Retina: An approachable Part of the Brain.* Harvard University Press, Cambrdge, MA.

Fabbri, E., Brighenti, L., & Ottolenghi, C. (1991). Inhibition of adenylate cyclase of catfish and rat hepatocyte membranes by 9-(tetrahydro-2-furyl)adenine (SQ 22536). *J. Enzyme Inhib.*, Vol. 5, No. 2, 87-98.

Gaasterland, D., & Kupfer, C. (1974). Experimental glaucoma in the rhesus monkey. *Invest. Ophthalmol. Vis. Sci.*, Vol. 13, No. 6, 455-457.

Harada, T., Harada, C., Nakamura, K., Quah, H.M., Okumura, A., Namekata, K., Saeki, T., Aihara, M., Yoshida, H., Mitani, A., & Tanaka, K. (2007). The potential role of glutamate transporters in the pathogenesis of normal tension glaucoma. *J. Clin. Invest.*, Vol. 117, No. 7, 1763-1770.

Hare, W.A., & Wheeler, L. (2009). Experimental glutamatergic excitotoxicity in rabbit retinal ganglion cells: block by memantine. *Invest. Ophthalmol. Vis. Sci.*, Vol. 50, No., 6, 2940-2948.

Hare, W.A., WoldeMussie, E., Lai, R.K., Ton, H., Ruiz, G., Chun, T., & Wheeler, L. (2004). Efficacy and safety of memantine treatment for reduction of changes associated with experimental glaucoma in monkey, I: Functional measures. *Invest. Ophthalmol. Vis. Sci.*, Vol. 45, No. 8, 2625-2639.

Heijl, A., Leske, M.C., Bengtsson, B., Hyman, L., Bengtsson, B., Hussein, M. & Early Manifest Glaucoma Trial Group. (2002). Reduction of intraocular pressure and glaucoma progression: results from the Early Manifest Glaucoma Trial. *Arch. Ophthalmol.*, Vol. 120, No. 10, 1268-1279.

Hernández, M., Urcola, J.H., & Vecino, E. (2008). Retinal ganglion cell neuroprotection in a rat model of glaucoma following brimonidine, latanoprost or combined treatments. *Exp. Eye Res.* Vol. 86, No. 5, 798-806.

Hestrin, S., Nicoll, R.A. (1990). Properties of excitatory postsynaptic currents recorded in vitro from rat hippocampal interneurones. *J. Physiol.*, Vol. 430, No. 11, 605-616.

Ito, Y., Nakamura, S., Tanaka, H., Shimazawa, M., Araie, M., & Hara, H. (2008). Memantine protects against secondary neuronal degeneration in lateral geniculate nucleus and superior colliculus after retinal damage in mice. *CNS Neurosci Ther.*, Vol. 14, No. 3, 192-202.

Johnsona, T.V., & Tomareva, S.I. (2010). Rodent models of glaucoma. *Brain Res. Bull.*, Vol. 81, 349–358.

Ju, W.K., Kim, K.Y., Angert, M., Duong-Polk, K.X., Lindsey, J.D., Ellisman, M.H., & Weinreb, R.N. (2009). Memantine blocks mitochondrial OPA1 and cytochrome c release and subsequent apoptotic cell death in glaucomatous retina. *Invest. Ophthalmol. Vis. Sci.*, Vol. 50, No. 2, 707-716.

Kalapesi, F.B., Coroneo, M.T., & Hill, M.A. (2005). Human ganglion cells express the alpha-2 adrenergic receptor: relevance to neuroprotection. *Br. J. Ophthalmol.*, Vol. 89, No. 6, 758-763.

Kass, M.A., Hart, W.M. Jr., Gordon, M., & Miller, J.P. (1980). Risk factors favoring the development of glaucomatous visual field loss in ocular hypertension. *Surv. Ophthalmol.*, Vol. 25, No. 3, 155-162.

Krupin, T., Liebmann, J.M., Greenfield, D.S., Ritch, R., Gardiner, S.; Low-Pressure Glaucoma Study Group. (2011). A Randomized Trial of Brimonidine Versus Timolol in Preserving Visual Function: Results From the Low-pressure Glaucoma Treatment Study. *Am. J. Ophthalmol.* Vol. 151, No. 4, 671-681.

Lagrèze, W.A., Knörle, R., Bach, M., Feuerstein, T.J. (1998). Memantine is neuroprotective in a rat model of pressure-induced retinal ischemia. *Invest Ophthalmol Vis Sci.*,Vol. 39, No. 6,1063-1066.

Lai, R.K., Chun, T., Hasson, D., Lee, S., Mehrbod, F., & Wheeler, L. (2002). Alpha-2 adrenoceptor agonist protects retinal function after acute retinal ischemic injury in the rat. Vis. Neurosci., Vol. 19, No. 2, 175-185.

Lambert, W.S., Ruiz, L., Crish, S.D, Wheeler, L.A., & Calkins, D.J. (2011). Brimonidine prevents axonal and somatic degeneration of retinal ganglion cell neurons. *Mol. Neurodegener.*, Vol. 6, No. 1, 4.

López-Herrera, M.P.L., Mayor-Torroglosa, S., de Imperial, J.M., Villegas-Pérez, M.P. & Vidal-Sanz, M. (2002). Transient ischemia of the retina results in altered retrograde axoplasmic transport: neuroprotection with brimonidine. *Exp. Neurol.*, Vol. 178, No. 2, 243-258.

Lukasiewicz, P.D., Lawrence, J.E., & Valentino, T.L. (1995). Desensitizing glutamate receptors shape excitatory synaptic inputs to tiger salamander retinal ganglion cells. *J. Neurosci.*, Vol. 15, No. 9, 6189-6199.

MacDermott, A.B., Mayer, M.L., Westbrook, G.L., Smith, S.J., & Barker, J.L. (1986). NMDA-receptor activation increases cytoplasmic calcium concentration in cultured spinal cord neurones. Nature, Vol. 321, No. 6069, 519-522.

Matsui, K., Hosoi, N., & Tachibana, M. (1998). Excitatory synaptic transmission in the inner retina: paired recordings of bipolar cells and neurons of the ganglion cell layer. *J. Neurosci.*, Vol. 18, No. 12, 4500-4510.

Maze, M., & Tranquilli, W. (1991). Alpha-2 adrenoceptor agonists: defining the role in clinical anesthesia. *Anesthesiol.*, Vol. 74, No. 3,581-605.

Moore, D., Harris, A., WuDunn, D., Kheradiya, N., & Siesky, B. (2008). Dysfunctional regulation of ocular blood flow: A risk factor for glaucoma? *Clinical. Ophthalmol.*, Vol. 2, No. 4, 849–861.

Morgans, C.W., Bayley, P.R., Oesch, N.W., Ren, G., Akileswaran, L., & Taylor, W.R. (2005). Photoreceptor calcium channels: insight from night blindness. *Vis. Neurosci.*, Vol. 22, No. 5, 561-8.

Pan, Z.H. (2000). Differential Expression of High- and Two Types of Low-Voltage-Activated Calcium Currents in Rod and Cone Bipolar Cells of the Rat Retina. *J. Neurophysiol.*, Vol. 83, 513-527.

Pan, Z.H. (2001). Voltage-activated Ca2+ channels and ionotropic GABA receptors localized at axon terminals of mammalian retinal bipolar cells. *Vis. Neurosci.*, Vol. 18, No. 2, 279-288.

Pivovarova, N.B., & Andrews, S.B. (2010). Calcium-dependent mitochondrial function and dysfunction in neurons. FEBS J., Vol. 277, 3622-3636.

Quigley, H.A. (2005). Glaucoma: macrocosm to microcosm, the Friedenwald lecture. *Invest. Ophthalmol. Vis. Sci.*, Vol. 46, No. 8, 2662-2670.

Quigley, H.A., Enger, C., Katz, J., Sommer, A., Scott, R., & Gilbert, D. (1994). Risk factors for the development of glaucomatous visual field loss in ocular hypertension. Arch. Ophthalmol., Vol. 112, No. 5, 644-649.

Reid, C.A., Bekkers, J.M., & Clements, J.D. (2003). Presynaptic Ca2+ channels: a functional patchwork. *Trends Neurosci.*, Vol. 26, No. 12, 683-687.

Rodieck (1973). *The Vertebrate Retina: Principles of Structure and Function*. W.H. Freeman. San Francisco, CA.

Rodieck, R.W., & Watanabe, M. (1993). Survey of the morphology of macaque retinal ganglion cells that project to the pretectum, superior colliculus, and parvicellular laminae of the lateral geniculate nucleus. *J. Comp. Neurol.*, Vol. 338, No. 2, 289-303.

Sattler, R., Xiong, Z., Lu, W.Y., Hafner, M., MacDonald, J.F., & Tymianski, M. (1999). Specific coupling of NMDA receptor activation to nitric oxide neurotoxicity by PSD-95 protein. *Science*. Vol. 284, No. 5421, 1845-1848.

Sattler, R., & Tymianski, M. (2001). Molecular mechanisms of glutamate receptor-mediated excitotoxic neuronal cell death. *Mol. Neurobiol.*, Vol. 24, No. 1-3, 107-129.

Sharma, A.K., & Rohrer, B. (2004). Ashish K. Calcium-induced Calpain Mediates Apoptosis via Caspase-3 in a Mouse Photoreceptor Cell Line. *J. Biol. Chem.*, Vol. 279, No. 34, 35564–35572.

Siliprandi, R., Canella, R., Carmignoto, G., Schiavo, N., Zanellato, A., Zanoni, R, & Vantini, G. (1992). N-methyl-D-aspartate-induced neurotoxicity in the adult rat retina. *Vis. Neurosci.*, Vol. 8, No. 6, 567-573.

Starke, K. (2001). Presynaptic autoreceptors in the third decade: focus on alpha2-adrenoceptors. *J. Neurochem.*, Vol. 78, No. 4, 685-693.

Starkov, A.A., Chinopoulos, C., & Fiskum, G. (2004). Mitochondrial calcium and oxidative stress as mediators of ischemic brain injury. Cell Calcium, Vol. 36, No. 3-4, 257-264.

Stout, A.K., Raphael, H.M., Kanterewicz, B.I., Klann, E., & Reynolds, I.J. (1998). Glutamate-induced neuron death requires mitochondrial calcium uptake. *Nat. Neurosci.* Vol. 1, No. 5, 366-373.

Tachibana, M., Okada, T., Arimura, T., Kobayashi, K., Piccolino, (1993). M. Dihydropyridine-sensitive calcium current mediates neurotransmitter release from bipolar cells of the goldfish retina. *J. Neurosci.*, Vol. 13, No. 7, 2898–2909.

Teixeira, M.M., Gristwood, R.W., Cooper, N., Hellewell, P.G. (1997). Phosphodiesterase (PDE)4 inhibitors: anti-inflammatory drugs of the future? *Trends. Pharmacol. Sci.*, Vol. 18, No. 5, 164-171.

Thompson, W.J., Anderson, P.S., Britcher, S.F., Lyle, T.A., Thies, J.E., Magill, C.A., Varga, S.L., Schwering, J.E., Lyle, P.A., & Christy, M.E. (1990). Synthesis and pharmacological evaluation of a series of dibenzo[a,d]cycloalkenimines as N-methyl-D-aspartate antagonists. *J. Med. Chem.*, Vol. 33, No. 2, 789-808.

Tsai, J.C., & Kanner, E.M. (2005). Current and emerging medical therapies for glaucoma. *Expert Opin. Emerg. Drugs*. Vol. 10, No. 1, 109-118.

Vaney, D.I. (1984). 'Coronate' amacrine cells in the rabbit retina have the 'starburst' dendritic morphology. *Proc. R. Soc. Lond. B Biol. Sci.*, Vol. 220, No. 1221, 501-508.

Vaney, D.I., Peichi, L., & Boycott, B.B. (1981). Matching populations of amacrine cells in the inner nuclear and ganglion cell layers of the rabbit retina. *J. Comp. Neurol.*, Vol. 199, No. 3, 373-391.

Vasudevan, S.K., Gupta, V., & Crowston, J.G. (2011). Neuroprotection in glaucoma. *Indian J. Ophthalmol.*, Vol. 59, Suppl., S102-113.

Virtanen, R. (1989). Pharmacological profiles of medetomidine and its antagonist, atipamezole. Acta. Vet. Scand. Suppl. Vol. 85, 29-37.

Waxman, S.G., Black, J.A., Ransom, B.R., & Stys, P.K. (1994). Anoxic injury of rat optic nerve: ultrastructural evidence for coupling between Na+ influx and Ca(2+)-mediated injury in myelinated CNS axons. *Brain Res.* Vol. 644, No. 2, 197-204.

WoldeMussie, E., Ruiz, G., Wijono, M., & Wheeler, L.A. (2001). Neuroprotection of retinal ganglion cells by brimonidine in rats with laser-induced chronic ocular hypertension. *Invest. Ophthalmol. Vis. Sci.* Vol. 42, No. 12, 2849-2855.

WoldeMussie, E., Yoles, E., Schwartz, M., Ruiz. G, & Wheeler, L.A. (2002). Neuroprotective effect of memantine in different retinal injury models in rats. *J. Glaucoma.* Vol. 11, No. 6, 474-480.

Yoles, E., Wheeler, L.A., & Schwartz, M. (1999). Alpha2-adrenoreceptor agonists are neuroprotective in a rat model of optic nerve degeneration. *Invest. Ophthalmol. Vis. Sci.* Vol. 40, No. 1, 65-73.

# Glaucoma Genetics – Regulation of Cell Surviving and Death in the Retina

Maria D. Pinazo-Durán[1], Roberto Gallego-Pinazo[2], Vicente Zanón-Moreno[3,4], and Manuel Serrano[5]

[1]*Ophthalmic Research Unit "Santiago Grisolia", Valencia,*
[2]*Ophthalmology Department, University and Polytechnic Hospital La Fé, Valencia,*
[3]*Preventive Medicine and Public Health Department. Medical School, University of Valencia,*
[4]*CiberOBN - Biomedical Research Center Network of Pathophysiology of Obesity and Nutrition,*
[5]*Spanish National Cancer Research Center (CNIO), Madrid, Spain*

## 1. Introduction

Primary open-angle glaucoma (POAG) is a leading cause of various degrees of visual impairment and blindness worldwide, affecting in a disproportional manner women Afroamericans and Asians. In the Canadian Glaucoma Study, a recent multicenter prospective longitudinal study carried out in 258 participants (131 men versus 127 women; median age, 65.0 years), patients were followed up at 4-month intervals with perimetry, optic disc imaging, and a standardized interventional protocol for intraocular pressure (IOP) control. Univariate and proportional hazards models were used by the authors, in order to identify factors that predicted glaucoma progression. Data from this study showed that higher baseline age (HR per year, 1.04; 95% CI, 1.01-1.07), female sex (HR, 1.94; 95% CI, 1.09-3.46), and higher mean follow-up IOP (HR per 1 mm Hg, 1.19; 95% CI, 1.05-1.36) were associated with progression of glaucomatous disease (Chauhan et al., 2008).

It was estimated that over 8.4 million people were bilaterally blind from glaucoma in 2010, rising to 11.1 million by 2020. (Quigley & Broman, 2006). Moreover, approximately 50% of patients with POAG remain undiagnosed in most communities.

A wide spectrum of etiopathogenic theories have been proposed in relation to glaucoma. In the 19$^{th}$ century, Müller described that the elevated IOP caused a compression in the eye tissues, whereas chronic heightened IOP led subsequently to the neuronal death (*elder mechanical theory*), while simultaneously von Jaeger (1858) suggested that vascular alterations were responsible of the optic atrophy (*vascular theory*). Schnabel (1892) reported that it were created empty spaces during the process of atrophy of neural elements, which bowing back of the lamina cribrosa and posteriorly cupping the nervehead (*cavernous atrophy theory*). In 1925, La Grange and Beauvieux established that glaucomatous optic neuropathy was secondary to ischaemia (*ischaemic theory*). Changing criteria in the seventies pointed to the role of altered axoplasmic flow in glaucomatous optic neuropathy. In fact, monkey eyes with a lesser elevation of IOP and shorter duration of glaucoma, showed changes sharply localized to the axon bundles in the scleral lamina cribrosa. Accumulation of mitochondria was detected anterior and posterior to collagenous septae. These changes co-localized to the sites of axoplasmic transport blockage, as identified by autoradiographic studies. It was speculated that these cytologic changes reflect interruption of axoplasmic flow in the optic nerve of glaucoma eyes, which raised the *new mechanical theory* (Gasterlaand et al., 1978).

The resistance of the trabecular meshwork (TM) to aqueous humour outflow increases as an ageing change, leading to increased IOP (Levin 1997). Therefore, elevated IOP is considered the main factor responsible for the glaucomatous optic neuropathy, this latter involving death of retinal ganglion cells and their axons. Clinically it is characterized by morphologic/morphometric changes of the optic disc, visual field defects (Agarwal et al., 2002) and increased rate of retinal nerve fiber layer thinning (Lee et al., 2011).

New extensive investigations into glaucoma pathophysiology contribute to our understanding of the role of a high variety of factors in the retinal ganglion cells damage and death. External and internal factors, as those within the retina and optic nerve ultrastructure, are important in the development and progression of primary open-angle glaucoma (POAG) (Lutjen-Drecoll et al., 1986; Hernandez et al., 1991; Triviño et al., 1996). More recent scientific knowledge revealed a complex situation in which other factors, as the circulatory (Yanagi et al., 2010), inflammatory (Kumarasamy et al., 2006), toxicologic (Schori et al., 2001), biochemical and molecular (Zanón-Moreno & Pinazo-Durán, 2008; Zanón-Moreno et al., 2008, 2009; Ray & Mookherjee, 2009, Osborne, 2010), are likely to be involved in the pathogenesis of glaucomatous optic neuropathy.

Whatever may be the real factors involved in glaucoma pathogenesis, the glaucomatous eyes suffer the dysfunction and death of the retinal ganglion cells leading to optic atrophy and irreversible visual loss. This may be the consequence of the association of multiple factors rather than only one functioning individually. In this context one question arises as to whether the molecular and cellular POAG basis, can be closely related to cell cycle abnormalities, leading to cell surviving and death involutionary processes, as a response to a cell stressor: the increased IOP.

### 1.1 The cell cycle

The cell-division cycle, are recognized as the events occurring in a cell that leads to its division and duplication (replication). The cell cycle consists of four phases: Gap 1 (G1) phase is the interval between mitosis and DNA synthesis, DNA synthesis (S) phase, Gap 2 (G2) phase (interphase) during which growth and preparation for cell division occurs, and finally the mitosis and cytokinesis (M) phase, as shown in the Fig. 1. During the cell cycle progression, activation of each phase is strictly dependent on the proper completion of the previous one. It has also to be stated that the cells that have temporarily stopped dividing have entered a stage of quiescence named the G0 phase.

Cell cycle is positively regulated by holoenzymes formed by a regulating subunit called cyclin (cyc), and cyclin-dependent kinases (cdk) (Ivanova et al., 2011). These complexes cyc/cdk become activated or inhibited sequentially in different phases of the cell cycle. Cell cycle progression is the result of the interaction between cyclins and their cdks, and a high variety of inhibitory proteins, the corresponding cdk inhibitors (cdki) (Lee et al., 2005). As

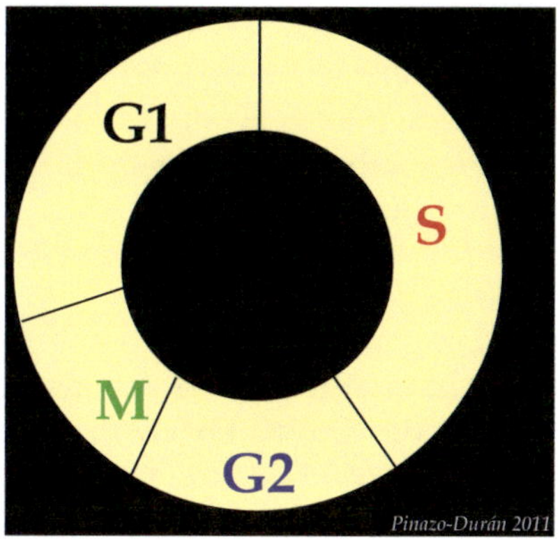


Fig. 1. The cell-division phases

shown in the following scheme, the cycD and the corresponding cdk4/6 activities regulate the early progression of the cell cycle, through the G1 phase. Then, cycE can be expressed, and in association with cdk2 controls the G1-S transition step. Finally, cell cycle arrest is achieved by the negative regulation of cdks, exerted either by antiproliferative signals or by the specific cdki activities (Serrano et al., 1993) (Fig. 2). Following growth arrest cells undergo senescence or apoptosis (Chen et al., 2000). The cip/kip family of cdki includes the genes p21CIP1/WAF (p21), p27 and p57, which halt cell cycle in G1 phase and inhibit several cyc/ckd complexes. The Inhibitor of Kinase 4/Alternative Reading Frame (INK4a/ARF) family prevent the progression of the cell cycle, and includes p16INK4a (p16), p15, p18, and p19, which specifically inhibit ccyc/dk4/6 activities (Serrano et al., 1993; Dean et al., 2010).

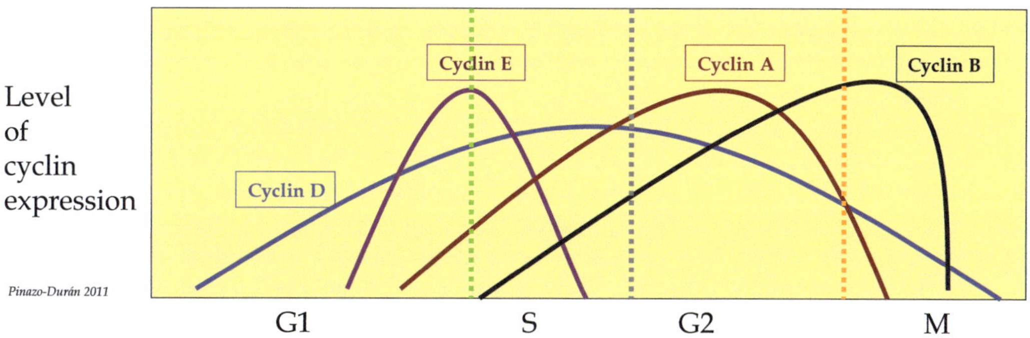


Fig. 2.

### 1.2 Genetics of glaucoma

Glaucoma is a multifactorial disease in which genetic and environmental factors are involved. Advancing knowledge in glaucoma is slow and insidious, because the polygenic character of the disease makes more difficult to progress through the genetic studies. However, genetics of glaucoma are the key for get preventing the glaucomatous blindness. It is necessary to deepen inside the influence of polymorphisms of each gene with the disease and, likewise, analyze the interactions among these genes (gene-gene) and through them with the environment (gene-environment).

Currently, there are some genes which have been associated to glaucoma, as myocilin/trabecular meshwork inducible glucocorticoid response **(MYOC/TIGR)** gene, that was identified in the latter nineties (Stone et al., 1997). The MYOC gene encodes an extracellular glycoprotein called **myocilin**. This protein is expressed in different human organs, among them the TM, ciliary body, retina and optic nervehead. Mutations in this gene result in juvenile glaucoma. The MYOC gene is altered in approximately 4% of cases of POAG (Lopez-Martinez et al., 2007).

Subsequently, other genes related to glaucoma were identified. Another causative gene was localized on chromosome 10p14 in a study of 54 families with autosomal dominantly inherited adult-onset POAG. It was designated **OPTN** (by its related protein, **optineurin**). The OPTN gene codes for a conserved 66-kilodalton protein of unknown function that has been implicated in the tumor necrosis factor-alpha signaling pathway and that interacts with diverse proteins including Huntingtin, Ras-associated protein RAB8, and transcription factor IIIA. Optineurin is expressed in the TM, nonpigmented ciliary epithelium, retina, and brain, and it was speculated that it plays a neuroprotective role (Rezaie et al., 2002). Moreover, sequence alterations in OPTN were found in 16.7% of families with hereditary POAG, including individuals with normal intraocular pressure

The WD repeat domain 36 (**WDR36**) gene that encodes a member of the **WDR protein family** was also found to be associated with glaucoma disease. WDR36 gene expressed in lens, iris, sclera, ciliary muscles, ciliary body, TM, retina and optic nerve, as established by real time-PCR. WDR36 is a novel causative gene for adult-onset POAG at the open-angle glaucoma (GLC1G) locus. Specific ocular expressions and observed mutations are consistent with WDR36 role in aetiology of both high- and low-pressure glaucoma (Monemi et al., 2005).

The **CYP1B1** gene encodes a dioxin inducible member of subfamily I of the **cytochrome p450** protein superfamily. The human CYP1B1 gene consists of three exons of which the first is non-coding. The putative open reading frame starts in the second exon and is 1629 bp in length, and the CYP1B1 gene has been related to 20-80% of primary congenital glaucoma cases (GLC3A) (Sitorus et al., 2003).

In addition to these four genes (MYOC, OPTN WDR36, CYP1B1) alterations in many others and their possible association with some type of glaucoma have been analyzed. There are studies involving the apolipoprotein E (ApoE) gene polymorphisms in the glaucomatous optic neuropathy. Copin et al., (2002) indicate that single nucleotide polymorphisms on the promoter region of the ApoE gene is associated with increased optic nerve and visual field damage in glaucomatous patients. This study also demonstrates that another single nucleotide polymorphism interacts with the recently reported MYOC single nucleotide polymorphism (mt1) that, in turns results in increased IOP, suggesting that may be involved in the limited effectiveness of IOP-lowering treatments among POAG patients. More recently it has been shown that heterozygous non-synonymous variants of the retinitis pigmentosa GTPase regulator interacting protein 1 (RPGRIP1) gene also may cause, or increase, the susceptibility to various forms of glaucoma (Fernández-Martínez, 2011).

At the same time, we shouldn't ignore epigenetics, which regards to the study of those heritable changes in phenotype or gene expression caused by processes different to variations in the DNA sequence. Epigenetic information modulates gene expression without alter the DNA sequence, by several mechanisms: 1) DNA methylation, 2) Genomic imprinting and 3) Histone modifications –acetylation, methylation, phosphorylation-. Therefore, epigenetics does refer to the mechanisms that utilize the organism for translating the genetic

information of a generation. The clinical effects that arise from the disease-associated sequence changes in gene might be influenced by modifier genes, as well as by endogenous factors that could alter pathogenic mechanisms affected by the mutations. Therefore, it could potentially explain some variations in the observed clinical signs and symptoms and also in the progression rates of the POAG patients (Lam et al. 2000).
Moreover, from a nutrition and health viewpoint, preventive strategies from population-based recommendations to personalized nutritional advice are detected as an attractive topic. Biomedical studies may help in understanding how genetic variation and epigenetic events may change requirements and responses to nutrients, and developing outstanding techniques for identifying patients at risk because of its own nutrigenetic profile (Zeisel, 2007). A discipline that is gaining importance in glaucoma studies is the nutritional genetics, which has two main branches: nutrigenetics and nutrigenomics. Nutrigenetics focuses on the study of genetic variations in the body's response to nutrients. Otherwise, nutrigenomics investigates the influence of nutrients on gene expression. In relation to these two concepts especial attention has to be paid to the emergence of nutrigenetic tests, which use genetic information to identify food products that suited or not suited to the personalized nutrigenetic profile, allowing us to define individual dietary advice (Haga et al, 2003).

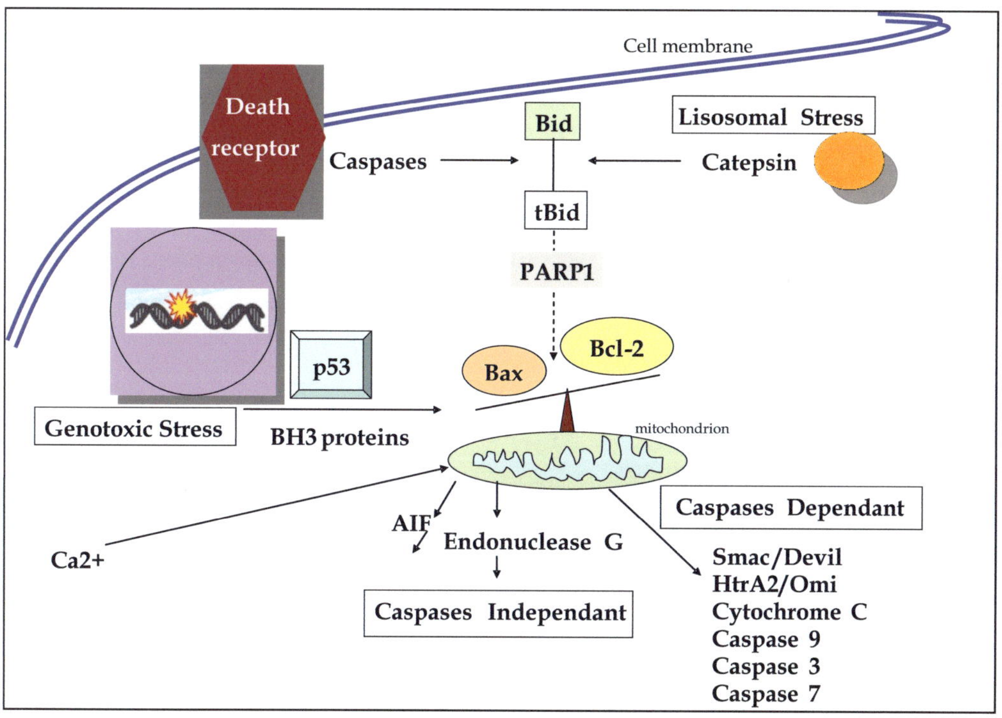


Fig. 3.

Numerous studies on gene alterations that encode proteins related to cell survival and death in relation to glaucoma have been conducted through the past twenty years, in order to stop or prevent apoptosis of retinal ganglion cells and optic nerve degeneration. In this regard, it has been analyzed mutations in genes of the B-cell lymphoma 2 (bcl-2) family such as the B-cell lymphoma 2-associated X (BAX) gene, which encodes a pro-apoptotic X protein. The circuits involved in these cell pathways are shown below (Fig. 3). If the BAX protein is not present, or there are BAX limited availability, ganglion cell somas are capable to resist indefinitely an optic nerve insult. In the presence of BAX the damage cannot be blocked and cell death program reaches an irreversible point (Nickells, 2008).

### 1.3 The p53 gene

Another key protein in the regulation processes of cell survival and death is p53. It was identified in 1979 and encodes the transcription factor also named p53, a phosphoprotein (MW 53 kD). The p53 gene comprises 20 kb of DNA and is located on the short arm of chromosome 17p13.1 (Levine and Finlay 2004). It has been called the "guardian of the genome" (Lane 1992). Its expression and function has been related to apoptosis, cell proliferation and/or angiogenic processes.
The p53 protein is located in the cytoplasm as an inactive monomer, but upon stimulation by a variety of cellular stresses, p53 forms a tetramer from double dimers. The p53 protein binds DNA (see the figure 4) and, among other target genes, induces the expression of the p21 gene to synthetize the p21 protein that, in turns, inhibits the cycE/cdk2 complexes. The complex p21/cycE/cdk2 inactivates cell division by stopping the cell cycle. p53 is an essential molecule in cell proliferation and apoptosis (Guevara et al., 1999). Inactive, as a good guardian, p53 only starts functioning when a genetic damage appears in a cell (Fig. 3,4). Only then, it activates a system with two main programs: 1) The cell suicide, 2) A process of cellular senescence by which the cell remains alive but unable to proliferate. The p53 gene detects almost any alteration in the cell, oncogenes and other DNA alterations, lack of nutrients, and abnormalities that occur during the proliferative and angiogenic processes. Therefore, p53 is a multifunctional "star" gene, involved in a wide spectrum of biomedical facts (Boesten et al., 2009; Gallego-Pinazo et al., 2008, 2010; Jeong et al., 2009). The tumour suppressor p53 mediates the cellular response to a variety of stresses mainly by regulating

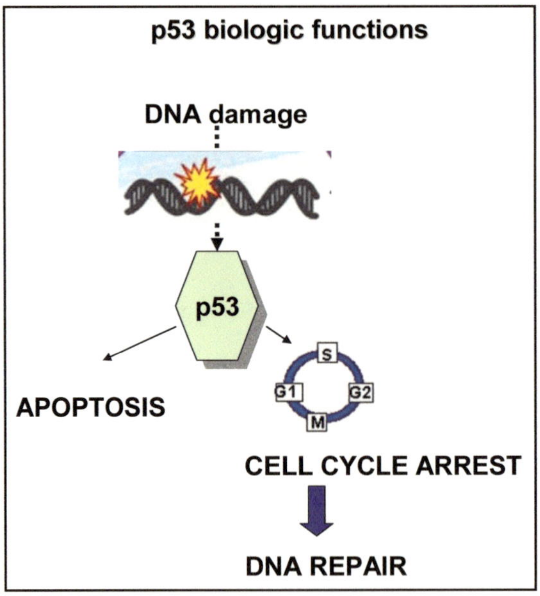


Fig. 4.

the transcription of over 150 genes (Jeong et al, 2009). Active p53 gene can induce reversible growth arrest in the cell cycle G1 or G2 phases, as well as cellular senescence or apoptosis. As such, p53 acts as a sensor of damage to the genome (Lane 1992). Main biologic functions of p53 are shown in the scheme below.

### 1.4 Glaucoma, visual loss and apoptosis

In a first clinic-pathologic report Levin and Louhab (1996) identified retinal ganglion cells undergoing apoptosis in one of the eyes of a 70-year-old man with anterior ischaemic optic neuropathy. These authors speculated that the affected eye underwent a functional optic nerve axotomy. A wide variety of clinical and experimental studies strongly indicate that retinal ganglion cells and optic axons demise represents the final pathway of vision loss in glaucoma patients (Quigley et al., 2000; Agar et al., 2006; Ju et al., 2007; Agarwal et al., 2009, Lee et al., 2011) and that the intrinsic pathogenic mechanism is the ganglion cell death by apoptosis (Nickells 1999; Osborne et al., 1999; Osborne, 2011; Zhang & Bhavnani 2005; Levkovitch-Verbin 2009; Tatton, 2011). Although there are compelling evidences showing apoptosis as the primary and early mechanism of ganglion cell death in glaucoma (Levkovitch-Verbin 2006), necrosis is also a contributory mechanism in the late phase of glaucoma progression, evidence to which was observed in rats subjected to optic nerve transection (Cordeiro et al., 2010).

When managing glaucoma patients, ophthalmologists consider individualized therapy for lowering IOP, as well as the true IOP-lowering efficacy of each drug that is given to any patient, and the compliance degree, with the final goal of maintaining the adequate IOP levels and subsequently the vision and the quality of life (Levin 1997; Agarwal et al., 2009). However, the anti-hypertensive therapy is clearly unable to properly maintain the visual function. Further research and translation of knowledge to the clinical practice in urgently needed to improve glaucoma prognosis.

Apoptosis (Kerr et al., 1972) is a regulated manner to destroy a cell. During development apoptosis is a pivotal process. In addition, apoptosis performs essential functions in morphogenesis and tissue remodelling, homeostasis, removal of damaged or infected cells, and others. Although it is essential for normal development and health, an aberrant activation contributes to the pathogenesis of ischemic or neurodegenerative diseases and other processes (Walker et al., 1988). On the contrary, the apoptosis failure is a key factor in the pathogenesis of cancer or autoimmune disorders (Wyllie 1974). Apoptosis, is caused by the production of an endonuclease that destroys the DNA and induces cell phagocytosis by the neighboring elements, but without stimulating inflammation (Birge & Ucker 2008). In this context, visual impairment and blindness in glaucoma patients is attributed to the retinal ganglion cell damage and death (McKinnon, 1997).

Apoptosis is a genetically coded cell suicide program that activates when any cell has been profoundly damaged or the cell is no longer needed. Microscopic findings of apoptotic cells include: 1) cytoplasmic organelles compaction, 2) nuclear chromatin condensation, and 3) membrane blebbing (Meagher et al., 1992).

Furthermore, neurotrophin withdrawal and cytotoxic neurotransmitters release have also been involved in ganglion cell and optic fibers damage and death by apoptosis, in glaucoma (Carmignoto et al., 1997). Among the neurotrophic factors the BDNF is a pivotal molecule for neuron survival, in the developing and mature visual system (Snider 1994; Carmignoto et al., 1997). The BDNF was investigated in rats and monkeys regarding the retinal ganglion cells neurotrophin transport in experimental glaucoma, by using acute and chronic IOP elevation and immunohistochemical assays with antibodies directed against the tyrosine kinase receptors (TrkA, B, C) and against BDNF, as well as by autoradiography to identify retrograde axonal transport of 125I-BDNF injected into the superior colliculus. The authors concluded that the interruption of BDNF retrograde transport and the accumulation of TrkB at the optic nervehead in acute/chronic glaucoma models strongly suggest a role for neurotrophin deprivation in the pathogenesis of glaucomatous ganglion cell death (Pease et al., 2000).

Recently it has been stressed the importance of identifying molecular biomarkers or inducers of apoptosis for better glaucoma managing (Golubnitschaja & Flammer, 2007; Zanón-Moreno & Pinazo-Durán, 2008). Therefore, different classes of molecular anomalies can be detected and utilized for glaucoma progression, among them specific molecules closely related to cell survival and apoptosis, as follows.

**Caspase-3** is one of the cysteine proteases family that plays a role in apoptosis by cleaving a high variety of key proteins such as the poly (ADP-ribose) polymerase 1 (PARP-1), protein kinase C (PKC), DNA-dependent protein kinase, DNA-fragmentation factor (DFF) and others (see the drawn schematic on figure 3). Zang and Bhavnani (2005) described that up-regulation of caspase-3 expression preceded neuronal cell death, supporting the possibility that glutamate-induced apoptotic cell death was the consequence of up-regulation of caspase-3 gene in cortical neurons. These observations are consistent with up-regulation of precursor caspase-3 in frontal neuronal cortex of subjects with Alzheimer's disease. This enzyme has been proposed to activate death effector molecules resulting in the fragmentation of genomic DNA and was associated with morphological and structural changes characteristic of apoptosis.

**Poly-Adenil Ribose Polymerase 1 (PARP1)** is a reversible post-translational protein modification that is involved in the regulation of several biological functions. Whereas an 18 member superfamily of PARP enzymes synthesize poly (ADP-ribose) (PAR), a single protein, PAR glycohydrolase (PARG) is responsible for the catabolism of the polymer. PARP-1 accounts for more than 90% of the poly (ADP-ribosyl)ating capacity of the cells (Viraq 2005). PARP-1 activated by DNA breaks cleaves NAD(+) into nicotinamide and ADP-ribose, and uses it to synthesize long branching PAR polymers covalently attached to acceptor proteins including histones, DNA repair enzymes, transcription factors and PARP-1 (Aguilar-Quesada et al., 2007). Activation of PARP-1 by mild genotoxic stimuli may facilitate DNA repair and cell survival. However irreparable DNA damage triggers apoptotic or necrotic cell death (as reflected in figure 3). In apoptosis, early PARP activation may assist the apoptotic cascade, by stabilizing p53, by mediating the translocation of apoptosis inducing factor (AIF) from the mitochondria to the nucleus or by inhibiting early activation of DNases. In most severe oxidative stress situations, excessive DNA damage causes over activation of PARP-1, which blocks the apoptotic elements and switches the mode of cell death from apoptosis to necrosis. In addition to serving as a cytotoxic mediator, PARP-1 is also implicated in transcriptional regulation processes, most notably in the NF kappaB and AP-1 driven expression of inflammatory mediators (Viraq 2005). In the case of pharmacological blockage or genetic inhibition of PARP-1 provided remarkable protection from tissue injury in various oxidative stress-related disease models ranging from endothelial dysfunction, myocardial ischaemia-reperfusion, stroke, shock, diabetes mellitus, Parkinson's disease, arthritis, and uveitis. These beneficial effects are attributed to inhibition of the PARP-1 mediated suicidal pathway and to reduced expression of inflammatory cytokines and other molecules (Quiles-Perez et al., 2010).

Despite former glaucoma statements, it has been suggested that within the retina, other cell phenotypes that the ganglion cells may be implicated. There is also increasing evidence that neuronal changes occur both in retina and central visual pathways in glaucoma and other neurodegenerative diseases. Axonal projections can be distinguished from dendrites by the shape, length and function. Dendrites are fine neuronal processes which support postsynaptic contact elements and are responsible for receiving synaptic signals. The morphological and functional integrity of dendrites has important effects on integrating neuronal input to the CNS from the peripheral targets. Axonal and dendritic changes have been detected in neurodegenerative processes, including those occurring in development, ageing and diseases. Therefore, axonal and dendritic pathology are early signs in disease and providing new insights into therapeutic strategies. Increased latency and reduced amplitude of visual evoked potentials, frequently encountered in ocular hypertension or POAG, suggest slowed neural conduction in the visual pathways (Parisi 1997; Bach and Hoffmann 2008). Recent research in monkeys demonstrated that the glaucomatous damage extends from the retina to the visual centers in the brain, but being the primary region of damage the optic nervehead, with the lateral geniculate nucleus being secondarily affected. These findings indicate that in Japanese monkeys, damage to neurons in the geniculate can be detected in a very early phase (first weeks) after an IOP elevation occurs, as can damage to optic nervehead (Itoa et al., 2009). By utilizing neuroimaging techniques such as diffusion tensor magnetic resonance imaging, functional magnetic resonance imaging, and magnetic resonance spectroscopy it has been evaluated the microstructural integrity of white-matter fibers and the functional activity of gray matter. They have been widely employed to investigate various diseases of the central nervous system, as glaucoma. It has been demonstrated alterations involving the human visual cortex that are consistent with clinically documented losses of visual function. These data support the use of imaging techniques as reliable, noninvasive tools for monitoring the progression of human glaucoma (Garacci et al., 2008)

In this context, there may be new opportunities to develop treatments directed at the retina and the brain, such as those that promote healthy ocular tissues, the neurotrophic factors.

Neurotrophic factors includes: 1) neurotrophins (NGF, BDNF, NT-3, NT-4), 2) neurokines (CNTF), and glial cell line-derived neurotrophic factor (GDNF) family ligands (GFLs) (Bespalov and Saarma, 2007). Neurotrophic factors and their receptors regulate the development and physiology of neurons, but their roles in the CNS are far from complete. Among the neurotrophins, the brain derived neurotrophic factor (BDNF) (Snider 1994; Osborne et al., 1999; Harada et al., 2011) may help retinal ganglion cells to survive themselves; may increase axon outgrowth in the optic nerve, and may improve the environment in which the dying retinal ganglion cells and the surrounding elements are placed within the retina, optic nerve and visual pathway.

Considering that the cell surviving and death mechanisms play a pivotal role in glaucoma progression, we propose that the p53 gene, as the outstanding cell cycle regulator, can be involved in the pathogenic processes of glaucoma in the retina and optic nerve. Therefore, we deal with examining the events that take place in the retina at the molecular level, after overexpressing p53 gene, with the inhibition of the cell cycle progression and the induction of the apoptosis-related pathway.

## 2. The super p53 mice

The C57BL6 strain is the most commonly used for genetic manipulation and biomedical research. Transgenic mice of the Charles River C57BL6/J strain were generated by addition of two extra copies of p53 gene (García-Cao et al., 2002; Effeyan et al., 2006). Our main purpose is to characterize molecules involved in cell surviving and death in mice retina-choroid.

### 2.1 Animal and tissue handling

All procedures were performed to minimize animal suffering in accordance with the European Community guidelines for the use of animals in research (609/1986). The Research Committee and Animal Research Committee of the participating centers approved the study. Mice were sacrificed and utilized by several investigators in our working area. For the purposes of the present study we utilized 24 mice that were distributed into two groups 1) super p53 (sp53; n=12) and wild type (CG; n=12).

Eyes with the retrobulbar optic nerves were microsurgically dissected, in a Nikon SM2 1500 microscope. Briefly, after performing an "ab externo" enucleation, the eyes were washed in bidistilled water and placed on a Petri dish to be immobilized by means of a Barraquer forceps to perform an anterior segment paracentesis with a micro sharp blade angled 15°. By using the Vannas scissors a complete peritomy was performed, to separate the cornea and lens from the posterior eyecup (with the optic nerve attached), as previously described (Pinazo-Durán et al., 1993, 1997, 2005, 2011). The retina-choroid was obtained, and frozen and stored at -80° until processing. Homogenates of the retina-choroid were used to perform two main techniques:

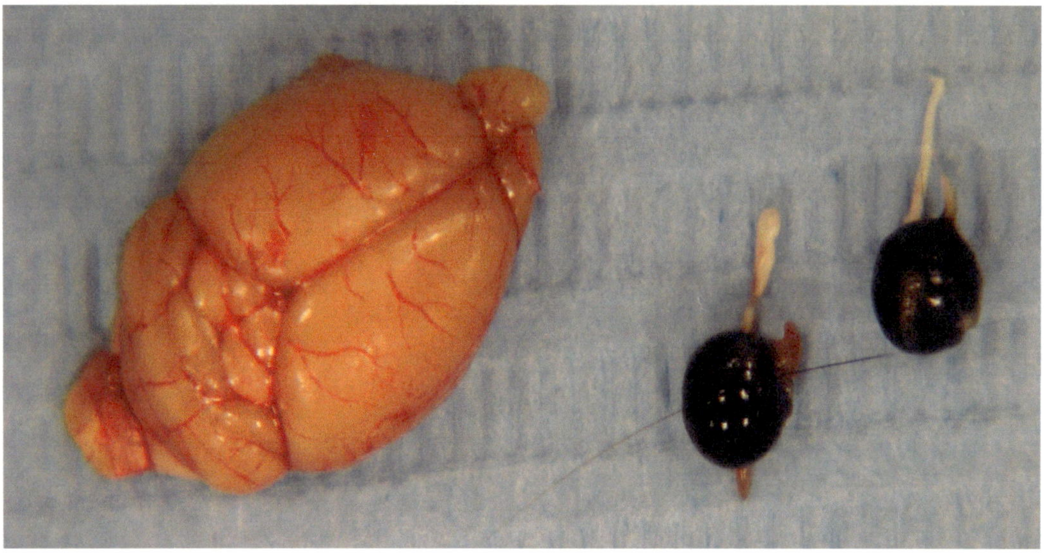

Fig. 5. The super p53 mice brain, eyeballs and optic nerves

1) Enzyme-Linked ImmunoSorbent Assay (ELISA) for determining the BDNF levels in the ocular tissues, and 2) Western blot and immunoblotting procedures by determining the total protein concentration in the eye tissues, and SDS Page with transferring to nitrocellulose membranes, incubating alternatively with anti PARP1 and anti CS3 antibodies, as previously described by Laemmli (1970) and with some respectful modifications for the eye tissue processing by Pinazo-Durán et al., (1996). The expression bands of both molecules were alternatively examined and quantified by laser densitometry.

### 2.2 Expression of the BDNF, PARP1 and CS3 in the sp53 retina-choroid

The ELISA assay allowed us to detect the BDNF concentration in the retina-choroid of both groups of mice. It was observed that the BDNF expression was significantly higher in the sp53 tissues than in the corresponding controls, as reflected in the Table 1.

| Molecules | Sp53G | WTG | p-value |
|---|---|---|---|
| **BDNF** (pg/mL) | 121,13 ± 2,72 | 108,16 ± 4,43 | 0,00250 |
| **PARP-1** (laser rdu) | 143,28 ± 5,38 | 105,46 ± 3,91 | 0,00003 |
| **CS-3** (laser rdu) | 169,20 ± 3,17 | 167,22 ± 1,40 | 0,29600 |

Table 1.

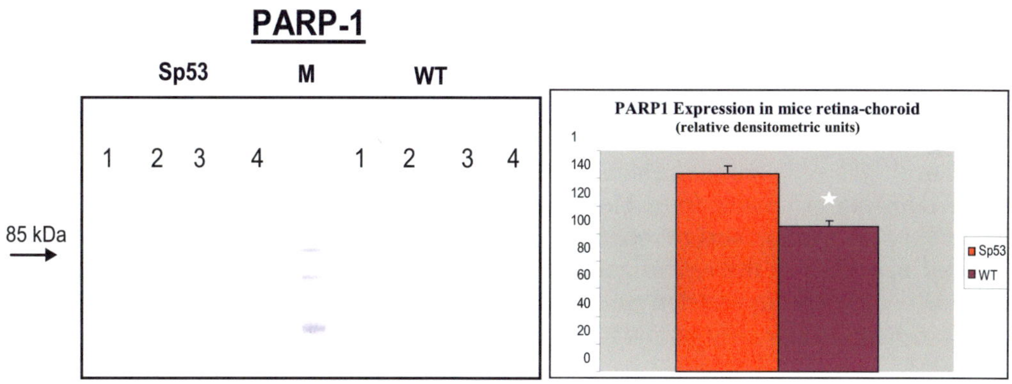


Fig. 6. Immunobloting in mice retina choroid for PARP1 expression and the corresponding quantitative results by laser spectrometry

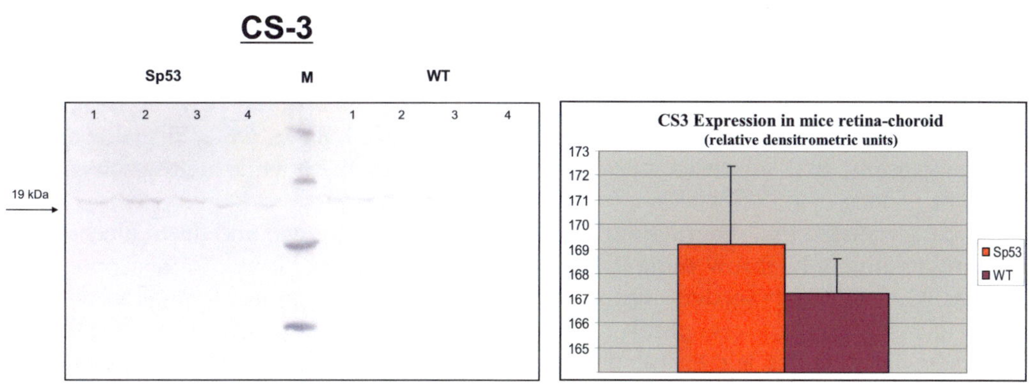


Fig. 7.

The results showed that the two enzymes involved in the apoptotic cascade, PARP1 and CS 3 expressed differently in the retina-choroid of the two groups of mice, depending on the genetic background. When the nitrocellulose membranes were incubated, revealed and examined, the corresponding bands of the PARP1 and CS3 expression were more noticeable in the sp53G than in the wtG eyes, data confirmed by the quantification analysis performed by laser densitometry (relative densitometric units), as can also be observed in the above table 1. CS3, although there was more noticeable in mouse tissue samples sp53, showed no significant differences with the wild mouse having normal p53 genetic load (figures 6 and 7).

## 3. Cell surviving and death

As mentioned previously, several mechanisms have been implicated in initiating the apoptotic cascade in glaucoma. These mechanisms and their potential therapeutic effects include inflammation, ischaemia, excitotoxicity, oxidative stress, mitochondrial dysfunction, and neurotrophin deprivation. Taking into consideration that apoptosis significantly contributes to ganglion cell loss in glaucoma, and in the case that the specific apoptosis signalling pathways for glaucoma can be known (Ray & Mookherjee 2009), any agent that can help to block or interrupt the specific signalling, may have the potential to slowing or stopping glaucoma progression and visual loss.

Charles et al., (2005) investigated the apoptosis-related signaling pathways in a cultured rat retinal ganglion cell (RGC-5) line deprived of growth factors after serum withdrawal from the culture medium. The authors described that serum withdrawal induces apoptotic cell death in RGC-5 cells, via mitochondrial pathways, leading to the speculation that growth factor deprivation arising from blockade of retrograde transport of neurotrophins, may involve similar mechanisms of retinal ganglion cell death in glaucoma. Khalyfa et al., (2007) induced apoptosis in the retinal ganglion cells in transformed rats in order to generate a genome-wide gene expression in cultures of retinal ganglion cells, following serum deprivation and to identify candidate genes that may be involved in the signal transduction pathways.

Thus, the genes identified in microarray data and validated by real-time RT-PCR may play an important role in retinal ganglion cell death. Among the validated genes, C3 and C1s showed significant upregulation of the complement component pathway. The results further indicate that components of the complement pathway are present in neurons of the rat retina.

It would be appropriate also in the context to cite that Erythropoietin modulates erythropoiesis by inhibiting apoptosis in erythrocyte progenitors. This molecule has been demonstrated to be protective in experimental models of trauma, cerebral and retinal ischaemia and neuroinflammation. Moreover, it was described that erythropoietin promoted retinal ganglion cell survival, without affecting IOP, in DBA/2J glaucomatous mice, suggesting that erythropoietin may be a potential therapeutic neuroprotectant in glaucoma (Zhong et al. 2007).

It may be speculated that determining the regulation of cell survival and death mechanisms in the retina it may be throw some light on the pathogenesis of POAG. In this context, the elevated IOP leads to molecular events that are destructive to the retinal ganglion cells and optic axons, but also induces specific changes that are potentially protective against cellular injury and death. If this is the case, then the glaucomatous retinal ganglion cell death and subsequent axonal loss would result not only from initiation of apoptosis, but also from failure of intrinsic cell protective mechanisms.

Consequently, it should therefore be theoretically probable to act on the regulation processes of these two classes of responses, and improving ganglion cells survival when glaucoma develops, as well as in glaucoma progression. Since the transgenic mouse used in the present work, which has 4 copies of the p53 gene, displayed a significantly higher expression of molecules involved in cell surviving and death in the retina, we suggest that p53 may be involved in regulation of these processes. Our findings may open new diagnostic and therapeutic possibilities by the p53 related biomedical and biotechnological applications in glaucoma.

## 4. References


Agar A, Li S, Agarwal N, Coroneo MT, Hill MA, Retinal ganglion cell line apoptosis induced by hydrostatic pressure, *Brain Res.* 2006; 1086:191-200.

Agarwal R, Gupta SK, Agarwal P, Saxena R, Agrawal SS. Current concepts in the pathophysiology of glaucoma. *Indian J Ophthalmol* 2009 57:257-266

Aguilar-Quesada R, Muñoz-Gámez JA, Martín-Oliva D, Peralta-Leal A, Quiles-Pérez R, Rodríguez-Vargas JM, Ruiz de Almodóvar M, Conde C, Ruiz-Extremera A, Oliver FJ Modulation of transcription by PARP-1: consequences in carcinogenesis and inflammation. *Curr Med Chem.* 2007; 14:1179-87.

Bach M, Hoffmann MB. Update on the pattern electroretinogram in glaucoma. *Optom Vis Sci.* 2008; 85:386-395.

Baltmr A, Duggan J, Nizari S, Salt TE, Cordeiro MF. Neuroprotection in glaucoma -Is there a future role? *Exp Eye Res.* 2010 ; 91:554-566.

Bespalov M & Saarma M. (2007). GDNF receptor complex is an emerging drug target. *Trends in Pharmacol Sci* 28: 68-74.

Birge RB, Ucker DS. Innate apoptotic immunity: the calming touch of death. *Cell Death Differ* 2008 15, 1096–1102

Boesten LS, Zadelaar AS, van Nieuwkoop A, Hu L, Teunisse AF, Jochemsen AG, Evers B, van de Water B, Gijbels MJ, van Vlijmen BJ, Havekes LM, de Winther MP. Macrophage p53 controls macrophage death in atherosclerotic lesions of apolipoprotein E deficient mice. *Atherosclerosis.* 2009; 207:399-404.

Carmignoto G, Pizzorruso T, Tia S, Vicini S. Brain derived neurotrophic factor and nerve growth factor potentiate excitatory synaptic transmission in the rat visual cortex. *J Physiol* 1997; 498 153-164.

Charles I, Khalyfa A, Kumar DM, Krishnamoorthy RR, Roque RS, Cooper N, Agarwal N. (2005) Serum deprivation induces apoptotic cell death of transformed rat retinal ganglion cells via mitochondrial signaling pathways. *Invest Ophthalmol Vis Sci* ; 46 :1330-1338.

Chauhan BC, Mikelberg FS, Balaszi AG, LeBlanc RP, Lesk MR, Trope GE; Canadian Glaucoma Study Group. (2008). Canadian Glaucoma Study: 2. risk factors for the progression of open-angle glaucoma. *Arch Ophthalmol;* 126:1030-1036.

Chen QM, Liu J, Merret JB. (2000). Apoptosis or senescence-like growth arrest: influence of cell-cycle position, p53, p21 and bax in H2O2 response of normal human fibroblasts. *Biochem J* 347: 543-551

Copin B, Brézin AP, Valtot F, Dascotte JC, Béchetoille A, Garchon HJ. (2002) Apolipoprotein E-promoter single-nucleotide polymorphisms affect the phenotype of primary open-angle glaucoma and demonstrate interaction with the myocilin gene. *Am J Hum Genet*;70(6):1575-81.

Cordeiro F, Guo L, Coxon KM, Duggan J, Nizari S, Normando EM, Sensi SL, Sillito AM, Fitzke FW, Salt TE,E Moss SE. (2010). Imaging multiple phases of neurodegeneration: a novel approach to assessing cell death in vivo. *Cell Death and Disease.*

Dean JL, Thangavel C, McClendon AK, Reed CA, Knudsen ES. (2010) Therapeutic CDK4/6 inhibition in breast cancer: key mechanisms of response and failure. *Oncogene;* 29:4018-4032

Efeyan A, Garcia-Cao I, Herranz D, Velasco-Miguel S, Serrano M. (2006) Tumour biology: Policing of oncogene activity by p53. *Nature;* 443(7108):159

Fernández-Martínez L, Letteboer S, Mardin CY, Weisschuh N, Gramer E, Weber BHF, Rautenstrauss B, Ferreira PA, Kruse FE, Reis A, Roepman R, Pasutto F. (2011) Evidence for RPGRIP1 gene as risk factor for primary open angle glaucoma. *Eur J Human Genetics* 19: 445–451

Gallego-Pinazo R, Zanón-Moreno V, Sanz S, Andrés V, Serrano M, García-Cao I, Pinazo-Durán MD. (2008) Biochemical characterization of the optic nerve in mice overexpressing the P53 gen. Oxidative stress assays. *Arch Soc Esp Oftalmol;* 83:105-111

Gallego-Pinazo R, Pinazo-Durán MD, Serrano M. (2010). The cell cycle and gene p53. An approach to molecular ophthalmology. *Arch Soc Esp Oftalmol.* 85:229-231.

Garaci FG, Cozzolino V, Nucci C, Gaudiello F, Ludovici A, Lupattelli T, Floris R, Simonetti G. (2008) Advances in neuroimaging of the visual pathways and their use in glaucoma. *Prog Brain Res;* 173:165-77.

García-Cao I, García-Cao M, Martín-Caballero J, Criado LM, Klatt P, Flores JM, Weill JC, Blasco MA, Serrano M. (2002). "Super p53" mice exhibit enhanced DNA damage response, are tumor resistant and age normally. *EMBO* ; 21:6225-6235.

Gaasterland D, Tanishima T, Kuwabara T. (1978). Axoplasmic flow during chronic experimental glaucoma. 1. Light and electron microscopic studies of the monkey optic nervehead during development of glaucomatous cupping. *Invest Ophthalmol Vis Sci;* 17:838-846.

Guevara NV, Kim HS, Antonova EI, Chan L. (1999). The absence of p53 accelerates atherosclerosis by increasing cell proliferation in vivo. *Nat Med;* 5:335-339.

Golubnitschaja O & Flammer J. (2007). What are the biomarkers for glaucoma? Survery Ophthalmology; 52:S155-S161

Harada Ch, Guo X, Namekata K, Kimura A, Nakamura K, Tanaka K, Parada L, Harada T (2011) Glia- and neuron-specific functions of TrkB signalling during retinal degeneration and regeneration. *Nature Communications.*

Hernández MR, Wang N, Hanley NM, Neufeld AH. (1991) Localization of Collagen Types I and IV mRNAs in

Human Optic Nerve Head by In Situ Hybridization. Investigative Ophthalmol Vis Sci. 32:2169-2177

Ivanova T, Gómez-Escoda B, Hidalgo E, Ayté J. (2011) G1/S transcription and the DNA synthesis checkpoint: Common regulatory mechanisms. *Cell Cycle* 10: 912-915

Jeong B-S, Hu W, Belyi V , Rabadan R, Levine AJ. (2009) Differential levels of transcription of p53-regulated genes by the arginine/proline polymorphism: p53 with arginine at codon 72 favors apoptosis. *FASEB J.* 24: 1347-1353

Ju WK, Liu Q, Kim KY, Crowston JG, Lindsey JD, Agarwal N, Ellisman MH, Perkins GA, Weinreb RN (2007), Elevated hydrostatic pressure triggers mitochondrial fission and decreases cellular ATP in differentiated RGC-5 cell. *Invest Ophthalmol Vis Sci.;* 48:2145-51.

Haga SB, Khoury MJ, Burke W (2003) Genomic profiling to promote a healthy lifestyle: not ready for prime time. *Nat Genet* 34:347–350.

Khalyfa A, Chlon T, Qiang H, Agarwal N, Cooper NG. (2007) Microarray reveals complement components are regulated in the serum-deprived rat retinal ganglion cell line. *Mol Vis;* 13:293-308.

Kerr JF, Wyllie AH, Currie AR (1972) Apoptosis: a basic biological phenomenon with wide-ranging implications in tissue kinetics. *Br J Cancer;* 26:239-57.

Kumarasamy NA, Lam FS, Wang AL, Teoharides TC. (2006) Glaucoma: Current and developing concepts in inflammation, pathogenesis and treatment. *Eur J Inflammation;* 4:129-137

Itoa Y, Shimazawaa M, Chenc YN, Tsurumaa K, Yamashimad T, Araiec M, Haraa H. (2009) Morphological changes in the visual pathway induced by experimental glaucoma in Japanese monkeys Exp Eye Res; 89:246-255

LaGrange, F, Beauvieux, J (1925). Anatomie de I'excavation glaucomateuse, *Arch Opthalmol (Paris)* 42:129.

Lam DS, Leung YF, Chua JK, Baum L, Fan DS, Choy KW, Pang CP. Truncations in the TIGR gene in individuals with and without primary open-angle glaucoma. *Invest Ophthalmol Vis Sci.* 2000: 41:1386-91.

Lane DP (1992) p53, guardian of the genome. *Nature;* 358:15-16.

Lee KM, Miklos I, Du HY, Watt S, Szilagyi Z, Saiz JE, Madabhushi R, Penkett CJ, Sipiczki M, Bahler J, Fisher R P (2005) Impairment of the TFIIH-associated CDK-activating kinase selectively affects cell cycle-regulated gene expression I in fission yeast. *Mol Biol Cell* 16:2734 - 2745

Lee EJ, Kim TW, Weinreb RN, Park KH, Kim SH, Kim DM. (2011). {beta}-zone Parapapillary Atrophy and the Rate of Retinal Nerve Fiber Layer Thinning in Glaucoma. *Invest Ophthalmol Vis Sci.* 2011

Levin LA, Louhab AB (1996). Apoptosis of retinal ganglion cells in Anterior Ischaemic Optic Neuropathy. *Arch Ophthalmol;* 114:488-491

Levin, LA (1997). Mechanisms of optic neuropathy . *Curr Opin Ophthalmol ;* 78:9-15

Levin LA (1999) . Intrinsic survival mechanisms for retinal ganglion cells. *Eur J Ophthalmol;* 9 Suppl 1:S12-6.

Levine AJ, Finlay (2004) CA. P53 is a tumour suppressor gene. *Cell;* S116: 67-69

Levkovitch-Verbin H, Dardik R, Vander S, Nisgav Y, Kalev-Landoy M, Melamed S. (2006) Experimental Glaucoma and Optic Nerve Transection Induce Simultaneous Upregulation of Proapoptotic and Prosurvival Genes. *Invest Ophthalmol Vis Sci* 47: 2491-2497

Lopez-Martinez F, Lopez-Garrido MP, Sanchez-Sanchez F, Campos-Mollo E, Coca-Prados M, Escribano J (2007) Role of MYOC and OPTN sequence variations in Spanish patients with primary open-angle glaucoma. *Mol Vis;* 13:862-72.

Lutjen-Drecoll E, Shimizu T, Rohrbach M, Rohen JW (1986). Quantitative analysis of 'plaque material' in the inner- and outer wall of Schlemm's canal in normal- and glaucomatous eyes. *Exp Eye Res;* 42:443-55.

McKinnon SJ (1997); Glaucoma, apoptosis, and neuroprotection. *Curr Opin Ophthalmol;* 8:28-37

Meagher LC, Savill JS, Baker A, Fuller RW, Haslett C. (1992) Phagocytosis of apoptotic neutrophils does not induce macrophage release of thromboxane B2. *J Leuk Biol* ; 52: 269-272

Monemi S, Spaeth G, DaSilva A, Popinchalk S, Ilitchev E, Liebmann J, Ritch R, Héon E, Crick RP, Child A, Sarfarazi M. (2005). Identification of a novel adult-onset primary open-angle glaucoma (POAG) gene on 5q22.1. *Hum Mol Genet* 14:725-733.

Muller H (1858). Anatomische Beitrge zur Qphthalmologie: Ueber Nervean-Veranderungen an der Eintrittsstelle'des Schnerven. *Arch Ophthalmol*; 41:1.

Nickells RW. (1999) Apoptosis of the retinal ganglion cells in glaucoma: an update of the molecular pathways involved in cell death. *Surv Ophthalmol* 43: S151-161

Osborne N, Wood J, Chidlow G, Bae J, Melena J, Nash N, (1999) Ganglion cell death in glaucoma: what do we really know?, *Br J Ophthalmol.*; 83: 980-986.

Osborne NN. (2010) Mitochondria: Their role in ganglion cell death and survival in primary open angle glaucoma. *Exp Eye Res*; 90:750-757.

Parisi V. (1997) Neural conduction in the visual pathways in ocular hypertension and glaucoma. *Graefes Arch Clin Exp Ophthalmol.*; 235:136-142.

Pease ME, McKinnon SJ, Quigley HA, Kerrigan-Baumrind LA, Zack DJ. (2000) Obstructed axonal transport of BDNF and its receptor TrkB in experimental glaucoma. *Invest Ophthalmol Vis Sci.*; 41:764-774.

Pinazo-Durán MD, Renau Piqueras J, Guerri C (1993). Developmental changes in the optic nerve related to ethanol consumption in pregnant rats. Analysis of the ethanol-exposed optic nerve. *Teratology* 48:305-322.

Pinazo-Durán, M.D., Vallés, S., Guerri, C., Renau- Piqueras, J. (1996). Gestational-ethanol-induced changes in the developing optic nerve. *Int J Dev Biol*; Suppl 1:141S-142S.

Pinazo-Durán MD, Renau Piqueras J, Guerri C, Strömland K (1997) Optic nerve Hypoplasia in fetal alcohol syndrome: An update. *Eur. J. Ophthalmol.*; 50:100-111.

Pinazo-Durán MD, Gallego-Pinazo R, Pons Vazquez S, Muñoz A. (2005) Postnatal thyroid hormone supplementation rescues the retinal abnormalities in a rat model of congenital neonatal hypothyroidism. *Ophthalmic Res* ; 37: 225-234

Pinazo-Durán MD, Pons-Vázquez S, Gallego-Pinazo R, Galbis Estrada C, Zanón-Moreno V, Vila-Bou V, Sanz-Solana P. (2011) Thyroid hormone deficiency disrupts rat eye neurodevelopment. *Brain Res* .

Quigley HA, McKinnon SJ, Zack DJ, Pease ME, Kerrigan-Baumrind LA, Kerrigan DF, Mitchell RS, (2000) "Retrograde axonal transport of BDNF in retinal ganglion cells is blocked by acute IOP elevation in rats", *Invest Ophthalmol Vis Sci.*; 41:3460-6.

Quigley HA, Broman AT. (2006) The number of people with glaucoma worldwide in 2010 and 2020. *Br J Ophthalmol.*; 90: 262–267.

Quiles-Perez R, Muñoz-Gámez JA, Ruiz-Extremera A, O'Valle F, Sanjuán-Nuñez L, Martín-Alvarez AB, Martín-Oliva D, Caballero T, Muñoz de Rueda P, León J, Gonzalez R, Muntané J, Oliver FJ, Salmerón J. (2010) Inhibition of poly adenosine diphosphate-ribose polymerase decreases hepatocellular carcinoma growth by modulation of tumor-related gene expression. *Hepatology.* ; 51:255-266.

Ray K, Mookherjee S. (2009) Molecular complexity of primary open angle glaucoma. Current concepts. *J. Genetics* ; 88: 451-467.

Rezaie T, Child A, Hitchings R, Brice G, Miller L, Coca-Prados M, Heon E, Krupin T, Ritch R, Kreutzer D, Crick RP, Sarfarazi M (2002) Adult-onset primary open-angle glaucoma caused by mutations in optineurin. Science 295:1077-1079.

Schori H, Kipnis J, Yoles E et al., (2001) Vaccination for protection of retinal ganglion cells against death from glutamate citotoxicity and ocular hypertension: implications for glaucoma. *Proc Natl Acad Sci USA*; 98:3398-3403

Schnabel, J (1892). Das glaucomatose Sehnervenleiden. *Archiv fur Augenheikunde;* XXIV: 18.

Serrano M, Hannon GJ, Beach D. (1993) A new regulatory motif in cell cycle control causing specific inhibition of cyclin D/CDK4. Nature 366:704–707.

Snider WD. (1994) Functions of the neurotrophins during nervous system development: what the knockouts are teaching us. *Cell* ; 77:627-638

Sitorus R Ardjo M, Lorenz B, Preising M. (2003) CYP1B1 gene analysis in primary congenital glaucoma in Indonesian and European patients. *J Med Genet* 40: 1-6

Stone EM, Fingert JH, Alward WL, Nguyen TD, Polansky JR, Sunden SL, et al. (1997) Identification of a gene that causes primary open angle glaucoma. *Science.* 275:668–70.

Tatton WG, Chalmers-Redman RM, Tatton NA. (2011) Apoptosis and anti-apoptosis signalling in glaucomatous retinopathy. *Eur J Ophthalmol. Suppl* 2:S12-22.

Trivino A, Ramirez JM, Salazar JJ, Ramirez AI, Garcia-Sanchez J. (1996). Immunohistochemical study of human optic nerve head astroglia. Vision Res; 36:2015–2028

von Jaeger E Ueber Glaucom und seine Heilung durch Iridectomie. *Z Ges der Aerzte zu Wien* 1858; 14:465- 484.

Walker NI, Harmon BV, Gobé GC, Kerr JF (1974) Patterns of cell death. *Methods Achiev Exp Pathol.* 1988; 13:18-54.

Wyllie AH. Death in normal and neoplastic cells. *J Clin Pathol Suppl.*; 7:35-42.

Yanagi M, Kawasaki R, Wang JJ, Wong TY, Crowston J, Kiuchi Y. (2010) Vascular risk factors in glaucoma: a review. *Clin Exp Ophthalmol*

Zanón-Moreno V, Pinazo-Durán MD. Impact of biomarkers in primary open-angle glaucoma. *Arch Soc Esp Oftalmol* 2008; 83: 465-468

Zanon-Moreno V, Garcia-Medina JJ, Zanon-Viguer V, Moreno-Nadal MA, Pinazo-Duran MD. (2009) Smoking, an additional risk factor in elder women with primary open-angle glaucoma. *Mol Vis.*; 15:2953-2959.

Zanón-Moreno VC, Pinazo-Durán MD. (2008) Impact of biomarkers in primary open-angle glaucoma. *Arch Soc Esp Oftalmol.*; 83:465-8

Zanon-Moreno V, Marco-Ventura P, Lleo-Perez A, Pons-Vazquez S, Garcia-Medina JJ, Vinuesa-Silva I, Moreno-Nadal MA, Pinazo-Duran MD. (2008) Oxidative stress in primary open-angle glaucoma. *J Glaucoma.*; 17:263-268.

Zhang Y, Bhavnani BR. Glutamate-induced apoptosis in primary cortical neurons is inhibited by equine estrogens via down-regulation of caspase-3 and prevention of mitochondrial cytochrome c release. *BMC Neurosci.* 2005; 6:13.

Virág L (2005) Structure and function of poly(ADP-ribose) polymerase-1: role in oxidative stress-related pathologies. *Curr Vasc Pharmacol.*; 3:209-214.

Zeisel SH (2007) Nutrigenomics and metabolomics will change clinical nutrition and public health practice: insights from studies on dietary requirements for choline. *Am J Clin Nutr* 86:542–548

Zhong L, Bradley J, Schubert W, Ahmed E, Adamis AP, Shima DT, Robinson GS, Ng YS. (2007) Erythropoietin promotes survival of retinal ganglion cells in DBA/2J glaucoma mice. *Invest Ophthalmol Vis Sci*. 48:1212-1218.

# 10

# A Vascular Approach to Glaucoma

Luís Abegão Pinto[1] and Ingeborg Stalmans[2]
[1]*Department Ophthalmology, CHLC Lisbon,*
[2]*Department Ophthalmology, UZ Leuven,*
[1]*Portugal*
[2]*Belgium*

## 1. Introduction

Despite the tremendous impact of glaucoma on the vision of our elderly population, the mechanisms of glaucomatous neuropathy have not been fully elucidated. Intra-ocular pressure (IOP) has been convincingly identified as the main risk factor for glaucoma development and progression, and IOP lowering, therefore, is the hallmark of glaucoma therapy. However, a certain proportion of glaucoma patients continue to show disease progression despite "optimal" IOP control. This observation has been a great motivation for the quest for discovering pathogenic mechanisms beyond IOP.
Besides IOP, glaucomatous optic neuropathy has also been associated with various causes of impaired blood flow, such as hypotension, migraine or peripheral vasospasm, and laboratory evidence of ocular and systemic vasodysregulation. These observations support the idea that the eye being treated for glaucoma is likely part of a wider systemic dysfunction, particularly blood flow dysregulation. The ophthalmologist with interest in glaucoma is thus confronted with the need to know what to recognise as a vascular risk factor, how to diagnose vascular dysfunction, which tools are available to study it and what the possibilities for improving such blood flow impairment are. To better understand the complexity and systemic nature of this multifactorial neuropathy, ophthalmologists must look beyond the eye.

## 2. Anatomic considerations and clinical relevance

The need for extensive knowledge about the vascular anatomy of the eye and especially the optic nerve is universal to all ophthalmologists. The complexities of the arterial branching and supply network for each anatomical compartment in the eye have a number of clinical implications that result from the eye's unique vascularisation tree.
All blood to the optic nerve comes from the carotid artery through its ophthalmic artery branch. This ophthalmic artery follows a tortuous path inside the orbit towards the anterior nasal orbital wall, crossing the optic nerve as the short posterior ciliary arteries, the long posterior ciliary arteries and the central retinal artery branch off. The anatomical proximity between the optic nerve and major pulsating arteries, such as the carotid artery, has been proposed as a risk factor for optic nerve damage in some normotensional glaucoma patients due to optic nerve compression (Ogata N., 2005).

Glaucomatous neuropathy is characterised by structural damage to the optic nerve head (ONH) and a decrease in the thickness of the retinal nerve fiber layer. While the retinal nerve fiber layer blood supply derives exclusively from the central retinal artery, the ONH blood supply is divided into four anatomic compartments (see table 1). The most anterior, named surface nerve fiber layer, is also supplied by the retinal arteries. The prelaminar and laminar compartments are supplied by branches of the short posterior ciliary artery, which sometimes encircle the ONH, creating the Zinn-Haller ring. A functional anastomosis could theoretically protect the optic nerve from occlusion or hypoperfusion of a single short posterior ciliary artery. The most posterior compartment, the retrolaminar region, is mostly supplied by pial vessels that give off centripetal branches into the septa of the optic nerve.

| Arterial vascularisation of the different compartments of the optic nerve head | |
|---|---|
| Retinal nerve fiber layer | Central retinal artery |
| Prelaminar | Short posterior ciliary artery |
| Laminar | Short posterior ciliary artery |
| Retrolaminar | Pial arteries |

Table 1. Overview of main arterial branches supplying the optic nerve head

Regulation of blood flow is also different in the various ocular compartments. As elsewhere in the body, blood flow in the eye should be under the control of the autonomic nervous system. However, as this innervation stops at the level of the lamina cribosa, the retinal circulation is not regulated by sympathetic output. Instead, retinal arteries have the ability through autoregulation to constrict or dilate in response to changes in oxygen or pH and thus maintain a constant metabolic environment despite exposure to conditions that might upset this equilibrium. The choroidal circulation, on the contrary, is under the control of the autonomic nervous system and has no intrinsic ability to adapt to these stimuli. It is able to decrease or increase blood flow in response to cervical sympathetic stimulation, but it cannot adapt to sudden changes in IOP, for example. A clinical consequence of this inability to self-regulate its flow is the uveal effusion that can be seen when opening the eye during surgery. As a consequence of these differences in vasoreactive mechanisms, the response to medical therapy also differs between these vascular beds. Phosphodiesterase inhibitors, for example, clearly enhance choroidal flow by increasing nitric oxide concentration, whereas the retinal circulation does not significantly change in response to this drug (Harris A., 2008).

ONH circulation has particularities that make its study particularly challenging. Like its retinal counterparts, the ONH capillaries lack pre-capillary sphincters; they have pericytes instead. As in the retinal circulation, these pericytes respond to metabolic and neuro-endocrine factors that regulate their contractility. However, while there is no consistent evidence of autonomic nervous system directly regulating ONH blood flow, the lack of a cellular barrier separating the ONH from the choroid tissues could make the ONH susceptible to autonomic stimulations. As both are supplied by the same vessels, imbalances in the choroidal blood flow could redirect blood flow away from the ONH.

The venous drainage of the entire retina and ONH takes place through the central retina vein. Although not directly involved in aqueous humour drainage, the central vein has been

studied for glaucoma progression purposes. Indeed, there seems to be a relationship between spontaneous venous pulsations and glaucoma progression, suggesting the lack of spontaneous pulsations as a risk factor for progression visual field damage (Balaratnasingam C., 2007) (Nicolela, 2007).
The aqueous humour, however, is drained from Schlemm's canal through the episcleral veins. Therefore, an increase in venous pressure leads to a decrease in drainage due to passive diffusion. Altered vein reactivity or systemically increased vein pressure can lead to an increase in IOP. Increased episcleral venous pressure in glaucoma patients may be one mechanism behind the nocturnal rise in IOP many of these patients present (Liu JH., 1999).

## 3. Tools to study ocular blood flow

There are an increasing number of tools that can provide insight into different aspects of ocular blood flow (OBF) in various vascular beds in and around the eye. A full description of all the techniques is beyond the scope of this book, and thus, we will focus on succinctly describing the most commonly used methods.
*Colour Doppler imaging (CDI)* is a non-invasive ultrasound-based technology that uses the Doppler effect to measure blood velocities. This technique can provide information on the ophthalmic artery, short posterior ciliary arteries (divided into temporal and nasal groups) and the central retinal artery (figure 1). It describes peak systolic velocities (PSV), end-diastolic velocities (EDV), resistance index (RI) (Pourcelot, 1975) and, in some devices, the mean flow velocities (MFV) and the pulsatility index (PI) (Gosling, 1971). These two indices can be calculated using the following formulas: RI = (PSV-EDV)/PSV and PI = (PSV-EDV)/MFV. CDI is not dependent on optical transparency or pupil size. The downside of this technology, however, is that it provides only blood velocities. To calculate blood flow from these velocities, the vessel diameter would have to be known. However, the diameter of the retrobulbar vessels cannot be measured with high precision with this technique, making blood flow calculations uncertain (Zeitz, 2006). As with any ultrasound-based technique, it is highly observer-dependent, and good reproducibility requires an experienced technician. A consensus is needed to define standard operating procedures, thus reducing such bias, so that valid comparisons can be made between the results from different centers.

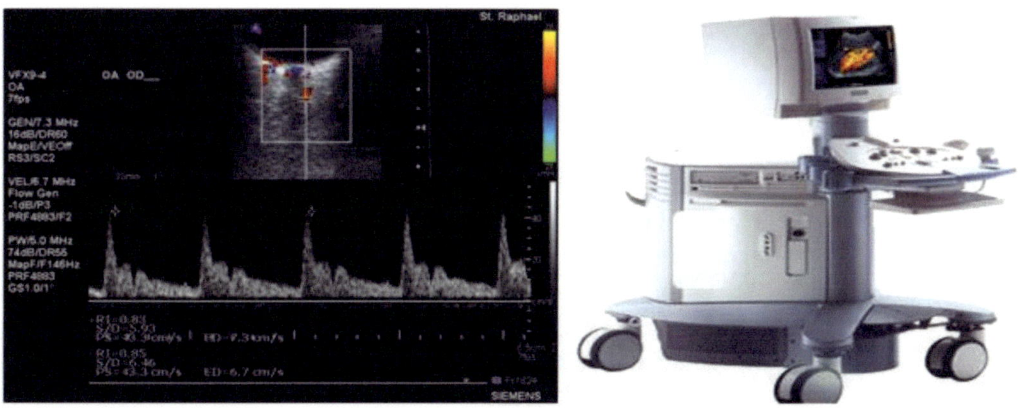


Fig. 1. CDI data printout (left); CDI device (right)

*Laser Doppler flowmetry* (LDF) utilises a fundus camera and non-invasive confocal laser flowmetry using the Doppler effect to measure retinal capillary blood flow. This confocal system provides individual data points from each analysed vessel, allowing the information to be interpreted on a pixel-to-pixel level by several different types of automated software, all of which have a very good coefficient of reproducibility (figure 2). Although this technique provides volumetric measurements, it does so in arbitrary units, which is the major drawback of this technology. As with any fundoscopic-based evaluation, it is dependent on clear optical media, pupil size and the fixation capability of the patient.

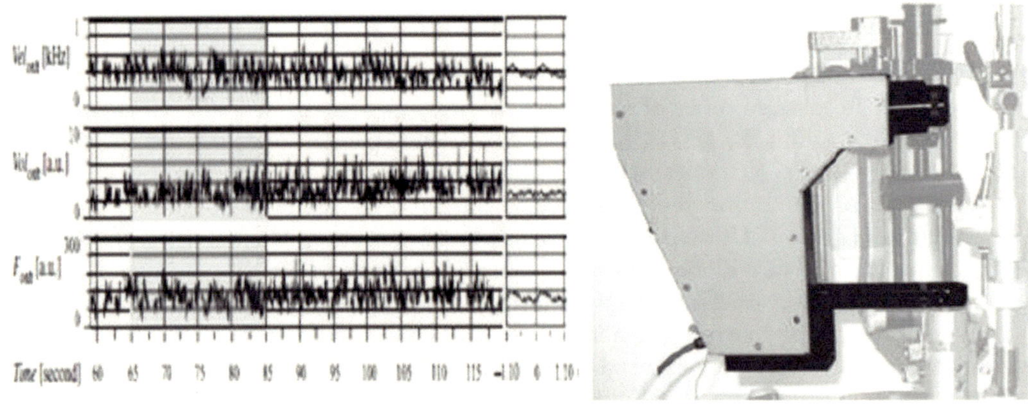

Fig. 2. LDF printout data (left); LDF device (right) (courtesy of Charles Riva; reproduced with permission from Acta Ophthalmologica)

*Doppler optical coherence tomography (OCT)* is another device that uses the Doppler frequency shift. Recent technological advances have allowed this technology to be added to Fourier-domain OCT, making it possible to determine the velocity of the blood inside the major retinal vessels and the cross-sectional diameter of these vessels throughout the cardiac cycle. This allows for a volumetric assessment of the flow rate while taking into account background motion, beam incidence angle and pulsation (figure 3). However, this device is still under further development and has currently a limited clinical application.

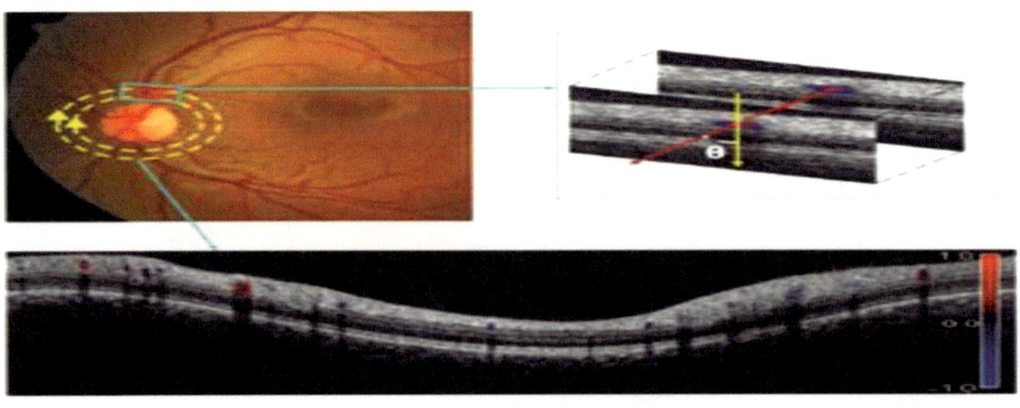

Fig. 3. Doppler OCT image printout (courtesy of David Huang)

The *retinal vessel analyser* (RVA) also relies on a fundus camera and uses vessel diameter analysis software. It allows for real-time retinal vessel diameter measurements with a maximum frequency of 50 Hz (figure 4). Although it provides measurements in arbitrary units, an approximation can be made to microns. The main advantage of this technique is the real-time acquisition, which allows for the simultaneous investigation of different vessels and vascular segments. In contrast to CDI, this technology can measure vessel diameter but not the velocity of the blood within the vessel. It is again influenced by optical media transparency and requires pupil dilation, which may affect blood flow itself.

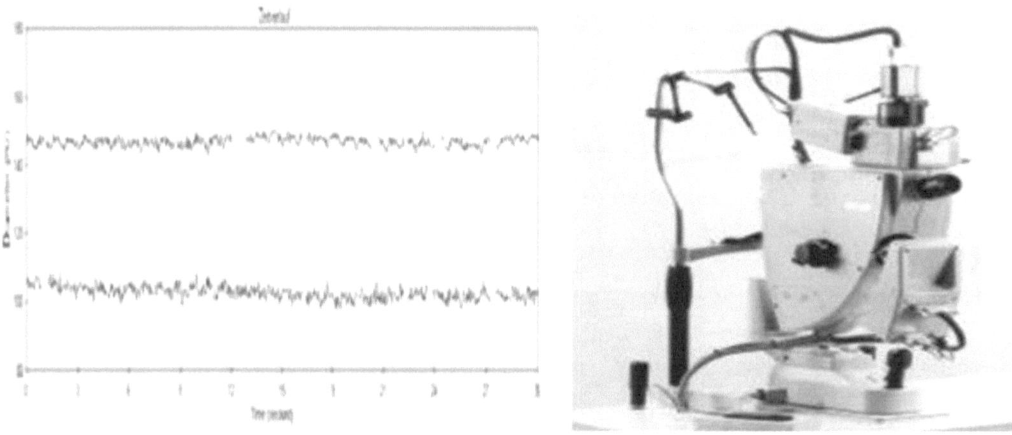

Fig. 4. RVA data printout (left); RVA device (right) (courtesy of Gerhard Garhofer; reproduced with permission from Acta Ophthalmologica)

*Retinal oximetry* is a non-invasive method for assessing the haemoglobin oxygen saturation in the retinal vessels. It relies on digital fundus photography coupled with a beam splitter and a filter that discriminates different bandwidths. Using both an oxygen-sensitive and an oxygen-insensitive bandwidth, it can determine the oxygen saturation of the retinal vessels in comparison to the retinal background (figure 5). It is used to study *in vivo* the metabolic needs of the retina and its ability to react to stimuli, either pharmacological or physiological. Its drawbacks are related to the lack of information about the oxygenation of the optic nerve itself, as only retinal vessels are analysed, and the need for pupil dilation and clear optic media.

*Dynamic contour tonometry (DCT)* represents a device for non-invasive continuous measurement of IOP. Contrary to applanation tonometers, its concave contact surface allows for the equal distribution of forces between the device and the cornea as the pressure applied by the observer equals the pressure inside the eye. Because it allows for a continuous reading, a sinusoidal variation can be registered (figure 6). The difference between the highest and the lowest IOP is called the ocular pulse amplitude (OPA) (figure 3). This parameter probably relates to the blood volume that is pumped into the eye during each cardiac cycle, and it may represent choroidal blood flow or the pulsatile component itself. It has an acceptable intra- and inter-observer variability. Factors modulating this amplitude are not fully understood. It is not dependent on corneal thickness, but it positively correlates with IOP and negatively with axial length. An algorithm that transforms this pressure amplitude into blood flow is not yet available.

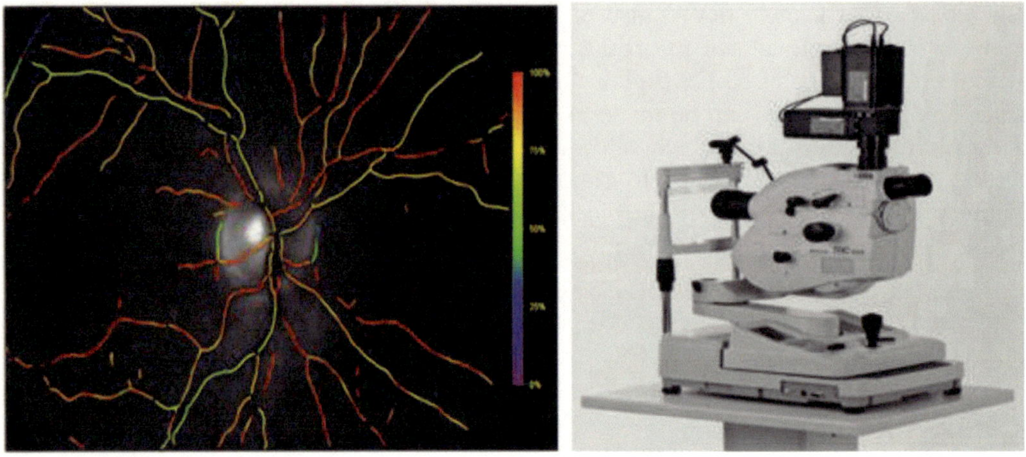

Fig. 5. Retinal oximetry data printout (left); retinal oximetry device (right) (reproduced with permission from Oxymap ©)

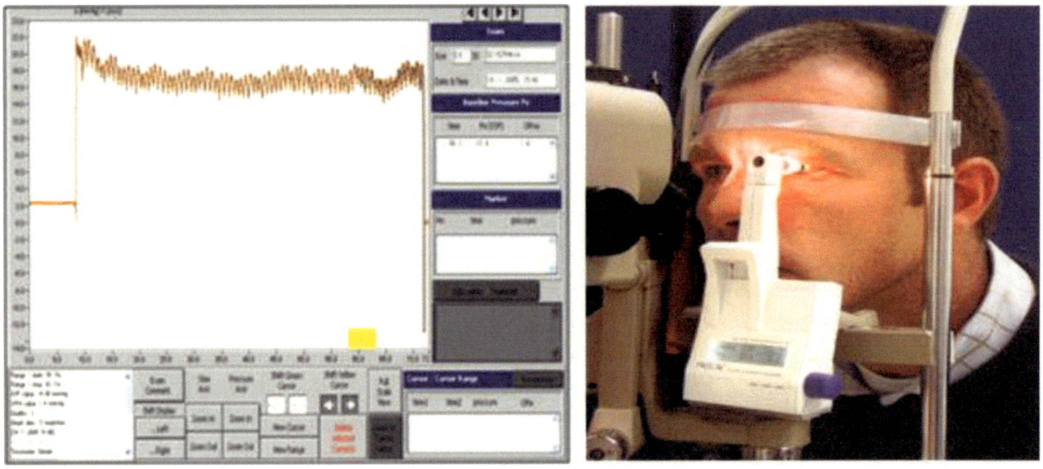

Fig. 6. DCT data printout (left) (courtesy of C. Marques-Neves); DCT device (right) (reproduced with permission from Ziemer Ophtalmic ©)

*The pulsatile ocular blood flow (POBF)* analyser is a modified pneumotonometer that also measures ocular pulse. As with DCT, this device also allows for digital recording of the sinusoidal intra-ocular pressure curve throughout the cardiac cycle (figure 7). However, this device actually indents the cornea instead of adapting to its surface. Its similarities to DCT are reflected in its limitations. While changes in POBF measures are assumed to be related to choroidal blood flow, due to its greater significance to the overall OBF, this cannot be directly tested. Structurally, POBF also negatively correlates with axial length while still being more sensitive to changes in cornea thickness than DCT. It is nevertheless an inexpensive and simple to operate device that can produce data related to blood flow, such as changes in ocular pulse volume, duration of systole and diastole and the maximum speed of blood flowing into the eye (in µl/s).

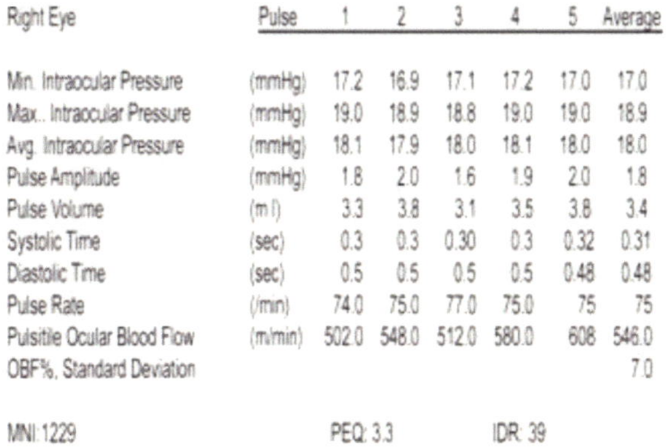

| Right Eye | Pulse | 1 | 2 | 3 | 4 | 5 | Average |
|---|---|---|---|---|---|---|---|
| Min. Intraocular Pressure | (mmHg) | 17.2 | 16.9 | 17.1 | 17.2 | 17.0 | 17.0 |
| Max.. Intraocular Pressure | (mmHg) | 19.0 | 18.9 | 18.8 | 19.0 | 19.0 | 18.9 |
| Avg. Intraocular Pressure | (mmHg) | 18.1 | 17.9 | 18.0 | 18.1 | 18.0 | 18.0 |
| Pulse Amplitude | (mmHg) | 1.8 | 2.0 | 1.6 | 1.9 | 2.0 | 1.8 |
| Pulse Volume | (m l) | 3.3 | 3.8 | 3.1 | 3.5 | 3.8 | 3.4 |
| Systolic Time | (sec) | 0.3 | 0.3 | 0.30 | 0.3 | 0.32 | 0.31 |
| Diastolic Time | (sec) | 0.5 | 0.5 | 0.5 | 0.5 | 0.48 | 0.48 |
| Pulse Rate | (/min) | 74.0 | 75.0 | 77.0 | 75.0 | 75 | 75 |
| Pulsitile Ocular Blood Flow | (m/min) | 502.0 | 548.0 | 512.0 | 580.0 | 608 | 546.0 |
| OBF%, Standard Deviation | | | | | | | 7.0 |

MNI 1229 PEQ 3.3 IDR 39

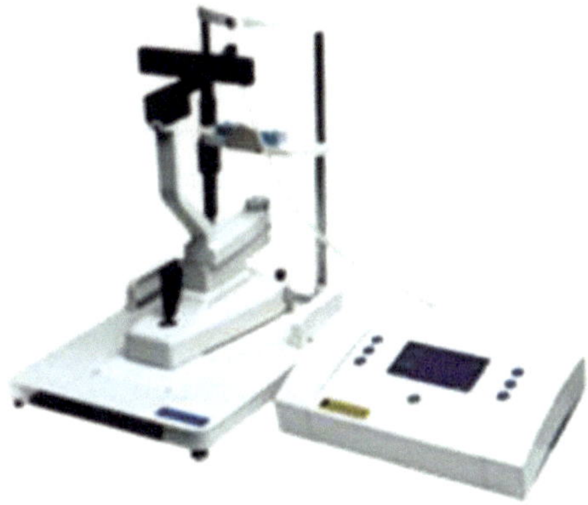

Fig. 7. POBF analyser data printout (left); POBF analyser device (right) (reproduced with permission from Paradigm Medical Industries Inc)

| | Anatomic region of blood flow studied | Contact | Arbitrary units | Clear media | Pupil dilation |
|---|---|---|---|---|---|
| CDI | Retrobulbar | Yes | No | No | No |
| Laser Doppler Flowmetry | Retinal | No | Yes | Yes | Yes |
| Doppler OCT | Retinal | No | No | Yes | Yes |
| Retinal vessel Analyser | Retinal | No | Yes | Yes | Yes |
| Retinal oximetry | Retinal | No | No | Yes | Yes |
| DCT | Choroid? | Yes | No | No | No |
| POBF analyser | Choroid? | Yes | No | No | No |

Table 2. Overall description of OBF measuring tools

## 4. Altered blood flow as a risk factor for glaucoma (progression)

There are a growing number of publications showing blood flow disturbances in glaucoma patients that emphasise the role for a vascular component in glaucoma pathogenesis. However, the nature of these disturbances in OBF is still under discussion, including weather such changes are part of the pathogenic mechanism or secondary to the underlying disease. When considering ocular diseases in which vascular mechanisms are involved, such as diabetic retinopathy or occlusion of the central retinal artery or vein, none of these diseases produce a characteristic glaucomatous cupping of the disc (Jonas, 1993) (Jonas, 1999). Therefore, hypoperfusion, as seen in those diseases, does not provide a full explanation for glaucomatous neuropathy. Should hypoperfusion alone represent the vascular risk factor for glaucoma (progression), one would expect a stronger relationship between glaucoma and known risk factors for atherosclerosis, such as C-reactive protein or dyslipidaemias. However, data on these variables is far from consistently pointing them out as risk factors for glaucoma (de Voogd, 2006). Alternatively, or in addition to hypoperfusion, there may be a vascular dysfunction that compromises the normal self-regulating mechanisms of the vessels supplying ONH in response to hypoperfusion (Sossi, 1983). Interestingly, the ONH, due to its unique anatomical condition, is exposed to circulating hormones in a way that the rest of the central nervous system is not. Not only is the barrier function decreased in the capillaries in this region (Grieshaber, 2007), but there is also diffusion from the choroid, where these mechanisms do not exist (Flage, 1977). Vasoconstrictive agents, such as angiotensin II and endothelin, could therefore have a greater impact in this region than elsewhere in the nervous system. Available data suggest that glaucoma patients may have an endothelial dysfunction with increased levels of endothelin and vasodilation impairment, thus increasing the risk for ONH injury.

Such dysfunction, as suggested by Flammer, would not lead to a stable reduction in OBF but rather to an instability of ocular perfusion, leading to a repeated mild reperfusion injury (Flammer, 2006) (Flammer J., 1999). This mechanism of ischaemia-reperfusion injury is associated with the generation of reactive oxygen species and cellular apoptosis. These reactive oxygen species induce changes in the trabecular meshwork, possibly resulting in decreased aqueous humour drainage and increased IOP (Saccà, 2007). Additionally, they alter nitric oxide metabolism. Indeed, mitochondrial malfunction due to hypoxia can lead to increased superoxide formation, a metabolite with high affinity for nitric oxide, in a reaction that creates peroxynitrite (Beckman, 1990). This process not only reduces nitric oxide availability but also the ability of this molecule to induce endothelial-dependent dilation (Aslan, 2007). The resulting increase in vasoconstriction and oxidative stress can lead to an activation of several apoptotic pathways through cellular dysfunction (Kim, 1999). It has been suggested that this oxidative stress could also occur as a result of elevated intra-ocular pressure in what seems to be an IOP-related mechanical stress event (Sacca, 2005). In humans, the role of this cellular hypoxia in glaucoma is further supported by increased staining of hypoxia-induced factor (HIF-1α) in the retina and optic nerve of patients with glaucoma compared with non-glaucomatous individuals (Tezel, 2004).

This endothelial dysfunction believed to exist in glaucoma can also have an impact on rheological factors. In addition to perfusion pressure and local vascular resistance, blood viscosity can also reduce OBF (Flammer, 2002). Glaucoma patients have been described as having decreased erythrocyte deformability (Ates, 1998), hyperaggregability of the erythrocytes (Hamard, 1994) and altered red blood cell membrane integrity (Carter, 1990). In addition, the presence of an activated coagulation cascade (O'Brien, 1997) and an increase in platelet aggregability (Hoyng, 1992) (Bojic, 1998) have been reported in glaucoma patients. It is also possible, however, that these rheological abnormalities are a consequence of the vascular changes. The endothelial cells not only release vasoactive factors abluminally, which influence vascular smooth muscle cells and pericytes, but they also release factors intraluminally that influence blood cells. For instance, nitric oxide, whose impairment in glaucoma patients has been widely described (see above), is a powerful inhibitor of platelet aggregation (Hampton, 1967) (Zhou, 2010).

This impaired self-regulation capacity of the vessels supplying the ONH may be clinically relevant. Recent studies have shown that fluctuations in perfusion pressure are particularly important in glaucoma progression, especially in patients with normotensional glaucoma (Sung, 2009). Glaucoma patients not only have a higher IOP, but they also show circadian vascular rhythms that can tip the balance of perfusion pressure to pathogenic levels. These abnormal circadian cardiovascular responses may be due to an underlying dysautonomic disturbance, as it is the autonomic nervous system's responsibility to regulate these daily rhythms (Appenzeller, 1997). Glaucoma patients seem to have a number of signs of autonomic dysfunction, from dysregulation of aqueous humour production and drainage (Curtis, 2002) to abnormal heart rate and blood pressure variability, both of which are associated with increased cardiovascular risk. This blood pressure variability is particularly prominent in patients with normotensional glaucoma, and a correlation between the extent of autonomic nervous system dysfunction and the severity of the disease has been suggested (Gherghel, 2004).

Blood pressure itself has been positively correlated with IOP, with a calculated average increase of 0.21 mmHg in IOP for every 10 mmHg increase in blood pressure (Klein, 2005). However, the literature is not conclusive on the impact that arterial hypertension may have on glaucoma. While there are studies showing a correlation between higher blood pressure and a higher prevalence of glaucoma (Tielsch, 1995) (Mitchell, 2004), this has not been the case in the Barbados Study, in which baseline hypertension actually decreased the risk for primary open-angle glaucoma (Leske, 2002). More consistently, a lower ocular perfusion pressure (perfusion pressure = blood pressure-IOP), in particular a lower diastolic OPP, has been associated with a significant increase in the risk for glaucoma (Leske, 2002) (Hulsman CA., 2007). Because measuring the local arterial pressure in the eye is not currently feasible, epidemiologic and other studies calculate ocular perfusion pressure from the brachial artery blood pressure and IOP. In the Baltimore Eye Survey (Tielsch, 1995), a perfusion pressure above 50 mmHg was a predictor for a low risk of optic nerve atrophy. This risk roughly doubled if the perfusion pressure was between 30 and 49 mmHg, and it increased more than 6-fold if the perfusion pressure fell below 30 mmHg. As both IOP and blood pressure show circadian variations, this ocular perfusion pressure can fluctuate during a 24-hour period (Bagga, 2009) (Millar-Craig, 1978). The night-time period, when there is an increase in IOP perfusion of the optic nerve head, may be a particularly vulnerable time for decreases in blood pressure. While the vast majority of the overall population shows a physiological decrease in blood pressure of less than 10%, there are a number of patients who have a decrease of over 20%. These patients are known as big dippers and are considered to be at a higher risk of developing cardiac ischaemia and silent brain damage (Pierdomenico, 1998). These patients may also have an increased risk for glaucoma due to ocular hypoperfusion and ischaemia-reperfusion damage.

Interestingly, deeper glaucomatous visual field defects are associated with a decreased arteriovenous difference in retinal oxygen saturation, possibly indicating decreased oxygen delivery to the retina. These data suggest a change in oxygen metabolism in the glaucomatous retina, possibly related to tissue atrophy (Olafsdottir, 2010). Whether these changes are causes or effects of damage to the retinal ganglion cells is still under debate. IOP is not likely a clinically relevant factor in oxygen saturation, as large decreases in IOP, such as after trabeculectomy, have almost no effect on retinal vessel oxygen saturation (Hardarson, 2009).

A number of studies have shown that this vascular dysfunction and impairment in normal blood flow associated with glaucoma is not restricted to the eye. Indeed, there are also indications of slower flow in peripheral capillary beds (Gasser, 1991) and signs of microvascular encephalopathy, such as white matter lesions (Stroman, 1995). This association between ocular circulation and systemic cardiovascular disease has been extensively studied, with changes in retinal vessel diameters having been shown to predict risk for coronary heart disease, stroke and stroke mortality (Wong, 2001) (Wong, 2002). Pooled data from the Beaver Dam Eye Study and the Blue Mountains Eye Study also show that smaller arterial diameters and larger retinal venous diameters are associated with increased risk for stroke mortality (Wang, 2007). As glaucoma patients also have similar disturbances in retinal arterial diameter (Jonas, 1989), there is clear reasoning for associating glaucoma with cardiovascular dysfunction.

One of the most striking disturbances of clinical importance happening in the ocular vessels is the splinter optic disk haemorrhage, a clinical feature that has been associated with glaucoma progression. These haemorrhages more frequently occur in patients with normotensional glaucoma and are strongly associated with altered circulation within the optic disc (Drance, 1977) (Bengtsson, 1990). Some authors have suggested that these splinter haemorrhages represent distressed small venules (Soares, 2004), as these thinner veins may reflect earlier lamina cribosa changes than their thicker arterial counterparts (Jonas, 2003). Data have indicated that an increased central vein pressure is associated with progressing glaucomatous damage (Balaratnasingam C., 2007), predicts optic disc excavation (Morgan, 2009) and is correlated with visual field defects (Morgan, 2005). This association between glaucoma and increased venous pressure and decreased pulse can help explain why glaucoma is a risk factor for central vein occlusion.

The changes in OBF are not restricted to the retinal vessels, as changes of clinical significance have also been found in the retrobulbar circulation. A number of CDI studies have found reduced peak systolic and diastolic velocities and increased resistivity indices in the retrobulbar vessels of glaucoma patients compared with healthy normal controls (Galassi, 1992), (Trible, 1994) (Harris A, 1994) (Michelson, 1995) (Kaiser, 1997). Interestingly, patients that progress seem to have a more important alteration in blood flow, namely, reduced PSV and EDV in short posterior ciliary arteries (Zeitz O, 2006). Moreover, a prospective study showed that within individuals, the eye with the more pronounced blood flow impairment also showed a faster progression (Drance, 1995). By helping determine patterns associated with a worst disease prognosis, CDI studies may be important in identifying glaucoma patients that are at greater risk for progression.

Other fundoscopic imaging techniques, such as fluorescein angiography, also provide data that are consistent with the CDI data. In normotensional glaucoma patients, for example, filling defects were correlated with lower EDV and increased RI of the short posterior ciliary arteries and with lower blood flow velocities of the central retinal arteries (Plange, 2003). Other imaging techniques have also been consistent in documenting these OBF disturbances in normotensional glaucoma patients. Laser Doppler flowmetry showed a decrease in retinal and optic nerve flow in glaucoma patients (Kerr, 1997) (Grunwald, 1998). Furthermore, measurements of pulsatile OBF showed it to be significantly lower in normotensional glaucoma eyes with or without field-loss than in normal subjects (Fontana, 1998). OPA, the alternative to study the pulsatile component of OBF, is reduced in both primary open angle and normotensional glaucoma patients (Schwenn O., 2002) (Stalmans I., 2008). Moreover, lower OPA values are associated with more advanced visual fields defects (Vulsteke C., 2008). OPA is positively correlated with IOP and negatively correlated with axial length. Its relationship with other blood flow-related parameters is still under discussion. In an initial study, blood pressure was found to be correlated with OPA (Pourjavan, 2007). Subsequent studies could not confirm an impact of blood pressure on OPA (Grieshaber MC., 2009) and found no correlation with the blood pressure amplitude itself (Choi J., 2010). However, there have been case reports of OPA being increased in patients with aortic insufficiency (McKee HD., 2004) and decreased in patients with carotid stenosis (Perkins, 1985). Further reports about increases in OPA after correcting upstream arterial stenosis (Kaufmann C., 2002) give support to the intuitive notion that blood pressure might yet be important. Of note, the studies that have ruled out a relationship between blood pressure and OPA were either performed in young healthy volunteers (Grieshaber MC., 2009) or in glaucoma patients with normal arterial blood pressure (Choi J., 2010).

Recently, it has been proposed that OPA can be related to blood pressure amplitude, specifically in glaucoma patients with arterial hypertension (Pinto, 2010). As mentioned above, choroidal blood flow may be capable of autoregulation (Schmidt KG., 1998). However, such mechanisms may be insufficient to maintain normal blood flow at both high and low extremes. This may result in the transmission of an abnormally high arterial pulse pressure to the choroidal vascular bed, leading to an increased OPA. Furthermore, as the choroid is supplied by the short posterior ciliary arteries, one could expect OPA to reflect changes in those arteries. A CDI study has shown a positive correlation between OPA and the RI in the short posterior ciliary arteries (and ophthalmic and central retinal arteries) in non-glaucomatous subjects. However, no correlation could be found in patients with primary open-angle or normotensional glaucoma, again suggesting a vascular dysregulation in glaucoma patients (Stalmans I., 2009). However, the mechanisms involved in such dysregulation in glaucoma are not yet completely understood.

Although the totality of these observations provides a strong indication for blood flow disturbances to be related to glaucoma, many uncertainties remain. One of the questions that remain to be answered is whether the decreased blood flow is actually involved in the aetiology of glaucoma or whether it is secondary to a loss of retinal ganglion cells and a decrease in the corresponding metabolic demand for oxygen and nutrients. There are indications that the reduction in OBF precedes the glaucomatous damage (Costa, 1994) (Kaiser, 1997), which contradicts the objection that the observed OBF impairment might be solely secondary to tissue atrophy.

The extent of the damage induced by OBF alone is difficult to determine. OBF changes *per se* might lead to glaucoma damage, but they could also synergistically act with other risk factors. For example, OBF disturbances might act as a sensitiser to IOP, making it possible for normal-range values of IOP to produce damage. Finally, while these vascular disturbances exist and are associated with (particularly progressive) glaucoma, there is still very little evidence that improving blood flow in glaucoma patients might change the course of their disease.

## 5. Clinical approach

When assessing possible vascular issues in glaucoma patients, it may be useful to consider the following two aspects: 1. systemic conditions that are associated with an overall vascular dysfunction and 2. external influences from lifestyle, diet or current medication that may negatively affect the patient's OBF.

### 5.1 A sick eye in a sick body

As referred to by Flammer, glaucoma may well be an ocular disease that is part of a wider systemic condition (Pache, 2006). As such, the ophthalmologist may inquire for signs of vascular dysfunction that have been associated with glaucoma, namely, peripheral vasospasm, Raynaud phenomenon and migraine. Other cardiovascular conditions, like blood pressure fluctuations, irregular heart rate and vascular resistance or obstruction, might influence OBF and are thus worth attention.

Blood pressure, for instance, has been extensively studied with regard to its impact on glaucoma. Changes in ocular perfusion pressure are well established as a risk factor for glaucoma progression (see above). On the one hand, high values of blood pressure can be deleterious to the retina and optic nerve (Caprioli, 2010). As it can be associated with an increase in overall mortality, blood pressure should remain below the 140/90 threshold or below 125/75 in a diabetic patient with microproteinuria (Chobanian, 2003). On the other hand, blood pressure values are subject to change during the 24-hour period. The combination of the otherwise physiological decrease in blood pressure during the night and the otherwise normal nocturnal increase in IOP can lead to a severe decrease in ocular perfusion pressure (Leske, 2002). The magnitude of this blood pressure nocturnal dip in glaucoma patients correlates with visual field progression, as greater nocturnal dips were associated with progressive visual field defects (Graham, 1999). Idiopathic blood pressure dippers exist, especially in patients with signs of autonomic dysfunction. Importantly, iatrogenic-induced blood pressure dipping due to over-medication for arterial hypertension should also be kept in mind as a possible cause of unexplained visual field progression despite good IOP control. Additionally, the quality of sleep can alter an individual's blood pressure dip status (Sei, 1999). Obstructive sleep apnoea syndrome, characterised by snoring, excessive daytime sleepiness, and insomnia, has been proposed as a glaucoma risk factor (Walsh, 1982). The incidence of glaucoma in patients with sleep apnoea syndrome has been described to range from 7.2 to up to 50% (Mojon, 1999) (Onen SH, 2000), with the latter figure likely corresponding to normotensional glaucoma patients (Mojon, 2002). Obstructive sleep apnea syndrome, which is due to intermittent collapse of the upper airway, leads to insufficient tissue oxygenation. Concomitantly, the produced negative intra-thoracic pressure leads to reflex activation of the adrenergic system with increased peripheral resistance (Gherghel, 2004). These combined actions may aggravate an underlying endothelial dysfunction and impair autoregulation by the vessels supplying blood to the eye (Dean, 1993). Data connecting sleep apnoea with glaucoma, especially normotensional glaucoma, is mounting, with authors claiming a correlation between sleep apnoea and a decrease in the retinal nerve fibre layer (Kargi, 2005) and with an increase in both perimetric mean defect and resistance index of the central retinal artery (Karakucuk, 2008).

Blood pressure dipping has been addressed in some patients by prescribing fludrocortisone (Gugleta, 1999) or salt tablets (Pechère-Betschi, 1998) as intra-vascular volume expanders. Fludrocortisone treatment in glaucoma patients may not only slightly increase blood pressure and reduce nocturnal dips but also improve the regulation of blood flow indirectly (Gugleta, 1999). Patients with sleep apnoea should be counselled towards weight loss and avoidance of alcohol and sedatives. Mechanical measures, including continuous or bilevel positive airway pressure devices, may also be used.

One of the clinical signs for the vascular impact of glaucoma is the presence of vasospasm. Not to be mistaken for Raynaud syndrome, patients with symptoms of cold hands, sometimes cold feet and a tendency towards low blood pressure should be investigated as whether they have primary vasodysregulation syndrome (Flammer, 2001). The vasospastic prototype patient has a low body mass index, is frequently intellectual and is a (pre-menopausal) female (Prunte-Glowazki, 1991) (Harada, 1991) (Flammer, 2006). They have different sensitivities to medications, such as beta blockers or calcium channel blockers. In such patients, the desired pharmacological effect may be achieved by a lower dosage of such drugs (Flammer, 2001). Patients presenting with this inborn dysfunction of vascular endothelium have inappropriate constriction or insufficient dilatation in the microcirculation (Flammer, 1996). This leads to ischaemia-reperfusion damage (see above) in what seems to be an endothelin-related phenomenon (Flammer J., 1999). Being a systemic condition, these patients are prone to ischaemia in other organs, not just the eye. The heart or the inner ear, for example, are likely to show signs of vascular dysfunction-related events, such as silent cardiac ischaemia (Waldmann, 1996) and benign positional vertigo (Ishiyama, 2000), respectively. Diagnostic procedures have been developed, including nailfold capillaromicroscopy combined with a cold provocation test (Gasser, 1990) or measuring serum endothelin-1 (Miyauchi, 1999). The syndrome is mostly harmless. However, if the patient has symptoms or if the optic nerve head turns pale or even starts to excavate, a clinical evaluation is warranted (Flammer, 2001).

Treatment for vasospasticity in glaucoma patients has tried to establish a safe way to prevent or reverse endothelin-induced vasoconstriction. Antivasospastic treatment with calcium channel blockers in glaucoma patients seems to be helpful, although its usefulness has not yet been firmly established (Yamamoto, 1998) (Tomita, 1999). Short-term studies indicate that calcium channel blockers diminish the effect of increased levels of endothelin-1 on ocular perfusion (Strenn, 1998) and improve visual field defects (Gasser, 1990) (Gaspar, 1994). The same effect can be achieved by $CO_2$ inhalation, suggesting that the visual function improvements are in fact due to vasodilation (Niwa, 2000).

The blood-brain barrier prevents exposure of the brain to endothelin. Accordingly, brain-located vascular spasms are only slightly correlated with primary vasodysregulation. Nevertheless, migraine is also associated with vascular reactivity. This disease has been consistently pointed out as a risk factor for glaucoma. This evidence is mostly confined to normotensional glaucoma patients because cross-sectional population-based prevalence studies have generally found no significant association between migraine and glaucoma. Nevertheless, migraine was identified as an independent risk factor for progression in the Collaborative Normal-Tension Glaucoma Study (Drance, 2001). Migraine treatment is not only related to pain control but also to the use of vasoactive substances. Prophylaxis of migraine attacks can be achieved by the administration of beta-blockers, which act via a mechanism thought to down regulate the serotonergic and beta-receptor activity involved in initiating the attacks (Evers, 2006). Acute migraine treatment, however, involves drugs with powerful vasoconstrictive activity, such as ergot derivates and triptans (Silberstein, 2000). Although they produce preferential vasoconstriction of intracranial extracerebral blood vessels due to serotonin receptor binding activity, some have important peripheral activity and are formally contraindicated in patients with Raynaud phenomenon, for instance (Tfelt-Hansen P, 2000). Although there is not enough evidence to draw conclusions on its impact on ONH blood flow, the fact that serotonergic activity may play a significant role in modulating OBF should raise awareness of a possible hypoperfusion of the ONH.

Age is a known risk factor for developing glaucoma. As such, it has also been studied whether age has an impact on OBF. In healthy individuals, CDI showed a decrease in blood flow parameters in both the ophthalmic and central retinal arteries correlating with increasing age (Williamson, 1995) (Lam, 2003). The resistance index of the vessels seems to increase with age, as a possible sign of increased arterial stiffness (Groh, 1996). Different devices have also identified choroidal and optic nerve head blood flow decreases (Ravalico, 1996) (Boehm, 2005). These changes do not seem to stem from a decreased metabolic demand by retina neural cells, as there seems to be no significant correlation between perfusion parameters as measured by scanning laser Doppler flowmetry and retinal nerve fibre layer thickness (Kuba, 2001). However, gender may play a role in age-related changes in OBF, as short posterior ciliary arteries in males is less affected than that in females, with significant differences at EDV and RI levels (Harris, 2000). The Collaborative Normal-Tension Glaucoma trial showed that women were at risk of increased progression (odds ratio: 1.85) after correction for age and IOP (Drance, 2001). Age-related changes are of

particular importance in women, where menopause-induced changes in oestrogen levels induce a number of changes at the cardiovascular level, such as increasing blood pressure and heart rate. At the ocular level, there seems to be an increase in IOP in post-menopausal women but no significant changes in OBF (Siesky, 2000).
Finally, concerns over the optic nerve's OBF must also take into account what can happen upstream of the ophthalmic artery, namely, in the blood flow passing through the carotid artery. Even in unilateral carotid stenosis, there have been reports of bilateral decrease in OBF. Such changes would rely on a patent circle of Willis that would balance blood flow between the two carotid arteries, resulting in a reduced OBF in both eyes (Quaranta, 1997). In patients presenting with unilateral stenosis above 70%, endarterectomy improved PSV in all retrobulbar vessels of the operated side and the PSV in ophthalmic artery and short posterior ciliary arteries of the fellow eye. The perimetric median defect also bilaterally improved, thus supporting the above hypothesis of OBF in one eye influencing the fellow eye (Kozobolis, 2007).

### 5.2 Systemic medications and other measures

The ophthalmologist should be aware of the complete medical history and treatment of his glaucoma patients, as many systemic medications may have an impact on OBF. Systemic modulators of the cardiovascular responses, such as patient lifestyle or dietary habits, should also be considered.
Anti-hypertensive medications are particularly important because they can change perfusion pressure directly. Calcium channel blockers are one of the most well-studied groups of anti-hypertensive medications. Because they prevent smooth muscle contraction, they are vasodilators that reduce peripheral resistance (Braunwald, 1982). They have been used in glaucoma patients with primary vasodysregulation, where they have shown improvement not only in OBF (Schmidt, 1996) but also in visual field indices (Flammer, 1987). The widespread use of calcium channel blockers has been controversial because of the severe nocturnal hypotension they can induce. Such a hypotensive profile can have severe implications on ocular perfusion pressure. However, the impact on OBF does not seem to be a class effect. Generally speaking, centrally acting calcium channel blockers, such as nimodipine, appear to increase OBF, whereas peripheral agents, such as nifedipine, do not (Lesk, 2008). Magnesium, known as "nature's physiological calcium blocker" (Iseri, 1984), has also been studied regarding its impact on OBF. A small, non-randomised study has shown a statistically significant improvement in peripheral blood flow and a tendency to improve visual field scores in glaucoma patients (Gaspar, 1995). Other hypotensive medications, such as angiotensin-converting enzyme inhibitors or angiotensin receptor antagonists, have also been studied. Both trandolapril, (an angiotensin-converting enzyme inhibitor) (Steigerwalt, 1998), and losartan, (an angiotensin receptor antagonist)(Matulla, 1997), slightly improved OBF in healthy individuals.
Anti-platelet medications and statins are among the most widely prescribed cardiovascular drugs. As both of them have positive impacts on ischaemia-reperfusion damage and oxidative stress, researchers have tried to determine their impact, if any, on OBF and glaucoma. Dypiradamole, a known anti-platelet drug, acts by increasing the levels of adenosine and cyclic adenosine monophosphate. Both metabolites have vasoactive properties that increase coronary vasodilation (Alonso, 1967). In glaucoma patients and anterior ischemic optic neuropathy patients, dypiridamole induced increases in PSV and

EDV in the retrobulbar vessels (Kaiser, 1996). Other more common anti-platelet drugs, such as aspirin, may also have a role in glaucoma. Aspirin may stabilise OBF by decreasing platelet aggregation (Bell, 2004). It may have a neuroprotective role in glutamate-related apoptosis (Ritch, 2000) and may improve the efficiency of prostaglandin analogues in IOP lowering by up-regulating prostaglandin F receptors (Hardy, 1998). No studies, however, have proven these hypothesis. Statins, in contrast, have been the focus of many researchers in OBF. They are the mainstay treatment for hypercholesterolaemia, but thanks to their pleiotropic properties, their vasoactive effects extend beyond their cholesterol-lowering ability. They reduce the incidence of cerebrovascular and cardiovascular events, independently of a patient's blood cholesterol level at baseline (Everett, 2010) (Stroke Prevention by Aggressive Reduction in Cholesterol Levels (SPARCL), 2006). Statins upregulate endothelial nitric oxide synthase and possess antioxidant properties that may ameliorate ischemic oxidative stresses in the brain (Vaughan, 1999) (Cimino, 2007). This vascular endothelial protective effect may have an effect in OBF because statins have been shown to increase the retinal vasculature calibre (Nagaoka, 2006). One may postulate that this dilatation may affect the ONH vasculature as well. Although no study has yet tested for ONH blood flow improvements, a prospective study showed that simvastatin use may be associated with visual field defect stabilisation in patients with normotensional glaucoma (Leung, 2010).

While much controversy exists over the cardiovascular benefits for hormone-replacement therapy, it does not seem to significantly change ONH blood flow. While apparently reducing vascular resistance distal to the ophthalmic artery to levels matching those of younger women, oestrogen replacement has little impact on flow velocities in the short posterior ciliary arteries (Harris-Yitzhak, 2000). While oestrogen alone may not significantly change the risk of developing glaucoma, oestrogen-progestin hormone replacement therapy may be associated with a reduced risk of primary open-angle glaucoma (Pasquale, 2007).

Everyday life activities, food habits and other systemic medications may also affect OBF. Coffee, for example, has been studied regarding its impact on glaucoma and ocular circulation. Caffeine is a xanthine with known cardiovascular effects, such as increasing heart rate and increasing peripheral resistance by vasoconstriction (Bunker, 1979). A placebo-controlled trial in healthy individuals showed that the resistance index of ophthalmic; short posterior ciliary arteries and central retinal arteries were significantly increased after coffee ingestion (Ozkan, 2008). Despite its concomitant ability to mildly increasing IOP, a prospective study did not find an increased risk for primary open-angle glaucoma in average coffee drinkers (people consuming more than 5 cups a day had a small risk increase) (Kang, 2008). Alcohol, however, is associated with a mild IOP-lowering property while having known neurotoxicity. Its impact on glaucoma is not completely understood, but a link between alcohol consumption and glaucoma has not been found (Kang, 2007). Other dietary habits have also been studied in glaucoma. Diets favouring omega-3 fatty acids, such as soy oils, instead of omega-6 fatty acids, such as corn or sunflower oils, have been associated with an increased risk for glaucoma (Kang, 2004). Considering its OBF-related effects, fish oil (rich in omega-6) improves circulation in patients with Raynaud's phenomenon (DiGiacomo, 1989) by inhibiting the endothelin-1 effect (Nitta, 1998). A number of dietary anti-oxidative agents, such as ginkgo biloba (Ritch, 2000), might also improve OBF. A single, small study in normotensional glaucoma patients has suggested an improvement in visual field damage while on ginkgo (Quaranta, 2003). Vitamin E supplements, despite improving vasospastic angina by decreasing oxidative stress, have a still unknown impact on glaucoma (Motoyama, 1998). Nevertheless, the enthusiasm over such therapies must be balanced with the risks of overconsumption because high dosages are known to increase all-cause mortality (Miller, 2005). Another lifestyle activity is cigarette smoking. A meta-analysis has shown a significant increase in the risk of developing glaucoma in smokers (Bonovas, 2004). Smokers show a markedly reduced ability of retinal vessels and the choroid to adapt to stimuli, such as light exposure or a carbogen breathing environment, when compared with a non-smoker population (Havelius, 2005) (Wimpissinger, 2004). Physical fitness and cardiovascular health status probably also impact glaucoma. People who do regular exercise have lower baseline IOPs. However, upon the cessation of exercise, values return to pretraining levels within 1 month. In healthy subjects, moderate exercise has been known to increase endothelial shear stress, which improves nitric oxide release and therefore has a positive impact on blood flow, for instance, in the coronary arteries (Niebauer, 1996). OBF seems to be unchanged during exercise due to vascular autoregulation. This autoregulation fails at ocular perfusion pressures greater than 70% above baseline. Summarising, at this time, the consensus recommendations are that regular exercise is most likely beneficial in glaucoma patients and should be encouraged (Risner, 2009).

## 6. Ophthalmological therapies

Ophthalmologists today have a greater arsenal of drugs with IOP-lowering effects than ever before. The IOP-lowering effect of each medication is beyond the scope of this vascular approach to glaucoma and can be found elsewhere, particularly in the European Glaucoma Society guidelines (European Glaucoma Society, 2008). We shall therefore focus instead on what is currently known about their non-IOP-related vascular impact on OBF.

Carbonic anhydrase inhibitors act by specifically inhibiting the carbonic anhydrase-II isoform, which is concentrated in the ciliary body. This enzyme is responsible for producing bicarbonate, an important part of the aqueous humour, from the hydration of $CO_2$. This carbonic anhydrase blockade thus leads not only to a decrease of aqueous humour production but also to an increase in $CO_2$ and a lower tissue pH. In vessels with autoregulatory mechanisms, these last two changes can lead to vasodilation. Carbonic anhydrase inhibitors have been found to increase OBF when compared with other treatments with similar IOP reduction. A recent meta-analysis concluded that patients receiving topical carbonic anhydrase inhibitor treatment had a higher PSV and EDV in the central retinal and short posterior ciliary arteries, while their calculated vascular RI was reduced (Siesky, 2009). Increased blood flow velocities in both nasal and temporal short posterior ciliary arteries may improve blood flow in the ONH and possibly even the high-flow, low-resistance choroidal circulation. No statistically significant effects were seen in the ophthalmic artery. This improvement in blood flow has also been reported in retinal arteries, with dorzolamide accelerating the arteriovenous passage of fluorescein dye when compared with a beta-blocker (Harris, 2000). Topical carbonic anhydrase inhibitors may also play a role in retinal oxygenation because withdrawal of the drug leads to a decrease in arterial and venous saturation (Traustason, 2009). However, this class of drug is mostly used in association with other drugs, namely, beta-blockers. Studies comparing therapies combining beta-blockers with either carbonic anhydrase inhibitors or prostaglandins have shown that despite a similar lowering in IOP, patients taking carbonic anhydrase inhibitors/beta-blockers had a smaller RI in the retrobulbar vasculature (Siesky, 2006) (Januleviciene, 2009).

Systemic carbonic anhydrase inhibitors, such as acetazolamide, are not carbonic anhydrase-II specific and block both isoforms II and IV. Their ability to change vascular parameters is not only widely known but is clinically used in provocative tests to study cerebrovascular vasomotor reactivity. The cerebral vasodilatory effects of systemic carbonic anhydrase inhibitors are therefore well established and often utilised to test for vasodilative reserve potential. Unlike its topical counterparts, acetazolamide has also been reported to affect ophthalmic artery, decreasing RI (Dallinger, 1998). No additional effect seems to exist by combining both topical and systemic carbonic anhydrase inhibitors. Interestingly, a recent basic research study has offered a new perspective on the use of carbonic anhidrase inhibitors in glaucoma. As previously stated, the mechanisms behind glaucoma may be related to vascular endothelial dysfunction and impairment of nitric oxide activity (see above). Carbonic anhydrase inhibition by dorzolamide and acetazolamide may increase the affinity of the carbonic anhydrase for another substrate besides bicarbonate, namely, nitrite, in a reaction that produces nitric oxide. This IOP-independent activity would not only decrease reactive oxygen species activity by consuming nitrite but probably replenish nitric oxide, allowing for better endothelial function (Aamand, 2009). No multicentre, randomised study has reached a conclusion about the impact of these changes on glaucoma progression.

Beta-blockers are among the most prescribed IOP-lowering therapies. They reduce IOP by decreasing aqueous humour production by approximately 30–50%. The exact mechanism involved in this inhibition is unknown, although the β2 receptors in the non-pigmented ciliary body epithelium are the most likely target. However, the beta-blockers clinically in use are not a uniform group, ranging from non-selective beta-blockers (timolol) to β1-selective blockers (betaxolol) to non-selective beta-blockers with intrinsic sympathetic activity (carteolol). Because the non-selective beta-blockers could be associated with a vasoconstrictive effect, this impact on OBF has been extensively studied. A review on this potential effect concluded that neither primary open-angle nor normotensional glaucoma patients had a deleterious response to beta-blockers therapy in retinal, choroidal or retrobulbar vascular beds (Costa, 2003). Few reports have focused on the impact of carteolol on blood flow. Its intrinsic sympathetic activity would theoretically prevent the negative impact of blocking vasodilation-related β2 receptors. A small study comparing timolol with carteolol, in which the IOP lowering was not significantly different, showed that the RI of the short posterior ciliary arteries was significantly lower in the carteolol group (Montanari, 2001). Interestingly, a recent review has shown that the β1-selective blocker betaxolol has been associated with greater preservation of visual field defects when compared with other beta-blockers despite a smaller IOP reduction (Grieshaber, 2010). It also seems to have a different effect on OBF. When compared with other non-selective beta-blockers, it has been shown to reduce the RI of the ophthalmic artery while increasing both central retinal artery RI and diameter (Evans, 1999) (Collignon, 1997). One hypothesis about this probable non-IOP-related impact on visual field preservation is a positive impact on OBF because betaxolol has been demonstrated to have a calcium channel blocking activity (Grieshaber, 2010).

Prostaglandin analogues are a powerful tool in IOP-lowering therapy. Their activity on prostaglandin F receptors leads to an overall increase in the uveoscleral outflow of aqueous humour. As one of the most effective IOP-lowering agents, these drugs can improve ocular perfusion pressure by significantly decreasing IOP. Their direct impact on OBF in an IOP-independent manner is still controversial. As such, the majority of available data has shown a neutral effect on OBF by prostaglandin analogues therapy administration (Nicolela, 1996)

(Liu, 2002). However, there are some reports claiming that patients under prostaglandin analogues have an improvement in OBF, specifically at the level of the ONH (Ishii, 2001). Endothelin-1-induced vasoconstriction was successfully prevented *in vivo* by PA, most likely by blocking ET-1-induced capacitative calcium entry (Kurashima, 2010).

Of the alpha-2 agonists used in clinical practice, the only one with relevance for chronic IOP-lowering treatment in glaucoma is brimonidine. This drug is a potent alpha-adrenoceptor agonist that is 1000-fold more selective for the alpha-2 *versus* the alpha-1 adrenoceptor. Other than the IOP-lowering effect, this drug has been touted as having a potential in neuroprotection (Krupin, 2011). This first prospective clinical trial demonstrated that normotensional glaucoma patients showed a slower progression rate when treated with brimonidine when compared with their beta-blocker-treated, IOP-adjusted counterparts. This neuroprotective effect is, however, not likely related to changes in OBF. Despite its theoretic vasocontrictive properties, there seems to be no strong evidence on modulation, positive or negative, of OBF in either the retinal, or ONH vascular territories (Costa, 2003). It may, however, lead to decreased flow and increased resistance in the choroidal compartment, but further studies are warranted (Weigert, 2007).

Pilocarpine is a parasympathomimetic drug that stimulates the ciliary muscle contraction, which results in traction of the scleral spur, altering the configuration of the trabecular meshwork and leading to enhanced outflow and therefore reduced IOP. Its limited use in the clinical management of open angle glaucoma has also limited its study on the impact of OBF. The only study in glaucoma patients revealed no IOP-independent impact on blood flow (Claridge, 1993).

Glaucoma surgery has also been studied for OBF changes. Existing data on the subject is not only scarce but also conflicting. While some authors have described a neutral effect in retrobulbar and retinal artery flow velocities by trabeculectomy (Breusegem, 2010) (Cantor, 2001), others have found increases in OBF (Berisha, 2005) (Trible, 1994). Different measuring techniques and different experimental designs have precluded definitive conclusions as to whether surgery can significantly improve OBF. To the best of our knowledge, no study so far has focused on OBF and glaucoma laser therapy.

## 7. Future research

Glaucoma specialists still debate the mechanisms that initiate and perpetuate optic neuropathy. The growing evidence for a background vascular dysfunction in primary open angle glaucoma is transforming the clinical approach to these patients. However, and despite the recognition of disturbances in OBF, little is known about the impact of correcting such imbalances. A question still remains as to whether these OBF changes represent the cause or rather the end result of impaired neuron metabolism. Studies so far have not been able to answer these complex issues. There are still no available population-based studies on OBF and no randomised, multi-centre studies on long-term follow-up. Current data is nevertheless encouraging, with reports claiming that improving OBF might slow disease progression. Advances in the tools to study OBF, such as magnetic resonance imaging, or a more widespread clinical use of already existing devices, such as Doppler OCT, will most likely allow for a more thorough analysis of the ocular vascular system. Importantly, efforts to increase the standardisation of procedures and methodology in OBF research centres worldwide might lead to a more effective and rational use of currently available data. The Association for Ocular Circulation (http://www.obfra.org) is currently addressing this problem by outlining consensus reports on the subject.

## 8. References


Aamand, R., Dalsgaard, T., Jensen, FB., Simonsen, U., Roepstorff, A. & Fago, A. 2009. Generation of nitric oxide from nitrite by carbonic anhydrase: a possible link between metabolic activity and vasodilation. *Am J Physiol Heart Circ Physiol.* 2009, Vol. 297, pp. 2068-74.

Alonso, S. & O'Brian, GS. 1967. Enhancement of the coronary vasodilator action of adenosine tri-phosphate by dipyridamole. *Circ Res.* 1967, Vol. 20, pp. 403–408.

Appenzeller, O. & Orbie, E. 1997. *The Autonomic Nervous System: An introduction to basic and clinical concepts.* Amsterdam, The Netherlands : Elsevier Science, 1997. ISBN 0444825460.

Aslan, M., Freeman, BA. 2007. Redox-dependent impairment of vascular function in sickle cell disease. *Free Radic. Biol. Med.* 2007, Vol. 43, pp. 1469–1483.

Ates, H., Uretmen, O., Temiz, A. & Andac, K. 1998. Erythrocyte deformability in high-tension and normal tension glaucoma. *Int Ophthalmol.* 1998, Vol. 22, pp. 7–12.

Bagga H., Liu JH. & Weinreb RN. 2009. Intraocular pressure measurements throughout the 24 h. *Curr Opin Ophthalmol.* 2009, Vol. 20(2), pp. 79-83.

Balaratnasingam C., Morgan WH., Hazelton ML., House PH., Barry CJ., Chan H., Cringle SJ. & Yu DY. 2007. Value of retinal vein pulsation characteristics in predicting increased optic disc excavation. *Br J Ophthalmol.* 2007, Vol. 91, pp. 441-4.

Beckman, JS., Beckman, TW., Chen, J., Marshall, PA. & Freeman, BA. 1990. Apparent hydroxyl radical production by peroxynitrite: implications for endothelial injury from nitric oxide and superoxide. *Proc. Natl. Acad. Sci.* 1990, Vol. 87, pp. 1620–1624.

Bell, NP., Orengo-Nania, S., Pietz, K. & Gross, RL. 2004. Aspirin use in advanced uncontrolled glaucoma. *J Glaucoma.* 2004, Vol. 13, pp. 365–70.

Bengtsson, B. 1990. Optic disc haemorrhages preceding manifest glaucoma. *Acta Ophthalmol.* 1990, Vol. 68, pp. 450–454.

Berisha, F., Schmetterer, K., Vass, C., Dallinger, S., Rainer, G., Findl, O., Kiss, B. & Schmetterer, L. 2005. Effect of trabeculectomy on ocular blood flow. *Br J Ophthalmol.* 2005, Vol. 89, pp. 185-8.

Boehm, AG., Koeller, AU. & Pillunat, LE. 2005. The Effect of Age on Optic Nerve Head Blood Flow. *Invest Ophthalmol Vis Sci.* 2005, Vol. 46, pp. 1291–1295.

Bojic, L. & Skare-Librenjak, L. 1998. Circulating platelet aggregates in glaucoma. *Int. Ophthalmol.* 1998, Vol. 22, pp. 151–154.

Bonovas, S., Filioussi, K., Tsantes, A. & Peponis, V. 2004. Epidemiological association between cigarette smoking and primary open-angle glaucoma: a meta-analysis. *Public Health.* 2004, Vol. 118, pp. 256-61.

Braunwald, E. 1982. Mechanisms of action of calcium channel blocking agents. *N. Engl. J. Med.* 1982, Vol. 307, pp. 1618–1627.

Breusegem, C., Fieuws, S., Zeyen, T. & Stalmans, I. 2010. The effect of trabeculectomy on ocular pulse amplitude. *Invest Ophthalmol Vis Sci.* 2010, Vol. 51, pp. 231-5.

Bunker, ML. & McWilliams, M. 1979. Caffeine content of common beverages. *J Am Diet Assoc.* 1979, Vol. 74, pp. 28–32.

Cantor, LB. 2001. The effect of trabeculectomy on ocular hemodynamics. *Trans Am Ophthalmol Soc.* 2001, Vol. 99, pp. 241-52.

Caprioli, J., Coleman, AL., Blood Flow in Glaucoma Discussion Group. 2010. Blood Pressure, Perfusion Pressure, and Glaucoma. *Am J Ophthalmol.* 2010, Vol. 149, pp. 704–712.

Carter, CJ., Brooks, DE., Doyle, DL. & Drance, SM. 1990. Investigations into a vascular etiology for low-tension glaucoma. *Ophthalmology.* 1990, Vol. 97, pp. 49-55.

Chobanian, AV., Bakris, GL., Black, HR., Cushman, WC., Green, LA., Izzo, JL., Jones, DW., Materson, BJ., Oparil, S., Wright, JT., Rocella, EJ., JNC. 2003. The Seventh Report of the Joint National Committee on Prevention, Detection, Evaluation and Treatment of High Blood Pressure: the JNC7 report. *JAMA.* 2003, Vol. 289, pp. 2560-72.

Choi J., Lee J., Park SB., Lee KS., Sung KR. & Kook MS. 2010. Factors affecting ocular pulse amplitude in eyes with open angle glaucoma and glaucoma suspect eyes. *Acta Ophthalmol.* 2010, Vols. doi: 10.1111/j.1755-3768.2010.01954.x.

Cholesterol Treatment Trialists' (CTT), Collaborators. 2005. Efficacy and safety of cholesterol-lowering treatment: prospective metaanalysis of data from 90,056 participants in 14 randomized trials of statins. *Lancet.* 2005, Vol. 366, pp. 1267–78.

Cimino, M., Gelosa, P., Gianella, A., Nobili, E., Tremoli, E. & Sironi, L. 2007. Statins: multiple mechanisms of action in the ischemic brain. *Neuroscientist.* 2007, Vol. 13, pp. 208-13.

Claridge, KG. 1993. The effect of topical pilocarpine on pulsatile ocular blood flow. *Eye.* 1993, Vol. 7, pp. 507–510.

Collignon, NJ. & Collignon-Brach, JD. 1997. Effect of topical betablockers on human retinal vessels diameters. *Int Ophthalmol.* 1997, Vol. 21, pp. 199-203.

Costa, VP., Sergott, RC., Spaeth, GL., Moster, MR., Katz, LJ., Schmidt, CM., Wilson, RP. & Smith, M. 1994. Color Doppler imaging in glaucoma patients with asymmetric cups. *J Glaucoma.* 1994, Vol. 3, pp. S91–97.

Costa, VP., Harris, A., Stefánsson, E., Flammer, J., Krieglstein, GK., Orzalesi, N., Heijl, A., Renard, JP. & Serra, LM. 2003. The effects of antiglaucoma and systemic medications on ocular blood flow. *Prog Retin Eye Res.* 2003, Vol. 22, pp. 769-805.

Curtis, BM. & O'Keefe, JH. 2002. Autonomic tone as a cardiovascular risk factor: the dangers of chronic fight or flight. *Mayo Clin Proc.* 2002, Vol. 77, pp. :45-54.

Dallinger, S., Bobr, B., Findl, O., Eichler, HG. & Schmetterer, L. 1998. Effects of acetazolamide on choroidal blood flow. *Stroke.* 1998, Vols. 997-1001, p. 29.

de Voogd, S., Wolfs, RC., Jansonius, NM., Witteman, JC., Hofman, A. & de Jong PT. 2006. Atherosclerosis, C-reactive protein, and risk for open-angle glaucoma: the Rotterdam study. *Invest Ophthalmol Vis Sci.* 2006, Vol. 47, pp. 3772-6.

Dean, RT. & Wilcox, I. 1993. Possible atherogenic effects of hypoxia during obstructive sleep apnea. *Sleep.* 1993, Vol. 16, pp. S15–21.

DiGiacomo, RA., Kremer, JM. & Shah, DM. 1989. Fishoil dietary supplementation in patients with Raynaud's phenomenon: a double-blind, controlled, prospective study. *Am J Medicine.* 1989, Vol. 86, pp. 158–164.

Drance, SM., Fairclough, M., Butler, DM. & Kottler, MS. 1977. The importance of disc hemorrhage in the prognosis of chronic open angle glaucoma. *Arch Ophthalmol.* 1977, Vol. 95, pp. 226–228.

Drance, SM. & Rojanapongpun, P. 1995. The ophthalmic artery velocity in open-angle glaucoma. [book auth.] Drance SM. *Update to Glaucoma, Ocular Blood Flow, and Drug Treatment.* New York, NY : Kugler Publications, 1995.

Drance, S., Anderson, DR., Schulzer, M., Collaborative Normal-Tension Glaucoma Study Group. 2001. Risk factors for progression of visual field abnormalities in normal-tension glaucoma. *Am J Ophthalmol.* 2001, Vol. 131, pp. 699-708.

European Glaucoma Society. 2008. *Terminology and guidelines for glaucoma, 3rd Edition.* Savona, Italy : Dogma, 2008. ISBN - 978-88-87434-28-6.

Evans, DW., Harris, A. & Cantor, LB. 1999. Primary open-angle glaucoma patients characterized by ocular vasospasm demonstrate a different ocular vascular response to timolol versus betaxolol. *J Ocul Pharmacol Ther.* 1999, Vol. 15, pp. 479-87.

Everett, BM., Glynn, RJ., MacFadyen, JG. & Ridker, PM. 2010. Rosuvastatin in the prevention of stroke among men and women with elevated levels of C-reactive protein: justification for the Use of Statins in Prevention: an Intervention Trial Evaluating Rosuvastatin (JUPITER). *Circulation.* 2010, Vol. 121, pp. 143-150.

Evers, S., Afra, J., Frese, A., Goadsby, PJ., Linde, M., May, A. & Sándor, PS. 2006. EFNS guideline on the drug treatment of migraine - report of an EFNS task force. *Eur J Neurol.* 2006, Vol. 13, pp. 560-72.

Flage, T. 1977. Permeability properties of the tissues in the optic nerve head region in the rabbit and the monkey. An ultrastructural study. *Acta Ophthalmol (Copenh).* 1977, Vol. 55, pp. 652-64.

Flammer, J. & Guthauser, U. 1987. Behandlung chorioidaler vasospasmen mit kalziumantagonisten. *Klin. Mbl. Augenheilk.* 1987, Vol. 190, pp. 299–300.

Flammer, J. 1996. *To what extent are vascular factors involved in the pathogenesis of glaucoma?* Basel : Karger, 1996.

Flammer J., Haefliger IO., Orgül S. & Resink T. 1999. Vascular dysregulation: a principal risk factor for glaucomatous damage? *J Glaucoma.* 1999, Vol. 8(3), pp. 212-9.

Flammer, J., Pache, M. & Resink, T. 2001. Vasospasm, its role in the pathogenesis of diseases with particular reference to the eye. *Prog Retin Eye Res.* 2001, Vol. 20, pp. 319-49.

Flammer, J., Orgul. S, Costa, VP., Orzalesic, N. & Krieglsteind, GK. 2002. The impact of ocular blood flow in glaucoma. *Progress in Retinal and Eye Research.* 2002, Vol. 21, pp. 359–393.

Flammer, J. 2006. *Glaucoma; A Guide for the Patient; An Introduction for Care-Providers; A Quick Reference.* 3. Gottingen, Germany, Bern : Hogrefe and Huber Publishers, 2006.

Fontana, L., Poinoosawmy, D., Bunce, CV., O'Brien, C. & Hitchings, R.A. 1998. Pulsatile ocular blood flow investigation in asymmetric normal tension glaucoma and normal subjects. *Br. J. Ophthalmol.* 1998, Vol. 82, pp. 731-736.

Galassi, F., Nuzzaci, G., Sodi, A., Casi, P. & Vielmo, A. 1992. Color Doppler imaging in evaluation of optic nerve blood supply in normal and glaucomatous subjects. *Int. Ophthalmol.* 1992, Vol. 16, pp. 273–276.

Gaspar, AZ., Flammer, J. & Hendrickson, P. 1994. Influence of nifedipine on the visual foelds of patients with optic nerve head diseases. *Eur. J. Ophthalmol.* 1994, Vol. 1, pp. 24-8.

Gaspar, AZ., Gasser, P. & Flammer, J. 1995. The influence of magnesium on visual field and peripheral vasospasm in glaucoma. *Ophthalmologica.* 1995, Vol. 209, pp. 11–13.

Gasser, P. & Flammer, J. 1990. Short- and long-term effect of nifedipine on the visual field in patients with presumed vasospasm. *J. Int. Med. Res.* 1990, Vol. 18, pp. 334–339.

Gasser, P. & Flammer, J. 1991. Blood-cell velocity in the nailfold capillaries of patients with normal-tension and hightension glaucoma. *Am J Ophthalmol.* 1991, Vol. 111, pp. 585--8.

Gherghel, D., Hosking, LS. & Orgul, S. 2004. Autonomic Nervous System, Circadian Rhythms, and Primary Open-Angle Glaucoma. *Surv Ophthalmol.* 2004, Vol. 49, pp. 491–508.

Gosling, Rg., Dunbar, G., King, DH., Newman, DL., Side, CD., Woodcock, JP., Fitzgerald, DE., Keates JS. & Macmillan, D. 1971. The Quantitative Analysis of Occlusive Peripheral Arterial Disease By a Non-Intrusive Ultrasonic Technique. *Angiology.* 1971, Vol. 22, pp. 52-55.

Graham, SL. & Drance, SM. 1999. Nocturnal hypotension: role in glaucoma progression. *Surv Ophthalmol.* 1999, Vol. 43, pp. S10–16.

Grieshaber, MC. & Flammer, J. 2007. Does the blood--brain barrier play a role in glaucoma? *Surv Ophthalmol.* 2007, Vol. 52, pp. S115-21.

Grieshaber MC., Katamay R., Gugleta K., Kochkorov A., Flammer J. & Orgul S. 2009. Relationship between ocular pulse amplitude and systemic blood pressure measurements. *Acta Ophthalmol.* 2009, Vol. 87, pp. 329–334.

Grieshaber, MC. & Flammer, J. 2010. Is the medication used to achieve the target intraocular pressure in glaucoma therapy of relevance? – An exemplary analysis on the basis of two beta-blockers. *Prog Retin Eye Res.* 2010, Vol. 29, pp. 79-93.

Groh, MJ., Michelson, G., Langhans, MJ. & Harazny, J. 1996. Influence of age on retinal and optic nerve head blood circulation. *Ophthalmology.* 1996, Vols. 529-34, pp. 529-34.

Grunwald, JE., Piltz, J., Hriprasad, SM. & DuPont, J. 1998. Optic nerve and choroidal circulation in glaucoma. *Investig. Ophthalmol. Vis. Sci.* 1998, Vol. 39, pp. 2329-2336.

Gugleta, K., Orgul, S., Stumpfig, D., Dubler, B. & Flammer, J. 1999. Fludrocortisone in the treatment of systemic hypotension in primary open-angle glaucoma patients. *Int Ophthalmol.* 1999, Vol. 23, pp. 25-30.

Hamard, P., Hamard, H., Dufaux, J. & Quesnot, S. 1994. Optic nerve head blood flow using a laser Doppler velocimeter and haemorheology in primary open angle glaucoma and normal pressure. *Br. J. Ophthalmol.* 1994, Vol. 78, pp. 449–453.

Hampton, JR., Harrison, AJ., Honour, AJ. & Mitchell, JR. 1967. Platelet behaviour and drugs used in cardiovascular disease. *Cardiovasc Res.* 1967, Vol. 1, pp. 1-6.

Harada, N., Ueda, A. & Takegata, S. 1991. Prevalence of Raynaud's phenomenon in Japanese males and females. *J Clin Epidemiol.* 1991, Vol. 44, pp. 649-55.

Hardarson, SH., Gottfredsdottir, MS., Halldorsson, GH., Karlsson, RA., Benediktsson, JA., Eysteinsson, T., Beach, JM., Harris, A. & Stefansson E. 2009. Glaucoma filtration surgery and retinal oxygen saturation. *Invest Ophthalmol Vis Sci.* 2009, Vol. 50, pp. 5247-50.

Hardy, P., Bhattacharya, M., Abran, D., Peri, KG., Asselin, P. & Varma, DR. 1998. Increases in retinovascular prostaglandin receptor functions by cyclooxygenase-1 and -2 inhibition. *Invest Ophthalmol Vis Sci.* 1998, Vol. 39, pp. 1888–98.

Harris A, Sergott RC, Spaeth GL, Katz JL, Shoemaker JA, Martin BJ. 1994. Color Doppler analysis of ocular vessel blood velocity in normal-tensional glaucoma. *Am J Ophthalmol.* 1994, Vol. 118, pp. 642-9.

Harris, A., Arend, O., Chung, HS., Kagemann, L., Cantor, L. & Martin, B. 2000. A comparative study of betaxolol and dorzolamide effect on ocular circulation in normal-tension glaucoma patients. *Ophthalmology.* 2000, Vol. 107, pp. 430-4.

Harris, A., Harris, M., Biller, J., Garzozi, H., Zarfty, D., Ciulla, TA. & Martin, B. 2000. Aging affects the retrobulbar circulation differently in women and men. *Arch Ophthalmol.* 2000, Vol. 118, pp. 1076-80.

Harris-Yitzhak, M., Harris, A., Ben-Refael, Z., Zarfati, D., Garzozi, HJ. & Martin, BJ. 2000. Estrogen-replacement therapy: effects on retrobulbar hemodynamics. *Am J Ophthalmol.* 2000, Vol. 129, pp. 623-628 .

Harris A., Kagemann L., Ehrlich R., Ehrlich Y., Lopez CR. & Purvin VA. 2008. The effect of sildenafil on ocular blood flow. *Br J Ophthalmol.* 2008, Vol. 92, pp. 469–473.

Havelius, U. & Hansen, F. 2005. Ocular vasodynamic changes in light and darkness in smokers. *Invest Ophthalmol Vis Sci.* 2005, Vol. 46, pp. 1698-705.

Hoyng, P.F., de Jong, N., Oosting, H. & Stilma, J. 1992. Platelet aggregation, disc haemorrhage and progressive loss of visual fields in glaucoma. A seven year follow-up study on glaucoma. *Int. Ophthalmol.* 1992, Vol. 16, pp. 65–73.

Hulsman CA., Vingerling JR., Hofman A., Witteman JC. & de Jong Pt. 2007. Blood pressure, arterial stifness, and opena-angle glaucoma: the Rotterdan Study. *Arch Opthalmol.* 2007, Vol. 125, pp. 805-812.

Iseri, LLT. & French, JH. 1984. Magnesium: nature's physiologic calciumblocker. *Am. Heart J.* 1984, Vol. 108, pp. 188–193.

Ishii, K., Tomidokoro, A., Nagahara, M., Tamaki, Y., Kanno, M., Fukaya, Y. & Araie, M. 2001. Effects of topical latanoprost on optic nerve head circulation in rabbits, monkeys, and humans. *Invest Ophthalmol Vis Sci.* 2001, Vol. 42, pp. 2957-2963.

Ishiyama, A., Jacobson, KM. & Baloh, RW. 2000. Migraine and benign positional vertigo. *Ann. Otol. Rhinol. Laryngol.* 2000, Vol. 109, pp. 377–380.

Januleviciene, I., Ehrlich, R., Siesky, B., Nedzelskienė, I. & Harris, A. 2009. Visual function, optic nerve structure, and ocular blood flow parameters after 1 year of glaucoma treatment with fixed combinations. *Eur J Ophthalmol.* 2009, Vol. 19, pp. 790-7.

Jonas, JB., Nguyen, XN. & Naumann, GO. 1989. Parapapillary retinal vessel diameter in normal and glaucoma eyes. I. Morphometric data. *Invest Ophthalmol Vis Sci.* 1989, Vol. 30, pp. 1599-603.

Jonas, JB. & Xu, L. 1993. Optic disc morphology in eyes after nonarteritic anterior ischemic optic neuropathy. *Invest Ophthalmol Vis Sci.* 1993, Vol. 34, pp. 2260–5

Jonas, JB. & Hayreh SS. 1999. Optic disk morphology in experimental central retinal artery occlusion in rhesus monkeys. *Am J Ophthalmol.* 1999, Vol. 127, pp. 523–30.

Jonas, JB. 2003. Central retinal artery and vein collapse pressure in eyes with chronic open angle glaucoma. *Br J Ophthalmol.* 2003, Vol. 87, pp. 949-51.

Kaiser, HJ., Stumpfig, D. & Flammer, J. 1996. Short-term effect of dipyridamole on blood flow velocities in the extraocular vessels. *Int. Opthalmol.* 1996, Vol. 19, pp. 355–358.

Kaiser, HJ., Schoetzau, A., Stumpfig, D. & Flammer, J. 1997. Bloodflow velocities of the extraocular vessels in patients with hightension and normal-tension primary open-angle glaucoma. *Am J Ophthalmol.* 1997, Vol. 123, pp. 320–327.

Kang, JH., Pasquale, LR., Willett, WC., Rosner, BA., Egan, KM., Faberowski, N. & Hankinson, SE. 2004. Dietary fat consumption and primary open-angle glaucoma. *Am J Clin Nutr.* 2004, Vol. 79, pp. 755-64.

Kang, JH., Willett, WC., Rosner, BA., Hankinson, SE. & Pasquale, LR. 2007. Prospective study of alcohol consumption and the risk of primary open-angle glaucoma. *Ophthalmic Epidemiol.* 2007, Vol. 14, pp. 141-7.

Kang, JH., Willett, WC., Rosner, BA., Hankinson, SE. & Pasquale, LR. 2008. Caffeine consumption and the risk of primary open-angle glaucoma: a prospective cohort study. *Invest Ophthalmol Vis Sci.* 2008, Vol. 49, pp. 1924-31.

Karakucuk, S., Goktas, S., Aksu, M., Erdogan, N., Demirci, S., Oner, A., Arda, H. & Gumus, K. 2008. Ocular blood flow in patients with obstructive sleep apnea syndrome (OSAS). *Graefes Arch Clin Exp Ophthalmol.* 2008, Vol. 246, pp. 129-34.

Kargi, SH., Altin, R., Koksal, M., Kart, L., Cinar, F., Ugurbas, SH. & Ayoglu, F. 2005. Retinal nerve fibre layer measurements are reduced in patients with obstructive sleep apnea syndrome. *Eye.* 2005, Vol. 19, pp. 575–579.

Kaufmann C., Fierz A., Kollias SS. & Robert YC. 2002. Ocular pulse amplitude in a case of innominate steal syndrome. *Am J Ophthalmol.* 2002, Vol. 133(1), pp. 155-6.

Kerr, J., Nelson, P. & O'Brien, C. 1997. A comparison of ocular blood flow in untreated primary open-angle glaucoma and ocular hypertension. *Am. J. Ophthalmol.* 1997, Vol. 126, pp. 42-51.

Kim, Y M., Bombeck, CA. & Billiar, TR. 1999. Nitric oxide as a bifunctional regulator of apoptosis. *Circ. Res.* 1999, Vol. 84, pp. 253–256.

Klein BE., Klein R. & Knudtson MD. 2005. Intraocular pressure an systemic blood pressure: longitudinal perspective: the Beaver Dam Eye Study. *Br J Ophthalmol.* 2005, Vol. 89, pp. 284-287.

Kozobolis, PV., Detorakis, ET., Georgiadis, GS., Achtaropoulos, AA., Papas, TT. & Lazarides, MK. 2007. Perimetric and retrobulbar blood flow changes following carotid endarterectomy. *Graefe's Arch Clin Exp Ophthalmol.* 2007, Vol. 245, pp. 1639–1645.

Krupin, T., Liebmann, JM., Greenfield, DS., Ritch, R., Gardiner, S., Low-Pressure Glaucoma Study Group. 2011. A Randomized Trial of Brimonidine Versus Timolol in Preserving Visual Function: Results From the Low-pressure Glaucoma Treatment Study. *Am J Ophthalmol.* 2011, Vol. 151, pp. 671-81.

Kuba, GB., Pillunat, LE., Bohm, AG. & Klemm, M. 2001. Retinal nerve fiber layer thickness and peripapillary blood flow in glaucoma patients and healthy probands. *Ophthalmologe.* 2001, Vol. 98, pp. 41–46.

Kurashima, H., Watabe, H., Sato, N., Abe, S., Ishida, N. & Yoshitomi, T. 2010. Effects of prostaglandin F(2α) analogues on endothelin-1-induced impairment of rabbit ocular blood flow: comparison among tafluprost, travoprost, and latanoprost. *Exp Eye Res.* 2010, Vol. 91, pp. 853-9.

Lam, AK., Chan, ST., Chan, H. & Chan B. 2003. The effect of age on ocular blood supply determined by pulsatile ocular blood flow and color Doppler ultrasongraphy. *Optom Vis Sci.* 2003, Vol. 80, pp. 305-311.

Lesk, MR., Wajszilber, M. & Deschenes, MC. 2008. The effects of systemic medications on ocular blood flow. *Can J Ophthalmol.* 2008, Vol. 43, pp. 351-5.

Leske Mc., Wu SY., Nemesure B. & Hennis A. 2002. incident open-angle glaucoma and blood pressure. *Arch Ophthalmol.* 2002, Vol. 120, pp. 954-959.

Leung, DY., Li, FC., Kwong, YY., Tham, CC., Chi, SC. & Lam, DS. 2010. Simvastatin and disease stabilization in normal tension glaucoma: a cohort study. *Ophthalmology.* 2010, Vol. 117, pp. 471-6.

Liu JH., Kripke DF., Twa MD., Hoffman RE., Mansberger SL., Rex KM., Girkin CA. & Weinreb RN. 1999. Twenty-four-hour pattern of intraocular pressure in the aging population. *Invest Ophthalmol Vis Sci.* 1999, Vol. 40, pp. 2912-7.

Liu, CJ., Ko, YC., Cheng, CY., Chou, JC., Hsu, WM. & Liu, JH. 2002. Effect of latanoprost 0.005% and brimonidine tartrate 0.2% on pulsatile ocular blood flow in normal tension glaucoma. *Br J Ophthalmol.* 2002, Vol. 86, pp. 1236–1239.

Matulla, B., Streit, G., Pieh, S., Findl, O., Entlicher, J., Graselli, U., Eichler, HG., Wolzt, M. & Schmetterer, L. 1997. Effects of losartan on cerebral and ocular circulation in healthy subjects. *Br J Clin Pharmacol.* 1997, Vol. 44, pp. 369-75.

McKee HD., Saldaña M. & Ahad MA. 2004. Increased ocular pulse amplitude revealing aortic regurgitation. *Am J Ophthalmol.* 2004, Vol. 138(3), p. 503.

Michelson, G., Groh, MJ., Groh, ME. & Grundler, A. 1995. Advanced primary open-angle glaucoma is associated with decreased ophthalmic artery blood-flow velocity. *Ger. J. Ophthalmol.* 1995, Vol. 4, pp. 21–24.

Millar-Craig MW., Bishop CN. & Raftery EB. 1978. Circadian variation of blood-pressure. *Lancet.* 1978, Vol. i:, pp. 795-7.

Miller, ER., Pastor-Barriuso, R., Dalal, D., Riemersma, RA., Appel, LJ. & Guallar, E. 2005. Meta-analysis: high-dosage vitamin E supplementation may increase all-cause mortality. *Ann Intern Med.* 2005, Vol. 142, pp. 37-46.

Mitchell P., Lee AJ., Rochtchina E. & Wang JJ. 2004. Open-angle glaucoma and systemic hypertension: the Blue Mountains Eye Study. *J Glaucoma.* 2004, Vol. 13, pp. 319-326.

Miyauchi, T. & Masaki, T. 1999. Pathophysiology of endothelin in the cardiovascular system. *Annu. Rev Physiol.* 1999, Vol. 61, pp. 391–415.

Mojon, DS., Hess, CW., Goldblum, D., Fleischhauer, J., Koerner, F., Bassetti, C. & Mathis, J. 1999. High prevalence of glaucoma in patients with sleep apnea syndrome. *Ophthalmology.* 1999, Vol. 106, pp. 1009–1012.

Mojon, DS., Hess, CW., Goldblum, D., Boehnke, M., Koerner, F., Gugger, M., Bassetti, C. & Mathis, J. 2002. Normal-tension glaucoma is associated with sleep apnea syndrome. *Ophthalmologica.* 2002, Vol. 216, pp. 180–184.

Montanari, P., Marangoni, P., Oldani, A., Ratiglia, R., Raiteri, M. & Berardinelli, L. 2001. Color Doppler imaging study in patients with primary open-angle glaucoma treated with timolol 0.5% and carteolol 2%. *Eur. J. Ophthalmol.* 2001, Vol. 11, pp. 240–244.

Morgan, WH., Balaratnasingam, C., Hazelton, ML., House, PH., Cringle, SJ. & Yu, DY. 2005. The force required to induce hemivein pulsation is associated with the site of maximum field loss in glaucoma. *Invest Ophthalmol Vis Sci.* 2005, Vol. 46, pp. 1307-12.

Morgan, WH., Hazelton, ML., Balaratnasingamm, C., Chan, H., House, PH., Barry, CJ., Cringle, SJ. & Yu DY. 2009. The association between retinal vein ophthalmodynamometric force change and optic disc excavation. *Br J Ophthalmol.* 2009, Vol. 93, pp. 594-6.

Motoyama, T., Kawano, H., Kugiyama, K., Hirashima, O., Ohgushi, M., Tsunoda, R., Moriyama, Y., Miyao, Y., Yoshimura, M., Ogawa, H. and Yasue, H. 1998. Vitamin E administration improves impairment of endothelium-dependent vasodilation in patients with coronary spastic angina. *J. Am. Coll. Cardiol.* 1998, Vol. 2, pp. 1672-1679.

Nagaoka, T., Takahashi, A., Sato, E., Izumi, N., Hein, TW., Kuo, L. & Yoshida, A. 2006. Effect of systemic administration of simvastatin on retinal circulation. *Arch Ophthalmol.* 2006, Vol. 124, pp. 665-70.

Nicolela, MT., Buckley, AR., Walman, BE. & Drance, SM. 1996. A comparative study of the effects of timolol and latanoprost on blood flow velocity of the retrobulbar vessels. *Am J Ophthalmol.* 1996, Vol. 122, pp. 784–789.

Nicolela, MT. 2007. Retinal vein pulsation predicts increasing optic disc excavation. *Br J Ophthalmol.* 2007, Vol. 91, pp. 405-6.

Niebauer, J. & Cooke, JP. 1996. Cardiovascular effects of exercise: role of endothelial shear stress. *J Am Coll Cardiol.* 1996, Vol. 28, pp. 1652-60.

Nitta, K., Uchida, K., Tsutsui, T., Honda, K., Kawashima, A., Yumura, W. & Nihei, H. 1998. Eicosapentaenoic acid inhibits mitogen-induced endothelin-1 production and DNA synthesis in cultured bovine mesangial cells. *Am. J. Nephrol.* 1998, Vol. 18, pp. 164–170.

Niwa, Y., Yamamoto, T., Harris, A., Kagemann, L., Kawakami H. & Kitazawa, Y. 2000. Relationship between the effect of carbon dioxide inhalation or nilvadipine on orbital blood flow in normal-tension glaucoma. *J Glaucoma.* 2000, Vol. 9, pp. 262–267.

O'Brien, C., Butt, Z., Ludlam, C. & Detkova, P. 1997. Activation of the coagulation cascade in untreated primary open-angle glaucoma. *Ophthalmology.* 1997, Vol. 104, pp. 725–729.

Ogata N., Imaizumi M., Kurokawa H., Arichi M. & Matsumura M. 2005. Optic nerve compression by normal carotid artery in patients with normal tension glaucoma. *Br J Ophthalmol.* 2005, Vol. 89, 174-179.

Olafsdottir, OB., Hardarson SH., Gottfredsdottir, MS., Harris, A. & Stefánsson, E. 2010. Retinal Oximetry in Open-Angle Glaucoma. *ARVO.* [Online] 2010.

Onen SH, Mouriaux F, Berramdane L, Dascotte JC, Kulik JF Rouland JF. 2000. High prevalence of sleep-disordered breathing in patients with primary open-angle glaucoma. *Acta Ophthalmol Scand.* 2000, Vol. 78, pp. 638–641.

Ozkan, B., Yüksel, N., Anik, Y., Altintas, O., Demirci, A. & Cağlar Y. 2008. The effect of caffeine on retrobulbar hemodynamics. *Curr Eye Res.* 2008, Vol. 33, pp. 804-9.

Pache, M. & Flammer, J. 2006. A sick eye in a sick body? Systemic findings in patients with primary open-angle glaucoma. *Surv Ophthalmol.* 2006, Vol. 51, pp. 179-212.

Pasquale, LR., Rosner, BA., Hankinson, SE., & Kang, JH. 2007. Attributes of Female Reproductive Aging and Their Relation to Primary Open-angle Glaucoma: A Prospective Study. *J Glaucoma.* 2007, Vol. 16, pp. 598-605.

Pechère-Betschi, A., Nussberger, J., Biollaz, J., Fahti, M., Grouzmann, E., Morgan, T., Brunner, HR & Burnier, M. 1998. Circadian variations of renal sodium handling in patients with orthostatic hypotension. 1998, Vol. 54, pp. 1276-82.

Perkins, E.S. 1985. The ocular pulse and intraocular pressure as a screening test for carotid artery stenosis. *Br J Ophthalmol.* 1985, Vol. 69, pp. 676–680.

Pierdomenico SD., Bucci A., Costantini F., Lapenna D., Cuccurullo F. & Mezzetti A. 1998. Circadian blood pressure changes and myocardial ischemia in hypertensive patients with coronary artery disease. *J Am Coll Cardiol.* 1998, Vol. 31(7), pp. 1627-34.

Pinto, L. Leitão, P. Ferreira, J., Domingues, I., Vandewalle, E. & Fernandes, F. 2010. Diurnal variation of ocular pulse amplitude in primary open angle glaucoma patients. *Ophthalmologica.* 2010, pp. doi: 10.1111/j.1755-3768.2010.2356.x.

Plange, N., Remky, A. & Arend, O. 2003. Colour Doppler imaging and fluorescein filling defects of the optic disc in normal tension glaucoma. *Br J Ophthalmol.* 2003, Vol. 87, pp. 731–736.

Pourcelot, L. 1975. Indications de l'ultrasonographie Doppler dans l'etude des vaisseaux peripheriques. *Rev Prat.* 1975, Vol. 25, pp. 4671–4680.

Pourjavan, S., Boëlle, PY., Detry-Morel, M. & De Potter, P. 2007. Physiological diurnal variability and characteristics of the ocular pulse amplitude (OPA) with the dynamic contour tonometer (DCT-Pascal). *Int Ophthalmol.* 2007, Vol. 27, pp. 357-60.

Prunte-Glowazki, A. & Flammer, J. 1991. Ocular vasospasm. 4: Clinical examples. *Klin Monatsbl Augenheilkd.* 1991, Vol. 198, pp. 415-8.

Quaranta, L., Harris, A., Donato, F., Cassamali, M., Semeraro, F., Nascimbeni, G., Gandolfo, E. & Quaranta, CA. 1997. Color Doppler imaging of ophthalmic artery blood flow velocity: a study of repeatability and agreement. *Ophthalmology.* 1997, Vol. 104, pp. 653–658.

Quaranta, L., Bettelli, S., Uva, MG., Semeraro, F., Turano, R. & Gandolfo, E. 2003. Effect of Ginkgo biloba extract on preexisting visual field damage in normal tension glaucoma. *Ophthalmology.* 2003, Vol. 110, pp. 359-62.

Ravalico, G., Toffoli, G., Pastori, G., Croce, M. & Calderini, S. 1996. Age-related ocular blood flow changes. *Invest Ophthalmol Vis Sci.* 1996, Vol. 37, pp. 2645-2650.

Risner, D., Ehrlich, R., Kheradiya, NS., Siesky, B., McCranor, L. & Harris, A. 2009. Effects of exercise on intraocular pressure and ocular blood flow: a review. *J Glaucoma.* 2009, Vol. 18, pp. 429-36.

Ritch, R. 2000. Neuroprotection: is it already applicable to glaucoma therapy? *Curr Opin Ophthalmol.* 2000, Vol. 11, pp. 78–84.

Sacca, SC., Pascotto, A., Camicione, P., Capris, P. & Izzotti, A. 2005. Oxidative DNA damage in the human trabecular meshwork: clinical correlation in patients with primary open-angle glaucoma. *Arch. Ophthalmol.* 2005, Vol. 123, pp. 458–463

Saccà, SC., Izzotti, A., Rossi, P. & Traverso, C. 2007. Glaucomatous outflow pathway and oxidative stress. *Exp. Eye Res.* 2007, Vol. 84, pp. 389–399.

Schmidt, KG., Mittag, TW., Pavlovic, S. & Hessemer, V. 1996. Influence of physical exercise and nifedipine on ocular pulse amplitude. *Graefes Arch Clin Exp Ophthalmol.* 1996, Vol. 234, pp. 527-32.

Schmidt, KG., Mittag, TW., Pavlovic, S. & Hessemer, V.,. 1996. Influence of physical exercise and nifedipine on ocular pulse amplitude. *Graefes Arch. Clin. Exp. Ophthalmol.* 1996, Vol. 234, pp. 527–532.

Schmidt KG., Ruckmann A., Klingmuller V., Becker R., Pillunat LE. & Mittag TW. 1998. Ocular pulse amplitude during manipulation of systemic perfusion parameters. *Klin Monatsbl Augenheilkd.* 1998, Vol. 213, pp. 241–244.

Schwenn O., Troost R., Vogel A., Grus F., Beck S. & Pfeiffer N. 2002. Ocular pulse amplitude in patients with open angle glaucoma, normal tension glaucoma, and ocular hypertension. *Br J Ophthalmol.* 2002, Vol. 86, pp. 981–984.

Sei, H. & Morita, Y. 1999. Why does arterial blood pressure rise actively during REM sleep? *J Med Invest.* 1999, Vol. 46, pp. 11–7.

Shah, P., Whittaker, KW., Wells, AP. & Khaw, PT. 2001. Exercise-induced visual loss associated with advanced glaucoma in young adults. *Eye (Lond).* 2001, Vol. 15, pp. 616-20.

Siesky, BA., Harris, A., Patel, C., Klaas, CL., Harris, M., McCranor, LJ., Lauer, J. & Kaplan, B. 2000. Comparison of visual function and ocular hemodynamics between pre- and post-menopausal women. *Eur J Ophthalmol.* 2000, Vol. 18, pp. 320-3.

Siesky, B., Harris, A., Sines, D., Rechtman, E., Malinovsky, VE., McCranor, L., Yung, CW. & Zalish, M. 2006. A comparative analysis of the effects of the fixed combination of timolol and dorzolamide versus latanoprost plus timolol on ocular hemodynamics and visual function in patients with primary open-angle glaucoma. *J Ocul Pharmacol Ther.* 2006, Vol. 22, pp. 353-61.

Siesky, B., Harris, A., Brizendine, E., Marques, C., Loh, J., Mackey, J., Overton, J. & Netland, P. 2009. Literature review and meta-analysis of topical carbonic anhydrase inhibitors and ocular blood flow. *Surv Ophthalmol.* 2009, Vol. 54, pp. 33-46.

Silberstein, SD., Goadsby, PJ. & Lipton, RB. 2000. Management of migraine: an algorithmic approach. *Neurology.* 2000, Vol. 55, pp. 46-52.

Soares, AS., Artes, PH., Andreou, P., Leblanc, RP., Chauhan, BC. & Nicolela, MT. 2004. Factors associated with optic disc hemorrhages in glaucoma. *Ophthalmology.* 2004, Vol. 111, pp. 1653-7.

Sossi, N. & Anderson, DR. 1983. Blockage of axonal transport in optic nerve induced by elevation of intraocular pressure. Effect of arterial hypertension induced by angiotensin I. *Arch Ophthalmol.* 1983, Vol. 101, pp. 94--7,.

Stalmans I., Harris A., Vanbellinghen V., Zeyen T. & Siesky B. 2008. Ocular Pulse Amplitude in Normal Tension and Primary Open Angle Glaucoma. *J Glaucoma.* 2008, Vol. 17, pp. 403–407.

Stalmans I., Harris A., Fieuws S., Zeyen T., Vanbellinghen V., McCranor L. & Siesky B. 2009. Color Doppler imaging and ocular pulse amplitude in glaucomatous and healthy eyes. *European Journal of Ophthalmology.* 2009, Vol. 19, pp. 580-587.

Steigerwalt, RD., Belcaro, GV., Laurora, G., Cesarone, MR., De Sanctis, MT. & Incandela, L. 1998. Ocular and orbital blood flow in patients with essential hypertension treated with trandolapril. *Retina.* 1998, Vol. 18, pp. 539-45.

Strenn, K., Matulla, B., Wolzt, M., Findl, O., Bekes, MC., Lamsfuss, U., Graselli, U., Rainer, G., Menapace, R., Eichler, HG. & Schmetterer, L. 1998. Reversal of endothelin-1-induced ocular hemodynamic effects by low-dose nifedipine in humans. *Clin. Pharmacol. Ther.* 1998, Vol. 63, pp. 54–63.

Stroke Prevention by Aggressive Reduction in Cholesterol Levels (SPARCL), Investigators. 2006. High-dose atorvastatin after stroke or transient ischemic attack. *N Engl J Med.* 2006, Vol. 355, pp. 549 –59.

Stroman, GA., Stewart, WC., Golnik, KC., Curé, JK. & Olinger, RE. 1995. Magnetic resonance imaging in patients with low-tension glaucoma. *Arch Ophthalmol.* 1995, Vol. 113, pp. 168-72.

Sung, KR., Lee, S., Park, SB., Choi, J., Kim, ST., Yun, SC., Kang, SY., Cho, JW. & Kook, MS. 2009. Twenty-four hour ocular perfusion pressure fluctuation and risk of normal-tension glaucoma progression. *Invest Ophthalmol Vis Sci.* 2009, Vol. 50, pp. 5266-74.

Tezel, G. & Wax M. 2004. Hypoxia-inducible factor 1alpha in the glaucomatous retina and optic nerve head. *Arch Ophthalmol.* 2004, Vols. Tezel, G. and M. Wax, Hypoxia-inducible factor 1alpha in the glaucomatous retina and optic nerve head. Arch Ophthalmol, 2004. 122(9): p. 1348-56., pp. 1348-56.

Tfelt-Hansen P, Saxena PR, Dahlöf, C., Pascual, J., Láinez, M., Henry, P., Diener, H., Schoenen, J., Ferrari, MD. & Goadsby, PJ. 2000. Ergotamine in the acute treatment of migraine: a review and European consensus. *Brain.* 2000, Vol. 123, pp. 9-18.

Tielsch JM., Katz J., Sommer A., Quigley HA. & Javitt JC. 1995. Hypertension, perfusion pressure, and primary open angle glaucoma. A population-based assessment. *Arch Ophthalmol.* 1995, Vol. 113, pp. 216-221.

Tomita, K., Araie, M., Tamaki, Y., Nagahara, M., & Sugiyama, T. 1999. Effects of nilvadipine, a calcium antagonist, on rabbit ocular circulation and optic nerve head circulation in NTG subjects. *Invest. Ophthalmol.Vision Sci.* 1999, Vol. 40, pp. 1144–1151.

Traustason, S., Hardarson, SH., Gottfredsdottir, MS., Eysteinsson, T., Karlsson, RA., Stefánsson, E. & Harris, A. 2009. Dorzolamide-timolol combination and retinal vessel oxygen saturation in patients with glaucoma or ocular hypertension. *Br J Ophthalmol.* 2009, Vol. 93, pp. 1064-7.

Trible, JR., Costa, VP., Sergott, RC., Spaeth, GL., Smith, M., Wilson, RP., Katz, LJ., Moster, MR. & Schmidt, CM. 1994. The influence of primary open-angle glaucoma upon the retrobulbar circulation: baseline, postoperative and reproducibility analysis. *Trans. Am. Ophthalmol.* 1994, pp. 245–265.

Trible, JR., Sergott, RC., Spaeth, GL., Wilson, RP., Katz, LJ., Moster, MR. & Schmidt, CM. 1994. Trabeculectomy is associated with retrobulbar hemodynamic changes. A color Doppler analysis. *Ophthalmology.* 1994, Vol. 101, pp. 340-51.

Vaughan, CJ. & Delanty, N. 1999. Neuroprotective properties of statins in cerebral ischemia and stroke. *Stroke.* 1999, Vol. 30, pp. 1969 -73.

Vulsteke C., Stalmans I., Fieuws S. & Zeyen T. 2008. Correlation between ocular pulse amplitude measured by dynamic contour tonometer and visual field defects. *Graefes Arch Clin Exp Ophthalmol.* 2008, Vol. 246, pp. 559–565.

Waldmann, E., Gasser, P., Dubler, B., Huber, C. & Flammer, J. 1996. Silent myocardial ischemia in glaucoma and cataract patients. *Graefe's Arch. Clin. Exp. Ophthalmol.* 1996, Vol. 234, pp. 595–598.

Walsh, JT. & Montplaisir, J. 1982. Familial glaucoma with sleep apnoea: a new syndrome? *Thorax.* 1982, Vol. 37, pp. 845–9.

Wang, JJ., Liew, G., Klein, R., Rochtchina, E., Knudtson, MD., Klein, BE., Wong, TY., Burlutsky, G. & Mitchell, P. 2007. Retinal vessel diameter and cardiovascular mortality: pooled data analysis from two older populations. *Eur Heart J.* 2007, Vol. 28, pp. 1984-92.

Weigert, G., Resch, H., Garhofer, G., Fuchsjäger-Mayrl, G. & Schmetterer, L. 2007. Effects of topical clonidine versus brimonidine on choroidal blood flow and intraocular pressure during squatting. *Invest Ophthalmol Vis Sci.* 2007, Vol. 48, pp. 4220-5.

Williamson, TH., Lowe, GD. & Baxter, GM. 1995. Influence of ag, systemic blood pressure, smoking and blood viscosity on orbital blood velocities. *Br J Ophthalmol.* 1995, Vol. 79, pp. 17-22.

Wimpissinger, B., Resch, H., Berisha, F., Weigert, G., Schmetterer, L. & Polak, K. 2004. Response of choroidal blood flow to carbogen breathing in smokers and non-smokers. *Br J Ophthalmol.* 2004, Vol. 88, pp. 776-81.

Wong, TY., Klein, R., Couper, DJ., Cooper, LS., Shahar, E., Hubbard, LD., Wofford, MR. & Sharrett, AR. 2001. Retinal microvascular abnormalities and incident stroke: the Atherosclerosis Risk in Communities Study. *Lancet.* 2001, Vol. 358, pp. 1134-40.

Wong, TY., Klein, R., Sharrett, AR., Duncan, BB., Couper, DJ., Tielsch, JM., Klein, BE. & Hubbard LD. 2002. Retinal arteriolar narrowing and risk of coronary heart disease in men and women. The Atherosclerosis Risk in Communities Study. *JAMA.* 2002, Vol. 287, pp. 1153-9.

Yamamoto, T., Niwa, Y., Kawakami, H. & Kitazawa, Y. 1998. The effect of nilvadipine, a calcium-channel blocker, on the hemodynamics of retrobulbar vessels in normal-tension glaucoma. *J. Glaucoma.* 1998, Vol. 7, pp. 301–305.

Zeitz O, Galambos P, Wagenfeld L, Wiermann A, Wlodarsch P, Praga R, Matthiessen ET, Richard G, Klemm M. 2006. Glaucoma progression is associated with decreased blood flow velocities in the short posterior ciliary artery. *Br J Ophthalmol.* 2006, Vol. 90, pp. 1245-8.

Zeitz, O., Vilchez, SE., Matthiessen, ET., Richard, G. & Klemm, M. 2006. Volumetric colour Doppler imaging: a useful tool for the determination of ocular blood flow in glaucoma patients? *Eye (Lond).* 2006, Vol. 20, pp. 668-73.

Zhou, RH. & Frishman, WH. 2010. The Antiplatelet Effects of Nitrates: Is it of Clinical Significance in Patients With Cardiovascular Disease? *Zhou, Rui-Hai MD*†; Frishman, William H. MD‡.* 2010, Vol. 18, pp. 198-203.

# 11

# Corneal Viscoelastical Properties Related to Glaucoma

Horea Demea[1], Sorina Demea[1] and Rodica Holonec[2]
[1]*Ophthalmological Center - Review, Cluj-Napoca*
[2]*Technical University of Cluj-Napoca*
*Romania*

## 1. Introduction

Although elevated IOP is clearly the most frequent causative risk factor for glaucomatous optic nerve atrophy, it is not the only factor, and attempts to define glaucoma on the basis of ocular tension are no longer recommended. Considering IOP as a risk factor in the appearance of the glaucomatous lesions at the level of the optic nerve, it's important to establish the mechanisms which may enhance or reduce this risk. These complex processes refer to the way in which the IOP is transmitted from the ocular structures to the optic nerve head. (Downs et al., 2005)

For a better understanding of our work, some physical parameters must be defined and known. We found them used in materials physics: stress, stretch, strain, deformability, elastic and viscous materials, etc. A short special subchapter is dedicated to these mechanical characteristics.

The Reichert device named Ocular Response Analyzer (O.R.A.) is a special device used to measure intra ocular pressure correlated with the viscoelastic properties of the cornea - named IOPcc. In order to monitor the influence of IOPcc on the optic nerve we also made measurements on the Retinal Nerve Fiber Layers (RNFL). For that purpose, we used a Zeiss device named Stratus OCT on the Optical Coherence Tomography.

Using clinically measured values with Ocular Response Analyzer for IOPcc and the computed value which describes the performance, the efficiency (%) of eliminating the overpressure /for cycle of loading - named by us the specific damping capacity ($\varphi$) - we made a graphical representation of these two parameters, to grade the particular effort of the ocular structure and implicitly of the retinal nervous fibers layer of the studied patient. We named this graphic the Effort Staging System (ESS) (Demea et al., 2008) and we use it to classify glaucoma risk for our patients. In order to make our work easier we developed a computerized application which practically takes the data measured by us and calculates the specific damping capacity, so the patient is automatically introduced in the ESS scale. Consequently we obtain the class of the glaucoma risk, damage effort of RNFL, where that patient is situated.

The application has a user-friendly interface and helps the ophthalmologists in the clinical diagnosis.

## 2. Physical definitions – The dynamic of the expansion effort of the ocular structures

For a better understanding of the viscoelastic properties of the cornea we considered important to mention some elements from the material physics that help to characterize the properties of the ocular structures from the mechanical point of view.

### 2.1 Materials resistance to deformation

The Materials resistance to deformation is studied in accordance with two parameters: stress (σ) and strain (ξ).
The stress (σ) is defined as a measure of internal forces that arise in a body being deformed as a result of external forces and the stress intensity is given by the force which operates on the surface unity dF/dS =dP.
The strain can be characterized by more parameters. Thus, the stretch (dS) represents the expansion difference the material can reach, after the stress was applied. If the stretch ratio dS/S increases, the surface becomes elastic and can be deformed. If dS/S decreases, the surface becomes rigid and its deformability decreases as well.
At the same time, we can talk about the deformation effort dP/dS which can increase either due to the stress growth (dP), or due to the surface rigidity (dS decreases).

### 2.2 The viscoelasticity of the soft tissues

From the perspective of the stress factor, if we take into account the time factor (t) and its application frequency (f), the materials have an elastic or viscose behavior.
In the case of an elastic behavior the deformation is independent of the stress factors "t" and "f". For example, an elastic arch submitted to the compression is deformed in a linear way, according to the applied force size, and this deformation doesn't depend on the application time or on the behavior. The releasing of the tension takes place linearly as well, while the stress intensity decreases. Elastic materials strain instantaneously when stretched, and just as quickly return to their original state once the stress is removed.
In the case of a viscose behavior, the strain depends on the application time and/or on the application frequency. In this way, the applied stress resistance is mainly dynamically dependent on the force application speed, high speed means great resistance. Viscous materials resist shear flow and strain linearly with time when a stress is applied.
Viscoelasticity is the materials' property to exhibit both viscous and elastic characteristics when undergoing deformation. Cornea and all the soft tissues are viscoelastic and their response to the stress is a combination between an instantaneous response (elastic) and a response dependent on time (viscous - reaction time latency). Viscous-elastic materials have elements of both of these properties and exhibit time dependent strain (Jonas & Budde, 2000).

## 3. Ocular Response Analyzer (ORA) and the calculation of specific damping capacity

From the actual instruments for intraocular pressure measurement we chose the non-contact tonometer called Ocular Response Analyzer (Figure 1). This device determines 2 types of parameters:

- the ones related to the "stress" generated by the increase of the intraocular pressure named: IOP cc - intraocular pressure corrected and IOPg - intraocular pressure according to Goldman norms.
- the ones related to the "material behavior ", such as cornea, submitted to this stress, named: CH - Corneal Hysteresis and CRF - Corneal Resistance Factor

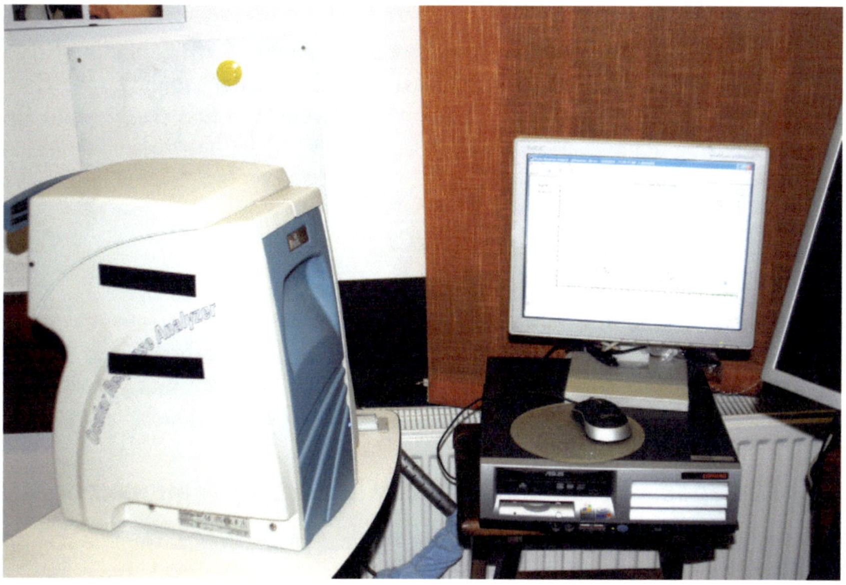

Fig. 1. Ocular Response Analyzer

The producer of ORA specified that:

1. IOPg- is the real IOP measured by the instrument, dependent on the cornea biomechanics.
2. IOPcc - this is the intraocular pressure measurement that is less affected by corneal properties than other methods of tonometry, such as Goldman. The instrument automatic adjusts the IOPg to IOPcc. The recommendation of Reichert Company is for use in clinical evaluation of intraocular pressure the value of IOPcc instead of IOPg.
3. CH - is the pressure lost during an upload cycle. This parameter is a measure of corneal tissue properties, a result of viscous damping in the corneal tissue.

The normal values for IOPcc and CH are shown in Table 1, as in (Allingham & al., 2005; Kevin & al., 2004; Luce &Taylor, 2006).

| | | | |
|---|---|---|---|
| IOPcc (mmHg) | Normal | | < 20 |
| | Pathologic | Suspect | 20 - 30 |
| | | Sure | > 30 |
| CH (mmHg) | Normal | | > 10 |
| | Pathologic | Suspect | 8 - 10 |
| | | Sure | < 8 |

Table 1. Normal values for IOPcc and CH

For example, the situation in which IOPcc < 20 mmHg and CH > 10 mmHg is a normal one, where cornea and the other ocular structures have functional reserves, which are able to absorb the loaded IOP and to reduce the tensional stress impact on the posterior pole (optic nerve). The situations where IOPcc reaches at values > 20 mmHg and CH ≤ 10 mmHg represent the "balance break point", that is, the moment where cornea loses the compensation capacity of the tensions and the "loaded stress" is transmitted to the ocular posterior pole.

To detect this situation of balance break point, we calculate the efficiency of eliminating the overpressure / cycle of loading and we named this: Damping capacity (φ). The damping capacity can specifically be calculated as the ratio between the lost energy and the stocked energy during a loading cycle.

$$\varphi = \frac{CH}{2IOPg} \tag{1}$$

Normal values for specific damping capacity (φ) are over 30 %.

O.R.A. may offer deductive, indirect data on the ocular structures strain (σ) characteristics. Thus, for instance, a low specific damping capacity (φ) is characteristic for the "rigid" viscoelastic systems, and this situation frequently occurs in glaucoma because of the non-enzymatic glycation of the glucose with the collagen fibers, which leads to sclera stiffness.

## 4. Cornea – The specific damping capacity in glaucoma etiopathogeny

It has been long suspected that corneal biomechanical properties influence the results and outcomes of various ocular measurements and procedures, and may hold clues to diagnosing and managing ocular diseases. Human corneal tissue is a complex viscouselastic structure (Ethier et al., 2004). Almost all known glaucoma evaluating systems consider an elastic ocular model, where IOP measured at the anterior eye segment is totally transmitted to the posterior eye pole. We consider the viscous-elastic ocular model (Sigal et al., 2004), where only a part of this IOP is considered to be transmitted toward posterior pole, because of the specific damping capacity or partial absorption of the pressure in the ocular walls and other ocular structures. A high damping capacity (more vascoelastic ocular structures) reduces the risk of the glaucoma, by decreasing the transmitted pressure toward optic nerve in the posterior pole. In reverse order, a reduced damping capacity (a more rigid eye, for example - an aged person) increases the risk of the optic nerve damage even at the medium IOP.

We studied the correlation between the most important factors in diagnosis and evaluating a glaucoma suspect patient: IOPcc – as a loading factor (stress) and CH – as unloading factor (protective). We noticed that it is most important to appreciate the efficiency of pressure elimination depending on each cycle of charging, reason for which we calculated the specific damping capacity (φ).

## 5. Evaluation method of the pressure risk in glaucoma

In order to quantify the mechanical risk of lesion in glaucoma we emphasized (Demea et al., 2008) the need to determine two important parameters from a pathophysiological point of view: the IOPcc - Compensated Intraocular Pressure and the CH - Corneal Hysteresis. We used O.R.A to measure these values, the most important factors in diagnosing and evaluating a patient suspected of glaucoma. The optical coherence tomography was also used to measure retinal nerve fiber layers around the head of the optic nerve. The risk of lesion for the retinal nerve fibers - implicitly the risk of glaucoma - is determined in any unbalance of these two factors.

Because the pressure loading (IOPcc) and unloading (CH) of the ocular system is fluctuant, we defined the efficiency [%] of eliminating the overpressure/cycle of loading as being the specific damping capacity (φ). This parameter is defined as the energy loss per cycle (D) divided by the stored peak energy (U), which, for a spring mass system, is the energy stored in the spring at maximum deflection (Stone, 2007). The energy loss per cycle is in our case a hysteretic damping factor (D) introduced and defined by the O.R.A. engineers as CH (Figure 2). In the same O.R.A. system, the peak energy stored (U) is 2xIOPg. The specific damping capacity is then $\varphi = D/U$

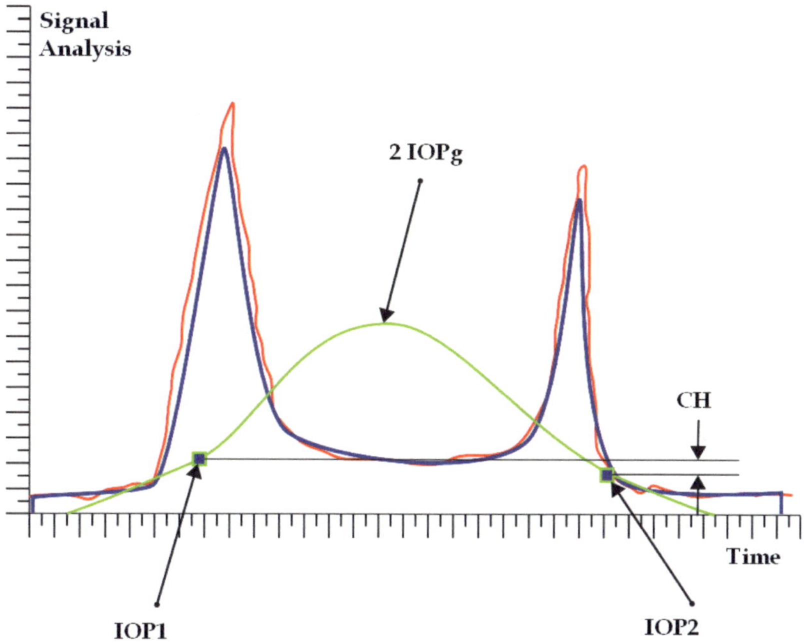


Fig. 2. Ocular Response Analyzer (O.R.A.) system signal response (CH - Corneal Hysteresis, CH = IOP1 - IOP2 , IOP1 and IOP2 are two determinations of intraocular pressure at two different moments of time : at the cornea inflection and at the corneal deflection, 2IOPg - is the peak of loading process delivered by O.R.A. , which is calculated at the double of IOPg)

A common basis for measuring damping involves energy loss and the determination of the energy lost per cycle. The normal and pathologic values for the specific damping capacity (φ) are specified in Table 2.

The condition of pressure protection and so the lack of risk of glaucoma is fulfilled when at any high value of the intraocular pressure (IOPcc) the system responds by a corresponding elimination of the overpressure (CH) and the efficiency of elimination (φ) is at least 30 %. The CH measurement is an indication of viscous damping in the cornea, or in other words, it represents the ability of the tissue to absorb and dissipate energy.

| Specific damping capacity | Clinical Evaluation |
|---|---|
| > 30 % | Normal |
| 18 – 30 % | Suspect |
| < 18 % | Pathologic |

Table 2. Specific damping capacity- values and clinical categories

Damping is the conversion of mechanical energy of a structure into thermal energy. Damping is most beneficial when used to reduce the amplitude of dynamic instabilities, or the resonance in a structure.
A viscous-elastic material is characterized by possessing both viscous and elastic behavior. A purely elastic material is one in which all the energy stored in the sample during loading is returned when the load is removed.
A complete opposite of an elastic material is a purely viscous material, which does not return any of the energy stored during loading. All the energy is lost as "pure damping", once the load is removed.
We call viscous-elastic material, and the eye is one of them, anything that does not fall into one of the above extreme classifications. Some of energy stored in a viscous-elastic system is recovered upon removal of the load, and the remainder is dissipated in the form of heat.
Structural engineering analysis tools have been used to improve the understanding of the biomechanical behavior of the cornea. These data were used to facilitate the construction of accurate finite-elements models, being adapted to study the response of the cornea to tonometry procedures used to measure the intra-ocular pressure as in (Kevin et all, 2004).
Normal and pathological values for corneal hysteresis (CH) are given in Table 1, and are calculated using formula (1). We used values that are considered statistically normal for CH and IOPcc in previous studies (Luce & Taylor, 2006).

## 6. The Effort Staging System (ESS)

Using clinically measured values with O.R.A. for IOPcc and the computed value for the specific damping capacity (φ), we made a graphical representation to grade the particular effort of the ocular structure and implicitly of the layer of nervous fibers (RNFL) in the studied patient (Figure 3). We named this graphic the Effort Staging System (ESS) and we use it to categorize glaucoma risk in our patients.
The ESS is the improved alternative of a previous study (Demea et al., 2008) and brings an original correlation between φ and IOPcc, resulted from Reichert Ocular Response Analyzer measurements.
We define stress as a physical factor (pressure in our case) which functions upon the studied material (the eye structures in our case. Mechanical stress is directly proportional to the IOPcc, and is inversely proportional to Specific Damping Capacity (φ).

### 6.1 ESS clinical approach

Using normal and pathological values indicated in (Kothecha et al., 2006), for the specific damping capacity (φ) and IOPcc we made a graphical representation to grade the particular effort of the ocular structures and implicitly of the layer of RNFL in the studied patient

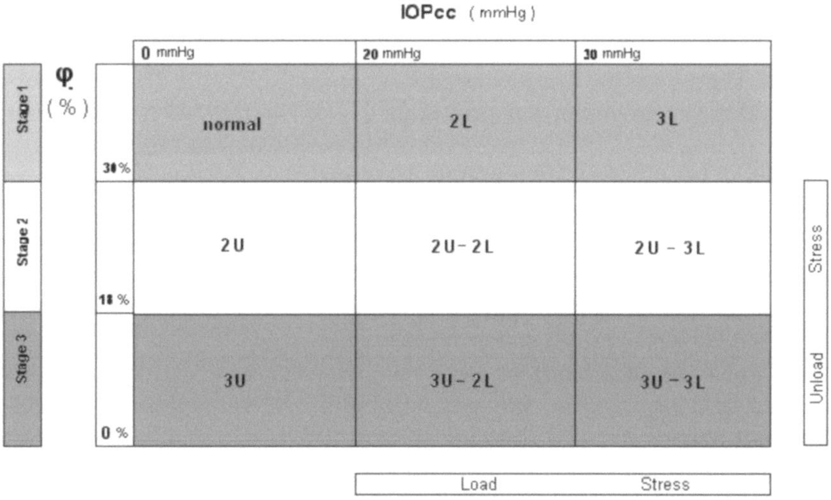


Fig. 3. The Effort Staging System (ESS) (L - Load Stress, U - Unload Stress, IOPcc-Compensated IOP, φ - specific damping capacity)

(Allingham et al., 2005;Brusini & Filacorda, 2006) as in Figure 3. We named this graphic the Effort Staging System (ESS) and it may be used in the automated calculation of the eliminating ocular pressure efficiency. We defined three types of stress (Table 3) and named them: L - Load stress (when IOPcc is high); U - Unload stress (when CH is low) and M - mixed stress (with IOPcc high and CH low). The defined types of the stress offer information about the pathophysiological mechanisms in glaucomatous nervous damage (Burgoyne et al. 2005): high intraocular pressure or low resistance in the optic nerve head.

| Type of stress | | IOPcc | CH | φ |
|---|---|---|---|---|
| Load stress | L | High | Normal | Normal or Low |
| Unload stress | U | Normal | Low | Low |
| Mixed stress | U-L | High | Low | Low |

Table 3. Type of stress correlated with IOPcc and φ

The effect of this mechanical stress upon the eye walls may be better understood if we introduce another physical parameter: the strain. During testing of a material sample, there is relationship between stress, derived from measuring the load applied on the sample, and strain, derived from measuring the deformation of the sample, i.e. elongation, compression, or distortion (McCrum et al., 2003; Mayers & Chawla, 1999; Roylance, 2001). In our case the material sample is the eye, IOPcc is the mechanical stress and the specific damping capacity φ is the equivalent of the strain.

To better understand the connection between IOPcc and damping capacity, the principle is this: "even if the structure is subjected to a high-loaded stress, measured by IOPcc, it will last as long as it has good damping capacity, over 30%, and will not appear optic nerve damage.

Corneal effort is defined by the stress and the strain, under different IOPcc.

We consider, clinically important, the following three different stages of ESS for the risk of lesion of Retinal Nerve Fiber Layer (RNFL) in glaucoma:

**Stage 1**: *Normal* - the system has an adequate efficiency, φ > 30 % in pressure elimination. CH is high enough to efficiently compensate any increase of IOPcc, both in medium (2L) and high quotas. There can be three alternatives: normal, 2L and 3L. For normal- both parameters CH and IOPcc are in normal quotas; for 2L- the system has normal efficiency but increased pressure demands (IOPcc increases at medium quotas ) and for 3L- the system has normal efficiency and much increased pressure demands (IOPcc increases at high quotas)
**Stage 2**: *Borderline* - The system has an medium efficiency, φ is between 18 - 29 % and the patient must be surveyed, different alternatives of pressure effort being possible: 2U - stress of unloading of medium severity (determined by the medium decrease of CH); 2U-2L - mixed stress of medium severity (determined by the medium increase of IOPcc and medium decrease of CH) and 2U - 3L - mixed stress of medium severity.
**Stage 3**: *Pathological* - the efficiency of the system is decreased, φ < 18 %, due to the decreased capacity of damping, the system can not efficiently compensate the increases in pressure efforts not even in normal charging quotas. There can also be three alternatives: 3U-stress of unloading of high severity (determined by the great decrease of CH); 3U-2L - mixed stress of high severity (determined by the great decrease of CH and medium increase of IOPcc ); 3U-3L- mixed stress of high severity with high pressure charges (determined by the great decrease of CH and great increase of IOPcc.

### 6.2 Effort Staging System computerized analysis application

To facilitate our work we developed a computerized application which automatically takes our measured data, calculates the specific damping capacity, and introduces it in the ESS scale. Therefore, we obtain the class of the glaucoma risk (damage effort of Retinal Nerve Fiber Layer) where the patient is situated. The application based on the Effort Staging System provides a better view of the clinical diagnosis and offers the physician a user-friendly interface for the patients' management and investigation, and also for the results' displaying and printing.

The application was implemented by using Visual Studio IDE (Integrated Development Environment) and a QT cross-platform application framework for developing the C++ code and the graphical user interface (GUI). The reasons for choosing these technologies are: C++ native implementation, which takes the best - when it comes to performance - from the available computing power and minimizes dependencies on other runtime application or components; QT technology, which provides a cross-platform powerful framework that gives access to multiple operating systems as target for future development. The application has some important features that make it an easier and quick way to diagnose. This way, there is the possibility to import and analyze CSV O.R.A. files and the patients' lists in order to be displayed.

An important feature of QT in development of this application is its international support, which means that the application can be translated in other languages, when required. Consequently, in the code, each displayed text was wrapped with the QT translation directives. For drawing the main ESS diagnose diagram, QT technologies are used in order to create scenes with graphic objects. In this way, a dynamical scene is obtained, which is easy to be modified and adapted to the other requirements. All the scene components are present as objects derived from CGraphicsObject with scale support according to the user's needs or to the custom printing mode. This approach allows the user to change the ESS values in the diagram without being necessary to step in the drawing code.

The application has a familiar native interface which is easier to be used by the operator (familiar controls, menus and user interface aspect). The application main window (Figure 4) is divided in four areas with different specific functions: toolbar, patients' lists, filter areas and results area. The patients' lists are displayed in two different ways: the principal tree list (above) which appears all the time and the list (below) which appears only when the user activates the filters. The tree list displays hierarchically all the available patients, with the possibility to expand this list for both right and left eyes. The files that contain the eyes information can be expanded as well, in order to have access to the patient measurement data.

The filters area is situated above the EES diagram and it contains two fields: patient condition and age intervals. The patient conditions can be selected by checking the "suspect" or/and "normal" and the age interval can be selected by using the available combined box-type control. In this way, under the main patients' list, the final list will include all the filtered patients that match the selected criteria. By clicking a certain result in this list, the name of the corresponding patient and his ESS diagram will be displayed:

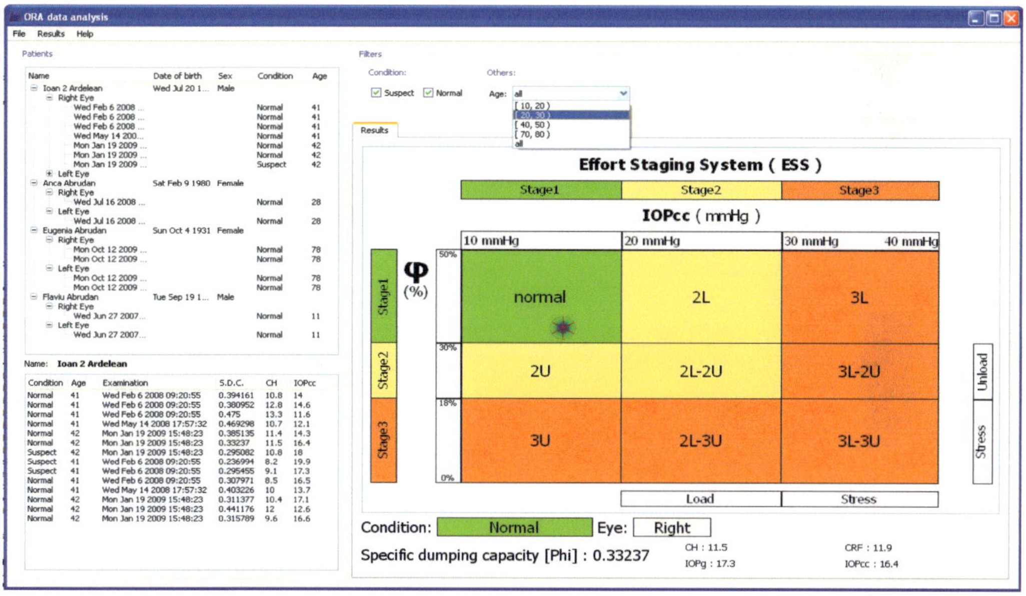


Fig. 4. The ESS application main window

The result area is represented mainly by the diagnose diagram (ESS) but it also contains the significant outcome values. For highlighting the risk region where the patient is situated, the application uses a cursor and pulsing animation. The diagram content changes dynamically and all the elements are recalculated, thus the user is the one who controls the displaying mode. The results and the patient's file can be previewed before printing and then they can be sent (including the ESS diagram) to a printer. The results can also be exported in a PDF file format.

The application's design is opened and improvements and changes can be made in the future. The filter zone is dynamically populated only with values found in the patients list. The supported file has a comma separated value format (CSV) as it is exported by the Ocular Response Analyzer application.

## 7. Clinical experimental

Once the ESS system was established as a quantifier of the pressure efficiency of the eye, we worked at the clinical validation of the method. Some experimental preliminary results are available (from Table 4 to Table 11) in a group of 150 eyes of the tested patients.
Our study sought to show the importance of protective factors to dissipate pressure. Therefore, efficiency calculation is very important to eliminate the pressure loaded at each loading cycle. We mention that in this clinical trial we studied the value of φ as a screening test in the cases in which we knew from preliminary studies that either they are healthy (with no lesions RNFLavg) or they have glaucoma (with damage to the RNFLavg).
All other pathological situations of optic nerve damage were excluded. The statistics presented here are focused on the relationships (Person index), clinical investigation and screening (sensitivity, specificity, PPV, NPV, PLR) analyses.

### 7.1 Preliminary results

To test out the glaucomatous damage in a person with certain IOPcc and φ, we focused on structural eye parameters like average Retinal Nerve Fiber Layers (RNFLavg) measured with Optical Coherence Tomography (OCT) (Figure 5).

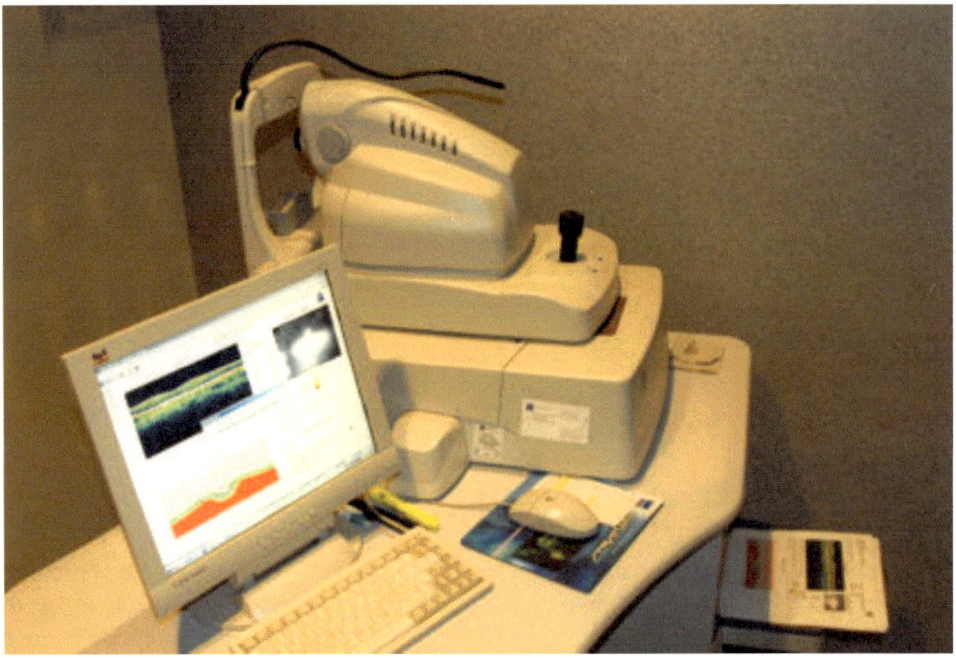

Fig. 5. Zeiss Status OCT

In order to validate the study we calculated a series of statistic parameters regarding the correlation between IOPcc and φ and avgRNFL values. So the positive values of avgRNFL represent the real positive values, and the negative values of avgRNFL represent the real negative values in this study. In defining the parameters we used the following abbreviations: RP = the number of the real positive cases; RN = the number of the real negative cases, FN = the number of the false negative cases; FP = the number of the false positive cases. The sensibility and specificity reflect the performance level of a test (in this case IOPcc and φ). The *sensitivity* of a test measures the degree to which a correct positive case is identified as being positive. On the other hand, the *specificity* represents the degree to which a correct negative case is identified as being negative. The ideal values of these parameters are of 100% or 1. The two parameters are calculated according to the relations (2) and (3).

$$Sensitivity = \frac{RP}{RN + FN} \quad (2)$$

$$Specificity = \frac{RN}{RN + FN} \quad (3)$$

The positive predictive value (PPV) represents the proportion of the correct cases identified as being positive from the total number of cases identified as being positive. In other words, PPV reflects the probability of a patient, diagnosed with a disease, to suffer of the respective disease. The negative predictive value (NPV) represents the proportion of the correct cases identified as being negative from the total number of cases identified as being negative. The two parameters are calculated according to the relations (4) and (5).

$$PPV = \frac{RP}{RP + FP} \quad (4)$$

$$NPV = \frac{RN}{RN + FN} \quad (5)$$

The Prequential Likelihood Ratio represents the probability of a positive test to indicate the presence of the disease. This is calculated according to the relation (6):

$$PLR = \frac{sensitivity}{1 - specificity} \quad (6)$$

The activity of medical research was structured as follows:

a. Initially the lot of 150 eyes was divided in normal and pathologic (Table 5) taking as indicator the average thickness of RNFL. As mentioned before, in these two groups we knew from previous studies, which are the healthy eyes (with RNFLavg normal) and which are the eyes with glaucoma (with damage of the RNFLavg).
   Using the criterion RNFLavg one case has been declared normal, without lesions, if RNFLavg thickness is higher than 94 μm, and pathologic if RNFLavg thickness is lower than 94 μm. The group of 150 eyes was divided in 69 % normal eyes and 31% pathologic eyes with RNFLavg in lesion quotas.

| Eye analyzed (150 eyes) | | RNFLavg | Glaucoma classification |
|---|---|---|---|
| Number | % | | |
| 103 | 69% | > 94 μm | Normal |
| 47 | 31% | < 94 μm | Pathologic |

Table 4. Classification of the eyes depending of RNFLavg

b. The group of 150 normal and pathologic eyes was also divided from the pressure stress point of view. According to the criterion IOPcc (Table 5) a case is declared normal (without risk of load pressure effort) if IOPcc is lower than 20 mmHg and pathologic (with risk) if IOPcc is higher than 20 mmHg. The studied group had a percentage distribution of 73 % eyes with IOPcc in normal quotas and 37 % eyes with IOPcc in pathologic quotas.

| | | | | | |
|---|---|---|---|---|---|
| IOPcc (mmHg) | Normal | | < 20 mmHg | 109 | 73% |
| | Pathologic | Suspect | 20 - 30 mmHg | 32 | 21% |
| | | Sure | > 30 mmHg | 9 | 6% |

Table 5. Classification of the eyes depending of IOPcc

According to the φ (Table 6) criterion, a case is declared normal (without risk of RNFL effort) if φ is higher than 30 % and pathological (with risk) if φ is lower than 30 %. The studied group had a percentage distribution of 75 % cases with φ normal and 25 % cases with pathologic φ.

| | | | | | |
|---|---|---|---|---|---|
| φ (%) | Normal | | > 30 % | 112 | 75% |
| | Pathologic | Suspect | 18 - 30 % | 17 | 11% |
| | | Sure | < 18 % | 21 | 14% |

Table 6. Classification of the eyes depending of φ

c. The next step was to study the predictive value of φ and IOPcc in assessing the risk of illness (quantified with the change of RNFLavg) through the correlation parameters: PPV, NPV, and PLR (Table 7).

| Statistical index | test | value |
|---|---|---|
| PPV | φ | 0.82 |
| | IOPcc | 0.79 |
| NPV | φ | 0.92 |
| | IOPcc | 0.91 |
| PLR | φ | 0.92 |
| | IOPcc | 0.91 |

Table 7. Positive Predictive Value (PPV), Negative Predictive Value (PPV), Positive Likelihood Ratio (PLR)

Collected data were analyzed and we observed that all these indicators are statistically significant, with strong correlations for tests φ and IOPcc: PPV being ≤ 0.8, NPV and PLR > 0.9.

d. The sensitivity and specificity odds of φ and IOPcc were also assessed; the results of the tests applied to the lot of 150 eyes are presented in detail in Table 8.

| Statistical index | test | value |
|---|---|---|
| Sensitivity | φ | 0.78 |
| | IOPcc | 0.74 |
| Specificity | φ | 0.94 |
| | IOPcc | 0.93 |

Table 8. Sensitivity and specificity odds

It can be noticed that the sensitivity (positive in disease) of the two tests is > 0.7 and the specificity ("negative in disease") is also very good, being > 0.9.

e. The capacity of correlation between the two performed tests (φ and IOPcc) and the value RNFL avg. (as indicator of disease) with Pearson correlation index ( r ) (Table 9) has also been determined.

| Statistical index | test | value |
|---|---|---|
| Pearson index (r) | φ | 0.56 |
| | IOPcc | - 0.45 |

Table 9. Pearson correlation index (r)

The values in Table 9 show a reasonable negative correlation of -0.45 between RNFLavg and IOPcc, meaning that higher IOPcc is associated to lower RNFLavg. There is also a reasonable positive correlation of 0.56 between RNFLavg and φ, meaning that a lower φ is associated to lower RNFLavg.

The calculation of this indicator: the specific damping capacity is important for a more realistic estimate of the risk-loaded. For example, there have been situations in which patients with pathologic IOPcc > 30 mmHg but with normal φ > 30% do not have any RNFLavg lesion, and situations where IOPcc is normal < 20 mmHg but with pathologic φ < 18% which have low RNFLavg.

f. In the final stage of our study the ESS computerized analysis application was used and a quick quantification of the studied eyes was obtained (Table 10).

| | |
|---|---|
| ESS stage I | normal type: 100 eyes (66.67 %) |
| | 2L type: 11 eyes (7.33 %) |
| | 3L type: 1 eye (0.66 %) |
| ESS stage II | 2U type: 8 eyes (5.33 %) |
| | 2U-2L type: 6 eyes (4 %) |
| | 2U-3L type: 3 eyes (2 %) |
| ESS stage III | 3U type: 1 eye (0.66 %) |
| | 3U-2L type: 15 eyes (10 %) |
| | 3U-3L type: 5 eyes (3.33%) |

Table 10. The ESS computerized analysis results

### 7.2 Discussions

This study is the first clinical investigation that calls into question the system's efficiency to eliminate ocular pressure. The purpose of calculating the yield is a better estimate of the risk-loaded to prevent glaucomatous damage.

The statistic analysis on the presented lot showed a good correlation between specific damping capacity (φ) and the occurrence of lesions in the layer of retinal nervous fibers (indicator: RNFLavg). Considering the elements above, it is possible to make a complex clinical evaluation of the patients. After they were measured with the Reichert Ocular Response Analyzer, we found IOPcc and calculated specific damping capacity (φ). Introducing these data in the mentioned graphic, we established a certain stage and type of the stress for their eyes. We verified other clinical, structural or functional parameters to appreciate the presence or absence of glaucoma.

We propose ESS computerized analysis to be used in clinical daily practice to appreciate the φ as a very good indicator of the RNFL effort for an eye in a glaucoma suspect patient. There are many parameters to look for, when we try to distinguish between a normal and a glaucomatous patient. The variability between individuals and within an individual over a lifetime makes it difficult to appreciate the situation of a patient at one moment. The biomechanical properties of the eye structures are very important in assessing a glaucoma suspect, and there are many studies focused on these properties (Burgoyne et al., 2005). Measurements of the corneal biomechanical properties with the Ocular Response Analyzer give us an additional parameter for a better assessment of the glaucoma risk in a patient with a high IOP.

By now, nearly everyone recognizes that the current gold standard for measuring IOP, the Goldmann tonometer, has considerable flaws. The measured IOP is affected by corneal properties including rigidity, thickness, structure, hydration curvature and perhaps other factors not yet identified. The Ocular Response Analyzer is capable to provide pressure measurements that are less affected by corneal properties and give us additional information. O.R.A. is more accurate, faster and easier to use in clinical practice. The parameters determined by this device: IOPcc, CH, CRF, IOPg and the proposed specific damping capacity (φ) allow us a better appreciation of the risk-loaded. The main disadvantage of this device is the high price compared to applanation tonometer, and not his lack of reliability.

Taking into account the above-mentioned aspects, we make a step forward to introduce these data into our daily medical practice.

Recent studies (Sigal et al., 2005) show that IOP induces a certain amount of stress and strain on the optic nerve head and leads to apoptosis of the ganglion cells; this process depends on biomechanical properties of sclera and lamina cribrosa. Our stress grading system takes these findings into consideration and tries to contribute to a better assessment of the patient's glaucoma risk.

ESS computerized system represents an original contribution, complementary in glaucoma diagnosis; compared to previously reported methods, this grading ocular stress resulted from IOPcc and specific damping capacity values.

## 8. Conclusions

Our clinical algorithm for a glaucoma suspect patient includes the next steps:

1. The gathering of personal and clinical data

2. The IOP measurement with ORA
3. The automatic data acquisition in the proposed application
4. The classification of patients according to the ESS system (risk group / stage)
5. The decision regarding further surveillance / investigation / treatment

Further studies on corneal biomechanics and its clinical importance are indicated. We actually consider three research directions:

a. Validation of the method in a statistically representative number of patients. After O.R.A. measurements, patients are categorized using ESS grading system: normal, borderline and pathological indices. Each of them will follow a standardized protocol of investigation: optic nerve head photography, visual field and OCT - retinal nerve fiber layers, optic nerve head scan; this structural and functional analysis will show or not glaucomatous typical damages. The results and their statistical analyses will be in further papers.
b. Other factors responsible for a reduced damping capacity will be in study (Oncel et al., 2009). Besides referring to the increase/decrease of the rigidity in the ocular structures, which modify CH and φ, there are other specific illnesses responsible for this, as: keratoconus, endothelial corneal dystrophy Fuchs (Spoerl et al., 2005). Therefore, reduced CH or φ may be considered structural normal variation or possible signs of corneal pathology and other investigations are useful to be considered, such as: Specular Endothelial Corneal Microscopy (SEM), corneal topography or pachimetry, Zernike analysis.

Generally, increases of the corneal thickness will determine the increase of the damping capacity (CH), but this study does not take into consideration the establishment of correlations between φ and the amount of corneal thickness (CCT).

c. ESS system offers a dynamic model for treatment efficiency follow-up, because both IOPcc and φ are important to be normalized, to reach at a minimum stage in ESS. For example, patients with low φ : 18- 30 % , IOPcc over 20-25 mmHg, ESS stage over 2 have a greater risk for glaucomatous damages. On the other hand, patients with the same IOPcc, but greater φ over 30 %, ESS stage 1, have no risk for glaucomatous damage. The last described situation is necessary to be considered for an appropriate anti-glaucomatous treatment.

The proposed ESS computerized analysis method enhances the possibility to categorize automatically the examined patients as normal, borderline, or a pathologic. The two studied parameters: IOPcc and specific damping capacity φ are useful in daily clinical practice and reliable indicators of this disease.

Using the Effort Staging System (ESS) we have an objective and quantifiable instrument to categorize our patients' glaucoma suspects. We have the possibility to have an objective assessment of stress related to their eyes; for example - a high IOPcc associated with a high specific damping capacity is not as stressful for the eye as a medium IOP associated with a low specific damping capacity. The defined type of stress offers valuable information about the pathophysiological mechanisms in glaucomatous nervous damage (Kothecha et al., 2006)

## 9. References

Allingham R.R., K. Damji , S. Freedman, Moroi S. & Shafranov,G., (2005), *Shields' Textbook of Glaucoma Textbook of glaucoma – fifth edition*, pp 116-143, pp. 191-197, pp.328-347 Lippincott Williams & Wilkinspp, ISBN 9780781739399

Brusini P & Filacorda S. (2006), Enhanced glaucoma staging system (GSS2) for classifying functional damage in glaucoma, *Journal of Glaucoma*, Volume: 15, Issue: 1, pp 40-46, Lippincott Williams & Wilkinspp, ISSN 1057-0829

Burgoyne, C. F., Downs J. C., Bellezza, A. J., Suh, J.K. & Hart, R. T., (2005), The optic nerve head as a biomechanical structure: a new paradigm for understanding the role of IOP-related stress and strain in the pathophysiology of glaucomatous optic nerve head damage, Volume 24, Issue 1, pp 39-73, *Progress in Retinal and Eye Research*, Elsevier, ISSN: 1350-9462

Downs, C. J., Suh, J.K. F., Thomas, K. A.& Bellezza A. J., (2005) - Viscoelastic material Properties of the peripapillary sclera in normal and Early Glaucoma Monkey Eyes – *Investigative Ophthalmology & Visual science* Feb; 46(2):540-546, ISSN: 1552-5783

Demea, H., Demea, S., Holonec, R. (2008). A Corneal effort mapping system for glaucoma risk based on ocular response analyzer. *IEEE International Conference on Automation, Quality and Testing, Robotics*, Volume: 1, pp: 333-336, ISBN: 978-1-4244-2576-1, Cluj-Napoca, Romania

Spoerl, E., Boehm, A.G., Pillunat, L.E., (2005), The Influence of various substances on the biomechanical behaviour of Lamina cribrossa and peripapilary sclera, *Investigative Ophthalmology & Visual science*, 46(4), pp 1286-1290, ARVO, ISSN: 1552-5783

Ethier C.R., Johnson M. & Ruperti J. (2004)- Ocular Biomechanics and Biotransport: *Annual Review of Biomedical Engineering*,. Volume 6, pp. 249-273,

Jonas, J.B. & Budde, W.M., Diagnosis and pathogenesis of glaucomatous optic neuropathy: morphological aspects, (2000), Volume 19, pp 1-40 *Progress in Retinal and Eye Research*, Elsevier, ISSN: 1350-9462

Kevin, A., El-Sheikh, A. & Newson, T.(2004), Application of structural analysis to the mechanical behaviour of the cornea, Journal *of the Royal Society Interface*, Professor Leslie Dutton FRS, 1(1), pp 3-15,

Kothecha, A., Elscheikh, A., Roberts, C. R., Zhu, H. & Garway-Heath D. F., (2006), Corneal thickness and age related biomechanical properties of the cornea measured with ocular response analyzer, *Investigative Ophthalmology & Visual science*, 47(12), pp 5337- 5347; ISSN: 1552-5783

Luce D. & D. Taylor, (2006), Ocular Response Analyzer measures of corneal biomechanical properties and IOP, *Ocular Response Analyzer White Paper*, Retrieved from http://www.ocularresponseanalyzer.com/downloads.html.

McCrum, N. G., Buckley, C. P., Bucknall, C. B., (1997), Principles of polymer engineering, *Oxford University Press*, ISBN 0-19-856526-7.

Meyers M & Chawla K.K., (2008), Mechanical behavior of materials, *Cambridge University Press*, ISBN: 9780521866750

Oncel B., Dinc U.A., Gorgun E., Yalvaç B.I. Yeditepe (2009), Diurnal variation of corneal biomechanics and intraocular pressure in normal subjects. *European Journal of Ophthalmology*, 19(6), pp 798-803, ISSN 1120-6721

Sigal I. A., J. G. Flanagan, Inka Tertineeg and C. Ross Ethier, (2004), Finite Element Modeling of Optic nerve Head Biomechanics, Investigative Ophthalmology & Visual science, 45 (12), pp 4378-4387, ARVO, ISSN: 1552-5783

Sigal I. A., J. G. Flanagan, C.R. Ethier, (2005), Factors influencing optic nerve head biomechanics, Investigative Ophthalmology & Visual science, 46 (9), pp 4189-4199, ARVO, ISSN: 1552-5783

# 12

# Effects of High Altitude Related Oxidative Stress on Intraocular Pressure and Central Corneal Thickness – A Research Model for the Etiology of Glaucoma

Sarper Karakucuk
*Erciyes University Medical Faculty, Department of Ophthalmology, Kayseri*
*Turkey*

## 1. Introduction

Glaucoma is a progressive optic neuropathy resulting in axonal death and is a leading cause of blindness. Several factors play a role in this progressive cell loss.

Hypoxia and oxidative stress are among the risk factors for glaucomatous changes. Tissue stress is also very crucial in glaucoma. This fact is evidenced by stress proteins and heat shock proteins in glaucoma models (Tezel & Wax, 2007). A relatively undiscovered field, namely high altitude related oxidative stress has recently gained attention in glaucoma research.

High altitude, which is usually regarded as an altitude over 2,400m, has various effects on the human body. Mountaineers, outdoor sports enthusiasts, military as well as other personnel working at high altitudes are at risk and the detrimental effects caused by high altitude hypoxia can reduce their performance.

At high altitudes, atmospheric pressure gradually falls and the oxygen partial pressure decreases. The resultant hypobaric-hypoxia with an oxygen partial pressure < 60mmHg is the culprit for detrimental effects of high altitude. High altitude may lead to a constellation of symptoms including acute mountain sickness, or in extreme cases, high altitude pulmonary edema or high altitude cerebral edema. At high altitude, hypoxia, ultraviolet rays, cold and increased energy need are amongst other contributing factors.

The human eye is also affected by hypoxia at high altitude and extensive research is being carried out by various teams all around the world. Erciyes University Medical Faculty is located at the skirts of Erciyes Mountain (3,917m), Kayseri, Turkey. Inspired by the Turkish ophthalmic surgeon, Dr. Bozkurt Ergör (1927-2009), who had practised ophthalmology in Kayseri, served as the president of Turkish Mountaineering Federation and climbed to numerous peaks all over Turkey and the world, we carried research on high altitude ophthalmology at Erciyes University Medical Faculty Department of Ophthalmology (Ergör, 2011; Karakucuk et al., 2000, 2004, 2010). (Figures 1 & 2).

In this chapter, effects of high altitude on central corneal thickness and intraocular pressure will be reviewed and the topic discussed in the light of the relationship of these parameters with high altitude related oxidative stress.

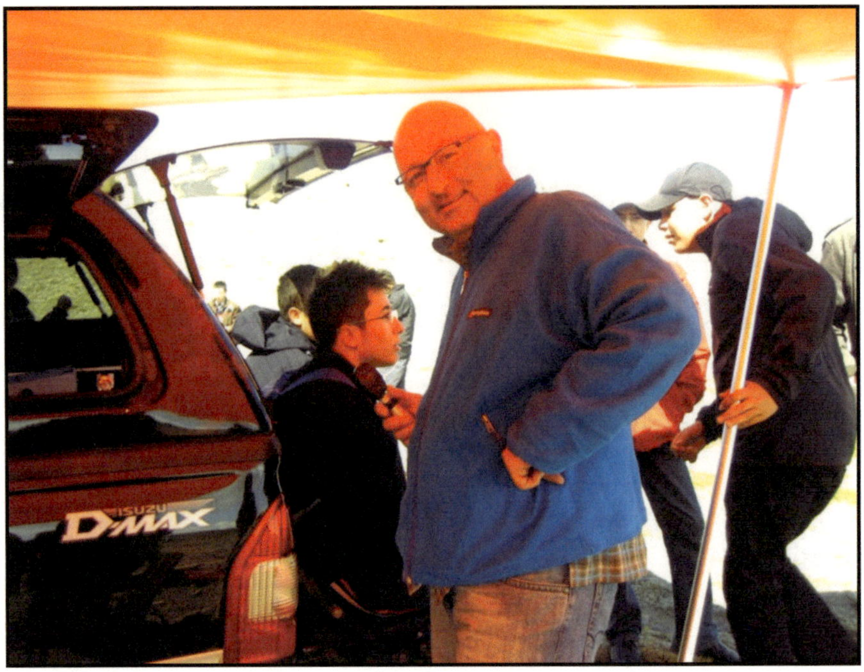


Fig. 1. Ophthalmoscopic examination is being made by the author at 2800m, (Mt. Erciyes, Kayseri, Turkey, Heine beta 200- direct ophthalmoscope). (Karakucuk et al., 2010)

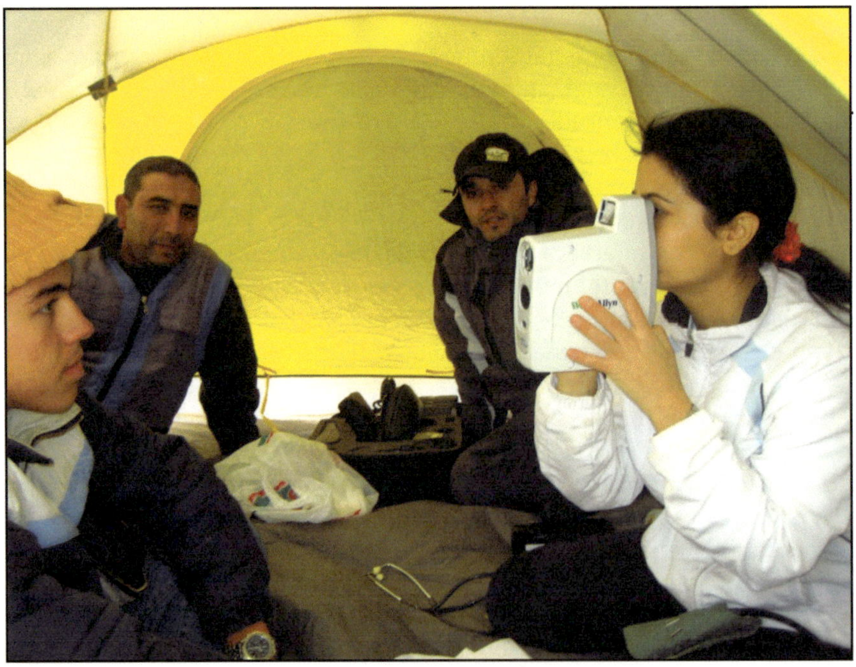

Fig. 2. Refractive changes are being evaluated inside the tent at 2800m (Mt. Erciyes, Kayseri, Turkey; Welch Allyn suresight). (Karakucuk et al., 2010)

The topic will be discussed as follows:

1. High altitude related oxidative stress and antioxidant defense mechanisms of the human body
2. Possible relationship of high altitude hypoxia with the etiopathogenesis of glaucoma
   i. Intraocular pressure changes at high altitude
   ii. Central corneal thickness changes at high altitude
   iii. Possible relationship of high altitude with pseudoexfoliation, cone cell sensitivity and visual fields
   iv. Future issues: Space travel and intraocular pressure

## 2. High altitude related oxidative stress and antioxidant defense mechanisms of human body

The capability of the defense network of the human body may be challenged by environmental conditions. High altitude related hypoxia is one of these great challenges. If the sea level O2 concentration is accepted as 100%, this ratio gradually decreases with increasing altitude. For example, in La Paz, Bolivia (3,660m), air pressure is 2/3 of the sea level, at Everest base camp, (around 6,000 m), air pressure is half the sea level and at the peak of Mt. Everest, the highest terrestial elevation (8,848m), air pressure is 1/3 of the sea level. In military or civil aviation, the performance of flight personnel heavily relies on the adaptive capacity of their body systems at high altitude. High altitude is usually regarded as an altitude over 2,400 m; cabin pressure during flight is usually kept around this 'safe' altitude. However, unpressurized flights, such as in small planes, military carriage aircrafts, or helicopters usually surpass this altitude and therefore occasionally detrimental effects can be seen on the personnel. There are several guidelines in worldwide aviation with regard to this matter; for example, according to the Turkish Airforce Commandership, only up to 2 hours of flying is allowed at 12,000 ft (3,657 m) when the cabin pressures are maintained at levels equivalent to the external atmospheric pressure (Bayer et al., 2004).

Despite well-defined regulations in aviation, hypoxia related incidents have been documented. A recent report stated that 3 fatal hypoxia incidents in US airforce have been observed during flights between 2001-2011 (Shender et al., 2011). In another study, hypoxic syncope in a helicopter pilot was reported at 18,000 feet (3,600 m). Although autonomic dysfunction did not cause any symptoms for this pilot during daily living, conduction block and vasovagal syncope developed at this high altitude (Chiang et al., 2011).

Temme et al., based on results from instructor pilots in a flight simulator, proposed that flight performance can be affected by hypoxia (Temme et al., 2010). This may necessitate oxygen monitoring via several methods such as pulse oximeter or near infrared spectroscopy during flight (O'Connor et al., 2004; Terry et al., 2004; Dillard & Bansal 2007). There are a number of guidelines for the pre-flight assessment of patients with pulmonary and/or cardiac diseases. However, these data are based on small studies. Therefore, Mortazavi et al. suggested that oxygen supplementation during air travel may be needed for individuals at risk (Mortazavi et al., 2003).

In light of the aforementioned facts, it is possible to say that the human body can be severely affected during flight even at moderate altitudes. In an attempt to reveal the effects of high altitude on the immune system, circulating cytokine levels were investigated by Burian et al. They searched for the changes in the levels of interleukin-1beta, interferon-gamma and tumor necrosing factor-alpha during flight, found that at a moderate altitude such as that felt inside the cabin, there is a subtle response compared to extreme altitudes (Burian et al., 2011).

Oxidative damage has also been the focus of interest at high altitude since high altitude also affects enzymatic as well as non-enzymatic systems in the body. (Chao et al., 1999; Imai et al., 1995). Reactive oxygen species are formed during stress conditions in the human body. When an extremely low availability of oxygen occurs, such as during ischemia or exposure to very low oxygen pressure, (for example at an altitude over 6,000 m), reactive oxygen species can exceed the capability of the defense mechanism, causing oxidative damage to lipids, proteins and to DNA. During heavy physical exercise such as mountaineering, different organ damage can occur as a result of oxidative challenge. High altitude exposure leads to altered activity of reactive oxygen species, which in turn leads to oxidative damage (Dosek et al., 2007).

When the human body is exposed to very low oxygen partial pressure (6,000m), cells tend to generate ATP. During this process, AMP is also generated but this AMP cannot be recycled; it is instead converted to hypoxanthine and via this pathway, xanthine dehydrogenase is converted to xanthine oxidase. Xanthine oxidase is a very potent reactive oxygen species generator and likely to occur during intermittent high altitude exposure. Reactive oxygen species increase in acute hypoxia but the balance is restored during the acclimatization process. This phenomenon may have relevance to the microcirculatory alterations associated with hypoxic exposure, including acute mountain sickness and high altitude pulmonary and cerebral edema. Despite our limited knowledge on acute mountain sickness, current information suggests that reactive oxygen species are active players in the process, however it is still not clear whether they are causative or associative agents. At high altitude, UV radiation is significantly increased and this also contributes to the overproduction of reactive oxygen species (Baconyi and Radák, 2004; Dosek et al., 2007).

It was found that 6 months of intermittent 4000 m exposure decreased mitochondrial superoxide dismutase in rat skeletal muscles (Radak et al., 1994). Nakanishi et al. reported that at 5,500m simulated altitude, superoxide dismutase immunoreactivity was increased in serum, whereas it was decreased in liver. This may suggest that liver may be sensitive to high altitude related oxidative stress (Nakanishi et al., 1995).

Highlanders may have lower gluthatione peroxidase levels than lowlanders; gluthatione peroxidase controls the thiol system. At high altitude, the capacity of enzymatic/non-enzymatic antioxidation systems is decreased. Ilavazhagan reported that Vitamin E supplementation reduced high altitude induced increase in lipid peroxidation during an experimental setting at 7,576 m (Ilavazhagan, 2001). Reactive oxygen species are not easy to measure because of reactivity, however, it is possible to measure them by several methods (Tarpey et al., 2004). For example, in a detailed experimental study by Maiti et al., rats were subjected to either 3 or 7 days of exposure to 6.100 m and increased reactive oxygen species and lipid peroxidation levels in brain tissue were detected (Maiti et al., 2006). Free radicals (mainly $H_2O_2$) were measured spectrofluorimetrically with the supernatant using 20,70-dichlorofluorescein-diacetate according to the modified method of Robinson et al. (Robinson et al., 1998); nitric oxide was measured by the accumulation of nitrites (NO2_) in supernatant from different brain regions, a method described elsewhere (Barrias et al., 2002; Mendoza et al., 1998); lipid peroxides are measured by quantitating the amount of malondialdehyde formed by 2-thiobarbituric acid reaction as thiobarbituric acid reactive substances using the method of Utley et al. (1967). It was also found that the magnitude of increase in oxidative stress was more in 7 day-exposure group as compared to 3 day-exposure group. (Maiti et al., 2006; Radák et al., 1994).

High altitude and strenuous exercise alone can result in oxidative challenge; the combined effect leads to aggravated oxidative damage. Increased physical activity at HA increases the

vulnerability of the body to oxidation (Bakonyi & Radák 2004). Møller exposed 12 healthy subjects to 4.559m; this caused significantly increased DNA strand breaks in urine. Another important factor is cold weather, which is frequently observed at high altitudes and this also increases the damage. For example, when people were simultaneously exposed to cold, the level of urinary lipid peroxides and DNA damage increased significantly (Møller et al., 2001).
In a study by Araneda, mountain bikers performing maximal cycloergometric exercise were first tested at 670m, then 2,160 m; soldiers climbing at 6,125 m in the Andes mountains of Northern Chile were also tested during the same study. In both groups, exhaled breath contained significantly more $H_2O_2$ levels and lipid peroxides compared to low altitudes. The pathology at the tissue level may be caused by localized free radical-mediated vascular damage, membrane permeability changes and the generated inflammation (Araneda et al., 2005).
On the other hand, at lower altitudes, for example at 1,860m, oxidative stress markers did not change in cyclists (Wilber et al., 2004). Lipid peroxides were found as elevated at high altitude; Joanny et al. reported that at 6,000m, lipid peroxides increased by 23% and at 8,848 m, by 79%. (Joanny et al., 2001). In experimental animal settings, it was found that a minimum of 3 months' exposure to high altitude was necessary to observe increased levels of lipid peroxides. At 13 months, the balance was found as normalized. (Dosek et al., 2007; Vij et al., 2005). Sinha et al. investigated antioxidant and oxidative stress responses of temporary residents at high altitude in different climatic temperatures. They found that oxidative stress markers exhibited higher levels in those with lower climatic temperature than the higher temperatures. They also concluded that chronic exposure to hypoxia in moderate climatic temperature has a potential preconditioning effect on the antioxidant system, but exposure to both cold and hypoxia causes greater oxidative stress due to altered metabolic rate. (Sinha et al., 2009).
Hagobian et al. researched the cytokine response at high altitude (4,300 m) and also investigated the effects of exercise and antioxidants at this altitude. They also aimed at detecting any alterations in plasma cytokine levels, such as interleukin 6 and C-reactive protein after antioxidant supplement, which composed of beta-carotene, alpha tocopherol, ascorbic acid, selenium, zinc, for three weeks. Although there was no increase in oxidative stress markers, elevated plasma levels of interleukin 6 and C-reactive protein was not attenuated by the antioxidant supplement, suggesting that this increase was independent from the oxidative stress pathway (Hagobian et al., 2006).
Kaur et al. found that a very short exposure of rats to 8,000m increased melatonin level in blood; it is important to note that melatonin acts as antioxidant (Kaur et al., 2002). On the other hand, natriuretic peptides were tested in 10 healthy lowlanders during an acute ascent to 5,200m Atrial natriuretic peptide levels did not changed significantly. (Toshner et al., 2008).
Magalhaes et al. investigated 6 mountaineers during a 3-week study. The study was carried out between 5,250-7,161 m. In their study, total antioxidant system, sulfhydryl groups, superoxide dismutase and glutathione peroxidase were studied. They concluded that a period of severe high altitude exposure during a Himalayan expedition constituted a systemic oxidative stress even to acclimatized climbers, with deleterious consequences such as quantitative changes in erythrocyte antioxidant enzyme activity and membrane fatty-acid profile. Erythrocyte antioxidant enzyme activity is determined by measuring superoxide dismutase, glutathione peroxidase and glutathione reductase; fatty acid profile is determined by measuring monounsaturated fatty acids, polyunsaturated fatty acids, saturated fatty acids and trans fatty acids (Magalhaes et al., 2005). It is known that

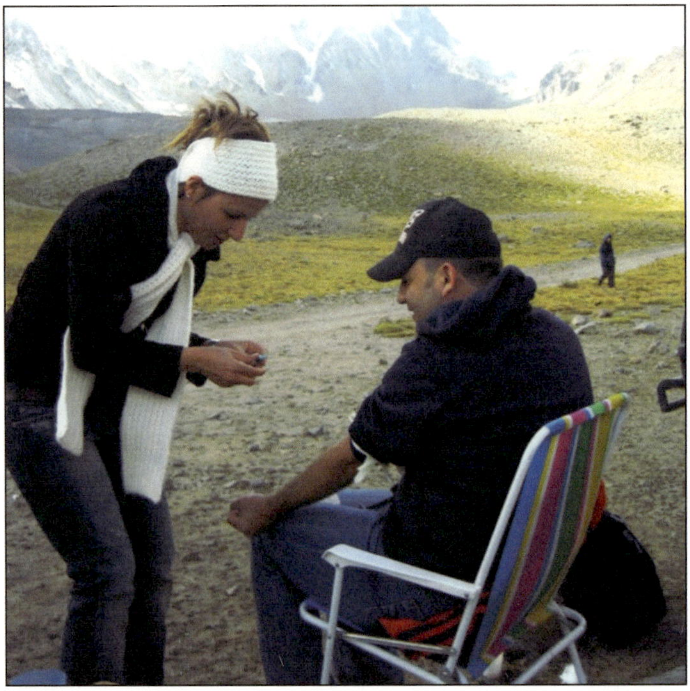

Fig. 3. Blood is drawn at 2800m, Mt. Erciyes. (Karakucuk et al., 2010)

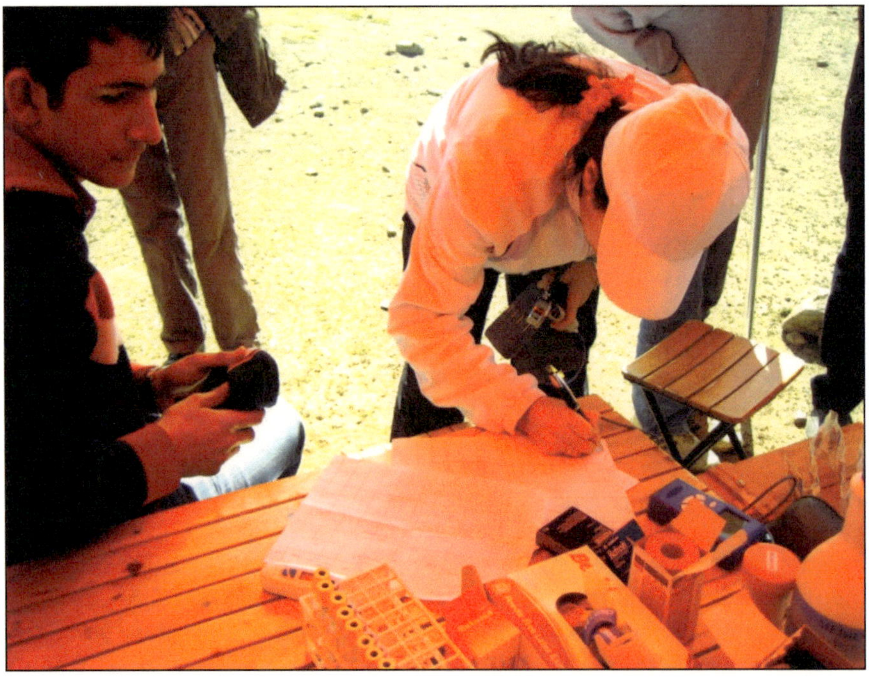

Fig. 4. Blood samples are analyzed and records made at 2800m; Mt. Erciyes. (Karakucuk et al., 2010)

although many Sherpas live at high altitudes for their entire lives, some of them surprisingly can manifest symptoms of acute mountain sickness during mountaineering at extremely high altitudes. Based on these findings, an interesting study was made by Droma et al.; they searched for the presence of hypoxia-inducible factor and von Hippel-Lindau tumor suppressor protein, which are putatively hypoxia sensors that control cellular responses to hypoxia. However, their study did not reveal such an association. Maybe another set of genes, or genetic mechanisms determines the susceptibility of individuals to high altitude (Droma et al., 2008).

Diet and oral antioxidant supplements may have a role in the body's response to high altitude. For example, Indians living at high altitude consume trichopus zeylanicus, which is an antioxidant, as a protection against the detrimental effects of high altitude (Tharakan et al., 2005). In one study, Schmidt et al. investigated the importance of antioxidant supplementation during high altitude related oxidative stress; they used a mixture of supplemented antioxidants such as Vitamin E, beta-carotene, ascorbic acid, selenium, alpha-lipolic acid, N-acetyl L-cysteine, catechin, lutein and lycopene at high altitude and reported that that this was effective (Schmidt et al., 2002). On the contrary, in some studies, antioxidant supplementation did not attenuate high altitude related oxidative stress (Subuthi et al., 2004).

Antioxidants in the human body can be measured from biological fluids which contain numerous compounds with chain breaking antioxidant activity, including urate, ascorbate, bilirubin, and thiols in the aqueous phase and alpha-tocopherol, carotenoids, and flavonoids in the lipid phase. Instead of measuring each antioxidant seperately, it is possible to measure the total antioxidant activity using the thiobarbituric acid reactive substances method described elsewhere (Koracevic et al., 2001). Total antioxidant level in normal healthy controls was reported as 2.42mmol/L in control subjects. (Olisekodiaka et al., 2009)

Since there is no single universal marker for protein oxidation, some macromolecules can be used as markers of oxidative stress; advanced oxidation protein products are among such macromolecules and can be analyzed using commercial kits with an Abbott C-16000 autoanalyzer, according to a method described elsewhere using spectrophotometry. Advanced oxidation protein products levels were expressed as micromolar chloramine-T equivalents (µmol/L) (Witko-Sarsat, et al., 1996; Baskol et al., 2008).

| | 1080m | 2800m | p |
|---|---|---|---|
| Total oxidative system | 3.32µmol H2O2 equiv/L (0.92-18.41) | 7.02µmol H2O2 equiv/L, (0.49-22.07) | 0.04* |
| Total antioxidative system | 2.13µmol H2O2 equiv/L (1.65-2.90) | 2.22µmol H2O2 equiv/L (1.72-2.77) | 0.30 |
| Advanced oxidative protein products | 195.58µmol/L, (84.77-663.16) | 220.74µmol/L, (103.81-667.35) | 0.03* |

Table 1. Oxidation and antioxidation parameters at normal (1,080) and high (2,800m) altitude; Mt. Erciyes. (Karakucuk et al., 2010; *statistically significant)

In one study, we measured blood levels of total antioxidant system, total oxidative system and advanced oxidative protein products as oxidative stress markers at 1,080 m and at 2,800 m in a group of 40 healthy individuals after an unacclimatized ascent to 2,800 m from 2,200 m at Erciyes Mountain. The results showed that there was a significant increase in levels of total oxidative system at 2,800m compared to 1,080 m ($p=0.04$). Advanced oxidative protein products also significantly increased at high altitude($p=0.03$). There was not a parallel increase in the total antioxidant system ($p=0.30$), suggesting that during acute unacclimatized ascent, antioxidant system cannot counterbalance the detrimental effects of the oxidant system (Karakucuk et al., 2010; Dolbun et al., 2010).

## 3. Possible relationship of high altitude hypoxia with the etiopathogenesis of glaucoma

Fast ascent during outdoor sports such as glacier skiing, heli-skiing, paragliding and parachuting has caused short acclimatization, making acute mountain sickness likely to occur with its consequences. This effect not only concerns skiers, skydivers, paragliders, and balloon travelers, but also participants in aviation and aerospace activities, particularly when unpressurized travel is to be made, such as helicopter or small aircraft flights. It is very important to note that results obtained in experimental settings, such as hypobaric high altitude chambers, do not always reflect geographical conditions; because in the real environment, strenuous exercise, cold and wind further complicate the issue.

### 3.1 Intraocular pressure changes at high altitude

Results with regard to the intraocular pressure (IOP) changes at high altitude are varying and somewhat confusing.

Ersanli et al. measured IOP in 34 healthy pilots at 792m and a simulated altitude of 9,144m. First, the subjects breathed 100% $O_2$ (hypobaric normoxia) at high altitude. Immediately after the measurement, the subjects removed their masks and IOP measurements were repeated with an inspired oxygen partial pressure of 47 mmHg (hypobaric hypoxia). Measurements were made by tonopen-XL. IOP at ground level in 68 eyes of 34 subjects was $12.31 \pm 2.98$ mmHg. It rose significantly to $16.75 \pm 4.14$ mmHg for hypobaric normoxia ($p = 0.003$). The value declined slightly to $14.37 \pm 3.44$ mmHg following mask removal at altitude, a value that was not significantly different from either the initial value ($p = 0.323$) or the mask-on value ($p = 0.195$). Following return to ground level, IOP was $12.81 \pm 1.74$ mmHg, statistically insignificant from the initial value. The authors concluded that healthy subjects whose baseline IOP is in the normal range experience only a small, temporary elevation of IOP during passive exposure to high altitude with either normoxia or acute hypoxia. The small rise in IOP seen in the healthy subjects might be much greater in older persons or those with limits on aqueous drainage, such as preexisting ocular hypertension or glaucoma. In addition, factors such as exercise and dehydration might alter the picture in mountains, especially when people are transported rapidly to a high elevation and then required to undertake various activities like heliskiing or paragliding. These results can also lead to the conclusion that during climbing to high altitude with oxygen masks, intraocular pressures can rise to significant levels and this may be important for climbers with ocular hypertension or glaucoma (Ersanli et al., 2006).

We also reported a nonsignificant rise in IOP at 3,932 m on Mount Kackar; in that study the measurements were made by Schiotz tonometer (Karakucuk & Mirza, 2000) (Figure 5). This type of tonometer is gravity dependent and therefore may not always be suitable for high altitude environments. The Tono-Pen XL, on the other hand, has been used in hypobaric environments and has been suggested to be unresponsive to changes in atmospheric pressure. In our following studies, we continued our intraocular pressure measurements with Tonopen and again obtained a similar rise (Karakucuk et al., 2010).

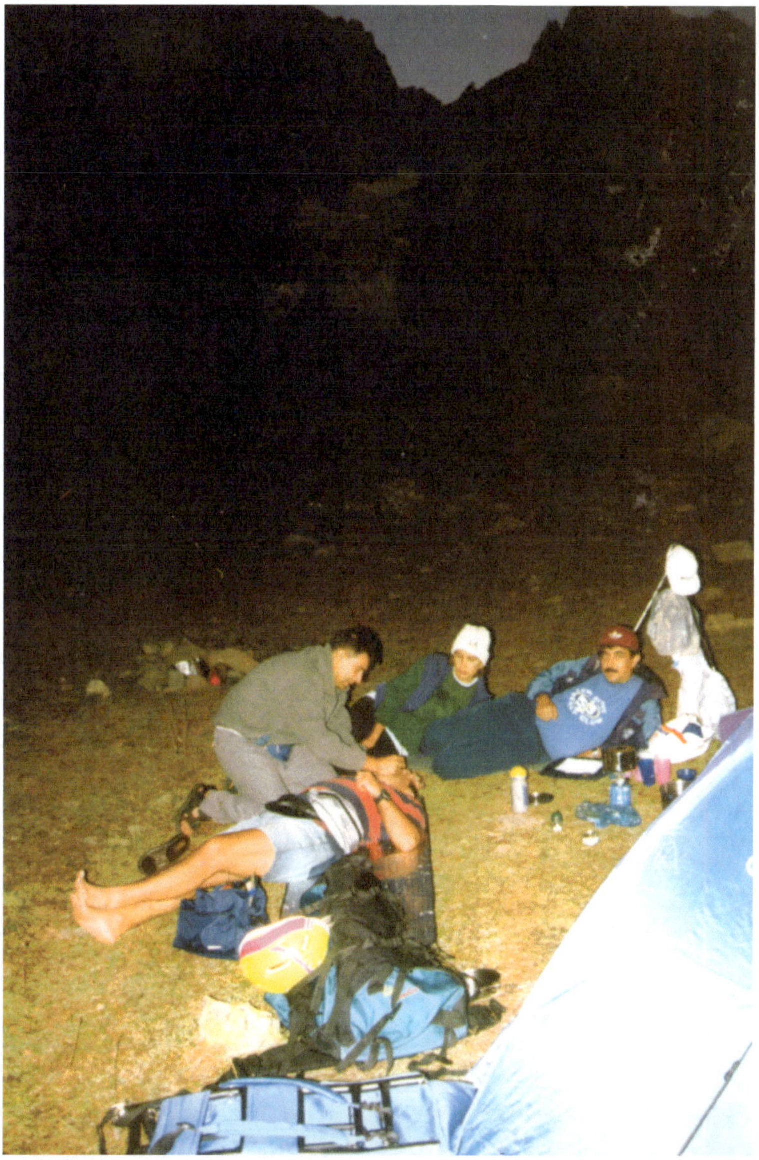

Fig. 5. IOP is being measured at Kaçkar mountains; Black Sea-Turkey. (Schiotz tonometer, Riester, Germany) (Karakucuk & Mirza, 2000)

Bayer et al. reported that in an unpressurized aircraft at 3,048 m, healthy subjects showed no significant change in IOP (Bayer et al., 2004). Another study also suggested that flying seems not to alter IOP in normal subjects. (Ayala et al., 2010).

Pavlidis et al. searched for intraocular pressure changes during high altitude acclimatization in healthy climbers between 500m and 5,050m. The mountaineers climbed with a gradual ascent, with rest stops and acclimatization days which were similar to that used by most trekkers in the Karakoram region to improve physiological acclimatization and reduce the incidents of serious acute high-altitude sickness. The climbing protocol of the expedition was as follows: day 1, from Skardu (2,286m) to Skardu lake (3,986m) by trekking and off road; day 2, transportation to Askole (2,900m); day 3, trek to Jola (3,100m); day 4, trek to Paju (3,350m); day 5, trek above Paju (3,850m) and return; day 6, trek to Urdukas (4,000m); day 7, trek to Goro II (4,220m); day 8, trek to Concordia (4,450m); day 9, trek to Ali camp (5,050m); day 10, ascent to Gondogoro La pass (5,650m). The authors reported that IOP decreased in sudden ascents of more than 200m/day and recovered, following acclimatization, for ascents up to 200m/day. They concluded that IOP changes may be related to hypoxia-induced respiratory alkalozis and that the IOP fall is proportional with the fall of oxygen partial pressure and acclimatization. They also suggested that IOP changes could reflect intracranial pressure variations and can be used for monitoring acute mountain sickness, high altitude cerebral or pulmonary edema (Pavlidis et al., 2006).

We also searched for the effects of high altitude on the IOP and various vital functions such as $SaO_2$, blood pressure, pulse and temperature. Systolic and diastolic arterial pressure and pulse rate increased whereas body temperature decreased and these findings were statistically significant ($p<0.05$). There were no correlations between these parameters and the IOP (Karakucuk et al., 2010) (Table 2).

| Parameters | 1080m (mean) (n=40) | 2800m (mean) (n=40) | p |
|---|---|---|---|
| Partial arterial oxygen pressure (%) | 96 | 92↓ | <0.001* |
| Systolic blood pressure (mmHg) | 105 | 114↑ | <0.001* |
| Diastolic blood pressure (mmHg) | 63 | 73↑ | <0.001* |
| Pulse rate (n/min ) | 83 | 96↑ | <0.001* |
| Body temperature (°C) | 35,9 | 35,7↓ | 0,05* |

Table 2. Vital parameters at low (1,080m) and high altitude (2,800m); Mt. Erciyes (Karakucuk et al., 2010; *statistically significant)

In one study, IOP was found as decreased at hyperbaric conditions. It was also suggested that swimming goggles significantly increase IOP at sea level since they may compress the eyeball (Van de Veire et al., 2008). The IOP increase observed in swimmers may be due to goggle/face area; in one study, IOP increased while wearing goggles by a mean pressure of 4.5 mm Hg ($p<0.001$) with this pressure rise being sustained for the duration of goggles wear. A smaller goggle/face area ($p = 0.013$) was consistently associated with greater IOP elevation (Morgan et al. 2008).

In a prospective study which involved 25 healthy mountaineers who were randomly assigned to two different ascent profiles at Mt. Muztagh Ata (7,546 m/24,751 ft); group 1 was assigned to a shorter acclimatization time before ascent than group 2. IOP in both groups showed small but statistically significant changes: an increase during ascent from 490 m/1,607 ft to 5,533 m/18,148 ft and then a continuous decrease during further ascent to 6,265 m/20,549 ft and on descent to 4,497 m/14,750 ft and to 490 m. The authors concluded that hypobaric hypoxia at very high altitude leads to small but statistically significant changes in IOP that are altered by systemic oxygen saturation (Bosch et al., 2010a).

Karadag et al. searched whether IOP changes at hypobaric hypoxic exposure are related to plasma pro-brain natriuretic peptide levels. They found that IOP increased at high altitude, however, proBNP levels did not have any significant differences (Karadag et al., 2010). Somner et al. reported that acute exposure to high altitude caused a statistically significant increase in IOP which returned to baseline levels with prolonged exposure to altitude. They concluded that observed changes in IOP may partially be explained by the change in central corneal thickness and are not predictive of symptoms of acute mountain sickness or development of high altitude retinopathy (Somner et al., 2007).

Karadag et al. reported that a short-term hypobaric hypoxic exposure caused a significant increase in IOP in healthy participants. As opposed to Somner et al., Karadag and associates concluded that this significant increase in IOP cannot be solely explained by a central corneal thickness-related overestimation error at high altitude. They also concluded that individuals with IOP-related disorders such as glaucoma should be cautious during high altitude exposure (Karadag et al., 2008).

### 3.2 Central corneal thickness changes at high altitude

Central corneal thickness is also shown to be affected by high altitude related hypoxia in many studies.

Bosch et al. investigated the effects of increasing altitude up to 6,265 m on healthy mountaineers. There was a statistically significant relationship between central corneal thickness increase and cerebral acute mountain sickness score. They found that adhering to a slower ascent profile results in less corneal edema. They concluded that corneal swelling is aggravated by low oxygen partial pressure. They also concluded that individuals with acute mountain sickness related symptoms had thicker corneas. Carbonic anhydrase is also found in cornea endothelium; they suggested that carbonic anhydrase inhibitors can negatively affect endothelial safety and must be cautiously used (Bosch et al., 2010b).

In our study at Erciyes Mountain, we also found a statistically significant increase in central corneal thickness at high altitude. There was a correlation with increased IOP on right eyes ($p=0.05$) whereas no such correlation was found on left eyes ($p>=0.05$; Fig. 6 & Table 3) There was not a significant correlation between central corneal thickness and any of the blood oxidation or antioxidation parameters studied (Karakucuk et al., 2010; Dolbun et al., 2010) (Fig. 6; Table 3).

Our results are in accordance with Morris et al. who also investigated central corneal thickness at high altitude in their Apex 2 study, during which an ascent was made to Chacaltaya cosmic research center (5,200m) and ultrasound pachymetry was made. Mean central corneal thickness increased significantly from 543 to 561 microns. Endothelial dysfunction causing stromal swelling was suggested as the causative agent for stromal edema. In their study, central corneal thickness increased 3.5% on day 1, 4% on day 3, 5% on day 7 (Morris et al., 2007). In an attempt to enlighten endothelium damage seen at altitude

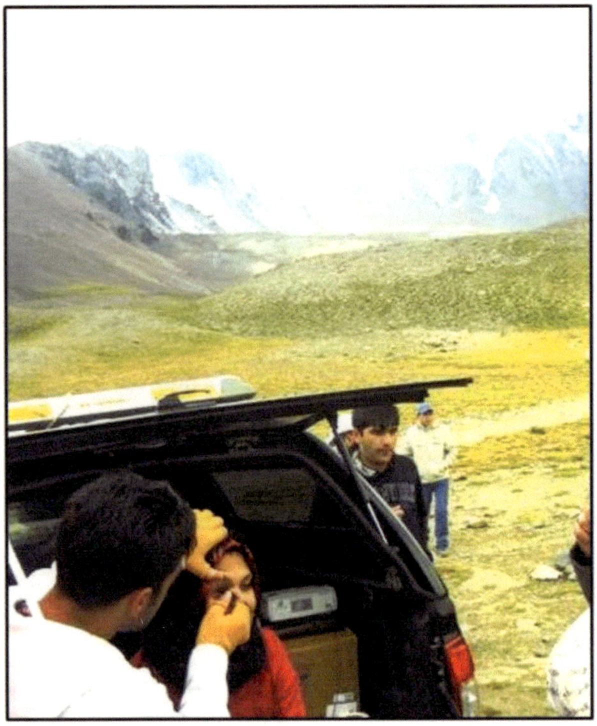

Fig. 6. Central corneal thickness measurements are made at 2800 m *(accutome-occupach5)* (Karakucuk et al., 2010)

| | 1080 m | 2800m | p |
|---|---|---|---|
| IOP-right eyes | 13.22±2.74 mmHg | 14.45±3.54mmHg | =0.05* |
| IOP-left eyes | 13.9± 3.0 mmHg | 14.3± 3.6 mmHg | >0.05 |
| Central corneal thickness-right eyes | 549±31.9µm | 555±31µm | <0.05* |
| Central corneal thickness-left eyes | 550±32.4µm | 554±30µm | <0.05* |

Table 3. IOP and central corneal thickness changes at low and high altitude. (Karakucuk et al., 2010; *statistically significant)

related hypoxia, ultrastructural analysis of the rat cornea revealed that a 30 day-stay at 5,500m brought about no changes on epithelium; on the other hand, stroma was hydrated, thickened and endothelium was damaged. Descemets membrane was also thickened (Mastropasqua et al. 1996). In another study, increased corneal vasoendothelial growth factor and cytochrome p450 were suggested as the causative factors (Mastyugin et al., 2001).

Karadag et al. investigated 70 eyes of 35 subjects from two different age groups. Measurements were carried at 792m and at a simulated altitude of 9,144m. A short term hypobaric hypoxia exposure increased central corneal thickness significantly in the older age group (Karadag et al., 2009).

Di Blasio et al. investigated central corneal thickness measurements in hypobarism and suggested treatment of corneal edema with hyperosmotic agents. They found evidence that after 20 min of staying at 25,000ft, the decrease of barometric pressure produces a significant stromal and epithelial edema and that this can be treated with a hyperosmotic solution (Di Blasio et al., 2011) which may be of practical importance for those exposed to high altitudes.

### 3.3 Possible relationship of high altitude with pseudoexfoliation, cone cell sensitivity and visual fields

Kozobolis et al. suggested that a correlation between increased pseudoexfoliation prevalence and high altitude may exist since they reported a higher incidence of pseudoexfoliation in Crete highlanders (Rethymnon 27%) as opposed to lowlanders (Heraklion %11.5, Chania 13.4% and Lasithi 16.9%) (Kozobolis et al., 1997). In another similar study, Jones et al. found an increased occurrence of pseudoexfoliation in males in a Spanish American population of New Mexico and proposed a geographic climatic theory that relates pseudoexfoliation to greater solar radiation levels due to a high overall altitude (Jones et al., 1992).

Horng et al. evaluated black-and-white visual field sensitivity during acute exposure to a simulated altitude of 7,620m in fifteen healthy male pilots with an age range of 26 - 39 yr. They measured arterial oxygen saturation using transdermal pulse oximetry with an oximeter clamped to the distal phalanx of the right middle finger of the subjects, while the visual field was measured within a 30° eccentricity in the right eye by using the quick mode of an SBP-3000 computerized perimeter. The pilots breathed 100% $O_2$ for 30 min before and during chamber ascent, then removed their masks while measurements were performed. Mean visual sensitivity was significantly reduced; peripheral sensitivity was significantly more diminished than central sensitivity. The different resistance of the cone cell system and the rod cell system functions to oxygen deprivation might account for this finding (Horng et al., 2008).

We also investigated the response of the cone cell system to altitude related hypoxia in sixteen healthy high school students, aged between 14 and 17 yr. Their color vision was examined with the Farnsworth-Munsell 100-Hue test at 1060 and 3000 m. It was found out that there was a statistically significant increase in the total number of errors ($p = 0.001$) as well as in the number of errors in sector 1 ($p = 0.007$) and sector 3 ($p = 0.013$) at 3,000 m when compared with 1,060m. We concluded that altitude related hypoxia resulted in a color vision deficit with a reduced cone sensitivity at the blue-yellow range (Karakucuk et al., 2004).

### 3.4 Future issues – Space travel and intraocular pressure

Microgravity is a term more or less a synonym for weightlessness and zero-gravity, but indicates that g-forces are not quite zero, just very small. It is a measure of the degree to which an object in space is subjected to acceleration. *Micro* indicates accelerations equivalent to one millionth ($10^{-6}$) of the force of gravity at Earth's surface. The symbol for microgravity, $\mu g$, was used on the insignia of Space Shuttle flight STS-87 because this flight was devoted to microgravity research (Harland 2011). Microgravity also has impacts on the IOP; it is known that IOP increases rapidly in microgravity. In an attempt to measure IOP through the eyelid during a space mission, a hardware, KARI was used (Jennings et al., 2010).

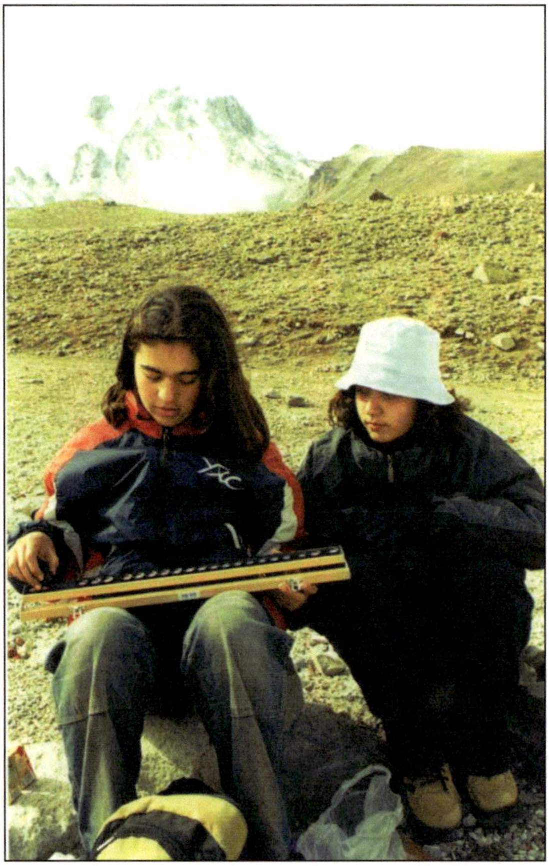

Fig. 7. Farnsworth-Munsell-100 Hue test is being performed on healthy young individuals at 3000m, Mt. Erciyes. (Karakucuk et al., 2004)

If a candidate for space travel has a potential risk for glaucoma, he or she may sustain significant glaucomatous damage during space flight likely to cause incapacitation. Currently, there is no established protocol to predict the possibility of glaucoma during space flight. Normally, head down posture, similar to that in space flight is demonstrated to increase IOP (Baskaran et al., 2006). Xu et al. modified a 'head down rest' test to predict the occurrence of ocular hypertension and glaucoma in astronaut and space tourist selection; they also investigated whether myopic subjects are more sensitive to microgravity than normal subjects. They concluded that myopes are more susceptible to the head down position and they may possess a risk factor for developing ocular hypertension and possibly glaucoma when exposed to microgravity (Xu et al., 2010).

## 4. Conclusion

It is clearly seen from the above mentioned studies that oxidative stress has a deep impact on the human body and the human eye is affected by altitudes over 2,400m, commonly regarded as high altitude. In an attempt to evaluate the effects of high altitude on antioxidant parameters and intraocular pressure, as well as central corneal thickness, we found that oxidative stress markers, total oxidative system and advanced oxidative protein products are increased, along with IOP during acute exposure to hypoxic environment at high altitudes and that antioxidant system may have a limited capacity to counterbalance this effect due to acute unacclimatized ascent (Karakucuk et al., 2010).

Taken all together, despite conflicting results from various centers, it is possible to say that intraocular pressure and central corneal thickness are affected by low atmospheric pressure at high altitudes. People with preexisting ophthalmological pathologies such as ocular hypertension or glaucoma must be very cautious when they are exposed to these altitudes. Acclimatization is crucial before strenuous high altitude activities. When acute unacclimatized ascent is inevitable, either in mountaineering or aviation, functions of the human eye which rely on the integrity of color vision, visual field, intraocular pressure and corneal thickness must be cautiously evaluated. In the next era when space flights will be more accessible to the inhabitants of our planet, effects of microgravity on intraocular pressure of the human eye will probably be the main topic of interest.

## 5. Acknowledgment

I am grateful to the academic personnel, residents, technicians and nurses of Erciyes University Medical Faculty Department of Ophthalmology. Valuable scientific support of EVER (European Association for Vision and Eye Research) and the research grant from the AAC (American Alpine Club) is greatly acknowledged. I thank my mountaineer friends from Kayseri Alpine Club and mountain guides from Mt. Erciyes region for their support and participation during related mountaineering activities. Finally, my thanks go to my daughters for their support during my studies.

## 6. References

Araneda OF., García C., Lagos N., Quiroga G., Cajigal J., Salazar MP & Behn C.(2005). Lung oxidative stress as related to exercise and altitude. Lipid peroxidation evidence in exhaled breath condensate: a possible predictor of acute mountain sickness. *Eur J Appl Physiol* 95: 383-90.

Ayala M., Högbeck IL & Chen E. (2010). Intraocular pressure changes during flight 9th European Glaucoma Society Congress, 12-17 September, 2010, Madrid.

Bakonyi T & Radák Z. (2004). High altitude and free radicals. Journal of Sports Science and Medicine 3: 64-69.

Barrias JAG., Escalante B., Valdes J., Bertha A., Chavez L & Fong DM. (2002). Nitric oxide and nitric oxide synthases in the fetal cerebral cortex of rats following transient uteroplacental ischaemia. *Brain Res.* 945:114–122.

Baskaran M, Raman K, Ramani KK, Roy J, Vijaya L & Badrinath SS. (2006). Intraocular pressure changes and ocular biometry during sirsasana (headstand posture) in yoga practitioners. *Ophthalmology* 113:1327-32.

Baskol G., Gumus K., Oner A., Arda H & Karakucuk S. (2008). The role of advanced oxidation protein products and total thiols in diabetic retinopathy. *Eur J Ophthalmol* 18(5):792-8.

Bayer A., Yumusak E., Sahin OF & Uysal Y. (2004). Intraocular pressure measured at ground level and 10,000 feet. Aviat Space Environ Med 75:543–5.

Bosch MM, Barthelmes D, Merz TM, Truffer F, Knecht PB, Petrig B, Bloch KE, Hefti U, Schubiger G & Landau K. (2010a). Intraocular pressure during a very high altitude climb. Invest Ophthalmol Vis Sci 51:1609-13.

Bosch MM, Barthelmes D, Merz TM, Knecht PB, Truffer F, Bloch KE, Thiel MA, Petrig BL, Turk AJ, Schoch OD, Hefti U & Landau K. (2010b). New Insights Into Changes in Corneal Thickness in Healthy Mountaineers During a Very-High-Altitude Climb to Mount Muztagh Ata. *Arch Ophthalmol* 128(2):184-189.

Burian D., Vicky WL., & McNeely E. (2011). Circulating cytokine levels during exposure to commercial aircraft cabin altitude oxygen levels. *Aviat Space Environ Med* 82: 278.

Chao WH., Askew EW & Roberts DE. (1999). Oxidative stress in humans during work at moderate altitude. J Nutr , 129: 2009-2012.

Chiang K., Chu H., Yang C & Chiou W. (2011). Case report: 18000 feet hypoxic syncope in a helicopter pilot. *Aviat Space Environ Med.* 82: 328.

Dillard TA & Bansal AK.(2007). Commentary: pulse oximetry during airline travel. *Aviat Space Environ Med* 78:143- 4.

Di Blasio D., Guadagno A., Appiani GC., Tomao E & Pescosolido N. (2011). *Aviat Space Environ Med.* 82: 333.

Dolbun K., Çakır I., Başkol G., Kılıç E., Müjdeci M., Arda H & Karaküçük S. (2010). Investigation Of The Relationship Between Central Corneal Thickness And Some Oxidation System Parameters At High Altitude. XXII nd National Biochemistry Congress, Eskişehir, 27-30 October 2010.

Dosek A., Ohno H & Acs Z. (2007). High altitude and oxidative stress. Respiratory Physiology & Neurobiology 158: 128–131.

Droma Y., Ota M., Hanaoka M., Katsuyama Y., Basnyat B., Neupane P., Arjyal A., Pandit A., Sharma D., Ito M & Kubo Kl. (2008). Two hypoxia sensor genes and their association with symptoms of acute mountain sickness in Sherpas. *Aviat Space Environ Med* 79: 1056 - 60.

Ergör B. (July 2011); Agri, Mount Ararat. In: *Republic of Turkey, Ministry of Culture and Tourism; Mountaineering.* Date of Access: 11th July, 2011; available from: http://www.kultur.gov.tr/EN/belge/2-17324/agri---mount-ararat.html

Ersanli D., Yildiz S., Sonmez M., Akin A., Sen A & Uzun G. (2006). Intraocular pressure at a simulated altitude of 9000 m with and without 100% oxygen. *Aviat Space Environ Med* 77:704–6.

Hagobian, T A., Jacobs KA & Subudhi AW. (2006). Cytokine Responses at High Altitude: Effects of Exercise and Antioxidants at 4300 m. *Med Sci Sports Exerc* 38:276–285.

Harland DM. Microgravity; In *Britannica.* Date of Access: 11th July, 2011; *available from:* http://www.britannica.com/EBchecked/topic/1133197/microgravity.

Horng C-T., Liu C-C., Wu D-M., Wu Y-C, Chen J-T., Chang C-J & Tsai M-L. (2008). Visual fields during acute exposure to a simulated altitude of 7620 m. *Aviat Space Environ Med* 79: 666 - 9.

Ilavazhagan G., Bansal A., Prasad D., Thomas P., Sharma SK., Kain AK., Kumar D & Selvamurthy W. (2001). Effect of vitamin E supplementation on hypoxia-induced oxidative damage in male albino rats. *Aviat Space Environ Med* 72:899-903.

Imai H., Kashiawazaki H., Suzuki T & Kabuto M. (1995). Selenium levels and gluthatione peroxidase activities in blood in an andean high-altitude population. J Nutr Sci Vitaminol (Tokyo) 41:349-361.

Jennings RT., Garriot OK., Bogomolov VV., Pochuev VI., Morgun VV & Garriott RA. (2010). The ISS flight of Richard Garriott: a template for medicine and science investigation on future space flight participant missions. *Aviat Space Environ Med* 81:133 - 5.

Joanny P., Steinberg J., Robach P., Richalet JP., Gortan C., Gardette B & Jammes Y. (2001). Operation Everest III (Comex'97): the effect of simulated sever hypobaric hypoxia on lipid peroxidation and antioxidant defence systems in human blood at rest and after maximal exercise. *Resuscitation* 49:307-14.

Jones W., White RE & Magnus DE. (1992). Increased occurrence of exfoliation in the male, Spanish American population of New Mexico. J Am Optom Assoc 63:643-8.

Karadag R., Sen A & Golemez H. (2008). The effect of short-term hypobaric hypoxic exposure on intraocular pressure. Curr Eye Res 33(10):864-7.

Karadag R., Sen A., Golemez H. (2009). Age-related differences in central corneal thickness alterations caused by short-term hypobaric hypoxia. Cornea. 28(2):136-9.

Karadag R., Sen A., Yildirim N., Basmak H., Golemez H., Cakir E & Akin A. (2010). The relation between intraocular pressure change and plasma natriuretic peptide under simulated hypobaric conditions. *Indian J Ophthalmol* 58(3):195-8.

Karakucuk S & Mirza GE. (2000). Ophthalmological Effects of High Altitude. Ophthalmic Res 32:30–40.

Karakucuk S., Oner AO., Goktas S., Siki E & Köse Ö. (2004). Color vision changes in young subjects acutely exposed to 3,000 m altitude. *Aviat Space Environ Med* 75:364–6.

Karakucuk S., Müjdeci M & Baskol G. (2010). Response of the human eye against oxidative stress at high altitudes. European Association for Vision and Eye Research (EVER) Annual Meeting; 6-9 October 2010; Crete; Greece.

Kaur C., Srinivasan KN., Singh J., Peng CM & Ling EA. (2002). Plasma melatonin, pinealocyte morphology, and surface receptors/antigen expression on macrophages/microglia in the pineal gland following a high-altitude exposure. J Neurosci Res 67(4):533-43.

Koracevic D., Koracevic G., Djordjevic V., Andrejevic S & Cosic V(2001). Method for the measurement of antioxidant activity in human fluids. *J Clin Pathol* 54:356–61.

Kozobolis VP., Papatzanaki M., Vlachonikolis IG., Pallikaris IG & Tsambarlakis IG. (1997). Epidemiology of pseudoexfoliation in the island of Crete (Greece). Acta Ophthalmol Scand 75:726-9.

Magalhaes J., Ascensa A., Marques F. (2005). Effect of a high-altitude expedition to a Himalayan peak (Pumori, 7,161 m) on plasma and erythrocyte antioxidant profile *Eur J Appl Physiol* 93: 726–732.

Maiti P., Singh SB., Sharma AK., Muthuraju S., Banerjee PK & Ilavazhagan G. (2006). Hypobaric hypoxia induces oxidative stress in rat brain. *Neurochem Int* 49: 709-16.

Mastropasqua L., Ciancaglini M., Di Tano G., Carpineto P., Lobefalo L., Loffredo B., Bosco D., Columbaro M & Falcieri E. (1998). Ultrastructural changes in rat cornea after prolonged hypobaric hypoxia.J Submicrosc Cytol Pathol 30 (2): 285-93.

Mastyugin V., Mosaed S., Bonazzi A., Dunn MW & Schwartzman ML. (2001). Corneal epithelial VEGF and cytochrome P450 4B1 expression in a rabbit model of closed eye contact lens wear. Curr Eye Res 23:1-10.

Mendoza SA., Hong E & Escalante B. (1998). The role of nitric oxide in angiotensin II induced renal vasoconstriction in reno vascular hypertension. *J Hypertens.* 16:697–703.

Morgan WH., Cunneen TS., Balaratnasingam C & Yu CY. (2008). Wearing swimming goggles can elevate intraocular pressure. *Br J Ophthalmol* 92(9): 1218-21.

Morris DS., Somner JEA., Scott KM., McCormick IJC., Aspinall P & Dhillon B. (2007). Corneal Thickness at High Altitude. *Cornea* 26:308–311.

Mortazavi A., Eisenberg MJ & Langleben D. (2003). Altitude-related hypoxia: risk assessment and management for passengers on commercial aircraft. *Aviat Space Environ Med* 74: 922–7.

Møller P., Loft S., Lundby C & Olsen NV. (2001). Acute hypoxia and hypoxic exercise induce DNA strand breaks and oxidative DNA damage in humans. *FASEB J* 15: 1181-6.

Nakanishi K., Tajima F., Nakamura A., Yagura S., Ookawara T., Yamashita H., Suzuki K., Taniguchi N & Ohno H. (1995). Effects of hypobaric hypoxia on antioxidant enzymes in rats. *J Physiol* 15: 869-76.

O'Connor T., Dubowitz G & Bickler PE. (2004). Pulse oximetry in the diagnosis of acute mountain sickness. High Alt Med Biol 5: 341-8.

Olisekodiaka MJ., Bello TO., Onuegbu AJ., Olowookere CJ., Lebi OM., Omotayo LO., Igbeneghu I & Olugbenga-Bello AI. (2009). Evaluation of the serum total antioxidant status level in health workers exposed to low radiation doses in a large Nigerian Hospital. International Journal of Research and Reviews in Applied Sciences 1 (2): 152-156.

Pavlidis M., Stupp T & Georgalas I. (2006). Intraocular pressure changes during high-altitude acclimatization. *Graefe's Arch Clin Exp Ophthalmol* 244: 298–304.

Radák Z., Lee K., Choi W., Sunoo S., Kizaki T., Oh-ishi S., Suzuki K., Taniguchi N., Ohno H & Asano K.(1994). Oxidative stress induced by intermittent exposure at a simulated altitude of 4000 m decreases mitochondrial superoxide dismutase content in soleus muscle of rats. *Eur J Appl Physiol Occup Physiol* 69:392-5.

Robinson JP., Bruner LH., Basoe CF., Hudson JL., Ward PA & and Phan SH. (1998). Measurement of intracellular fluorescence of human monocytes reactive to oxidative metabolism. *J Leukoc Biol* 43: 304–310.

Schmidt MC., Askew EW., Roberts DE., Prior RL., Ensign WY Jr & Hesslink RE Jr. (2002). Oxidative stress in humans training in a cold, moderate altitude environment and their response to a phytochemical antioxidant supplement. Wilderness Environ Med 13: 94-105.

Shender BS., Mattingly CW., Warren MB., Coleman SM & Askew GK. (2011). Determination of the time multitask performance degrades during exposure to 7620m normobaric hypoxia. *Aviat Space Environ Med* 82: 327.

Sinha S., Singh SN., Saha M., Kain TC & Tyagi AK. (2009). Antioxidant and oxidative stress responses of sojourners at high altitude in different climatic temperatures. *Int J Biometeorol* 54:85-92.

Somner JEA., Morris DS., Scott KM., MacCormick JC., Aspinall P & Dhillon B. (2007). What Happens to Intraocular Pressure at High Altitude? *Invest Ophthalmol Vis Sci* 48:1622–1626.

Subuthi AW., Jacobs KA., Hagobian TA, Fattor JA., Fulco CS., Muza SR., Rock PB., Hoffman AR., Cymerman A & Friedlander AL. (2004). Antioxidant supplementation does not attenuate oxidative stress at high altitude. *Aviat Space Environ Med* 75:881– 8.

Tarpey MM., Wink DA & Grisham MB. (2004). Methods for detection of reactive metabolites of oxygen and nitrogen: in vitro and in vivo considerations. *Am J Physiol Regul Integr Comp Physiol.* 286(3):R431-44.

Temme LA., Still DL., & Acromite MT. (2010). Hypoxia and flight performance of military instructor pilots in a flight simulator. Aviat Space Environ Med 81:654-9.

Terry, O., Dubowitz G & Bickler P. (2004). Pulse oximetry in the diagnosis of acute mountain sickness. *High Alt. Med. Biol.* 5:341-348.

Tezel G & Wax MB. (2007). Glaucoma. *Chem Immunol Allergy* 92: 221–227.

Tharakan B., Dhanasekaran M & Manyam BV. (2005). Antioxidant and DNA protecting properties of anti-fatigue herb Trichopus zeylanicus. *Phytother Res* 19: 669-73.

Toshner MR., Thompson AA., Irving JB., Baillie JK., Morton JJ & Peacock AJ. (2008). NT-proBNP does not rise on acute ascent to high altitude. High Alt Med Biol 9:307-10.

Utley HG., Bergheim F & Hochstein P. Effect of sulfydryl reagents on peroxidation of microsomes. (1967). *Arch Biochem Biophys.* 118:29–32.

Van de Veire S., Germonpre P., Renier C., Stalmans I & Zeyen T. (2008). Influences of Atmospheric Pressure and Temperature on Intraocular Pressure. Invest Ophthalmol Vis Sci. 49:5392–5396.

Vij AG., Dutta R., Satija NK. (2005). Acclimatization to oxidative stress at high altitude. High Alt Med Biol 6:301-10.

Wilber RL., Holm PL., Morris DM., Dallam GM., Subudhi AW., Murray DM & Callan SD. (2004). Effect of FIO2 on oxidative stress during interval training at moderate altitude. *Med Sci Sports Exerc* 36:1888-94.

Witko-Sarsat V., Friedlander M., Capeillère-Blandin C., Nguyen-Khoa T., Nguyen AT., Zingraff J., Jungers P & Descamps-Latscha B. (1996) Advanced oxidation protein products as a novel marker of oxidativestress in uremia. *Kidney Int* 49(5):1304–1313.

Xu X., Li L., Cao R., Tao Y., Guo Q., Geng J., Li Y & Zhang Z. (2010). Intraocular pressure and ocular perfusion pressure in myopes during 21 min head-down rest. *Aviat Space Environ Med* 81: 418–22.

# 13

# Sleep Apnea and Glaucoma – Greater Risk for Blacks?

Ferdinand Zizi[1,2,3], Adnan Mallick[1],
Monika Dweck[2], Douglas Lazzaro[2] and Girardin Jean-Louis[1,2,3]
[1]*Brooklyn Health Disparities Center, Department of Medicine,*
*SUNY Downstate Medical Center, NY;*
[2]*Department of Ophthalmology,*
*SUNY Downstate Medical Center, NY;*
[3]*Sleep Disorders Center, Department of Medicine,*
*SUNY Downstate Medical Center, NY*
*USA*

## 1. Introduction

Review of the extant literature indicates that both sleep apnea and glaucoma are highly prevalent in the Black population [1,2]. They tend to occur earlier among Blacks and are associated with other metabolic diseases (e.g., obesity and hypertension). that are also highly prevalent in that ethnic group [3,4]. While technology for early detection and evidence-based treatment regimens exist for sleep apnea and glaucoma, sadly Blacks underuse them. Consequently, Blacks in underserved communities continue to bear the burden of those conditions, which have remained largely undiagnosed [5,6].

Whereas prevalence data convincingly show the risks for expressing sleep apnea and glaucoma are higher among Blacks, they are, nevertheless, not as likely to seek medical care as do Whites, even where there is no disparity in adequate medical coverage [7]. Effort should be made to explore the reasons why so few Blacks participate in sleep apnea or ophthalmic screening programs or are receiving timely diagnoses [8,9]. This paper attempts to provide background information supporting greater prevalence of glaucoma and sleep apnea for Blacks in the US. Furthermore, it suggests that if these two conditions were causally associated Blacks would be at greater risk for related comorbidities.

## 2. Prevalence of sleep apnea and glaucoma – Is ethnicity an important factor?

There are no population-based prevalence studies documenting the relationship between glaucoma and sleep apnea. However, clinical and survey data strongly suggest that glaucoma is one of the ophthalmic diseases with a hypothesized link to sleep apnea [10-16]. Below, data supporting the link between sleep apnea and glaucoma are reviewed. However, since no published studies specifically ascertained effects of ethnicity on associations of sleep apnea with glaucoma, we first examined evidence supporting ethnic differences in the prevalence of sleep apnea and glaucoma.

## 3. Epidemiology of sleep apnea

Sleep apnea is a serious, potentially life-threatening condition, characterized by repeated cessation of breathing while sleeping, due mostly to complete or partial pharyngeal obstruction [6,17]. Obstructive sleep apnea, the most prevalent of the sleep-disordered breathing constellation, has several cardio-respiratory features (e.g., loud snoring, loud gasps, and daytime breathlessness). [18-20]. Sleep apnea is also associated with a number of metabolic diseases [21-28], cardiac arrhythmias [18,19], cardiovascular disease [18,20], decreased quality of life [17] and early mortality [18,28]. It causes significant sleep disturbances and excessive daytime sleepiness [18,29], which often lead to road traffic and industrial accidents [18,27,30] as well as cognitive deficits and poor performance [31]. Sleep apnea is also associated with numerous psychiatric comorbid diagnoses including depression (21.8%), anxiety (16.7%), posttraumatic stress disorder (11.9%), psychosis (5.1%), and bipolar disorders (3.3%). [32].

Sleep apnea is thought to be as prevalent as adult diabetes and might affect more than 18 million Americans [6,33]. Others view it as big a public health hazard as smoking [34], in part because of associated residual daytime sleepiness [18,29]. The National Commission on Sleep Disorders Research estimated that sleep apnea is probably responsible for 38,000 cardiovascular deaths yearly, with an associated 42 million dollars spent on related hospitalizations [35]. Evidence shows that sleep-disordered breathing not only increases the risk of cardiovascular related deaths, but increases risk of overall mortality [36].

Using a respiratory disturbance index* of 10 or greater, the Wisconsin Sleep Cohort Study, an epidemiological study conducted among the U.S. adult population, estimated that sleep apnea affects as much as 15% of men and 5% of women between the ages of 30 and 60 years [25]. Estimates are even higher in this age group when laboratory polysomnographic criteria are used. The largest population-based polysomnographic study conducted in the U.S. revealed that 24% of men and 9% of women had significant sleep apnea [37]. In the clinical setting, the proportion of sleep apnea cases rises to 68% [22]. Sleep researchers and public health advocates have become concerned over the lack of attention paid to ethnic disparities in sleep apnea, as several important epidemiological and clinical findings have shown greater rates for minority groups.

## 4. Sleep apnea – Ethnic variations

Sleep apnea is highly prevalent in the Black population [1]. A community-based study comparing older Blacks and Whites showed that Blacks experienced severe sleep apnea with a relative risk twofold as great as that of their White counterparts [38]. It is noteworthy that ethnicity is associated with the presence of sleep apnea (Respiratory Disturbance Index [RDI] ≥ 30). independently of age, sex, and body mass index, three of `the main risk factors for sleep apnea [6,39]. Blacks with sleep apnea are often more obese and have significantly greater prevalence of hypertension and glaucoma than their White counterparts [40] (see Table 1 and Figure 1).

---

* The apnea-hypopnea index (AHI). or respiratory disturbance index (RDI). refers to the total number of apneas (complete cessation of breathing lasting ≥ 10 s). and hypopneas (50% reduction in airflow lasting ≥ 10 s, followed by $SaO_2$ desaturations). divided by the patient's total sleep time. The AHI or RDI provides a measure of the severity of sleep apnea.

| Ethnicity | 1991 | 1995 | 1998 | 2001 | 2006-8 |
|---|---|---|---|---|---|
| Black | 19.3 | 22.6 | 26.9 | 31.1 | 35.7 |
| White | 11.3 | 14.5 | 16.6 | 19.6 | 23.7 |

data obtained from the Center for Disease Control; values represent percent of cases (http://www.cdc.gov/mmwr/PDF/wk/mm5827.pdf)

Table 1. Trends in obesity by ethnicity

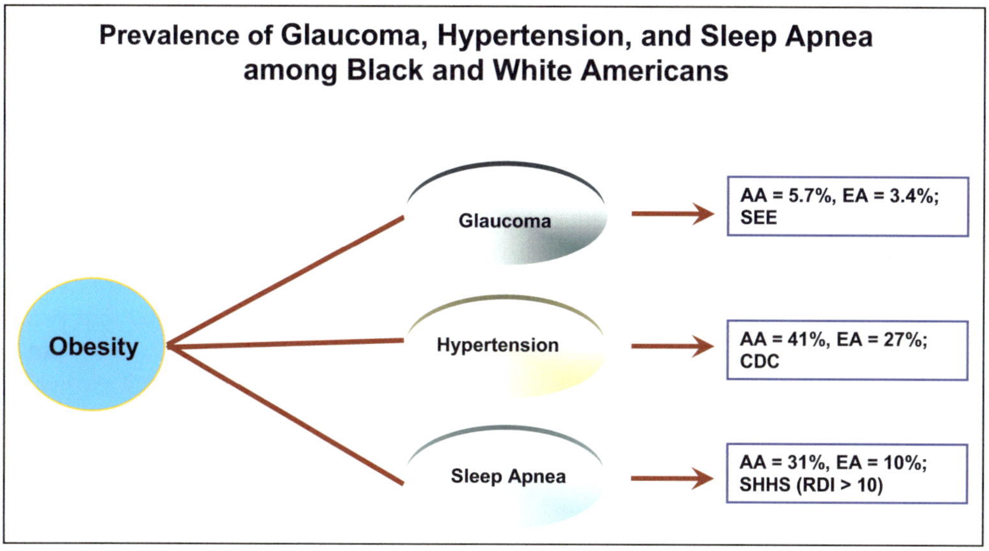


Fig. 1. Prevalence of glaucoma, hypertension, and sleep apnea for Blacks and Whites in the Salisbury Eye Study (SES), Center for Disease Control (CDC), and Sleep Heart Health Study (SHHS). All three conditions are linked to obesity, which is also more prevalent among Blacks (see Table 1)

This ethnic disparity is not observable only among adults who are 40 years old or older. A case-control family study of sleep apnea comparing 225 Blacks and 622 Whites, ages 2 to 86 years, indicated that 31% of Blacks versus 10% of Whites had RDI greater than 10 [1]. Also important in that study was the observation that Blacks may be at risk for sleep apnea at an earlier age. African-Americans with sleep-disordered breathing were younger than Caucasians with sleep-disordered breathing (37.2 +/- 19.5 years vs 45.6 +/- 18.7 years, $p < 0.01$). [1]. Observed ethnic differences in age of onset and anatomic risk factors for sleep apnea prompted the investigation of a possible racial/ethnic difference in the genetic underpinnings of this condition. Comparing Black and White families, investigators found evidence for segregation of a codominant gene with an allele frequency of 0.14; after adjusting for effects of Body Mass Index (BMI). and age, this accounted for 35% of the total variance in sleep apnea severity [41]. Other analyses by the same research group suggested genetic factors seem to underlie the susceptibility to sleep apnea and obesity among Blacks [42]; they suggest further that the severity of sleep apnea could modulate the genetic determinants of obesity in that ethnic group.

## 5. Epidemiology of glaucoma

Glaucoma is a disease defined by slow progressive loss of vision in association with characteristic signs of damage to the optic nerve. If left untreated, glaucoma leads to blindness, which could lead to sleep disturbances, diminished capacity in activities of daily living, reduced quality of life, and depressed moods [43-46]. Glaucoma is the leading cause of irreversible blindness among Blacks, and the second leading cause for all Americans [47,48]. Of the various forms of glaucoma (e.g., congenital, open-angle, closed-angle, secondary), primary open-angle glaucoma (OAG). is the most common, which affects almost 2.3 million Americans ages 40 and older, or about 1.9% of the U.S. population [49].

Glaucoma increases with age and is more common among Blacks than among Whites. According to data from the Center for Disease Control (CDC), ethnic differences in glaucoma for both men and women widened between 1984 and 1995 (see Figure 2). In the 65-69 age group, prevalence of glaucoma for White females is about 1.6%, while among Black females, prevalence is almost three times higher (4.6%). [49]. The Salisbury Eye Study showed that the prevalence of open-angle glaucoma for Blacks and Whites was 5.7% and 3.4%, respectively [2]. According to the Baltimore Eye Survey, which investigated a randomly selected, stratified, multistage cluster sample of 2395 Blacks and 2913 Whites (40 years of age and older), Whites were more likely to exhibit age-related macular degeneration, whereas Blacks primarily showed open-angle glaucoma [47]. This survey also showed that primary open-angle glaucoma accounted for 19% of all blindness among Blacks; this was six times as frequent among Blacks as among Whites and on average began 10 years earlier [47]. Interestingly, according to a population-based study the prevalence of glaucoma surgery among Blacks was 45% lower than the prevalence for Whites, although glaucoma is four times more prevalent among the former. [43]

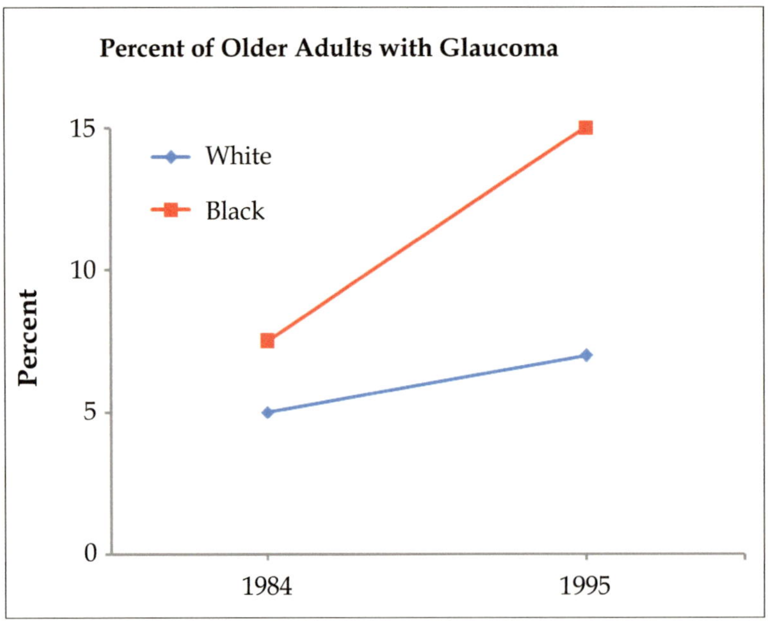


Fig. 2. Ethnic difference in glaucoma for both men and women is widened between 1984 and 1995; adapted from data obtained by the Center for Disease Control

## 6. Impaired regulation of ocular blood flow in glaucoma

The hypothesis that regulation of ocular blood flow might be impaired in glaucoma patients has received much attention since its inception in 1879. Principally, there are two competing theories purporting to explain the pathogenesis of glaucomatous optic neuropathy: the mechanical theory of glaucoma and the vascular theory of glaucoma. Technological advances have provided the impetus for several research studies examining the vascular theory. Essentially, it postulates that glaucomatous optic neuropathy results from inadequate blood flow caused by either increases in intraocular pressure or other risk factors that diminish ocular blood flow supply [50,51]. These two theories do not appear to be mutually exclusive. Both mechanical and vascular factors may converge to effectuate changes in intraocular pressure that might adversely impact perfusion of the retina and the optic nerve head [51,52]. It is equally likely that vascular dysregulations might increase the susceptibility to intraocular pressure (IOP).

Numerous clinical and epidemiologic studies converge to support the argument that deficits in ocular blood flow play a key role in the pathogenesis of glaucoma [50-55]. Indeed, population-based studies show an inverse relationship between ocular blood flow and intraocular pressure (Thessaloniki Eye Study). or associations between glaucoma and perfusion pressure (Barbados Eye Study, Baltimore Eye Study, and Neumarkt Glaucoma Study). [48,55,56]. A 9 year follow up to the Barbados Eye study indicated that lower ocular perfusion pressure [<40mmHg] more than doubled the risk for open angle glaucoma. (RR, 2.6; 95% CI, 1.4-4.6). [51]. With elevation of IOP, a linear and sensitive reduction in circulation through the short posterior ciliary arteries is commonly documented [55]. Some have argued that reduction of ocular blood flow often precedes reperfusion damage, and among glaucoma patients blood flow can also be reduced in other parts of the body.[53] Thus, ischemia and reperfusion damage do not seem to reflect hemodynamic changes only in vascular beds within the eye.

Numerous trials and reviews have discussed vascular dysregulation along with evidence for potential associations with Glaucoma. Dysfunction of both the autonomic nervous system and vascular endothelial cells might be a causal factor [52,54]. The underlying mechanism of the vascular dysregulations observed in glaucoma is not yet fully elucidated. Sleep apnea might also play a key role, as it produces myocardial infarction and/or nocturnal angina due to arterial vasospasm [57].

It is also important to note that even among patients with normal IOP, impaired blood flow may be observed. In addition, vascular compromise may occur in the presence of normal intraocular pressure if the lamina cribrosa, sclera, and cornea are thin [44]. A report by our colleagues at Indiana University indicated that glaucoma patients, who are otherwise characterized by normal pressure, exhibited prolonged retinal arteriovenous passage times in fluorescein angiography and color Doppler imaging, which suggests increased resistance downstream from the central retinal and posterior ciliary arteries [58]. This finding corroborates existing epidemiologic and clinical studies, evidencing that intraocular pressure may not be the only etiological factor in glaucoma [59]. Accumulating evidence points to ocular ischemia as a major factor as well [60]. Indeed, low perfusion pressure constitutes a significant risk factor for open-angle glaucoma, and most clinical studies comparing healthy and glaucoma patients demonstrate a reduction in perfusion pressure among the latter [50]. Authors of that review paper argue that the observed vascular dysregulation may be the principal element causing both low perfusion pressure and insufficient autoregulation. Newly available technology helps support this theory by allowing us to measure retinal blood flow rate. In a study of retinal blood flow in response to postural changes, patients with OAG were shown to have a very broad range of hemodynamic responses versus controls, suggesting dysregulation or no regulation of the retinal vasculature [54]. Thus, insufficient regulation could lead to low perfusion pressure as well as widely fluctuating perfusion pressures. Chronically low perfusion pressure and unstable, fluctuating pressures may in turn lead to ischemia and reperfusion damage [50].

## 7. Sleep apnea and glaucoma – Is there an association?

The link of sleep apnea to eye disorders has been reviewed recently [61]. Essentially, sleep apnea is linked to glaucoma [10-13], floppy eyelid syndrome [16,62], keratoconus [63], papilledema [64], and optic neuropathy [65]. In the present paper, we focus on glaucoma because it disproportionately affects individuals of the Black ethnicity, offering opportunities for research in its biologic and cultural underpinnings.

Examination of published reports on the link between glaucoma and sleep apnea has indicated that the prevalence of glaucoma among patients with sleep apnea ranges from 2% to 7.2% [11,14,15]. A recent cross-sectional case series suggested that as much as 27% of patients with moderate to severe sleep apnea might have glaucoma [66]. There is a lack of consensus whether the prevalence of glaucoma among patients with sleep apnea is greater than observed in the general population [15]. The discrepancy in reported findings amply demonstrates the need for random and representative, population-based studies to determine whether in fact patients with sleep apnea are at increased risks for developing glaucoma. Results of previous studies have limited generalizability because of selection bias, non-representative sampling, and small sample sizes. A recent Chicago study using a relatively larger sample size of 247 indicated the prevalence of glaucoma among patients with sleep apnea to be 5.7% [10].

Regarding the prevalence of sleep apnea itself among patients with glaucoma, no large-scale representative studies have been undertaken. Available estimates of the prevalence of sleep apnea among patients with glaucoma (ages 45 years and older). range from 20.0% to 57% [12,13]. Within glaucoma subtypes, approximately half of the patients with normal-tension glaucoma and one-third of those with primary open-angle glaucoma exhibit sleep apnea syndrome [67]. As noted previously, these results have not been replicated in the general population. If confirmed, this would support the argument that a sleep history should be recommended for patients with glaucoma [16].

## 8. Complex relationships between sleep apnea and glaucoma

The relationships between glaucoma and sleep apnea are somewhat complex. Several systematic studies are necessary to explicate fully the nature of those relationships. Clinical studies typically show that sleep apnea is associated with several glaucoma indices including intraocular pressure, visual field mean deviation, cup-to-disk ratios, and retinal nerve fiber layer thickness [68-70]. Additionally, evidence from a treatment study using ocular oxymetry recording, a novel tool utilized to measure ocular oxygen tension [71], suggests an association between finger blood flow and optic nerve head blood flow among patients with glaucoma. [72] Other preliminary data show reduction in intraocular pressure among glaucoma patients following a regimen of continuous positive airway pressure [73].

Hence, observational and clinical data converge to support an association between sleep apnea and glaucoma. Nonetheless, systematic studies are needed to establish the causal relationships between these two conditions. Though a direct relationship has not yet been established, data from a recent study makes an effort to imply some correlation. The study splits Sleep apnea patients up into a normal/mild group and a moderate/severe group. The prevalence of Glaucoma in the moderate/severe group was estimated to be 7.1%, significantly higher (p=.033). than the normal/mild group [10]. This study also suggested the severity of obstructive sleep apnea to be inversely correlated with the retinal nerve fiber layer thickness.

Delineating the nature of relations between sleep apnea and ophthalmic diseases remains a challenge. It is worth examining whether there is a direct influence of sleep apnea and glaucoma on ocular blood flow. Conceivably, glaucoma and sleep apnea have an interactive effect on ocular blood flow dysregulations. Preliminary data obtained from 31 patients with sleep apnea undergoing orbital doppler ultrasonography suggests a positive correlation between the ophthalmic artery resistivity index and the mean visual field defect, pointing to the possibility that visual field defects might be due to optic nerve perfusion defects [74]; of note 12.9% of the patients with glaucoma in that study had sleep apnea. These data are consistent with a previous study indicating that blood flow parameters in the orbital vessels were significantly different between patients with sleep apnea and those without the condition [75]. Specifically, among patients with mild sleep apnea, peak systolic velocity and end diastolic velocity in the posterior ciliary arteries were significantly higher than those observed for the control group [75]. In the next two sections, we discuss the effects of hypertension and obesity on the relationships between glaucoma and sleep apnea and the hypothesized effects of sleep apnea on ocular blood flow.

Since available studies do not permit an examination of ethnic effects on associations between sleep apnea and glaucoma, we rely on prevalence data to determine whether Blacks are at greater risk for related comorbidity. Epidemiologic evidence strongly supports the notion that both sleep apnea and glaucoma are highly prevalent among Blacks, and younger Black individuals are particularly more vulnerable [1,40,41]. Although not yet verified, data from two independent lines of clinical investigation have provided support for the idea that ethnicity influences associations between sleep apnea and glaucoma. The first line of study showed that retinal nerve fiber layer is thinner among patients with sleep apnea [69,76,77], which parenthetically generated the hypothesis that reduced ocular perfusion related to hypoxia and vasospasm observed in sleep apnea may cause nerve fiber layer thinning. The second line of investigation showed that retinal nerve fiber layer is typically thinner among Black patients [78]. Plausibly, Blacks with sleep apnea could have even thinner nerve fiber layers. Future large-scale, population-based studies should investigate some of the nuances in the link between glaucoma and sleep apnea and explore the reasons why blacks tend to show worse outcomes for these conditions.

## 9. Sleep apnea and glaucoma – Role of hypertension

One of the complexities permeating relations between glaucoma and sleep apnea relates to the fact that both conditions are potentially characterized by similar pathogenetic mechanisms. Both sleep apnea and glaucoma are linked to hypertension [25,40,79-82], which is more prevalent among Blacks (44% vs. 23%). based on a multi-site study of medically underserved patients [3]. Available data suggests that approximately 40% of patients with sleep apnea suffer from hypertension, whereas 30% of hypertensive patients have occult sleep apnea [79]. Data from the Wisconsin Sleep Cohort Study, sampling 1060 women and men ages 30 to 60 years showed a dose-response relationship between sleep apnea and blood pressure, independent of several confounding factors [25]. Furthermore, clinical evidence suggests that continuous positive airway pressure treatment for sleep apnea results in a diminution of daytime and nighttime arterial blood pressure [80].

Concerning linkage between glaucoma and hypertension, studies have shown that patients with normal-tension glaucoma exhibited increased variability of night-time blood pressure compared with healthy controls [82]. This is important since increased fluctuation of blood pressure may lead to ocular reperfusion damage and may cause ischemic episodes at the optic nerve head. According to a case-control study, hypertension was significantly more common among patients with glaucoma relative to age- and gender-matched individuals with healthy eyes (OR: 1.29 [81]. Investigators concluded that common pathogenetic mechanisms in ciliary and renal tubular epithelia might explain co-occurrence of glaucoma and systemic hypertension. It is important to mention that a few epidemiologic studies found mixed results. A recent review of studies discussing the association between glaucoma and hypertension acknowledges these studies that found weak or no relationships [52]. The same review acknowledges that blood pressure is likely related to intraocular pressure, but not necessarily the incidence of glaucoma.

## 10. Sleep apnea and glaucoma – Role of obesity

One might also conjecture another viable hypothesis that would suggest that both sleep apnea and glaucoma are caused by a defect in a common pathway potentially resulting from obesity (see Figure 1). Obesity is the strongest predictor of sleep apnea, with estimates suggesting that 60-90% of patients with sleep apnea are obese (defined as BMI >28 $kg/m^2$); data also suggests that a BMI of 28 $kg/m^2$ has a sensitivity of 93% and a specificity of 74% for sleep apnea [83]. Data analyzed from the National Health and Nutrition Examination Survey estimated the prevalence of sleep apnea in persons without obesity to be 3% in men and 0.7% in women ($p<0.01$), while in persons with obesity to be 12.1% in men and 7% in women ($p<0.01$). [24]. On balance, it is noteworthy that not all patients with sleep apnea are obese, suggesting the involvement of other explanatory factors. Mixed results have been found regarding effects of obesity on intraocular pressure, the widely accepted marker for glaucoma [84]. It may be that body mass index, the most commonly utilized obesity measure, is inadequate when predicting eye disorders [85].

It is likely that sleep apnea and glaucoma represent manifestations of what is referred to as the metabolic syndrome. Metabolic syndrome is defined as a cluster of interrelated risk factors of metabolic origin that increase chances of developing heart disease, stroke, and diabetes. The risk factors include raised blood pressure, dyslipidemia (raised triglycerides and lowered high-density lipoprotein cholesterol), raised fasting glucose, and central obesity. Metabolic syndrome is an emerging public health concern, affecting 25% of adult Americans [86]. According to data from the third National Health and Nutrition Examination Survey of adults (ages ≥ 20 years), the age-adjusted prevalence was similar for men (24.0%). and women (23.4%), but Black women had approximately a 57% higher prevalence than did Black men [4]. Individuals with the metabolic syndrome have several co-occurring disorders of the body's metabolism: obesity, hypertension, dyslipidemia, and hypercholesterolemia [87].

A direct link between metabolic syndrome and sleep apnea has not been systematically established. However, preliminary evidence from the Mayo Clinic indicates that the metabolic syndrome might be more prevalent among patients with sleep apnea. Clinical data shows that 60% of patients with sleep apnea had metabolic syndrome, compared with 40% of patients without sleep apnea [23]. Evidently, the components of the metabolic syndrome each correlate highly with sleep apnea [87]. Clinical evidence also suggests that the metabolic syndrome is associated with glaucoma; intraocular pressure is higher among individuals with this disease [88].

If indeed obesity was the final common pathway, this might explain the greater prevalence of sleep apnea and glaucoma among Blacks. Blacks are at greater risk for associated metabolic diseases because they are disproportionately more obese compared with Whites (see Table 1). According to data from the National Center for Health Statistics, about two-thirds of American adults are either overweight (BMI > 25; 33%). or obese (BMI > 30; 31%). [89]. The age-adjusted prevalence of overweight/obesity in ethnic minorities, especially minority women, is higher than in Whites in the U.S., reaching a critical level of greater than two-thirds of the female minority population [90].

## 11. Sleep apnea and ocular blood flow

No conclusive evidence exists for a cause-and-effect relationship between sleep apnea and glaucoma, although it is believed that various physiologic factors produced by sleep apnea may play a significant role in the pathogenesis of glaucoma [91,92]. Sleep apnea is widely recognized for its adverse vascular sequelae: acute myocardial infarction and/or nocturnal angina caused by arterial vasospasm [57]. These may be particularly harmful among patients with glaucoma because at night, ophthalmic artery flow velocities decrease commensurate with reductions in arterial blood pressure[82]. This is considered a vulnerable period when the risk of disease progression is heightened. It should also be noted that intraocular pressure increases, especially in glaucoma patients in the supine position [44] and may further influence the progress of glaucoma.

Optic nerve vascular dysregulation might be secondary to sleep apnea-induced arterial hypertension and arteriosclerosis [93]. Plausibly, impaired optic nerve-head blood flow autoregulation is a sequela of repetitive apnea events [93]. One study suggested that repetitive deep hypoxia, a phenomenon commonly observed during apneic events, might directly damage the optic nerve [13]. It is not certain whether repetitive hypoxia would cause increased intraocular pressure among patients with normal-tension glaucoma, based on data from a case study involving 3 patients [94]. This discrepancy may be explained by age differences in the sample studied; preliminary data suggested that effects of sleep apnea are more pronounced among older patients with normal-tension glaucoma [13]. Investigators argue that both chronic hemodynamic changes and recurring severe hypoxia may contribute to anoxic optic nerve damage observed in glaucoma [67].

Thus, sleep apnea might offer one explanation for the increased prevalence of glaucoma among Blacks. Since sleep apnea and hypertension are worse among Blacks [1,3], this might augur greater impairment of optic arterial blood supply for Blacks. Notwithstanding, the knowledge that Blacks might be at greater risk for morbidity related to untreated sleep apnea and glaucoma, little has been done to investigate the clinical presentation and course of these two diseases in that population. In effect, studies reported to date have only considered group analyses, making it difficult to ascertain racial/ethnic effects on the association between sleep apnea and glaucoma.

## 12. Link among sleep apnea, glaucoma, obesity, hypertension and blood flow

The aforementioned associations do not seem to be fortuitous, judging from the consistency across studies. Whether obesity is the final common pathway has not been convincingly demonstrated, although it is involved in all the disease entities herein discussed (see Figures 1 and 3). Obesity, glaucoma, and hypertension are all associated with sleep apnea, perhaps bi-directionally. This gives rise to the need for empirical studies testing causal models to explain links among obesity, hypertension, sleep apnea, blood flow, and glaucoma. One could imagine the difficulties inherent in performing experimental tests of cause-and-effects relationships of those factors. Such linkage analyses could benefit from the application of path analysis using available national data. Only through costly, systematic, empirical studies can we arrive at definitive explanations of causal models.

To date, no systematic linkage analyses have been performed to elucidate relations between sleep apnea and ocular blood flow dysregulation. If it can be demonstrated that sleep apnea is a mediating factor in the associations between glaucoma and ocular blood flow, this would lead to enhanced strategies to treat glaucoma. Identification and characterization of the relationship between sleep apnea and glaucoma would assist in the diagnosis and treatment of patients with glaucoma whose disease progresses despite medical intervention to lower intraocular pressure.

In formulating a glaucoma diagnosis, the clinician may have to consider the status of the autonomic nervous system in its relations to systemic hemodynamic parameters that might be dysfunctional. In addition, this information will assist the clinician in formulating novel treatment strategies for glaucoma that focus on enhancing end-tissue oxygenation. Since Blacks are at increased risks for developing both glaucoma and sleep apnea, special efforts should be made to target interventions to Blacks in underserved communities.

## 13. Conclusions

Most of the initial studies reported to date have used relatively small sample sizes, offering little definitive explanation of the link between sleep apnea and glaucoma or whether ethnicity influences such associations. Epidemiologic evidence shows that both glaucoma and sleep apnea are more prevalent among Blacks, and that their onset is earlier in that population. Glaucoma and sleep apnea are potentially characterized by similar pathogenetic mechanisms, as they are both linked to hypertension and obesity. Obesity and hypertension are highly prevalent in the Black population and are widely recognized for their involvement in numerous vascular diseases. Efforts are underway to ascertain whether one condition has a direct effect on the other or whether their co-occurrence engenders worse physiologic and behavioral outcomes among at-risk individuals. Plausibly, individuals with glaucoma show ocular hemodynamic changes and blood flow deficits due to untreated sleep apnea, which is more common among Blacks [7-9]. Systematic studies exploring reasons why Blacks don't participate in screening events or are not receiving timely diagnoses are needed. It may be assumed that the reasons for low participation in screening are probably lack of awareness and occupation with other issues.

Along with further epidemiological investigation, genetic research could also be explored. Genome scanning has already suggested genetic factors linking sleep apnea to obesity, diabetes, and insulin resistance [26,41,42]. More recent analysis of mRNA expression, protein interaction, and results from genome-wide association studies has made an attempt to connect some of the known pathways between these known co-morbidities [16]. This approach could be used in the future to better explain the potential link between sleep apnea and glaucoma.

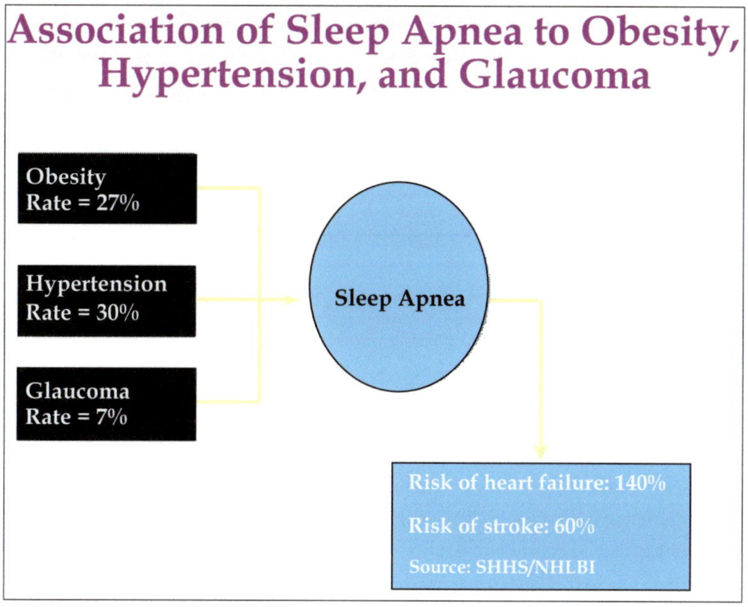


Fig. 3. Prevalence of individuals with obesity, hypertension, and/or glaucoma who also carry a diagnosis of sleep apnea; sleep apnea is itself a strong risk factor for cardiovascular disease

## 14. Acknowledgements

This research was supported by funding from the NIH (R25HL105444 and R01MD004113).

## 15. References

[1] Redline S, Tishler P, Hans M, Tosteson T, Strohl K, Spry K (1997). Racial differences in sleep-disordered breathing in African-Americans and Caucasians. Am J Respir Crit Care Med 155: 186-192.

[2] Friedman DS, Jampel HD, Muñoz B, West SK (2006). The prevalence of open-angle glaucoma among blacks and whites 73 years and older: the Salisbury Eye Evaluation Glaucoma Study. Arch Ophthalmol 124: 1625-1630.

[3] Lackland DT, Lin Y, Tilley BC, Egan BM (2004). An assessment of racial differences in clinical practices for hypertension at primary care sites for medically underserved patients. J Clin Hypertens (Greenwich ). 6: 26-31.

[4] Ford ES, Giles WH, Dietz WH (2002). Prevalence of the metabolic syndrome among US adults: findings from the third National Health and Nutrition Examination Survey. JAMA 287: 356-359.

[5] Jean-Louis G, von Gizycki H, Zizi F, Dharawat A, Lazar JM, Brown CD (2008). Evaluation of sleep apnea in a sample of black patients. Journal of Clinical Sleep Medicine

[6] Young T, Finn L (1998). Epidemiological insights into the public health burden of sleep disordered breathing: sex differences in survival among sleep clinic patients. Thorax 53 Suppl 3: S16-S19.

[7] Jones HL, Walker EA, Schechter CB, Blanco E (2010). Vision is precious: a successful behavioral intervention to increase the rate of screening for diabetic retinopathy for inner-city adults. Diabetes Educator 6:118-26.

[8] Basch CE, Walker EA, Howard CJ, Shamoon H, Zybert P (1999). The effect of health education on the rate of ophthalmic examinations among African Americans with diabetes mellitus. Am J Public Health 89: 1878-1882.
[9] DiPalma J, Jean-Louis G, Zizi F, Cohen C, Casimir G, Bobb L, Mukherji R, Felix K, Wolintz A (2002). Screening and Treatment of Obstructive Sleep Apnea in a Brooklyn-Based Minority Sample. Sleep 25: 185.
[10] Lin PW, Friedman M, Lin HC, Chang HW, Wilson M, Lin MC (2010). Normal Tension Glaucoma in Patients With Obstructive Sleep Apnea/Hypopnea Syndrome. Journal of Glaucoma 10:1097
[11] Batisse JL, Vix J, Swalduz B, Chave N, Mage F (2004). Sleep-related breathing disorders and normal or high-tension glaucoma: 35 patients with polysomnographic records. J Fr Ophtalmol 27: 605-612.
[12] Mojon DS, Hess CW, Goldblum D, Bohnke M, Korner F, Mathis J (2000). Primary open-angle glaucoma is associated with sleep apnea syndrome. Ophthalmologica 214: 115-118.
[13] Mojon A, Hess CW, Goldblum D, Boehnke M, Koerner F, Gugger M, Bassetti C, Mathis J (2002). Normal-tension glaucoma is associated with sleep apnea syndrome. Ophthalmologica 216: 180-184.
[14] Mojon DS, Hess CW, Goldblum D, Fleischhauer J, Koerner F, Bassetti C, Mathis J (1999). High prevalence of glaucoma in patients with sleep apnea syndrome. Ophthalmology 106: 1009-1012.
[15] Geyer O, Cohen N, Segev E, Rath EZ, Melamud L, Peled R, Lavie P (2003). The prevalence of glaucoma in patients with sleep apnea syndrome: same as in the general population. Am J Ophthalmol 136: 1093-1096.
[16] Mojon DS, Goldblum D, Fleischhauer J, Chiou AG, Frueh BE, Hess CW, Gugger M, Bassetti C, Boehnke M, Mathis J (1999). Eyelid, conjunctival, and corneal findings in sleep apnea syndrome. Ophthalmology 106: 1182-1185.
[17] Silva GE, An MW, Goodwin JL, Shahar E, Redline S, Resnick H, Baldwin CM, Quan SF (2009). Longitudinal evaluation of sleep-disordered breathing and sleep symptoms with change in quality of life: the Sleep Heart Health Study (SHHS). Aug 1; 32:1049-57
[18] Wright J, Johns R, Watt I, Melville A, Sheldon T (1997). Health effects of obstructive sleep apnoea and the effectiveness of continuous positive airways pressure: a systematic review of the research evidence. BMJ 314: 851-860.
[19] Mehra R, Benjamin EJ, Shahar E, Gottlieb DJ, Nawabit R, Kirchner HL, Sahadevan J, Redline S (2006). Association of Nocturnal Arrhythmias with Sleep-Disordered Breathing: The Sleep Heart Health Study. Am J Respir Crit Care Med.
[20] Shah NA, Yaggi HK, Concato J, Mohsenin V (2010). Obstructive sleep apnea as a risk factor for coronary events or cardiovascular death. Sleep & Breathing 14:131-6
[21] Lavie P, Herer P, Hoffstein V (2000). Obstructive sleep apnoea syndrome as a risk factor for hypertension: population study. BMJ 320: 479-482.
[22] Yaggi HK, Concato J, Kernan WN, Lichtman JH, Brass LM, Mohsenin V (2005). Obstructive sleep apnea as a risk factor for stroke and death. N Engl J Med 353: 2034-2041.
[23] Parish JM, Adam T, Facchiano L (2007). Relationship of metabolic syndrome and obstructive sleep apnea. J Clin Sleep Med 3: 467-472.
[24] Li C, Ford ES, Zhao G, Croft JB, Balluz LS, Mokdad AH. Prevalence of self-reported clinically diagnosed sleep apnea according to obesity status in men and women: National Health and Nutrition Examination Survey, 2005-2006. Preventive Medicine 51:18-23

[25] Young T, Peppard P, Palta M, Hla KM, Finn L, Morgan B, Skatrud J (1997). Population-based study of sleep-disordered breathing as a risk factor for hypertension. Arch Intern Med 157: 1746-1752.
[26] Liu Y, Patel S, Nibbe R, Maxwell S, Chowdhury SA, Koyuturk M, Zhu X, Larkin EK, Buxbaum SG, Punjabi NM, Gharib SA, Redline S, Chance MR (2011). Systems biology analyses of gene expression and genome wide association study data in obstructive sleep apnea. Pacific Symposium on Biocomputing 2011: 14-25.
[27] Tregear S, Reston J, Schoelles K, Phillips B (2009). Obstructive sleep apnea and risk of motor vehicle crash: systematic review and meta-analysis. J Clin Sleep Med 5(6):573-81.
[28] Lavie P, Herer P, Peled R, Berger I, Yoffe N, Zomer J, Rubin AH (1995). Mortality in sleep apnea patients: a multivariate analysis of risk factors. Sleep 18: 149-157.
[29] Pagel JF (2007). Obstructive sleep apnea (OSA). in primary care: evidence-based practice. J Am Board Fam Med 20: 392-398.
[30] Stoohs RA, Guilleminault C, Itoi A, Dement WC (1994). Traffic accidents in commercial long-haul truck drivers: the influence of sleep-disordered breathing and obesity. Sleep 17: 619-623.
[31] El Ad B, Lavie P (2005). Effect of sleep apnea on cognition and mood. Int Rev Psychiatry 17: 277-282.
[32] Sharafkhaneh A, Giray N, Richardson P, Young T, Hirshkowitz M (2005). Association of psychiatric disorders and sleep apnea in a large cohort. Sleep 28: 1405-1411.
[33] Omnibus Sleep in America Poll. National Sleep Foundation. 1-51. 2005. National Sleep Foundation. Ref Type: Report
[34] Report of the Scientific Committee on tobacco and Health. http://www.doh.gov.uk /public/scoth.htm. Accessed on 8-05-02. 8-5-2002. Ref Type: Internet Communication
[35] The National Commission on Sleep Disorders Research. Wake up America: a national sleep alert. Washington DC: US Government Printing Office, 1993. 2002. Ref Type: Report
[36] Punjabi NM, Caffo BS, Goodwin JL, Gottlieb DJ, Newman AB, O'Connor GT, Rapoport DM, Redline S, Resnick HE, Robbins JA, Shahar E, Unruh ML, Samet JM (2009). Sleep-disordered breathing and mortality: a prospective cohort study. PLoS Med. Aug6:e1000132
[37] Young T, Palta M, Dempsey J, Skatrud J, Weber S, Badr S (1993). The occurrence of sleep-disordered breathing among middle-aged adults [see comments]. N Engl J Med 328: 1230-1235
[38] Ancoli-Israel S, Klauber MR, Stepnowsky C, Estline E, Chinn A, Fell R (1989). Sleep-disordered breathing in African-American elderly. J Gerontol 44: M18-M21.
[39] Gottlieb DJ, Whitney CW, Bonekat WH, Iber C, James GD, Lebowitz M, Nieto FJ, Rosenberg CE (1999). Relation of sleepiness to respiratory disturbance index: the Sleep Heart Health Study. Am J Respir Crit Care Med 159: 502-507.
[40] Meetze K, Gillespie MB, Lee FS (2002). Obstructive sleep apnea: a comparison of black and white subjects. Laryngoscope 112: 1271-1274.
[41] Buxbaum SG, Elston RC, Tishler PV, Redline S (2002). Genetics of the apnea hypopnea index in Caucasians and African Americans: I. Segregation analysis. Genet Epidemiol 22: 243-253.
[42] Palmer LJ, Buxbaum SG, Larkin EK, Patel SR, Elston RC, Tishler PV, Redline S (2004). Whole genome scan for obstructive sleep apnea and obesity in African-American families. Am J Respir Crit Care Med 169: 1314-1321.

[43] Javitt JC, McBean AM, Nicholson GA, Babish JD, Warren JL, Krakauer H (1991). Undertreatment of glaucoma among black Americans. N Engl J Med. 325(20):1418-22.
[44] Schacknow P, Samples J (2010). The Glaucoma Book: A Practical, Evidence-Based Approach to Patient Care. New York, NY: Springer:399-420
[45] McKean-Cowdin R, Varma R, Hays RD, Wu J, Choudhury F, Azen SP; Los Angeles Latino Eye Study Group (2010). Longitudinal changes in visual acuity and health-related quality of life: the Los Angeles Latino Eye study. Opthalmology 117: 1900-7
[46] Zizi F, Jean-Louis G, Magai C, Greenidge K, Wolintz A, Heath-Phillip O (2002). Sleep Complaints and Visual Impairment Among Older Americans: A Community-based study. J Gerontol A Biol Sci Med Sci 57: M691-M694.
[47] Sommer A, Tielsch JM, Katz J, Quigley HA, Gottsch JD, Javitt JC, Martone JF, Royall RM, Witt KA, Ezrine S (1991). Racial differences in the cause-specific prevalence of blindness in east Baltimore. N Engl J Med 325: 1412-1417.
[48] Hennis AJ, Wu SY, Nemesure B, Hyman L, Schachat AP, Leske MC; Barbados Eye Studies Group (2009). Nine-year incidence of visual impairment in the Barbados Eye Studies. Ophthalmology. 2009 116:1461-8
[49] National Eye Institute Vision Report. Vision Problems in the U.S.: Prevalence of adult vision impairment and age-related eye disease in America, update to the fourth edition (2008). http://www.preventblindness.org/vpus/2008_update/VPUS_2008_update.pdf Accessed 04/20/11. 2008. Ref Type: Internet Communication
[50] Flammer J, Orgul S, Costa VP, Orzalesi N, Krieglstein GK, Serra LM, Renard JP, Stefansson E (2002). The impact of ocular blood flow in glaucoma. Prog Retin Eye Res 21: 359-393.
[51] Leske MC, Wu SY, Hennis A, Honkanen R, Nemesure B; BESs Study Group (2008). Risk factors for incident open-angle glaucoma: the Barbados Eye Studies. Opthalmology 115:85-93
[52] Deokule S, Weinreb RN. (2008). Relationships among systemic blood pressure, intraocular pressure, and open-angle glaucoma. Can J Ophthalmol. 43(3):302-7
[53] Harris A, Rechtman E, Siesky B, Jonescu-Cuypers C, McCranor L, Garzozi HJ (2005). The role of optic nerve blood flow in the pathogenesis of glaucoma. Ophthalmol Clin North Am 18: 345-53, v.
[54] Feke GT, Pasquale Lr (2008). Retinal blood flow response to posture change in glaucoma patients compared with healthy subjects. Ophthalmology 115:246-52
[55] Joos KM, Kay MD, Pillunat LE, Harris A, Gendron EK, Feuer WJ, Steinwand BE (1999). Effect of acute intraocular pressure changes on short posterior ciliary artery haemodynamics. Br J Ophthalmol 83: 33-38.
[56] Bonomi L, Marchini G, Marraffa M, Morbio R (2001). The Relationship between Intraocular Pressure and Glaucoma in a Defined Population. data from the egna-neumarkt glaucoma study. Ophthalmologica 215: 34-38.
[57] Fletcher EC (2000). Cardiovascular effects of continuous positive airway pressure in obstructive sleep apnea. Sleep 23 Suppl 4: S154-S157.
[58] Arend O, Remky A, Plange N, Martin BJ, Harris A, Garzozi HJ, Shoham N, Chung HS, Kagemann L, Harris A (2002). Capillary density and retinal diameter measurements and their impact on altered retinal circulation in glaucoma: a digital fluorescein angiographic study Ocular blood flow measurements and their importance in glaucoma and age-related macular degeneration. Br J Ophthalmol 86: 429-433.

[59] Garzozi HJ, Shoham N, Chung HS, Kagemann L, Harris A (2001). Ocular blood flow measurements and their importance in glaucoma and age-related macular degeneration. Isr Med Assoc J 3: 443-448.

[60] Harris A, Jonescu-Cuypers CP (2001). The impact of glaucoma medication on parameters of ocular perfusion. Curr Opin Ophthalmol 12: 131-137.

[61] McNab AA (2007). The eye and sleep apnea. Sleep Med Rev 11: 269-276.

[62] McNab AA (2000). Reversal of floppy eyelid syndrome with treatment of obstructive sleep apnoea. Clin Experiment Ophthalmol 28: 125-126.

[63] Culbertson WW, Tseng SC (1994). Corneal disorders in floppy eyelid syndrome. Cornea 13: 33-42.

[64] Purvin V, Kawasaki A, Yee RD (2000). Papilledema and obstructive sleep apnea syndrome. Arch Ophthalmol 2000 118: 1626-1630.

[65] Mojon DS, Hedges TR, III, Ehrenberg B, Karam EZ, Goldblum D, Abou-Chebl A, Gugger M, Mathis J (2002). Association between sleep apnea syndrome and nonarteritic anterior ischemic optic neuropathy. Arch Ophthalmol 120: 601-605.

[66] Bendel RE, Kaplan J, Heckman M, Fredrickson PA, Lin SC (2007). Prevalence of glaucoma in patients with obstructive sleep apnoea-a cross-sectional case-series. Eye.

[67] Onen SH, Mouriaux F, Berramdane L, Dascotte JC, Kulik JF, Rouland JF (2000). High prevalence of sleep-disordered breathing in patients with primary open-angle glaucoma. Acta Ophthalmol Scand 78: 638-641.

[68] Sergi M, Salerno DE, Rizzi M, Blini M, Andreoli A, Messenio D, Pecis M, Bertoni G (2007). Prevalence of normal tension glaucoma in obstructive sleep apnea syndrome patients. J Glaucoma 16: 42-46.

[69] Lin PW, Friedman M, Lin HC, Chang HW, Pulver TM, Chin CH (2010). Decreased retinal nerve fiber layer thickness in patients with obstructive sleep apnea/hypopnea syndrome. Graefes Arch Clin Exp Ophthalmol 10.1007/s00417

[70] Tsang CS, Chong SL, Ho CK, Li MF (2006). Moderate to severe obstructive sleep apnoea patients is associated with a higher incidence of visual field defect. Eye 20: 38-42.

[71] Stefansson E, Pedersen DB, Jensen PK, la Cour M, Kiilgaard JF, Bang K, Eysteinsson T (2005). Optic nerve oxygenation. Prog Retin Eye Res 24: 307-332.

[72] Hafez AS, Bizzarro R, Descovich D, Lesk MR (2005). Correlation between finger blood flow and changes in optic nerve head blood flow following therapeutic intraocular pressure reduction. J Glaucoma 14: 448-454.

[73] Kremmer S, Niederdraing N, Ayertey HD, Steuhl KP, Selbach JM, Kremmer S, Niederdraing N, Ayertey HD, Steuhl KP, Selbach JM (2003). Obstructive sleep apnea syndrome, normal tension glaucoma, and nCPAP therapy--a short note Obstructive sleep apnea syndrome, normal tension glaucoma, and nCPAP therapy--a short note. Sleep 26: 161-162.

[74] Karakucuk S, Goktas S, Aksu M, Erdogan N, Demirci S, Oner A, Arda H, Gumus K (2008). Ocular blood flow in patients with obstructive sleep apnea syndrome (OSAS). Graefes Arch Clin Exp Ophthalmol Jan;246(1):129-34. Epub 2007 Aug 4.

[75] Erdem CZ, Altin R, Erdem LO, Kargi S, Kart L, Cinar F, Ayoglu F (2003). Doppler measurement of blood flow velocities in extraocular orbital vessels in patients with obstructive sleep apnea syndrome. J Clin Ultrasound 31: 250-257.

[76] Shimmyo M, Ross AJ, Moy A, Mostafavi R (2003). Intraocular pressure, Goldmann applanation tension, corneal thickness, and corneal curvature in Caucasians, Asians, Hispanics, and African Americans. Am J Ophthalmol 136: 603-613.

[77] La Rosa FA, Gross RL, Orengo-Nania S (2001). Central corneal thickness of Caucasians and African Americans in glaucomatous and nonglaucomatous populations. Arch Ophthalmol 119: 23-27.
[78] Jean-Louis G, Zizi F, Dweck M, McKenzie D, Lazzaro DR (2007). Ophthalmic dysfunction in a community-based sample: influence of race/ethnicity. J Natl Med Assoc 2007 Feb ;99 (2):141 -4, 147 -8 99: 141-148.
[79] Fletcher EC (1995). The relationship between systemic hypertension and obstructive sleep apnea: facts and theory. Am J Med 98: 118-128.
[80] Becker HF, Jerrentrup A, Ploch T, Grote L, Penzel T, Sullivan CE, Peter JH (2003). Effect of nasal continuous positive airway pressure treatment on blood pressure in patients with obstructive sleep apnea. Circulation 107:68-73
[81] Langman MJ, Lancashire RJ, Cheng KK, Stewart PM (2005). Systemic hypertension and glaucoma: mechanisms in common and co-occurrence. Br J Ophthalmol 89: 960-963.
[82] Plange N, Kaup M, Daneljan L, Predel HG, Remky A, Arend O (2006). 24-h blood pressure monitoring in normal tension glaucoma: night-time blood pressure variability. J Hum Hypertens 20: 137-142.
[83] Kushida CA, Efron B, Guilleminault C (1997). A predictive morphometric model for the obstructive sleep apnea syndrome. Ann Intern Med 127: 581-587.
[84] Cheung N, Wong TY (2007). Obesity and eye diseases. Surv Ophthalmol 52: 180-195.
[85] Klein BE, Klein R, Lee KE, Jensen SC (2001). Measures of obesity and age-related eye diseases. Ophthalmic Epidemiol 8: 251-262.
[86] Zimmet P, Magliano D, Matsuzawa Y, Alberti G, Shaw J (2005). The metabolic syndrome: a global public health problem and a new definition. J Atheroscler Thromb 12: 295-300.
[87] Jean-Louis G, Zizi F, Clark LT, Kossotis J: Associations of Sleep Apnea to Cardiovascular Diseases: Role of Diabetes and Metabolic Syndrome. In *In Cardiovascular Disease and Diabetes: Contemporary Management*. Edited by Clark LT. New York: McGraw-Hill.; 2007:472-505.
[88] Oh SW, Lee S, Park C, Kim DJ (2005). Elevated intraocular pressure is associated with insulin resistance and metabolic syndrome. Diabetes Metab Res Rev 21: 434-440.
[89] National Center for Health Statistics Health, United States, 2006. 1-543. 2006. National Center for Health Statistics. Ref Type: Internet Communication
[90] Kumanyika SK, Gary TL, Lancaster KJ, Samuel-Hodge CD, Banks-Wallace J, Beech BM, Hughes-Halbert C, Karanja N, Odoms-Young AM, Prewitt TE, Whitt-Glover MC (2005). Achieving healthy weight in African-American communities: research perspectives and priorities. Obes Res 13: 2037-2047.
[91] Marcus DM, Lynn J, Miller JJ, Chaudhary O, Thomas D, Chaudhary B (2001). Sleep disorders: a risk factor for pseudotumor cerebri? J Neuroophthalmol 21: 121-123.
[92] Marcus DM, Costarides AP, Gokhale P, Papastergiou G, Miller JJ, Johnson MH, Chaudhary BA (2001). Sleep disorders: a risk factor for normal-tension glaucoma? J Glaucoma 10: 177-183.
[93] Kato M, Roberts-Thomson P, Phillips BG, Haynes WG, Winnicki M, Accurso V, Somers VK (2000). Impairment of endothelium-dependent vasodilation of resistance vessels in patients with obstructive sleep apnea. Circulation 102: 2607-2610.
[94] Goldblum D, Mathis J, Bohnke M, Bassetti C, Hess CW, Gugger M, Mojon DS (2000). [Nocturnal measurements of intraocular pressure in patients with normal-tension glaucoma and sleep apnea syndrome]. Klin Monatsbl Augenheilkd 216: 246-249.

14

# Quality of Life (QoL) in Glaucoma Patients

Georgios Labiris[1,2], Athanassios Giarmoukakis[2] and Vassilios P. Kozobolis[1,2]
[1]*Department of Ophthalmology, University Hospital of Alexandroupolis,*
[2]*Eye Institute of Thrace, Alexandroupolis,*
*Greece*

## 1. Introduction

The interest of clinicians and researchers concerning the quality of life (QoL) assessment in chronic diseases increases constantly. Many definitions have been proposed for the term quality of life, but it is commonly accepted that a universal definition of QoL is rather infeasible to be given. Furthermore, Aaronson has noted the multidimensionality of QoL in terms of physical (symptoms of a disease and treatment), functional (activities of daily living, mobility), social (interpersonal contacts and relationships) and psychological (mental health, emotional balance) parameters that compose it.[1]

Since the first research efforts that tried to examine QoL in glaucoma[2], serious advancement has been accomplished in this field, offering a better understanding of how and to what extend glaucoma influences QoL of individuals suffering from the disease. In addition, glaucoma QoL research yielded important insights with regard to the domains of daily living that are mostly affected by the disease.

It is well documented that glaucoma is a leading cause of visual impairment and blindness. Epidemiologic studies demonstrate that 2% of adults over the age of 40 suffer from glaucoma, with the disease prevalence increasing significantly with age.[3,4] Vision loss exerts a negative impact on physical ability of patients to perform activities of daily living (reading, adapting to different levels of light, outdoor mobility, avoiding obstacles, etc.), despite maintenance of central visual acuity in less advanced stages of the disease.[5] Furthermore, literature suggests that patients with impaired QoL form a more severe burden on health-care resources.[6,7]

Knowledge and information regarding the QoL of glaucoma patients could be useful in several aspects. It can help 'decision making' concerning customized disease management of individuals with glaucoma and promote alterations and guidelines regarding patients' daily living and safety (i.e. adjustment of home environment), in order to avoid problems concerning adaptation to variable lighting conditions, avoiding obstacles, near activities, outdoor mobility/activities (walking, driving) and other tasks that glaucoma patients seem to give the greatest importance and are significantly correlated with their QoL.[8,29] The diagnosis of glaucoma impacts individuals differently, with the majority of cases having little understanding of the need for adherence to their daily therapeutic regimen and the disease natural course and progress.[9] Towards this direction, information gained from QoL studies could improve the education of newly diagnosed patients and help them realize the severity of the disease and the importance of the adherence to daily treatment, despite the fact that symptoms are absent in early stages.

Deterioration of quality of life due to glaucoma can occur because of many reasons. The diagnosis itself, the progressive visual field loss, the intolerance of daily treatment, the side effects of topical anti-glaucoma medication (i.e. allergic conjunctivitis, dry eye, blepharitis), the constrictions concerning daily activities and the need of intensive and long-lasting observation and monitoring on an outpatient basis are some of these causes. In addition QoL is a more subjective rather than objective assessment,[10] since individuals with common visual deterioration due to glaucoma may estimate their QoL state differently. It is then obvious why QoL is considered to be subjective and multidimensional,[1] and why its assessment and the extent of the impact that glaucoma exerts on it is difficult to be accomplished and evaluated.

In general, QoL can be estimated by means of a series of instruments-questionnaires. In specific, generic health-related [the Short Form Health Survey-36 (SF-36), the Sickness impact Profile (SIP)], vision-specific (VS) [ the Visual Function-14 (VF-14), the National Eye Institute Visual Function Questionnaire-25 (NEIVFQ-25)] and glaucoma-specific [the Glaucoma Symptom Scale (GSS), the Glaucoma Quality of Life-15 (GQL-15)] QoL instruments (Table 1) have been employed to better rate glaucoma's impact on patients' daily living and enlighten clinicians about how patients experience the effect of glaucoma in their quality of life.

## 2. Validation of QoL instruments

Proper validation of a questionnaire's basic psychometric properties is considered a prerequisite (before it is administrated to subjects and implemented to studies), in order its' efficacy to be established. Psychometric properties indicate the quality status of an instrument and can be assessed by the classic test theory and/or by Rasch analysis. Both methods provide significant information about item selection, subscale structure and interpretability of an instrument.

The basic psychometric properties that are based on classic test theory are the 'content validity' and the 'internal consistency', the 'construct validity', the 'reproducibility' and the 'respondent burden' of an instrument.

'Content validity' evaluates if the items of the questionnaire measure the basic parameter (i.e. QoL) that is purported to measure and is necessary during the development of the tool.[11] It consists from 3 phases: item collection phase, item reduction phase and segregation of items in subscales phase that is accomplished by factor analysis or principal component analysis. 'Internal consistency' assesses the affinity of both the questionnaires' items and subscales. It is measured by calculation of the Cronbach α value. Cronbach α should range between 0.70-0.90.[12]

'Construct validity' expresses the associations of an instrument with other measurements or questionnaires (i.e. visual field (VF) scores, visual acuity). No specific measurement or value evaluates construct validity.

'Reproducibility' evaluates the extent to which the instrument's scores have limited fluctuations after repetition (test-retest reproducibility) or between observers (inter-observer reproducibility). The intraclass correlation coefficient (ICC) and the Bland-Altman analysis are the most common measures of reproducibility.[12-14]

'Respondent burden' demonstrates the questionnaire's demands from the respondents (i.e. time needed to respond to the instrument, emotional burden placed on respondents, the ratio of missing items). Andresen suggested that 15 min is the maximum temporal limit of a questionnaire's completion regarding disabled people.[15]

| QoL Instruments | Features |
|---|---|
| *Generic Health-related* | |
| SF-36 | 36 items, 8 subscales: general health, mental health, physical functions, social functions, role limitations by physical/mental disability, vitality and pain |
| MOS-20 | Shorter version of SF-36. 20 items, 6 subscales: physical functioning, social functioning, role functioning, mental health, health perceptions, pain |
| SIP | 136 items, 12 subscales, implemented by CIGTS after modification |
| *Vision-Specific* | |
| VF-14 | 14 items/vision-related activities, originally designed to evaluate functional impairment in cataract patients |
| ADVS | 20 items, 5 subscales: distance vision, near vision, day driving, night driving and glare, originally designed to evaluate functional impairment in cataract patients |
| NEI-VFQ | 51 items, 12 subscales; NEI-VFQ 25: 25 items, 12 domains, shorter and more practical tool from NEI-VFQ |
| IVI | 32 items, 5 subscales: leisure and work, consumer and social interaction, household and personal care, mobility and emotional reaction to vision loss |
| VAQ | 30 items, 8 subscales: acuity/spatial vision, peripheral vision, visual search, visual processing speed, color discrimination, glare disability, light/dark adaptation and depth perception. |
| *Glaucoma-Specific* | |
| GSS | 10 items, 2 subscales: (non-visual) symptom and visual ability |
| GQL-15 | 15 (glaucoma-specific) items demonstrating significant association with visual field loss |
| SIG | 43 items, 4 subscales: visual ability, local eye, systemic and psychological, developed for the CIGTS |
| GHPI | 6 items addressing the 'physical', 'emotional', 'social' and the 'stress' and 'worry of blindness associated with glaucoma' effects on QoL, developed for the CIGTS |

Table 1. Prevalent QoL questionnaires used in glaucoma-related studies

On the other hand, Rasch analysis provides interval ratings regarding the items' difficulty (item measures), the response choices (of an item) (response measures) and the persons' ability (person measures),[16] usually by means of fit (infit/outfit) meansquare (MNSQ) statistics.[17] Fit statistics calculate errors in the item, response and person measures that can occur because of redundancy or inappropriate construction during item and response choices selection. MNSQ values between 0.7 and 1.3 are considered acceptable. Items or response choices with MNSQ values outside these limits are considered misfitting and should be rephrased or omitted during the instrument's development.[18] When items 'fit' the model, then the instrument measures the underlying trait (i.e QoL).

In addition, another basic component of Rasch analysis is the 'person separation' measure. 'Person separation' measures the ability of an instrument to distinguish subgroups of individuals (or items).[19] The higher the (person separation) reliability coefficient, the more subgroups can be discriminated. In order a questionnaire to be considered acceptable the reliability coefficient should be at least 0.8 (it is able to discriminate 3 groups).[19]

## 3. Generic health-related instruments

Health-related tools try by nature to estimate the overall quality of life of subjects, without taking into account separate coexisting diseases or assessing how they individually impact QoL. It is rather difficult to attribute possible decreased QoL scores recorded by general health-related instruments only to glaucoma, without taking into account other co-morbidities that may also affect results. Thus, it is not surprising that general health-related tools lack sensitivity in the glaucoma QoL assessment domain.

### 3.1 The medical outcomes study (MOS-20) and the short form-36 (SF-36)

The SF-36 questionnaire contains 36 questions that are divided into eight subscales.[20] It has been used widely and administrated to patients with different diseases, it is suitable for self-administration and is considered reliable.[21] The MOS-20 composes a shorter form of the SF-36.[22]

The administration to glaucoma patients showed ambiguous results. A study found that glaucoma patients provided the lowest scores among three groups (glaucoma patients, glaucoma suspects and healthy subjects),[23] while another study indicated similar SF-36 scores between glaucoma and normal individuals. Furthermore, glaucoma seemed to greater affect vitality, mental health, bodily pain and social functioning domains.[2,24] Nevertheless, correlations between SF-36 subscales and visual acuity or visual field impairment have been found relative week, and therefore it is considered unsuitable for the QoL assessment in glaucoma.[2,25] Glaucoma subjects presented significantly lower scores than healthy individuals in all MOS-20 subscales except pain.[26] General health, physical and role functioning MOS-20 domains demonstrated the most significant differences between the two groups (-22%, -20% and -43%, respectively).[26]

### 3.2 The sickness impact profile (SIP)

The SIP questionnaire was initially developed in order to provide a measurable instrument of general health status that would be able to record the impact of different disease states. It includes 136 items categorized in 12 domains and showed good test-retest reliability and internal consistency. It takes more than 30 minutes to complete, is not user friendly and is unsuitable for implementation in daily clinical practice.[27]

The SIP instrument was employed by the Collaborative Initial Glaucoma Treatment Study (CIGTS) and after modification it was administrated to newly diagnosed glaucoma patients. Although showing good psychometric properties, the correlations between QoL measurements and clinical parameters were found weak but significant. In addition, glaucoma exerted a slightly stronger impact on the patients' psychological domain than the physical one.[28-30]

## 4. Vision specific instruments

Vision specific tools belong to the category of QoL instruments that try to directly link the quality of life status of individuals with a certain human function. These questionnaires have been commonly administered to ophthalmic patients, trying to assess the QoL status in a wide range of ocular diseases, including glaucoma.

### 4.1 The visual function-14 (VF-14)

The VF-14 was constructed to assess vision-specific functional activities in cataract patients. It consists of 14 vision-related activity questions.[31] Studies suggest that VF-14 has good internal consistency and that VF-14 scores correlate with visual acuity stronger than health-related instruments.[32]

After administration to glaucoma patients, the VF-14 showed moderate correlation with visual field loss and visual acuity.[2,40] However VF-14 proved incapable to distinguish normal from glaucoma subjects (P=0.07)[40] In another publication, glaucoma patients presented worse weighted mean VF-14 scores than cataract subjects but better than AMD patients.[33] Furthermore, it doesn't assess colour vision and other significant factors indicating optic nerve damage, making it inappropriate for QoL rating in glaucoma and in optic neuropathies in general.

### 4.2 The activities of daily vision scale (ADVS)

The ADVS includes 20 items categorized in the following subscales: near vision, far vision, day and night vision/driving, glare and overall vision. It is a cataract-oriented tool with good psychometric properties and is easy to use.[34]

ADVS was able to discriminate glaucoma patients from healthy subjects and ADVS scores showed significant correlation with visual acuity and visual field scores in patients with glaucoma.[26] Furthermore, individuals with bilateral glaucoma reported more difficulty (3 times greater probability) on the ADVS than normal subjects, while more advanced binocular VF impairment was correlated with a greater probability of selecting the most difficulty (response scale) on the instrument.[35] Patients with unilateral glaucoma in the study demonstrated an average mean defect VF index (MD) in the worse eye of -6.5 dB, while the average MD for the bilateral glaucoma group was -12.0 dB. The study could not elucidate whether the greater perceived difficulty found was due to bilaterality or greater VF loss.[35] However the questionnaire doesn't evaluate the parameter of peripheral field and therefore is less relative to glaucoma patients.

### 4.3 The national eye institute visual function questionnaire -51 (NEI-VFQ) and -25 (NEI-VFQ 25)

The NEI-VFQ and NEI-VFQ 25 instruments are used as benchmarks in the vision-related QoL evaluation and many disease-specific tools are compared with them in order their efficacy to be established. The NEI-VFQ is a fully validated, 51 item, 12-domain tool that has been widely used in several ocular morbidities. The NEI-VFQ 25 is a 25 item, 12 domain instrument that is a shorter and more practical version of its predecessor, designed mainly for clinical settings, with its validity proven to be similar with that of the NEI-VFQ.[36,37]

Studies agree that the domains affected greater in glaucoma subjects are mainly general health, general vision, mental health, expectations, driving and near activities both for NEI-VFQ and NEI-VFQ 25 questionnaires.[2,24,33,38-39] Both tools are shown to be capable of distinguishing glaucoma from normal control subjects, with the scores of glaucoma patients being significantly poorer on most subscales. In addition, lower scores correlated well with visual field loss of glaucoma patients in the eye with the least visual field deterioration.[40]

### 4.4 The impact of vision impairment (IVI)

The IVI questionnaire is a vision-specific QoL instrument that consists of 32 queries divided in 5 subscales: leisure and work, consumer and social interaction, household and personal care, mobility, and emotional reaction to vision loss.[41]
After administration to patients with glaucoma or age related macular degeneration (AMD), responses from glaucoma patients were greater (indicating more difficulty to a certain domain) in most subscales, including emotional reaction to vision loss, leisure, mobility, household and social interaction domains. [41] Only the social interaction subscale score was found greater for AMD subjects (indicating more difficulty in this domain).[41] When it was administered only to glaucoma subjects, responses to the subscale 'mobility' were the most limited and were proved to correlate significantly with binocular (Esterman) visual field deterioration.[42]

### 4.5 The visual activities questionnaire (VAQ)

The VAQ instrument consists of 33 items that assess the difficulty of individuals in performing common visual activities. A 1-5 rating score for each item is used regarding the frequency of each visual-related problem. A score of 1 indicates 'never', whereas 5 indicates 'always'. It provides a total score and VAQ items are further organized in 8 subscales: acuity/spatial vision, peripheral vision, visual search, visual processing speed, color discrimination, glare disability, light/dark adaptation and depth perception.[43]
Concerning glaucoma, the instrument was also employed by the CIGTS demonstrating good psychometric features.[28] The total VAQ and subscale scores, correlated weakly but significantly with visual acuity and VF scores of the better eye.[28,30] Particularly the peripheral vision subscale showed the strongest correlations with clinical measures (i.e. VA, MD, CIGTS scores).[28,30] The instrument was found to associate less strongly with glaucoma-related clinical measures than the NEI-VFQ.[44]

## 5. Glaucoma specific instruments

Glaucoma specific tools belong to the disease specific QoL instruments category. It has been demonstrated that they perform a better discriminating ability between glaucoma and normal subjects (specificity for glaucoma). Most of these instruments evaluate both symptoms that are relevant to glaucoma and instillation of anti-glaucoma medications (i.e. blurry/dim vision, difficulty in seeing in daylight, halos around lights, itching, dryness, tearing) and difficulty in performing daily activities.

### 5.1 The glaucoma symptom scale (GSS)

It includes 10 items, grouped into 2 domains: the non-visual symptoms (six items) and the visual ability (four items) subscales.[45] The instrument was found to demonstrate a good internal consistency (Cronbach $\alpha > 0.70$ for both domains), while GSS visual ability subscale showed good correlations with many NEI-VFQ subscales.[45] Furthermore, it is short and easy to use and thus, very practical for implementing in daily clinical practice.

Both GSS subscale responses were rated lower for glaucoma patients, when compared with normal control individuals. The GSS visual ability domain served as a better discriminator between glaucoma and non-glaucoma subjects.[45] However, GSS scores did not demonstrate significant correlation with Esterman (binocular) visual field alterations and visual acuity was found to associate only moderately with few GSS scores.[42,45] Furthermore, the instrument excludes treatment related effects on QoL assessment.

### 5.2 The glaucoma quality of life-15 (GQL-15)

GQL-15 was constructed after administration of 50 questions to 47 glaucoma patients who were divided into three groups according to the degree of their visual field loss (mild (n = 18), moderate (n = 19), and severe visual field loss (n = 10)) and 19 normal controls.[46]
Fifteen questions demonstrated significant association with vision field loss and finally were included in the GQL questionnaire. [46] Six questions were relevant to glare, six questions were relevant to peripheral vision, two questions were relevant to the central-near vision, and finally one question was associated with the outdoor mobility. All three glaucoma groups exhibited significantly lower scores compared with the normal control group. However, glaucoma subjects with moderate and severe visual field deterioration had similar responses to the instrument.[46] GQL-15 showed excellent validation features (Internal consistency: Cronbach alpha = 0.95, test-retest reliability: r = 0.87), while significant correlations were found between GQL-15 responses and a number of psychophysical measurements: Esterman (binocular) visual field (r = -0.39), dark adaptation (r = 0.34), perimetric mean deviation (MD) values (r = -0.6), Pelli-Robson contrast sensitivity (r = -0.45, $P < 0.001$), glare disability (r = -0.41, $P < 0.001$) and stereopsis (r = 0.26, P = 0.04).[46]
Increasing disease severity led to a poorer QoL status, as demonstrated by means of the instrument.[56] Central and near vision, peripheral vision, and outdoor mobility were the most affected domains among individuals with glaucoma.[56]

### 5.3 The symptom impact glaucoma score (SIG) and glaucoma health perceptions index (GHPI)

Both instruments were designed and developed for the Collaborative Initial Glaucoma Treatment Study (CIGTS). The SIG consists of 43 queries that are categorized into four subscales: visual ability, local eye, systemic and psychological domains. The GHPI contains 6 queries that try to explore the impact of glaucoma on emotional, physical and social aspects of QoL. In addition, the items of GHPI address the stress and worry about blindness domains that are in association with living with glaucoma.[28]
Both instruments exhibited good internal consistency and reproducibility (Cronbach α and ICC > 0.70).[28]
After administration to glaucoma subjects, both the SIG visual function subscale and the GHPI associated significantly with visual field scores of the worse eye. However the coefficients of correlation were found poor (r = 0.136 and 0.165, respectively).[28,30] These instruments are efficient tools for research settings but seem to have a limited role in clinical practice, since a 10-hour training course was necessary before being administered to individuals.

## 6. Measures of visual function and activities of daily living in glaucoma

QoL studies suggest tasks requiring central/near vision (i.e. reading), outdoor mobility and driving as the most deteriorated activities of daily living among glaucoma subjects.[9,49,56]

Furthermore, the presence of bilateral glaucoma and worse VF impairment seem to be the most significant predictors of functional ability regarding glaucoma individuals.[48]
Regarding central/near vision activities such as reading, in the Salisbury Eye Evaluation (SEE) bilateral glaucoma was associated strongly with reporting the most difficulty on the near vision subscale of the ADVS tool (odds ratio 4.57), while the presence of unilateral glaucoma was not correlated with any ADVS subscales.[35] Furthermore, other relative studies regarding glaucoma patients have revealed an association between Esterman binocular VF deterioration and both difficulty of finding the next line or following a line in a text and reading speed.[50,51]
With regard to outdoor mobility, glaucoma patients demonstrated slower walking speed when compared with age-matched non-glaucoma subjects, whereas walking speed was found to correlate significantly with MD in the worse eye.[52] In addition visually impaired glaucoma patients were found more prone to accidents and falls compared to glaucoma subjects without severe VF loss (odds ratio: 1.6)[6], whereas glaucoma subjects presented a 2-4 time greater probability of falling compared to normal control subjects.[53,54]
Concerning driving limitations, glaucoma patients tend to self-report more difficulties in driving, while this self reported difficulty correlates with deteriorating VF scores.[2,40] The SEE study demonstrated that patients with bilateral glaucoma had significantly poorer scores on the night driving subscale of ADVS compared to patients with unilateral glaucoma and normal control subjects.[35] Subjects with bilateral glaucoma were also more likely to report the most difficulty on the night driving subscale (odds ratio: 4.19).[35] In the same study the association between binocular VF and night driving subscale was found marginal, while VA and contrast sensitivity (which is a measure that surely deteriorates by glaucoma) were associated strongly with lower scores on the aforementioned subscale.[35]
Most of the aforementioned results are in accordance with analogous literature reports using other QoL assessment instruments such as the NEI-VFQ and NEI-VFQ-25 questionnaires.[40,55] Furthermore, there are a series of studies confirming the negative impact of visual field deterioration expressed by means of scores such as MD, pattern standard deviation (PSD), Advanced Glaucoma Intervention Study (AGIS) and CIGTS on the total QoL status of individuals with glaucoma.[30,39,46,57-62] These findings are further supported by the presence of the correlation between QoL and VF scores even among individuals who were unaware of having glaucoma.[62]

## 7. Conclusion

QoL is a multidimensional, subjective and dynamic sense. An effort to capture the patients' perceptions and feelings regarding their QoL is difficult to accomplish only by means of an artificial construct (i.e QoL questionnaires) and that is because no one can fully comprehend exactly how an individual perceives his own QoL state and eventually how he feels.
An ideal glaucoma QoL assessment tool should be multidimensional (comprise physical, social and mental components), enable self-administration, demonstrate good psychometric properties and include items that are directly correlated with glaucoma-related clinical measurements and are more glaucoma-specific (i.e. GQL-15). In addition, it should be in state to discriminate glaucoma patients from healthy individuals and provide responses that correlate sufficiently with clinical parameters related to the disease (visual acuity, VF scores, contrast sensitivity).
A great variety of instruments has been administered to glaucoma patients in order to evaluate their QoL. All of them have advantages and constraints. Generic health-related

tools are useful to make comparisons of QoL in a wide disease spectrum (ocular or not), but their generic character limits their specificity for glaucoma. Nevertheless, vision-specific tools enable comparisons between glaucoma and other ocular diseases, whereas they are more able to distinguish glaucoma patients from normal subjects and correlate better with clinical parameters than generic tools.[32] Furthermore, they have been used more frequently in glaucoma than other QoL instruments. The NEI-VFQ and NEI-VFQ 25 remain the benchmark in the vision-related QoL evaluation, with the domains of 'general health', 'expectations', 'mental health', 'near activities' and 'driving' being the most affected by glaucoma.[33] Glaucoma-specific tools are usually composed of items regarding (glaucoma-related) symptoms and activities of daily living that are more likely to be affected by the disease. Furthermore, they try to evaluate the importance that the patients place to their QoL deterioration because of the disease.[47] Although having specificity for glaucoma and correlating strongly with clinical measurements, they do not enable comparisons between QoL in glaucoma and other ophthalmic diseases.

Research of QoL in glaucoma in recent years has demonstrated significant progress and has provided important insights regarding how and to what extend glaucoma impacts on patients' daily living. Studies suggest that glaucoma patients with bilateral VF deterioration demonstrate worse performances in activities of daily living, especially in the domains of mobility and driving.[48] In a literature review that tried to compare QoL in glaucoma and other ocular morbidities, glaucoma proved to exert a stronger impact on mental aspects of QoL rather than physical ones.[33] The authors suggested the asymptomatic (in early stages) nature of the disease as a possible explanation. Glaucoma unlike other ophthalmic diseases respects the central visual acuity and therefore the ability of individuals suffering from the disease to perform certain physical activities could be maintained to a greater extent. Finally they concluded that the insufficient education of glaucoma patients regarding their disease combined with their worry of possible blindness may lead to a further deterioration of mental QoL.[33]

There is no ideal glaucoma QoL instrument, mainly due to the complexity and subjectivity of QoL. Further research efforts are needed that will address the weaknesses of QoL tools with regard to their construction and analysis of the data that are acquired.

## 8. References


[1] Aaronson N. K. Quality of Life: what is it? How should it be measured? Oncology (Huntingt) 1988;2:69-76.

[2] Parrish RK 2nd, Gedde SJ, Scott IU, et al. Visual function and quality of life among patients with glaucoma. Arch Ophthalmol 1997;115:1447–1455.

[3] Friedman DS, Wolfs RC, O'Colmain BJ, et al. Prevalence of open-angle glaucoma among adults in the United States. Arch Ophthalmol 2004;122:532–538.

[4] Friedman DS, Jampel HD, Munoz B, West SK. The prevalence of open-angle glaucoma among blacks and whites 73 years and older: the Salisbury Eye Evaluation Glaucoma Study. Arch.Ophthalmol 2006;124:1625–1630.

[5] Sahel JA, Bandello F, Augustin A, Maurel F, Negrini C, Berdeaux GH. Health-related quality of life and utility in patients with age-related macular degeneration. Arch Ophthalmol. 2007;125(7):945–951.

[6] Bramley T, Peeples P, Walt JG, et al. Impact of vision loss on costs and outcomes in medicare beneficiaries with glaucoma. Arch.Ophthalmol 2008;126:849–856.

[7] Lotery A, Xu X, Zlatava G, Loftus J. Burden of illness, visual impairment and health resource utilisation of patients with neovascular age-related macular degeneration: results from the UK cohort of a five-country cross-sectional study. Br J Ophthalmol. 2007;91(10):1303–1307.
[8] Aspinall PA, Johnson ZK, Azuara-Blanco A, et al. Evaluation of quality of life and priorities of patients with glaucoma. Invest.Ophthalmol.Vis.Sci 2008;49:1907–1915.1915.
[9] Pfeiffer N, Krieglstein GK, Wellek S. Knowledge about glaucoma in the unselected population: a German survey. J Glaucoma 2002;11:458–463.
[10] Hayry M. Measuring the quality of life: why, how, and what? Theor Med Bioeth 1991; 12: 97-116.
[11] Guyatt G.H., Feeny D.H., Patrick D.L. Measuring health-related quality of life. Ann. Intern. Med. 1993;118:622-629.
[12] Streiner D.L, Norman G.R. Health measurements scales: A practical guide to their development and use. Oxford University Press New York 1995.
[13] Lohr K.N., Aaronson N.K, Alonso J., Burnam M.A., Patrick D.L., Perrin E.B., Robert J.S. Evaluating quality-of-life and health status instruments: development of scientific review criteria. Clin. Ther. 1996;18:979-992.
[14] Bland J.M., Altman D.G. Statistical methods for assessing agreement between two methods of clinical measurement. Lancet 1986;1:307-310.
[15] Andersen E.M. Criteria for assessing the tools of disability outcomes research. Arch. Phys. Med. Rehabil. 2000;81(Suppl. 2):15-20.
[16] Velozo CA, Kielhofner G, Lai JS. The use of Rasch analysis to produce scale-free measurement of functional ability. Am J Occup Ther 1999; 53:83–90
[17] Smith EV Jr. Detecting and evaluating the impact of multidimensionality using item fit statistics and principal component analysis of residuals. J Appl Meas 2002; 3:205–231
[18] Wright BD, Linacre JM. Reasonable mean-square fit values.Rasch Meas Trans 1994; 8:370.
[19] Pesudovs K, Burr JM, Harley C, Elliott DB. The development, assessment, and selection of questionnaires. Optom Vis Sci 2007; 84:663–674.
[20] Ware JE Jr, Sherbourne CD. The MOS 36-item short-form health survey (SF-36): I, conceptual framework and item selection. Med Care 1992;30:473- 483.
[21] McHorney CA, Ware JE Jr, Lu JF, Sherbourne CD. The MOS 36-item Short-Form Health survey (SF-36): III, tests of data quality, scaling assumptions, and reliability across diverse patient groups. Med Care 1994;32:40–66.
[22] Ware JE Jr, Sherbourne CD. The MOS 36-item short-form health survey (SF-36): I, conceptual framework and item selection. Med Care 1992;30:473- 483.
[23] Wilson MR, Coleman AL, Yu F, et al. Functional status and well-being in patients with glaucoma as measured by the Medical Outcomes Study Short Form-36 questionnaire. Ophthalmology 1998;105:2112–2116.
[24] Parrish RK, 2nd. Visual impairment, visual functioning, and quality of life assessments in patients with glaucoma. Trans Am Ophthalmol Soc. 1996;94:919–1028.
[25] Jampel HD, Schwartz A, Pollack I, Abrams D, Weiss H, Miller R. Glaucoma patients' assessment of their visual function and quality of life. J Glaucoma 2002;11:154 -163.
[26] Sherwood MB, Garcia-Siekavizza A, Meltzer MI, Hebert A, Burns AF, McGorray S. Glaucoma's impact on quality of life and its relation to clinical indicators: a pilot study. Ophthalmology 1998;105:561–566.
[27] Bergner M, Bobbitt RA, Carter WB, Gilson BS. The Sickness Impact Profile: development and final revision of a health status measure. Med Care 1981;19:787- 805.

[28] Janz NK, Wren PA, Lichter PR, Musch DC, Gillespie BW, Guire KE. Quality of life in newly diagnosed glaucoma patients: The Collaborative Initial Glaucoma Treatment Study. Ophthalmology 2001;108(5):887-897

[29] Janz NK, Wren PA, Lichter PR, et al. The Collaborative Initial Glaucoma Treatment Study: interim quality of life findings after initial medical or surgical treatment of glaucoma. Ophthalmology. 2001;108(11):1954-1965.

[30] Mills RP, Janz NK, Wren PA, Guire KE. Correlation of visual field with quality-of-life measures at diagnosis in the Collaborative Initial Glaucoma Treatment study (CIGTS) J Glaucoma 2001;10:192-198.

[31] Steinberg EP, Tielsch JM, Schein OD, et al. The VF-14: an index of functional impairment in patients with cataract. Arch Ophthalmol 1994;112:630-638.

[32] Damiano AM, Steinberg EP, Cassard SD, et al. Comparison of generic versus disease-specific measures of functional impairment in patients with cataract. Med Care 1995;33:120-130.

[33] Keith Evans, Simon K Law, John Walt, Patricia Buchholz, Jan Hansen. The quality of life impact of peripheral versus central vision loss with a focus on glaucoma versus age-related macular degeneration. Clinical Ophthalmology 2009:3 433-445.

[34] Mangione CM, Phillips RS, Seddon JM, et al. Development of the "activities of daily vision scale": a measure of visual functional status. Med Care 1992;30:1111-1126.

[35] Freeman E.E, Munoz B., West S.K, Jampel H.D., Friedman D.S. Glaucoma and Quality of Life. The Salisbury Eye Evaluation. Ophthalmology 2008;115:233-238.

[36] Mangione CM, Lee PP, Pitts J, Gutierrez P, Burry S, Hays RD: Psychometric properties of the National Eye Institute Visual Function Questionnaire (NEI-VFQ). Arch Ophthalmol 1998; 166:1496-504.

[37] Mangione CM, Lee PP, Pitts J, Gutierrez PR, Spritzer K, Burry S, Hays RD, et al.: Development of the 25-item National Eye Institute Visual Function Questionnaire. Arch Ophthalmol 2001;119:1050-8.

[38] Labiris G, Katsanos A, Fanariotis M, Tsirouki T, Pefkianaki M, Chatzoulis D, Tsironi E. Psychometric properties of the Greek version of the NEI-VFQ 25. BMC Ophthalmol 2008; 8:4.

[39] Labiris G, Katsanos A, Fanariotis M, Zacharaki F, Chatzoulis D, Kozobolis VP. Vision-specific quality of life in Greek glaucoma patients. J Glaucoma. 2010 Jan;19(1):39-43.

[40] Gutierrez P, Wilson MR, Johnson C, et al. Influence of glaucomatous visual field loss on health-related quality of life. Arch Ophthalmol 1997;115:777-784.

[41] Keeffe JE, McCarty CA, Hassell JB, Gilbert AG. Description and measurement of handicap caused by vision impairment. Aust N Z J Ophthalmol 1999;27:184 -186.

[42] Noe G, Ferraro J, Lamoureux E, Rait J, Keeffe JE. Associations between glaucomatous visual field loss and participation in activities of daily living. Clin Experiment Ophthalmol 2003;31:482-486.

[43] Sloane ME, Ball K, Owsley C, Bruni JR, Roenker DL. The Visual Activities Questionnaire: developing an instrument for assessing problems in everyday visual tasks. In: Noninvasive Assessment of the Visual System Technical Digest. Washington, DC, Optical Society of America, 1992; 1:26-29

[44] Wren PA, Musch DC, Janz NK, Niziol LM, Guire KE, Gillespie BW; CIGTS Study Group. Contrasting the use of 2 vision-specific quality of life questionnaires in subjects with open-angle glaucoma. J Glaucoma. 2009 Jun-Jul;18(5):403-11

[45] Lee BL, Gutierrez P, Gordon M, Wilson MR, Cioffi GA, Ritch R, Sherwood, M, Mangione CM. The Glaucoma Symptom Scale. A brief index of glaucoma-specific symptoms. Arch Ophthalmol 1998; 166:861-6.

[46] Nelson P, Aspinall P, Papasouliotis O, Worton B, O'Brien C. Quality of life in glaucoma and its relationship with visual function. J Glaucoma 2003;12:139 –150.

[47] Spaeth G, Walt J, Keener J. Evaluation of Quality of Life for Patients with Glaucoma. Am J Ophthalmol 2006;141:3–14.

[48] Pradeep Ramulu. Glaucoma and Disability: Which tasks are affected, and at what stage of disease? Curr Opin Ophthalml.2009;20(2):92-98.

[49] Burr JM, Kilonzo M, Vale L, Ryan M. Developing a preference-based Glaucoma Utility Index using a discrete choice experiment. Optom. Vis. Sci 2007;84:797–808.

[50] Altangerel U, Spaeth GL, Steinmann WC. Assessment of function related to vision (AFREV). ) Ophthalmic Epidemiol 2006;13:67–80.

[51] Viswanathan AC, McNaught AI, Poinoosawmy D, et al. Severity and stability of glaucoma: patient perception compared with objective measurement. Arch. Ophthalmol 1999;117:450–454.

[52] Turano KA, Rubin GS, Quigley HA. Mobility performance in glaucoma. Invest Ophthalmol Vis Sci 1999;40:2803–2809.

[53] Lamoureux EL, Chong E, Wang JJ, et al. Visual impairment, causes of vision loss, and falls: the singapore malay eye study. Invest.Ophthalmol.Vis.Sci 2008;49:528–533.

[54] Ivers RQ, Cumming RG, Mitchell P, Attebo K. Visual impairment and falls in older adults: the Blue Mountains Eye Study. J.Am.Geriatr.Soc 1998;46:58–64.

[55] Broman AT, Munoz B, Rodriguez J, et al. The impact of visual impairment and eye disease on vision-related quality of life in a Mexican-American population: Proyecto VER. Invest Ophthalmol Vis Sci 2002;43:3393– 8.

[56] Goldberg I, Clement CI, Chiang TH, Walt JG, Lee LJ, Graham S, Healey PR. Assessing quality of life in patients with glaucoma using the Glaucoma Quality of Life-15 (GQL-15) questionnaire. J Glaucoma. 2009 Jan;18(1):6-12.

[57] van Gestel A, Webers CA, Beckers HJ, van Dongen MC, Severens JL, Hendrikse F, Schouten JS. The relationship between visual field loss in glaucoma and health-related quality-of-life. Eye (Lond). 2010 Dec;24(12):1759-69.

[58] Ringsdorf L, McGwin G Jr, Owsley C. Visual field defects and vision-specific health-related quality of life in African Americans and whites with glaucoma. J Glaucoma. 2006 Oct;15(5):414-8.

[59] Roberta McKean-Cowdin, Rohit Varma, Joanne Wu, Ron D. Hays, Stanley P. Azen, and The Los Angeles Latino Eye Study Group. Severity of Visual Field Loss and Health-related Quality of Life. Am J Ophthalmol 2007;143:1013–1023.

[60] Carrasco-Font C, Lorenzo-Martinez S, Gilli-Manzanaro P, et al. Influence of visual function on quality of life in patients with glaucoma. Arch Soc Esp Oftalmol. 2008;4:249-256.

[61] Magacho L, Lima FE, Nery AC, et al. Quality of life in glaucoma patients: regression analysis and correlation with possible modifiers. Ophthalmic Epidemiol. 2004;4:263-270.

[62] Roberta McKean-Cowdin, Ying Wang, Joanne Wu, Stanley P. Azen, Rohit Varma. Impact of Visual Field Loss on Health-Related Quality of Life in Glaucoma. The Los Angeles Latino Eye Study. Ophthalmology 2008;115:941–948.

# 15

# Glaucoma Animal Models

Elena Vecino[1] and Sansar C. Sharma[2]
*[1]Departament of Cell Biology and Histology, Faculty of Medicine, Science and Technology University of the Basque Country UPV/EHU, Leioa, Vizcaya,*
*[2]Departament of Ophthalmology, NY Medical College, Valhalla,*
*[1]Spain*
*[2]USA*

## 1. Introduction

### 1.1 Glaucoma is a progressive neuropathy

Glaucoma is an optic neuropathy that is considered to be the second leading cause of blindness worldwide. This disease is characterized by selective death of retinal ganglion cells (RGC) and a progressive loss of vision. Elevation of intraocular pressure (IOP) is a critical risk factor for glaucoma progression, and its lowering has become a major focus of intervention. However, many patients continue to lose vision despite IOP management. Additionally, some patients develop what is known as normal tension glaucoma, which is not associated with increased IOP. Taken together, the continued deterioration of some patients' vision despite IOP management as well as the incidence of normal tension glaucoma illustrate that several pressure-independent mechanisms are responsible for the development and progression of glaucomatous neuropathy (Pinar-Sueiro & Vecino, 2010).

Glaucoma is difficult to study in humans. The damage present at the time of diagnosis precludes the study of disease development from onset. Additionally, obtaining retinas at equivalent pathologic states is rare, confounding comparisons and limiting conclusions. For these reasons, the development of animal models has been necessary for the study of the pathophysiology of glaucoma.

Animal studies have articulated the mechanisms of the formation and evacuation of aqueous humour as well as the maintenance of intra-ocular pressure, thereby informing glaucoma etiology and therapeutic development. In 1901, Lauber determined that blood from the anterior ciliary veins of dogs contained fewer erythrocytes per unit volume than did blood from their paws. As early as 1903, Leber noted a significant histological connection between the Schlemm´s canal and the episcleral veins. Numerous investigators then demonstrated that various dyes and tracer substances injected into the anterior chamber later appeared in the anterior ciliary veins. It was not until 1942, when Ascher first described the appearance of aqueous veins and their connections to the episcleral venus plexus, and a connection between Schlemm's canal and eipiscleral veins was demonstrated under normal conditions *in vivo*. Ascher compressed the episcleral veins using a fine glass rod, thereby inhibiting aqueous flow into them. This flow resumed when the rod was removed. He described two types of stratification: vessels with a superior layer of aqueous flow and an inferior layer of blood flow and vessels with a center of aqueous flow surrounded by layers of blood above and below. The detection of aqueous veins confirmed a continuous evacuation of aqueous from the eye and indirectly confirmed local formation of aqueous for homeostasis (Ascher, 1942).

Through a diversity of drainage angles and functional structures across species, comparative animal studies have broadened the understanding of glaucoma. Due to their contribution to the understanding of hypertension and spontaneous or induced glaucoma, animal models have also facilitated the development of therapeutic strategies, which could not have been developed otherwise.

## 2. Natural-occurring glaucoma models

A variety of natural-occurring glaucoma models have been described in different animal species. Kolker *et al.* (1963) described a group of albino New Zealand rabbits that exhibited spontaneous alterations in trabecular mesh development. These rabbits presented a reduction in the number of lamelles, increased inter-cellular spaces between lamelles, vacuolation of the endothelial cells, and fragmentation of the basal cell. The description of these alterations gave ground to the hypothesis that a reduction in the structural support of the trabeculae could be the cause of elevated IOP. In addition, high fibrin levels detected in the aqueous humor suggested that the obstruction of aqueous evacuation associated with elevated IOP could be a result of fibrin accumulation. However, the rabbit is an inadequate animal model for studying alterations in the retina or its vascularization in glaucoma due to the absence of a *lamina cribosa*, the partial myelinization of the optic axons within the retina, and the existence of a prominent vasculous sac.

Later observations by veterinary ophthalmologists led to the development of a dog model of closed angle glaucoma in Beagles, Cockers, and Basset hounds. Cockers develop glaucoma at an early age, whereas Beagles and Bassets begin to develop the disease between 6 and 12 months of age (Gelatt et al., 1977). Beagles expressing autosomal recessive phenotype present a pre-glaucoma stage characterized by increased IOP and an open angle. The angle begins to close within 2-3 years as the glaucoma develops. Chronic pressures of 30-40mmHg with transient peaks of up to 60 - 80 mmHg can induce excavation of the optic nerve head. In these animals, glaucoma can be treated pharmacologically with drugs utilized in humans including pilocarpine, epinephrine, acetazolamide, and dichlorphenamide.

In 1974, Gaasterland *et al.* developed the first laser model of glaucoma in non-human primates, predating the description of spontaneous glaucoma in dogs. In 1993, a group of Macque monkeys in quay Santiago was characterized by a maternal inheritance pattern associated with a 40% prevalence of increased IOP. Affected animals exhibited a loss of retinal ganglion cells, excavation of the optic nerve, and electrophysiological evidence of damages in the retina peripheral field (Dawson et al., 1993). Similar to humans, the disadvantage of a naturally occurring glaucoma model in non-human primates is the difficulty in controlling the onset of the disease, thus, obtaining a homogenous experimental group to observe cellular and molecular mechanisms or test possible treatments.

## 3. Induced glaucoma models

To create the proper conditions for controlled experiments, induced glaucoma models have been developed over the decades. These models have provided the ability to examine both the onset and the pathological progression in a controlled, reproducible manner.

### 3.1 Non-human primates

The earliest models of induced glaucoma were developed in non-human primates. The idea to induce elevated IOP via intraocular injections of the proteolytic enzyme alpha chymotrypsin was initially developed following cataract surgery in humans (Kalvin et al., 1966). Alpha chymotrypsin, however, produced highly variable IOP responses depending on the doses and region of the eye into which it was applied. These initial experiments suggested that the substrate underlying IOP elevation in this primate model primarily resided in the posterior chamber, and that the drug has direct, dose-dependent degenerative effects on the neural retina and vasculature. Observed atrophy of the ciliary body associated with the corneal lesions and dislocation of the lens in the presence of alpha chymotrypsin suggested that the most likely cause of elevated IOP in this primate model is blockage of the anterior chamber drainage channels by drug-induced lysates of the ciliary body (Lessell & Kuwabara, 1969).

In an attempt to overcome the difficulties associated with the alpha chymotrypsin model and to develop a primate model more analagous to human primary open glaucoma, Gaasterland & Kupfer (1974) developed laser induced scar formation of the trabecular meshwork (TM) using a gonio lens and a slit lamp equipped with an Argon laser. This model became the gold standard for laser-induced glaucoma in non-human primates. Quigley and Hohman (1983) investigated different combinations of laser treatment duration, power, and number of application spots. Recently, the use of laser to generate pressure-induced experimental glaucoma in non-human primates was implemented with a high-power diode laser (Wang et al., 1998).

The use of the laser technique requires access to skilled personnel with highly specialized ophthalmic equipment. Following a trabeculoplasty with Argon laser in humans and non-human primates, there is a temporary increase in IOP, which seems to be caused by the formation of fibrin meshes obstructing the spaces of the trabecula. In non-human primates, there is an additional fixed midriasis probably due to the damage suffered by the ciliary nerves. In some non-human primate cases, large fluctuations in IOP mandate repeated laser sessions to sustain high pressure, causing severe inflammation in the ocular globe and trabecular alterations that preclude pharmacological studies. In spite of these difficulties, non-human primates have been broadly used for improving clinical indicators of initial optic nerve damage in glaucoma.

To circumvent the negative effects of the laser techniques, other methods were explored to elevate IOP. Quigley and Addicks (1980) injected autologous fixed red blood cells or ghost blood cells into the anterior chamber of the monkeys, but this method did not allow the visualization of the ocular fundus. The injection of latex microspheres into the anterior chamber of the rhesus monkey eye introduced a new, inexpensive technique. The microspheres do not induce ocular inflammation and do not compromise visibility of the optic disc necessary for clinical assessment of disease onset and progression (Weber & Zelenak, 2001). Our group obtained reliable results by modifying this method by injecting hydroxyproopylmethylcellulose added to the microspheres in rats and in pigs (Urcola et al., 2006; Ruiz-Ederra et al., 2005b).

Non-human primate models of induced glaucoma are useful for understanding human glaucoma. These studies can evaluate RGC density from standard clinical perimetry. Examination of the retina, trabecular meshwork, lamina cribosa, and optic nerve head has been well reviewed, as has the improvement of non-invasive assessments of glaucoma onset and progression through *in vivo* measurements of neural structure and function (Weber & Viswanathan, 2008).

### 3.2 Pigs and minipigs

Though non-human primates make excellent animal models for studying human disease, ethical and economical factors negatively affect their availability. The pig model is more accessible than non-human primates in addition to being phylogenetically close to humans.

The pig eye/retina shares many similarities with that of the human (Ruiz-Ederra et al., 2005a; Ruiz-Ederra et al., 2005a). The retina is more similar to the human retina than that of other larger mammals such as the dog, goat, cow, or ox (Prince et al., 1960). In minipigs, the central venous ring is formed by various vessels and occupies the center of the optic disc, making visualization of the lamina cribosa more difficult than in humans (Galdos et al., 2011a). The pig has recently been used to genetically reproduce a retinitis pigmentosa condition similar to one found in human (Li et al., 1998). The diagnostic tools, such as optical coherence tomography, corneal topography imaging or multi-focal electroretinography can be applied to the pig, supporting its use as an excellent model for diseases of the eye (Vecino et al., 2011). Image analysis of the porcine retina has been characterized well (Lalonde et al., 2006) and is useful in developing human transplantation experiments (Klassen et al., 2008).

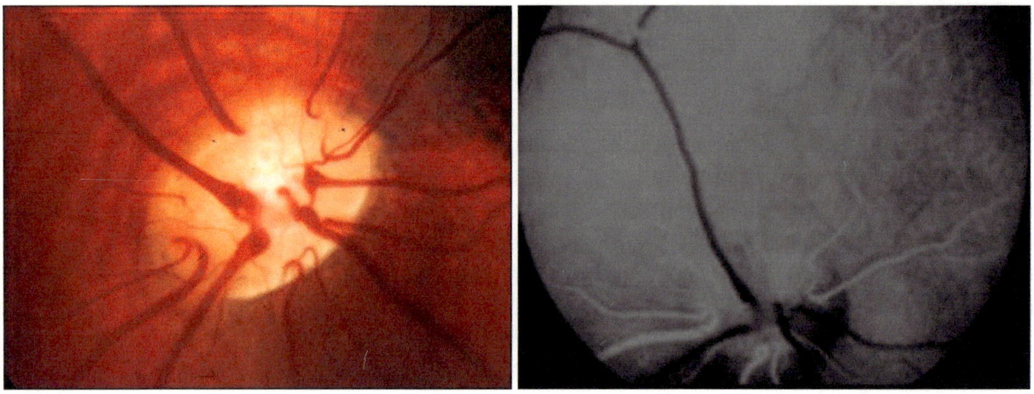

Fig. 1. Fundoscopy (left) and angiography (right) of a minipig eye. Note the lamina cribosa at the end of the optic nerve in the fundoscopic picture. In the angiography the veins appear dark and emerge from the optic nerve

The pig retina has been extensively studied. We have characterized three classes of RGCs (small, medium, and large) based on soma size (Garcia et al., 2002), and, in a detailed study of pig RGC topography, revealed that the distribution of the three classes is very similar in the porcine and human retina. This similarity may help elucidate the mechanisms implicated in the selective death of large RGCs generally accepted to be differentially vulnerable in human and experimental glaucoma (Glovinsky et al., 1991; Ruiz-Ederra et al., 2005a). We have found that porcine Müller cells *in vitro* secrete neuroprotective factors that facilitate the survival and axonal growth of large RGCs (Garcia et al., 2002). We have further described expression patterns of neurotrophins and their receptors in different RGC types *in vivo* and *in vitro*, suggesting that the expression of most of the molecules studied was preserved after either dissociation or regeneration *in vitro* (Garcia et al., 2003; Vecino, 2008b; Vecino, 2008a).

We have described the similarity of the two classes of astrocytes in the adult human and pig retina in terms of their expression of the high affinity neuronal growth factor receptor TrkA

(Ruiz-Ederra et al., 2003). The comparative description of the three neurofilament subunits were considered when describing the similarities between RGCs from human and pig (Ruiz-Ederra et al., 2004).

Considering the similarities between the porcine and human retinas, we used episcleral vein cauterization described by Sharma's group (Shareef et al., 1995) to induce elevation of IOP in the pig and minipig. Similarly, we used the injection of latex fluorospheres into the anterior chamber (Ruiz-Ederra et al., 2005b) to induce glaucoma in pigs and minipigs (Fig. 2). The use of minipigs facilitated the experiments because these animals are easy to handle and grow slowly (www.minipig.com). Glaucoma was identified by the presence of elevated IOP, altered eye fundus morphology, and RGC loss (Ruiz-Ederra et al., 2005a; Galdos et al., 2011a; Galdos et al., 2011b). Animals were kept for 21 weeks with up to a 1.4-fold increase of IOP in the operated eye versus the control fellow eye. Several factors that implicated in glaucoma etiology and development were analyzed in the pig and minipig models.

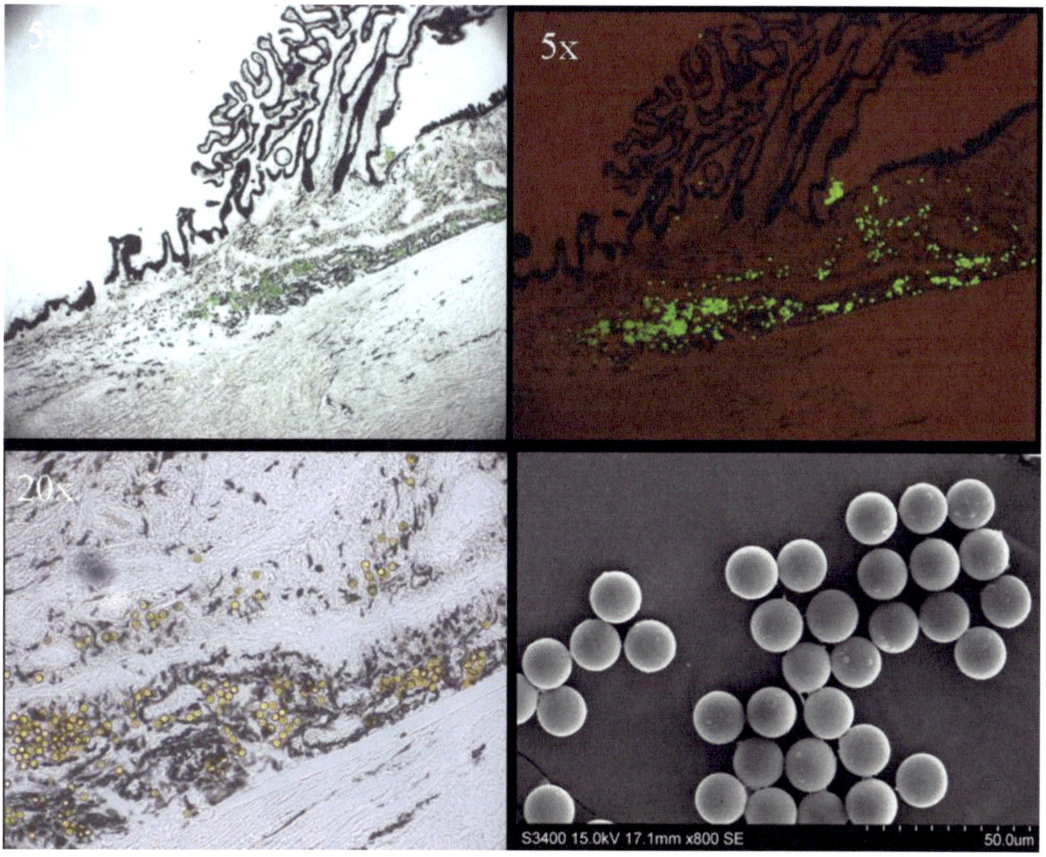


Fig. 2. Cryostat section of the minipig eye angle after Fluorospheres injection. Note the location of the latex fluorospheres in the trabecular meshwork and the aqueous humor evacuation channels. Upper left: light microscope picture. Upper right: fluorescent microscopic picture. Bottom left: higher magnification of the trabecular meshwork with fluorospheres. bottom right: scanning electronic microscopic picture of the injected 15 micrometres latex fluorospheres

*Angiographic and fundoscopic changes*

The minipig model of chronic, open-angle glaucoma induced by episcleral venous cauterization presented no angiopathic changes after elevation of the IOP. Therefore, neither surgery with episcleral vein cauterization nor elevated IOP induced changes in the chorio-retinal circulation. However, displacement of the vessels in the optic disc reflected significant differences in the neuroretinal ring that were also observed in humans with primary open angle glaucoma (POAG). In minipigs with experimental glaucoma, some arterioles were nasally displaced and incurved medially once outside of the optic disc. In minipigs, the central venous ring is formed by various vessels and occupies the center of the optic disc, making visualization of the lamina cribosa more difficult than in humans (see Fig. 1, Galdos et al., 2011a).

*Molecular and ultrastructural changes of the trabecular meshworks*

Increased resistance to aqueous humour outflow is generally accepted as a predominant risk factor for increased IOP in glaucomatous eyes. To date, neither the associated structures nor the pathophysiology of this increased resistance is well understood. In the pig model of glaucoma, we have reported the expression of the endothelial leukocyte adhesion molecule 1 (ELAM-1), which was identified as the first molecular marker for glaucomatous trabecular meshwork cells in humans (Wang et al., 2001). ELAM-1 was expressed by trabecular meshwork cells in eyes with various types of glaucoma, but not in non-glaucomatous controls. ELAM-1, also known as E-Selectin, is a 115 kDa cytokine endothelial cell surface glycoprotein that mediates the adhesion of neutrophils, monocytes, eosinophils, NK cells, and a subset of T cells to activated endothelium (Bevilacqua et al., 1989).

Based on our previous findings in the porcine trabecular meshwork, we propose that induced glaucoma begins when cauterization of three of the four episcleral veins produces a decrease in outflow of aqueous humor, leading to altered drainage in the front of the eye and subsequent elevation of IOP. The elevation of IOP induces ELAM-1 expression at the anterior chamber as a response to cellular stress (Suarez & Vecino, 2006). The finding that ELAM-1 is upregulated in the outflow pathway in pig and human experimental glaucoma will undoubtedly promote further studies about its treatment.

The induction of glaucoma by increasing the post-trabecular resistance to aqueous outflow allows the observation of ultrastructural changes in the trabecular meshwork secondary to increased IOP without chemically or mechanically changing the TM cells. The Gottingen minipig has a system with multiple vessels of the angular aqueous plexus contrasting with the unique Schelm's Canal of primates. In experimental eyes, ultrastructural differences were observed in the sub-endothelium of the inner wall of the juxta canalicular vessels, corresponding to the cribriform region in humans. Secondary ultrastructural changes in the optic disc in animals with induced elevation of IOP were noted.

In the animals that presented statistically significant chronic increase of the IOP and were then subject to ultrastructural analysis, changes were observed in vessels at the subendothelial region. The differences detected included: greater amounts of fibrillar material and elastic-like (EL) fibers, a smaller number of empty spaces (ES) and larger cisternae of the endoplasmic reticulum (ER) filled with electron-lucent material. Both in control and glaucomatous eyes, pores were observed in both the deepest and the most superficial vessels, although, pores were only present in the inner wall of the latter. Similarly, giant vacuoles were found in both the deepest the most superficial vessels, and could be seen in both the inner and outer wall of the vessels of the angular aqueous

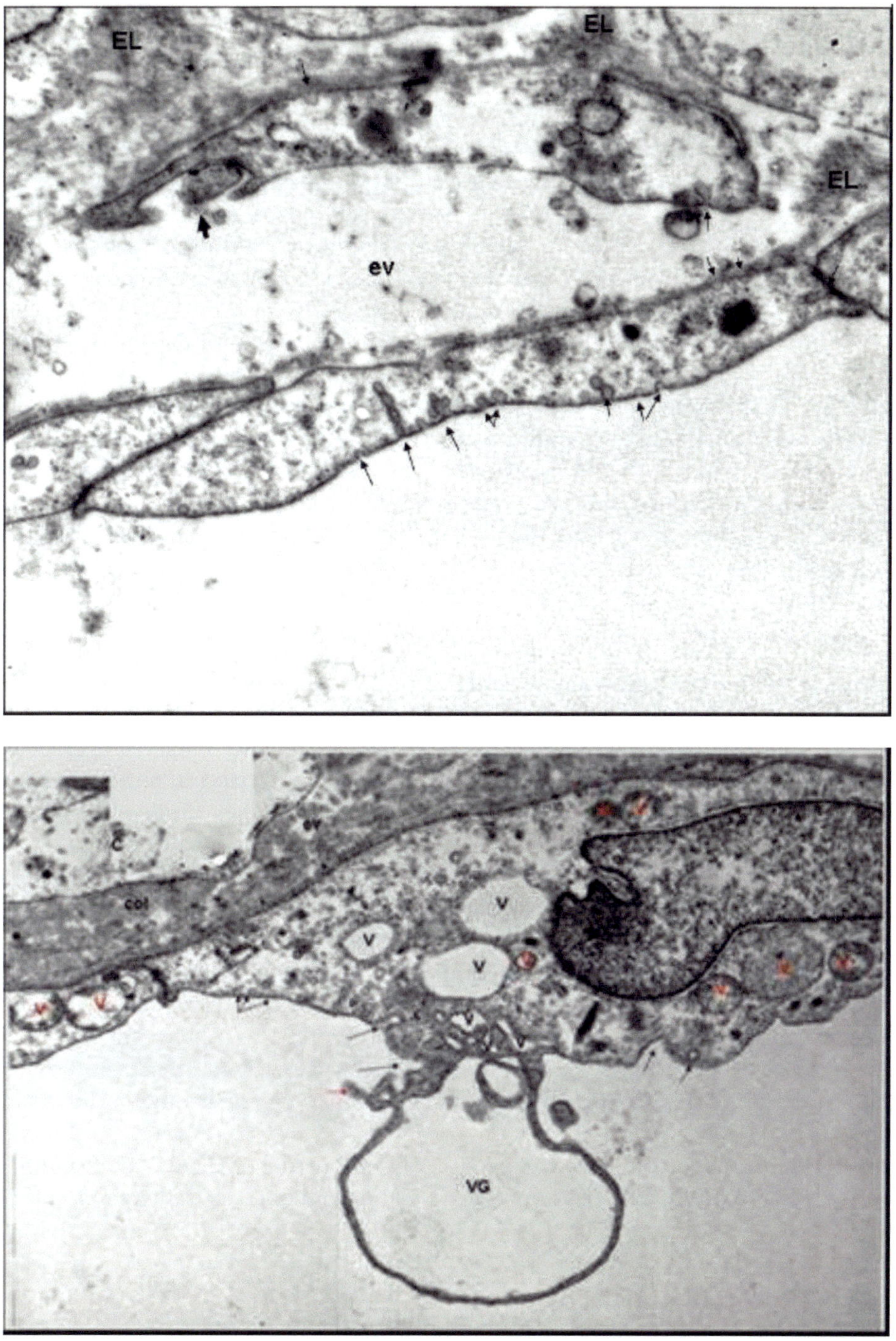


Fig. 3. Electron Microscopic pictures of different channals of the minipig trabeculum. Note transport of vesicles (arrows) and elastic like fibers (EL) in the upper picture. In the bottom picture the large vesicles (VG) are characteristic of the aqueous transport in the endothelial cells as well as the colagenous (col) fibres (v)vesicles, ev(external vessel)

plexus. We did not observe consistent differences in the number of vacuoles or pores in the inner and outer walls of the vessels of the angular aqueous plexus (Fig. 3) (Galdos et al., 2011b). Nevertheless, our findings suggest that the increase in IOP alone induces changes in the cribriform region. The increase in IOP seems to be a factor that increases the mechanical pressure on the subendothelial cribriform and juxtacanalicular cells. This pressure leads to a secondary release of stress factors, inducing changes in the extracellular matrix, that results in an increased resistance to the aqueous humor outflow, a mechanism that has been suggested by other authors as well. These morphological changes secondary to increased IOP would explain the progressive nature of this disease, characteristic of elderly people and requiring increasingly aggressive treatment.

On the basis of the results of this study, we suggest that the origin of POAG may initially be associated with an increase of the post-trabecular resistance to aqueous humor outflow and, subsequently, the increase in the IOP may cause changes in the trabecular meshwork. We cannot rule out that the changes start originally at the trabecular level in susceptible individuals, in whom peaks in lifelong physiological variations in IOP are sufficient to cause secondary changes in the cribriform region of the trabeculum. We propose that the obstruction of the trabecula could sometimes be the effect and not the cause, thereby initiating a vicious cycle that culminates in the chronic disease of glaucoma (Galdos & Vecino, 2011b).

*Retinal ganglion cell death*

IOP elevation led to RGC loss, which was significant in peripheral regions of the retina (the mid-peripheral retina). A greater loss of RGCs in the peripheral retina in monkey and rat models of experimental glaucoma has previously been reported (Laquis et al., 1998; Vickers et al., 1995). A more detailed analysis revealed that regions located in temporal quadrants showed a greater loss of RGCs (Ruiz-Ederra et al., 2005a). This finding correlates with previous reports of greater loss of visual function and RGC loss from temporal compared with the nasal human retina (Fortune et al., 2002; Garway-Heath et al., 2002; Takamoto & Schwartz, 2002). Moreover, we observed an increase in the mean area of RGC somata in those regions of the retina that presented significant RGC loss. The same phenomenon has been reported in a rat episcleral vein cauterisation glaucoma model, suggesting that the increment of RGC soma size intrinsically linked to soma density was probably a compensatory response to cell loss (Ahmed et al., 2001). It is possible that the remaining RGCs are stimulated to occupy the vacated areas after RGC death, increasing their soma area and/or dendritic field, as described by other authors (Perry & Linden, 1982; Kirby & Chalupa, 1986).

The similarities in glaucomatous changes in the minipig model of POAG and human POAG are necessary for the translation of an effective animal model to understand the human disease.

### 3.3 Corticosteroid model in rabbits

The use of corticosteroids to increase IOP as an effective model for glaucoma began in the 1960s. Many studies since have reported variable results. Beatty *et al.* (1984) found that topical steroid application produced dose-related increases in IOP in albino rabbits and humans, whereas Payne *et al.* (1990) noted that verapamil, diltiazem and nifedipine had no effect on IOP in rabbits. The corticosteroid-induced glaucoma mimics human chronic open-angle glaucoma. In contrast to most of the induced experimental models for glaucoma, corticosteroid glaucoma is also observed in ophthalmological practice after topical, periocular or systemic administration of corticosteroids, strengthening the parallel between the animal and human disease. It is important to remember that steroids can cause undesired secondary effects including cataracts and the accumulation of cellular debris at the trabecular meshwork. The increase in IOP is variable between species. Rabbits have been a common animal used by the pharmaceutical companies to test drugs; however, IOP measurements are difficult to standardize because the rabbit eye dries variably depending on the stress of the animal. In addition, the rabbit retina is partially myelinated by oligodendrocytes not present in human or other mammalian retina. Taken together, these reasons make the steroids treatment, as well as the rabbit, a sub-optimal model for studying glaucoma.

### 3.4 Rats and mice

Much of the progress in the study of glaucoma has been driven by the development of rat models. These animals offer advantages in economics and husbandry in addition to presenting fewer ethical restrictions. In 1995, the group of Dr. Sharma developed the cauterization of episcleral veins in rats as a model for obtaining chronically high intraocular pressures (Shareef et al., 1995). This model protects the trabecula structure, and it does not affect the ciliary nerve as the laser model does. In addition, elevated IOP can be maintained for up to 6 months (25% of a rat's lifetime). This animal model has allowed pharmacological trials of pressure-reducing and neuron-protecting drugs of different combinations and concentrations before subsequent studies in larger animals and clinical trials in humans. In this context, rats are making an enormous contribution to anti-glaucoma research. Also in 1995, the group of Dr. Sharma described, for the first time, the death of RGCs following a pattern or program known as apoptosis (Garcia-Valenzuela et al., 1995). This pattern involves cleavage enzymes known as caspases, which can conversely confer neuroprotection if inhibited at a specific time of the damage-inducing process. The main advantage of the rat as an animal model is that it can be generated in high numbers, so that many pharmacological tests can be performed simultaneously, but the small size of the rat eye limits its use in some areas of ophthalmology. The use of the episcleral vein cauterization model of glaucoma has been the most commonly used method to induce glaucoma since its inception (Shareef *et al.*, 1995). The method is less invasive than laser photocoagulation and induces no complications in the anterior chamber. Its efficacy and accessibility led to an explosion of research, and the majority of the molecular and functional studies in the experimental glaucoma field have used this method.

Other rat models for induced glaucoma have emerged. A few years after the episcleral vein cauterization was published, a hypertonic saline solution injection to the episcleral veins was developed as a variant (Morrison et al., 1997). The objective of this method was also to increase the IOP by reducing the drainage of the aqueous humour. One disadvantage of this method is that sequential hypertonic saline injections are needed to maintain chronic, elevated IOP (Ruduzinski & Saragovi H.U., 2005).

Laser energy has been employed in rats as a tool to perform burns directed at the trabecular meshwork alone (Ueda et al., 1998) and episcleral veins (Levkovitch-Verbin et al., 2002).

To compare the effects of IOP elevation on ganglion cell size and death, we used three experimental glaucoma models in rats: (i) injections of latex microspheres into the anterior chamber of the eye (ii) injections of microspheres and hydroxypropylmethylcellulose into the anterior chamber, and (iii) cauterization of three episcleral veins. A significant increase in IOP was found following each of the three methods (Urcola et al., 2006). Thirteen to 30 weeks later, RGCs were retrogradely labelled with fluorogold. Cell death was evident in the glaucomatous eyes when compared with controls, but no statistically significant effect was observed on the extent of cell death. The present results indicate that in animal groups subjected to the injection of microspheres alone and microsphres together with hydroxypropylmethylcellulose, nine and six injections, respectively, are necessary to achieve sustained, elevated IOP. The number of microsphere injections necessary to induce sustained, elevated IOP in rat is similar to that which has been reported for the monkey (Weber & Zelenak, 2001). Regarding episcleral vein cauterization, we observed IOP elevation more constant for at least 24 weeks as compared with the other two experimental glaucoma methods tested (Urcola et al., 2006). Similar results were observed when the three methods were compared in pigs (Ruiz-Ederra et al., 2005b).

Recently, it has been reported the induction of elevation of IOP in rats by using injection of magnetic microspheres to induce the same effect of the latex micropspheres but in this case the microspheres could be directed by an handheld magnet (Samsel et at., 2011).

Due to the small size of the mouse eye, injection of the latex microspheres (Fluo-Spheres, Molecular Probes) into the anterior chamber of mice has become a popular method to induce increase IOP. Authors that now use the spheres to increase IOP in rats and mice (Sappington et al., 2010) use the term "microbeads occlusion model" to refer to the same model that Urcola et al. published in 2006 in rats and Ruiz-Ederra et al., 2005b published in pigs.

To determine the effects of elevated IOP following episcleral vein cauterization, a detailed analysis of 15 different molecular markers was conducted for the different retinal cell types at different time points. The changes observed in the distribution of the immunoreactivity in the hypertensive rat retina were more severe in the inner retina than in the outer retina, especially in the AII amacrine cells. To our knowledge, we described for the first time that the rod bipolar cells pathway was also damaged in the hypertensive eye, as evidenced by changes in anti-PKC-α antibody. Changes in bipolar cells are not surprising when one considers that the RGCs lose their presynaptic connections. It is possible that the changes noticed may represent a plasticity mechanism in neuronal circuitry (Hernandez et al., 2009).

### 3.5 Transgenic mice

The appearance of the DBA/2J mouse, which develops a progressive increase in IOP leading to the death of retinal ganglion cells (John et al., 1998) resulted in a large amount of studies to establish the existence of homologies related to glaucoma in humans. The increase in IOP in these animals appears at 8 months of age, and the pressure remains chronically high until death. The limiting factors of these studies include the small globe and the absence of *lamina cribosa*. This animal model of spontaneous, chronic, high IOP is suitable for studying the causes of this pathology. However, with the exception of the DBA/2J mice, animals with glaucoma are difficult to obtain, especially at similar stages of pathology. More recently, other transgenic mouse models have emerged, including one with a targeted mutation in the gene for the alpha-1 subunit of collagen type 1, which demonstrates a gradual elevation of IOP and progressive optic nerve axon loss (Mabuchi et al., 2004). Another mouse, deficient in the glutamate transporters Glast or Eaac1, demonstrates retinal ganglion cell death and optic nerve degeneration without elevated IOP (Harada et al., 2007). The transgenic mouse expressing a mutant form of human myocilin protein has also been characterized (Senatorov et al., 2006; Zhou et al., 2008). Finally, mutations affecting a serine protease (PRSS56) cause a mouse phenotype resembling closed-angle glaucoma (Nair et al., 2011).

Just as progress in glaucoma diagnosis has been linked to developments in technology, progress in glaucoma treatment has been linked to the development of effective animal models. By using these animal models, we hope to continue the processes of glaucoma prevention as well as treatment.

| Mechanism | Procedure | Species | Reference |
|---|---|---|---|
| Pre-trabecular | Ghost red blood | Monkey | (Quigley & Addicks, 1980) |
| | Viscolastic | Human (*in vitro*) | (Benson et al., 1983) |
| | | Rabbit | (Torngren et al., 2000) |
| | Microspheres (beans) | Monkey | (Weber & Zelenak, 2001) |
| | | Pig/Minipig | (Ruiz-Ederra et al., 2005 a,b) |
| | | Rat | (Urcola et al., 2006) |
| | Microspheres + viscolastic | Pig/Minipig | (Ruiz-Ederra et al., 2005 a,b) |
| | | Rat | (Urcola et al., 2006) |
| | | Mouse | (Sappington et al., 2010) |
| Trabecular | Steroids | Rabbit | (Bonomi et al., 1978) |
| | Laser photocoagulation | Monkey | (Pederson & Gaasterland, 1984) |
| | | Rat | (Ueda et al., 1998) |
| Post-trabecular | Episcleral veins cauterization | Rat | (Shareef et al., 1995) |
| | | Pig/Minipig | (Ruiz-Ederra et al., 2005 a,b) |
| | Saline injection | Rat | (Morrison et al., 1995) |
| Genetic | DBA | mouse | (John et al., 1998) |
| | Myocilin | mouse | (Senatorov et al., 2006) |

Table 1.

## 4. Acknowledgments

Basque Government Grant Grupos Consolidados (IT43710), Red Patología Ocular RETICS (RD07/0062/2004), ONCE (Organization for Spanish blind persons).

## 5. References


Ahmed, F. A., Chaudhary, P., & Sharma, S. C. (2001). Effects of increased intraocular pressure on rat retinal ganglion cells. *Int. J. Dev. Neurosci.*, 19, 209-218.

Ascher, K. W. (1942). The aqueous veins. Physiological importance of the visible elimination of intraouclar fluid. 25[American Journal of Ophthalmology], 1174-1209.

Beatty, J. F., Krupin, T., Nichols, P. F., & BECKER, B. (1984). Elevation of intraocular pressure by calcium channel blockers. *Arch. Ophthalmol.*, 102, 1072-1076.

Benson, F. G., Patterson, M. M., & Einstein D.L. (1983). Obstruction of aqueous outflow by sodium hyaluronate in enucleated human eyes. *Am. J. Ophthalmol.*, 95, 668-672.

Bevilacqua, M. P., Stengelin, S., Gimbrone, M. A., Jr., & Seed, B. (1989). Endothelial leukocyte adhesion molecule 1: an inducible receptor for neutrophils related to complement regulatory proteins and lectins. *Science*, 243, 1160-1165.

Bonomi, L., Perfetti, S., Noya, E., Bellucci, R., & Tomazzoli, L. (1978). Experimental corticosteroid ocular hypertension in the rabbit. *Albrecht. Von. Graefes Arch. Klin. Exp. Ophthalmol.*, 209, 73-82.

Dawson, W. W., Brooks, D. E., Hope, G. M., Samuelson, D. A., Sherwood, M. B., Engel, H. M. et al. (1993). Primary open angle glaucomas in the rhesus monkey. *Br.J.Ophthalmol.*, 77, 302-310.

Fortune, B., Cull, G., Wang, L., Van Buskirk, E. M., & Cioffi, G. A. (2002). Factors affecting the use of multifocal electroretinography to monitor function in a primate model of glaucoma. *Doc. Ophthalmol.*, 105, 151-178.

Gaasterland, D. & Kupfer, C. (1974). Experimental glaucoma in the rhesus monkey. *Invest Ophthalmol.*, 13, 455-457.

Galdos, M., Bayon, A., Mico, C., & Vecino, E. (2010). Fundoscopic and ultrastructural evaluation in experimental glaucoma model in minipigs. ARVO e-abstract 6392.

Galdos, M., Bayon, A., Rodriguez, F. D., Mico, C., Sharma, S. C., & Vecino, E. (2011a). Morphology of retinal vessels in the optic disc in a Gttingen minipig experimental glaucoma model. *Veterinary Journal*, In press.

Galdos, M. & Vecino, E. (2011b). Ultraestructural changes in the travecular meshwork and IOP elevation. Which come first, the chicken or the egg? *Archivos de la Sociedad Espaöla de Oftalmologia*, In press.

Garcia, M., Forster, V., Hicks, D., & Vecino, E. (2002). Effects of muller glia on cell survival and neuritogenesis in adult porcine retina in vitro. *Investigative Ophthalmology and Visual Science*, 43, 3735-3743.

Garcia, M., Forster, V., Hicks, D., & Vecino, E. (2003). In vivo expression of neurotrophins and neurotrophin receptors is conserved in adult porcine retina in vitro. *Investigative Ophthalmology and Visual Science*, 44, 4532-4541.

Garcia-Valenzuela, E., Shareef, S., Walsh, J., & Sharma, S. C. (1995). Programmed cell death of retinal ganglion cells during experimental glaucoma. *Exp.Eye Res.*, 61, 33-44.

Garway-Heath, D. F., Holder, G. E., Fitzke, F. W., & Hitchings, R. A. (2002). Relationship between electrophysiological, psychophysical, and anatomical measurements in glaucoma. *Invest Ophthalmol. Vis.Sci.*, 43, 2213-2220.

Gelatt, K. N., Peiffer, R. L., Jr., Gwin, R. M., Gum, G. G., & Williams, L. W. (1977). Clinical manifestations of inherited glaucoma in the beagle. *Invest Ophthalmol.Vis.Sci.,* 16, 1135-1142.

Glovinsky, Y., Quigley, H. A., & Dunkelberger, G. R. (1991). Retinal ganglion cell loss is size dependent in experimental glaucoma. *Invest Ophthalmol.Vis.Sci.,* 32, 484-491.

Harada, T., Harada, C., Nakamura, K., Quah, H. M., Okumura, A., Namekata, K. et al. (2007). The potential role of glutamate transporters in the pathogenesis of normal tension glaucoma. *J.Clin.Invest,* 117, 1763-1770.

Hernandez, M., Rodriguez, F. D., Sharma, S. C., & Vecino, E. (2009). Immunohistochemical changes in rat retinas at various time periods of elevated intraocular pressure. *Molecular Vision,* 15, 2696-2709.

John, S. W., Smith, R. S., Savinova, O. V., Hawes, N. L., Chang, B., Turnbull, D. et al. (1998). Essential iris atrophy, pigment dispersion, and glaucoma in DBA/2J mice. *Invest Ophthalmol.Vis.Sci.,* 39, 951-962.

Kalvin, N. H., Hamasaki, D. I., & Gass, J. D. (1966). Experimental glaucoma in monkeys. I. Relationship between intraocular pressure and cupping of the optic disc and cavernous atrophy of the optic nerve. *Arch.Ophthalmol.,* 76, 82-93.

Kirby, M. A. & Chalupa, L. M. (1986). Retinal crowding alters the morphology of alpha ganglion cells. *J.Comp Neurol.,* 251, 532-541.

Klassen, H., Warfvinge, K., Schwartz, P. H., Kiilgaard, J. F., Shamie, N., Jiang, C. et al. (2008). Isolation of progenitor cells from GFP-transgenic pigs and transplantation to the retina of allorecipients. *Cloning Stem Cells,* 10, 391-402.

Kolker, A. E., Moses, R. A., Constant, M. A., & Becker, B. (1963). The Development of Glaucoma in Rabbits. *Invest Ophthalmol.,* 2, 316-321.

Lalonde, M. R., Chauhan, B. C., & Tremblay, F. (2006). Retinal ganglion cell activity from the multifocal electroretinogram in pig: optic nerve section, anaesthesia and intravitreal tetrodotoxin. *J.Physiol,* 570, 325-338.

Laquis, S., Chaudhary, P., & Sharma, S. C. (1998). The patterns of retinal ganglion cell death in hypertensive eyes. *Brain Res.,* 784, 100-104.

Lessell, S. & Kuwabara, T. (1969). Experimental alpha-chymotrypsin glaucoma. *Arch.Ophthalmol.,* 81, 853-864.

Levkovitch-Verbin, H., Martin, K. R., Quigley, H. A., Baumrind, L. A., Pease, M. E., & Valenta, D. (2002). Measurement of amino acid levels in the vitreous humor of rats after chronic intraocular pressure elevation or optic nerve transection. *J.Glaucoma.,* 11, 396-405.

Li, Z. Y., Wong, F., Chang, J. H., Possin, D. E., Hao, Y., Petters, R. M. et al. (1998). Rhodopsin transgenic pigs as a model for human retinitis pigmentosa. *Invest Ophthalmol.Vis.Sci.,* 39, 808-819.

Mabuchi, F., Lindsey, J. D., Aihara, M., Mackey, M. R., & Weinreb, R. N. (2004). Optic nerve damage in mice with a targeted type I collagen mutation. *Invest Ophthalmol.Vis.Sci.,* 45, 1841-1845.

McMenamin, P. G. & Steptoe, R. J. (1991). Normal anatomy of the aqueous humour outflow system in the domestic pig eye. *J.Anat.,* 178, 65-77.

Morrison, J. C., Fraunfelder, F. W., Milne, S. T., & Moore, C. G. (1995). Limbal microvasculature of the rat eye. *Invest Ophthalmol.Vis. Sci.*, 36, 751-756.

Morrison, J. C., Moore, C. G., Deppmeier, L. M., Gold, B. G., Meshul, C. K., & Johnson, E. C. (1997). A rat model of chronic pressure-induced optic nerve damage. *Exp.Eye Res.*, 64, 85-96.

Nair, K. S., Hmani-Aifa, M., Ali, Z., Kearney, A. L., Salem, S. B., Macalinao, D. G. et al. (2011). Alteration of the serine protease PRSS56 causes angle-closure glaucoma in mice and posterior microphthalmia in humans and mice. *Nat.Genet.* 43(6), 579-584.

Payne, L. J., Slagle, T. M., Cheeks, L. T., & Green, K. (1990). Effect of calcium channel blockers on intraocular pressure. *Ophthalmic Res.*, 22, 337-341.

Pederson, J. E. & Gaasterland, D. E. (1984). Laser-induced primate glaucoma. I. Progression of cupping. *Arch.Ophthalmol.*, 102, 1689-1692.

Perry, V. H. & Linden, R. (1982). Evidence for dendritic competition in the developing retina. *Nature*, 297, 683-685.

Pinar-Sueiro, S. & Vecino, E. (2010). Potential neuroprotective strategis for glaucoma. *J.Inherit.Metab Dis.*, 16, 1-38.

Prince, J. H., Diesem, C. C., Eglitis, I., & Ruskell, G. L. (1960). The pig. In C.C.Thomas (Ed.), *Anatomy and Histology of the Eye and Orbit in Domestic Animals* (pp. 210-230). Illinois.

Quigley, H. A. & Addicks, E. M. (1980). Scanning electron microscopy of trabeculectomy specimens from eyes with open-angle glaucoma. *Am. J. Ophthalmol.*, 90, 854-857.

Quigley, H. A. & Hohman, R. M. (1983). Laser energy levels for trabecular meshwork damage in the primate eye. *Invest Ophthalmol. Vis. Sci.*, 24, 1305-1307.

Ruduzinski, M. & Saragovi H.U. (2005). Glaucoma: validated and facile in vivo experimental models of a chronic neurodegenerative disease for drug development. *Current Med.Chem*, 5, 43-49.

Ruiz-Ederra, J., Garcia, M., Hernandez, M., Urcola, H., Araiz and Vecino E. (2005a). The pig eye as a novel model of glaucoma. *Exp Eye Res*, 81, 561-569.

Ruiz-Ederra, J., Garcia, M., Hicks, D., & Vecino, E. (2004). Comparative study of the three neurofilament subunits within pig and human retinal ganglion cells. *Mol Vis.*, 10, 83-92.

Ruiz-Ederra, J., Garcia, M., Martin, F., Urcola, H., Hernandez, M., Araiz, J. et al. (2005b). Comparison of three methods of inducing chronic elevation of intraocular pressure in the pig (experimental glaucoma. *Arch Soc.Esp Oftalmol.*, 80, 571-579.

Ruiz-Ederra, J., Hitchcock, P. F., & Vecino, E. (2003). Two classes of astrocytes in the adult human and pig retina in terms of their expression of high affinity NGF receptor (TrkA). *Neurosci Lett.*, 337, 127-130.

Samsel, P.A., Kisiswa L, Erichsen; J.T., Cross, S.D., & Morgan J. (2011) A novel method for the induction of experimental glaucoma using magnetic microspheres. *Invest Ophthalmol.Vis.Sci.*, 52, *1671-1675.*

Sappington, R. M., Carlson, B. J., Crish, S. D., & Calkins, D. J. (2010). The microbead occlusion model: a paradigm for induced ocular hypertension in rats and mice. *Invest Ophthalmol.Vis.Sci.*, 51, 207-216.

Senatorov, V., Malyukova, I., Fariss, R., Wawrousek, E. F., Swaminathan, S., Sharan, S. K. et al. (2006). Expression of mutated mouse myocilin induces open-angle glaucoma in transgenic mice. *J.Neurosci.*, 26, 11903-11914.

Shareef, S. R., Garcia-Valenzuela, E., Salierno, A., Walsh, J., & Sharma, S. C. (1995). Chronic ocular hypertension following episcleral venous occlusion in rats. *Exp.Eye Res.*, 61, 379-382.

Suarez, T. & Vecino, E. (2006). Expression of endothelial leukocyte adhesion molecule 1 in the aqueous outflow pathway of porcine eyes with induced glaucoma. *Mol Vis.*, 12, 1467-1472.

Takamoto, T. & Schwartz, B. (2002). Differences by quadrant of retinal nerve fiber layer thickness in healthy eyes. *J.Glaucoma.*, 11, 359-364.

Torngren, L., Lundgren, B., & Madsen, K. (2000). Intraocular pressure development in the rabbit eye after aqueous exchange with ophthalmic viscosurgical devices. *J.Cataract Refract.Surg.*, 26, 1247-1252.

Ueda, J., Sawaguchi, S., Hanyu, T., Yaoeda, K., Fukuchi, T., Abe, H. et al. (1998). Experimental glaucoma model in the rat induced by laser trabecular photocoagulation after an intracameral injection of India ink. *Jpn. J. Ophthalmol.*, 42, 337-344.

Urcola, J. H., Hernandez, M., & Vecino, E. (2006). Three experimental glaucoma models in rats: comparison of the effects of intraocular pressure elevation on retinal ganglion cell size and death. *Exp Eye Res*, 83, 429-437.

Vecino, E. (2008a). Neurotrophins:responsible for death and survival. In A. Mangas, R. Coveäs & Geffard M. *Brain Molecules: from vitamins to Molecules for Axon Guidance* (pp. 181-193).

Vecino, E. (2008b). Gene therapy against retinosis pigmentary. *Arch Soc. Esp Oftalmol.*, 83, 213-214.

Vecino, E., Bayon, A., Mico, C., & Palao C. (2011). Retrobulbar Optic Nerve Section in Pig: Optical coherence tomography an Multifocal Electroretinogram study. ARVO e-abstract 4683 .

Vickers, J. C., Schumer, R. A., Podos, S. M., Wang, R. F., Riederer, B. M., & Morrison, J. H. (1995). Differential vulnerability of neurochemically identified subpopulations of retinal neurons in a monkey model of glaucoma. *Brain Res.*, 680, 23-35.

Wang, N., Chintala, S. K., Fini, M. E., & Schuman, J. S. (2001). Activation of a tissue-specific stress response in the aqueous outflow pathway of the eye defines the glaucoma disease phenotype. *Nat Med*, 7, 304-309.

Wang, R. F., Schumer, R. A., Serle, J. B., & Podos, S. M. (1998). A comparison of argon laser and diode laser photocoagulation of the trabecular meshwork to produce the glaucoma monkey model. *J.Glaucoma.*, 7, 45-49.

Weber, A. J. & Viswanathan, S. (2008). The Primate Model of Experimental Glaucoma. In J.Tombran-Tink, C. J. Barnstable, & M. B. Shields (Eds.), *Mechanisms of the Glaucomas* (pp. 551-577). Humana Press.

Weber, A. J. & Zelenak, D. (2001). Experimental glaucoma in the primate induced by latex microspheres. *J. Neurosci. Methods*, 111, 39-48.

Zhou, Y., Grinchuk, O., & Tomarev, S. I. (2008). Transgenic mice expressing the Tyr437His mutant of human myocilin protein develop glaucoma. *Invest Ophthalmol. Vis. Sci.*, 49, 1932-1939.

# Part 2

## Clinical Concepts – Glaucoma Evaluation and Management

16

# Management of Glaucoma in the Era of Modern Imaging and Diagnostics

Anurag Shrivastava and Umar Mian
*Montefiore Medical Center: Albert Einstein COM*
*U.S.A.*

## 1. Introduction

In light of a rapidly expanding geriatric demographic worldwide, and the concomitant increased prevalence of glaucoma, the need for reliable and reproducible methods for disease progression has become increasingly necessary. Given the high costs and morbidity of treatment, whether medical, laser, or incisional, the ability to detect disease and to further demonstrate progression allows glaucoma specialists to make more informed decisions regarding both the initiation, and advancement of therapeutic modalities. Furthermore, our ability to image both the anterior segment and the optic nerve head has allowed for better elucidation of anatomic variants and mechanisms of secondary glaucomas, along with better detection of subtle glaucomatous optic neuropathies and progression of nerve fiber layer defects.

The treatment of glaucoma has advanced rapidly over the past decades, yet remains a chronic disease requiring life long control. The expansion of the armamentarium of interventions possible to help retard progression of disease has allowed us to cater treatments to the specific needs of an individual patient. As glaucomatous damage is essentially irreversible, the holy grail of glaucoma treatment, regardless of etiology, is early detection of a progressive disease state. Intraocular pressure (IOP) remains the only modifiable risk factor for glaucoma patients, and continues to serve as the metric by which the success of therapeutic intervention is judged. The need for accuracy of these measurements has led to a better understanding of ocular tissue properties, and potentially their relative effects on disease progression.

In terms of diagnosis and management of glaucoma, progress has been made since the days when visual field testing remained the only option for the detection and documentation of disease and its progression. As traditional perimetry provides a functional assessment of a patient's disease state, the need for reliable structural measurements has resulted in the development of a multitude of technologies. The relationship between structural damage and functional loss, however, is often complicated, and much remains to be elucidated at the current time. Since structural and functional assessments give us different information, both are often used in conjunction for the detection and treatment of glaucoma. Understanding the limitations of both assessments is tantamount when considering various therapeutic algorithms. Ultimately, it remains the role of the clinician to determine an individual patient's risk of progression. This is optimally achieved by determining the level of intervention necessary to prevent functional loss, balancing the risks, side effects, and costs of treatment.

## 2. Assessment and measurement of intraocular pressure

As intraocular pressure (IOP) remains the only modifiable risk factor for glaucoma, the importance of consistent and accurate measurements cannot be overstated. Reduction of IOP remains the cornerstone for the treatment of glaucoma, as adequate and reproducible data on neuroprotective agents is currently lacking. Given that all forms of tonometry have limitations, the reference standard for IOP assessment continues to be Goldmann applanation tonometry (GAT). A brief review of the principle behind IOP measurement is provided here. GAT relies on the Imbert-Fick principle, and is in part based upon a standardized GAT applanation diameter of 3.06mm. The IOP is inferred from the force needed to flatten this standardized area of the central cornea. Therefore, it is intuitive that central corneal pathologies and properties will affect these IOP measurements.

For patients with high corneal astigmatism, it is important to take the average of two measurements 90 degrees apart by adjusting the applanation tip accordingly. GAT measurements need to be furthermore adjusted according to standard corneal pachymetry nomograms, although no one nomogram that exists that is universally accepted. A range of IOP correction from 1.1 to 7.14mm Hg/100 microns of corneal thickness exists in the current literature[1]. It is of interest that the clinical utility of these adjustments remains somewhat controversial, and that other corneal biomechanical properties may be of higher utility (See Ocular Response Analyzer below). Regardless, it is likely that corneal pachymetry measurements below 500 microns underestimate IOP, and those over 600 microns overestimate the measurement. A variety of tonometers have been developed in response to these properties, and some are discussed within this section.

### 2.1 Tonopen (Reichert technologies depew, NY)

The Tonopen is a modified Mackay-Marg tonometer, and is commercially sold as the Tonopen XL, and more recently, the Tonopen Avia. Mackay-Marg tonometers work on the principle that the applanating force to flatten a cornea (transuducer with a 1.5 mm applanation tip) must be equivalent to the counteracting force from within the eye. The transducer only measures the pressures at the center of the applanator, in contrast to the GAT, and is theorized to be less dependent on intrinsic corneal properties. The Tonopen contains a micro strain gauge attached to a 1.0 mm transducer, sampling at a rate of 500 measurements per second. This high sampling rate allows the Tonopen to provide accurate and reproducible IOP measurements. The Tonopen has several major advantages over GAT. It does not require a slit lamp, and is therefore not dependent on patient positioning, allowing for easy use outside the examnination room setting.. It further provides objective results, and requires less skill and training than GAT to perform. The Tonopen is particularly useful in children and non-cooperative patients. The surface area of applanation is one-third that of the GAT, and the ability to measure IOP from a non-central location may be an advantage in patients with certain corneal pathologies.

A study done in the earlier years of the Tonopen on 15 eyes which needed corneal glue, or had band keratopathy, demonstrated that the Tonopen was equivalent to the GAT when the unaffected area was applanated The study further concluded that the Tonopen grossly overestimated the IOP when the affected area was tested[2]. A large cross-sectional study of over 2000 primary care patients who were screened for ocular hypertension (OHTN) with the Tonopen described no adverse effects of tonometry, and further determined the incidence of OHTN and primary open angle glaucoma (POAG) to be 4.89% and 1.04%

respectively. Broman, et al.[3], examined 230 glaucomatous eyes with the Tonopen, GAT, Ocular Response Analyzer (ORA- see below), and further obtained measurements of central corneal thickness (CCT), axial length, corneal curvature, corneal astigmatism, central visual acuity, and refractive error. The IOP measured was noted to be lowest by the Tonopen, and highest by the ORA. Interestingly, it was found that the GAT was least affected by corneal pachymetry, and corneal hysteresis (see ORA below) was correlated with CCT. The authors concluded that corneal parameters affect tonometers in different ways. Lester, et al.[4] in an analysis of 104 patients found that the Tonopen XL gave similar results to GAT in only 62% of patients, and in subgroup analysis, found that the Tonopen XL underestimates IOP when GAT was above 20mm Hg.

### 2.2 Ocular Response Analyzer (ORA: Reichert instruments, depew, NY)

The Ocular Response Analyzer is a modified non-contact tonometer, which measures previously un-recordable corneal biomechanical properties. These properties are thought to be the result of viscous damping of corneal tissue. The ORA utilizes a rapid air impulse, combined with a highly sensitive optical system, to record applanation pressures when the cornea is both maximally deformed inwards, and then once again on reformation. The *average* of the two IOP measurements is termed IOPg, to denote the fact that it is the equivalent of the correlated GAT. The *difference* between the two IOP measurements is termed corneal hysteresis (CH) (Figure 1-2). The ability to measure hysteresis allows for further derivations of other newer metrics, such as corneal-corrected IOP (IOPcc) and the corneal resistance factor (CRF). These derived metrics eliminate the need for corneal pachymetry compensation of IOP. The IOPcc is derived from a normative database of patients undergoing keratorefractive surgery, and "compensates" the IOP based on corneal properties, not corneal thickness. CRF is a measurement of the cumulative effects of both the viscous and elastic resistance encountered by the air jet while deforming the corneal surface, and is derived from CH measurements using various algorithms. ORA measurements have proven to be particularly useful in patients with corneal edema and some secondary glaucomas, where IOPg can serve as a surrogate for GAT when it is not possible. Patients with abnormal ORA hysteresis measurements may be at higher risk for corneal ectasia and possibly post keratorefractive surgery complications as well[5].

A study of 90 eyes (30 normal, 30 with POAG, 30 pseudoexfoliative) was recently performed with the ORA, and corneal hysteresis was found to be significantly lower in pseudoexfoliatives when compared to the controls and POAG patients[6]. Another recent review of 108 POAG patients demonstrated both lower corneal hysteresis and resistance factor measurements when compared to those of ocular hypertensives and controls[7]. In a prospective cross-sectional study of 117 POAG patients with asymmetric visual fields, Anand et al[8] demonstrated that abnormal ORA parameters were significantly associated with the eye with the greater visual field defect. Neither corneal pachymetry, nor GAT, were significantly different between the eyes. These findings suggest that the ORA is able to detect subtle differences in asymmetric glaucoma, when GAT and CCT measurements are symmetric.

Lastly, Ang et al performed a prospective comparative analysis of 40 patients with normal tension glaucoma (NTG) with 41 diagnosed with POAG, demonstrating higher hysteresis measurements in the NTG group. The highest recorded GAT measurement was also statistically significantly correlated with lower hysteresis and higher resistance factor values. These findings suggest that alterations in corneal biomechanical properties may occur in response to chronically elevated IOP[9]. It is clear that the ORA is able to distinguish corneal biomechanical properties that were previously undetectable. As our understanding of the clinical relevance of these parameters improves, the predictive and diagnostic utility of ORA will likely lead to a greater adoption of this technology.

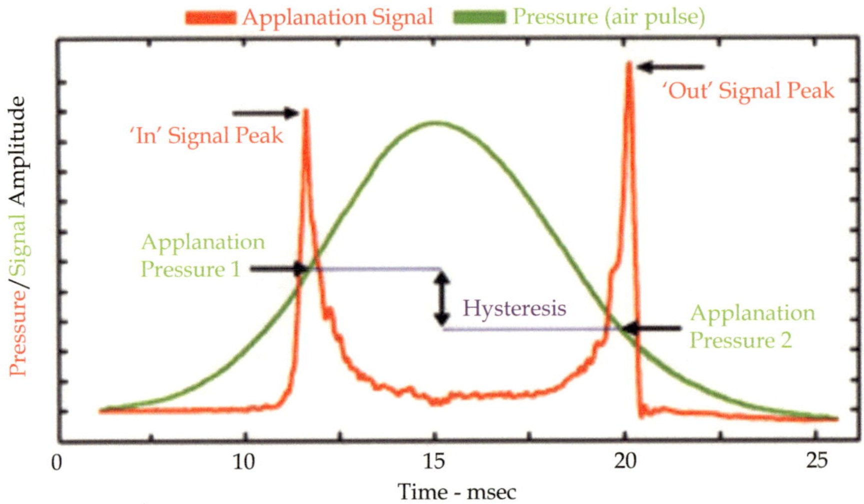


Ocular Response Analyzer(ocularresponseanalyzer.com), Reichert Industries website, 2011

Fig. 1. Ocular Response Analyzer (ORA). The ORA results from both eyes are displayed in graphical form, and are referred to as the "Signal Time Response" curves. The dynamic air puff to the cornea leads to two applanation events (inward and outwards), and the delays in these events are due to intrinsic corneal biomechanical properties. The Y-axis is the "Pressure/Signal Amplitude", and the X-axis is time in msec. The solid curve which peaks in the center of the plot is the pressure (air pulse). The bimodal peaked line represents the applanation signal. The first peak represents the "in-signal", when the cornea is flattened inwards by the air-puff. The second peak represents the "out-signal", when the cornea essentially "unflattens" back to its original state. The intersection of the pressure and signal plots at both peaks represents the two applanation measurements respectively. The average of the two pressures is the calculated IOPg, or Goldmann-correlated IOP. The difference between the two pressures is termed corneal hysteresis (CH), and is thought to be due to the viscous damping effects of the corneal tissue. The normal range of CH varies significantly from 8-16mm Hg, with the value of 11mm Hg considered normal. The IOPcc and CRF are derived from the CH. The IOPcc is the estimated IOP given the CH of a cornea, and is considered to be independent of pachymetry, etc. The CRF provides an estimate of the overall resistance of the cornea, and normal values range similar to the CH

### 2.3 Pascal dynamic contour tonomoter (DCT)

The Pascal DCT (Zeimer Ophthalmics, Port, Switzerland) was developed in response to the large degree of variability of IOP measurements obtained by GAT, with respect to various corneal properties and biomechanics. It further eliminates the subjective nature of GAT by providing a slit-lamp mounted digital readout of the IOP. The advantages of the digital readout, along with the resultant reductions in intra-observer variability, are intuitive in a busy clinical setting. Measurement of the ocular pulse amplitude (OPA) , a metric estimating the quality of ocular blood flow, is further displayed digitally. The SensorTip™ of the DCT is a concave applanator which houses a piezo resistant pressure sensor able to take approximately 100 measurements per second. A spring loaded Cantilever maintains a constant applanation force of 1 gram, reducing the likelihood of iatrogenic corneal injury as well. A major theoretical advantage of DCT, when compared to GAT, is that IOP measurements from DCT are not affected by corneal pachymetry. This difference is especially useful for keratorefractive and keratoconic[10]patients, where thin corneas and astigmatism greatly affect GAT measurements. The DCT clearly addresses many of the major shortcomings of standard GAT. DCT likely will play a larger role in glaucoma

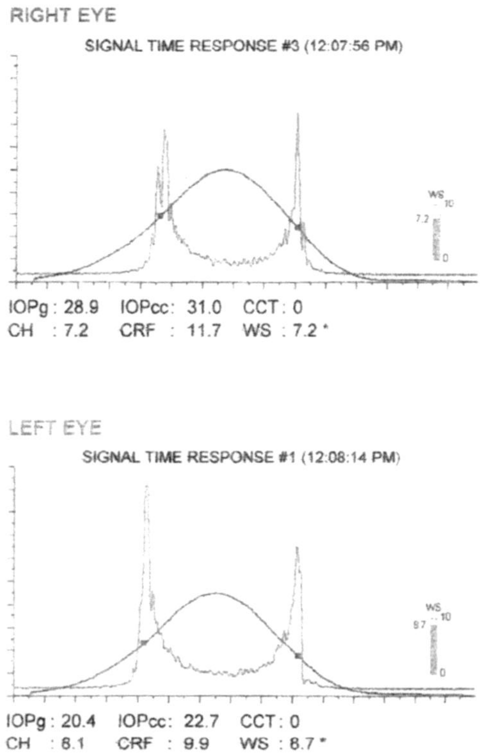


Fig. 2. ORA of glaucoma patient

The ORA scans of a patient show extremely an extremely high IOPg in both eyes, with the right eye being significantly higher than the Left (28.9 mm Hg, 20.4 mm Hg). CH values are low in both eyes, with an IOPcc even higher than IOPg (31.0 mm Hg OD, 22.7 mm Hg OS). The intraocular pressures of this patient by GAT have ranged from 12m Hg-18mm Hg on medical therapy, significantly lower than the measurements by the ORA. It is likely that the ORA is demonstrating a gross underestimation of this patient's IOP control. If functional and structural analysis continues to show progression, it is likely that this patient will need more aggressive IOP management than that being demonstrated by serial GAT. As with all testing, it is important to reproduce abnormal results prior to advancing to any therapeutic intervention management, especially given that data generated from the DCT can be wirelessly integrated into many electronic medical record (EMR) systems. A hand-held DCT has been developed recently, and results have been shown to be consistent with the slit-lamp mounted model[11]. The DCT has been widely studied, and the current body of literature supports its use clinically. A retrospective review of 200 patients by Ang, et al.[9] demonstrated poor correlation of DCT with GAT measurements that had been corrected with six different pachymetry compensation formulae. Gunvant, et al[12] examined 120 eyes, and demonstrated that the Ehlers formula for GAT correction actually reduced agreement with DCT measurements. This study demonstrates that simple GAT corneal correction factors may be inadequate to compensate for complex corneal biomechanics. Kotecha, et al[13], examined 100 patients with GAT, ORA, and DCT, and concluded that the DCT demonstrated the best repeatability and reproducibility. Interestingly, ORA and DCT generally measured the IOP to be 2 mm higher than GAT in this study. Sullivan-Mee, et al[14] performed a similar analysis on 126 eyes, and found that all three forms of tonometry (GAT, ORA, and DCT) had similar repeatability and reproducibility, concluding from their data that the ORA and DCT are acceptable alternatives to GAT in routine clinical practice.

### 2.4 Icare® rebound tonometry (IRT)

Rebound tonometry, commercially available as the Icare tonometer TA01i (Tiolat Oy, Helsinki, Finland), has shown tremendous promise in the realm of pediatric ophthalmology and community screenings in particular. The Icare tonometer does not require topical anesthesia, and is able to provide rapid digital IOP measurements painlessly. The handheld device is first stabilized on the patient's forehead, and a small disposable rebounding probe briefly applanates the cornea. It is able to measure the IOP in microseconds, obviating the need for anesthesia and prolonged measurements, making the technology especially useful for children and special needs patients. The probe is briefly magnetized by an induction coil prior to firing, and the tonometer calculates and digitally displays the IOP from the generated induction current. It is important to note that IRT is likely subject to the same constraints as GAT with respect to various corneal parameters.

Flemmons et al[15]collected GAT and IRT measurements from 71 pediatric glaucoma patients, and found that the IRT measurements were within 3mm Hg of GAT in 63% of patients. It was further noted that the IOP was higher by IRT than GAT in 75% of patients measured. Scuderi, et al,[16] in a clinical study of 93 patients, examined the validity and limitations of IRT. They concluded that IRT was comparable to other nonconventional tonometers, and can replace GAT when it is not available. Munkwitz, et al[17] similarly examined 75 patients with GAT and IRT, and found that the IRT performed well within 3mm Hg for normotensive patients. However, in patients with IOPs ranging from 22-60 mm Hg, the IRT was shown to have larger variability than the GAT. This result potentially reduces the validity of IRT measurements in ocular hypertensive patients.

One of the most challenging aspects of glaucoma management is an absence of IOP data between office visits. Compliance rates likely change in the days preceding office visits, and extrapolating IOP over time from limited data points has serious limitations. In diabetic and hypertensive patients, inter-visit monitoring of blood pressure and blood glucose offers internists a great deal of information regarding the efficacy of treatment for these diseases. The possibility of home monitoring of IOP by IRT was addressed in a recent study by Asrani, et al. They observed excellent inter- and intra-observer variability (less than 3mm Hg) in 100 patients that performed IRT on themselves, compared with IRT and GAT performed by a technician[18]. The possibility of home monitoring of IOP may have particular significance for patients where large diurnal IOP variability is suspected given normal measurements at office visits.

## 3. Standard automated perimetry (SAP) and short wavelength automated perimetry (SWAP) – Functional assessment of the glaucoma patient

SAP, or static perimetry, is most commonly performed by the Humphrey or Octopus perimeter. Alternately, manual (kinetic) perimetry, is most commonly performed with the Goldmann perimeter, although it is important to note that some automated perimeters do have kinetic testing functionality. SAP serves as a nonspecific assessment of visual function, and is designed to detect loss of sensitivity to light perception. This is traditionally done with a white stimulus on a standardized white background of uniform luminescence. However, newer testing paradigms which isolate specific wavelengths of light (see SWAP testing below) have been introduced for certain clinical indications. SAP serves as a global metric of functional loss. In clinical practice, this means that visual field deficits may represent a disease process anywhere from the ocular surface to the visual cortex. Characteristic patterns of deficit allow the practitioner to anatomically localize the site of injury, and are tremendously useful in the diagnosis and monitoring of many disease states. It is important to note that any visual field defect that is suspected to obey the vertical midline warrants further neurological assessment. The temporality and congruity of the field deficits further provide useful clues to the etiology of the defects. Bitemporal lesions generally localize pathology to the sella turcica adjacent to the optic chiasm, whereas homonomous defects are generally post-chiasmal. Highly congruous homonomous defects, especially with macular sparing, often localize to occipital pathology.

SAP testing relies on a variety of strategies, which ultimately determine the threshold necessary to reliably detect the presence of a stimulus in predetermined locations within the visual field. Algorithms and testing strategies have been constantly advancing to maximize sensitivity and specificity, while reducing test time and patient fatigue. Given the wide variety of options, it is imperative that the clinician not only chooses the correct test, but also furthermore accounts for an individual patient's ability to reliably perform that test.

The decision to advance treatment based on visual field analysis is inherently fraught with confounding factors. While the advent of structural analysis (see below) have allowed for some quantification of glaucomatous defect, the necessity for analysis and documentation of functional disease progression with perimetry remains a vital component of glaucoma management. This is especially the case when there are disparities between clinical examination, perimetry, and structural analysis. An improved understanding of the limitations of standard perimetry and structural analysis allows the astute clinician to avoid treatment errors. This is particularly important given the high levels of morbidity associated with many of the interventions presently available. The following sections aim to highlight the strengths and weaknesses of the wide range of testing modalities currently available.

### 3.1 Humphrey field analyzer (HFA)

One of the most commonly utilized perimetry devices is the HFA, with over 35,000 units in use currently worldwide. Indeed, many of the landmark glaucoma trials such as the Ocular Hypertensive Trial (OHTS)[19], Advanced Glaucoma Intervention Study (AGIS)[20], and Collaborative Initial Glaucoma Treatment Study (CIGTS)[21]to name a few, used this form of perimetry to diagnose and detect functional glaucomatous progression. HFA analysis is the current gold standard for clinical trials, allowing for older studies to be appropriately compared. Recent advancements in progression analysis software by multiple vendors have increased the clinical utility of serial SAP testing by allowing for greater detection of subtle changes.

The choice of the most appropriate HVF should be based upon a wide variety of considerations. Some of these considerations include the extent of the visual field that needs to be tested, the intensity and size of the stimulus needed, and the best suited testing strategy for the clinical question being analyzed (i.e. screening vs. monitoring progression, etc.). An important caveat is that once a reliable visual field is obtained, it is advisable to utilize the same testing strategy as much as possible to reliably detect disease progression over time.

### 3.1.1 Degrees of visual field tested

The major options on standard HVF perimetry are 10-2, 24-2, 30-2, and the less commonly performed 60-2. The first number refers to the number of degrees around the fovea that will be tested (i.e. a 10-2 test 10 degrees of the visual field centered at the fovea). The second digit which is currently always "2", refers to the protocol type which tests points on either side of the horizontal and vertical meridians, as opposed to points on the meridians themselves. Testing points directly on the meridia is denoted with a "1" as the second digit. The "1" strategy is particularly useful in neuro-ophthalmic evaluation, to highlight the presence of vertical midline defects, for example. In general, the use of 10-2 testing is reserved for patients with very advanced glaucoma to detect subtle progression in an extremely constricted field, and for patients with suspected maculopathy. The 60-2 strategy can be applied in patients where peripheral defects detected by smaller field analyses require further confirmation, however patient fatigue and artifacts may limit the clinical utility of this strategy.

The choice between 24-2 and 30-2 is somewhat variable between practitioners, and there are advantages and disadvantages to each test. Many glaucoma specialists follow patients with 24-2 testing in lieu of full 30-2 testing as it has been demonstrated that both tests have approximately equal sensitivity and specificity[19] in the detection of glaucomatous field damage. The 30-2 paradigm can lead to significantly more fatigue for patients given the additional test spots in the periphery of the visual field. The 30-2 tests one more row of points in the peripheral visual field compared to the 24-2. This area of the field is most sensitive to rim, lid, and other artifacts, thereby reducing its clinical utility in some cases. As the detection of subtle field changes necessitates accurate testing (see below: reliability indices), the choice of a 24-2 paradigm may allow for improved reliability and more clinically meaningful data. Some clinicians choose to order a 30-2 test as the baseline, and assuming that it is normal, will follow patients with 24-2 testing. It is important to note that often multiple tests need to be performed to set a reliable baseline, as field testing accuracy generally improves along a variable learning curve. In patients having difficulty with increased test time, it is appropriate to set a baseline with the most extensive test that a patient can reasonably tolerate (see below: testing strategies) Important testing specifications are reviewed below:

- 10-2: The points adjacent to the horizontal and vertical meridians test 1 degree of the visual field; points tested peripheral to these points are 2 degrees apart

- 24-2 and 30-2: The points adjacent to the horizontal and vertical meridians test 3 degrees of the visual field; points tested peripheral to these points are 6 degrees apart

In a patient with a subtle maculopathy, affecting only a few degrees of the central visual field, defects can easily be missed by the 24-2 and 30-2 based on the aforementioned testing specifications, as the scotoma could fall in the region between the tested points. Alternately, dense paracentral/arcuate scotomas characteristic of glaucomatous optic neuropathies can "blacken" out an entire 10-2 field, and the 24-2 or 30-2 paradigms are far better suited.

**a. Screening considerations**

Screening protocols are variable amongst practitioners and practices. Large volume screenings for glaucoma are often performed with Humphrey Matrix Analyzers/ (FDT) based on the test time needed to perform the analysis. It is appropriate for "high risk" patients being screened (eg Strong family history of glaucoma, ocular hypertensives, IOP/cup-to-disc asymmetry, etc.) to perform more extensive perimetry with SITA-fast protocols (see below). Patients with positive screening tests warrant further work-up, often with structural and corneal biomechanical analyses.

**b. Other considerations**

As HFA analyses are based on age-matched controls, it is imperative that the correct birth date is entered prior to testing. The age groups of patients in the database are stratified into 10 year increments. For example, a 59 year old patient will be compared to age matched controls between the ages of 50-60. It is common, therefore, for patients to have deterioration of their visual field as they progress through each decade of life. Alternately, "improvements" in the visual field can be seen immediately after the patient's age increases to the next decade stratification. Furthermore, assessment of the mental and physical status of an elderly patient to determine whether they will be able to tolerate the high levels of concentration required to perform the test.

Refractive errors, especially presbyopic errors, need to be neutralized with the appropriate loose lenses, and vertex distances/head positioning optimized. Astigmatic correction over 1.25D should be neutralized along with spherical aberration. The HVF will determine the optimal neutralization from manifest refractions accounting for a target distance of 30cm. Reassessing head position relative to refractive neutralization is critical during testing, as rim artifacts can be generated by the lenses if head positioning is not adequately monitored. Furthermore, prismatic deviation caused by high power lenses need to be accounted for when testing is analyzed, and peripheral rim defects discounted appropriately in these cases. Pupil size is able to be measured by HFA, and is displayed with the results. Pupil size generally less than 2-3mm can lead to artifactual loss of threshold sensitivity of both central and peripheral fields[22]. This is of particular importance in following patients on miotic therapy for glaucoma. Pharmacological dilation of the pupil in these cases may help limit the effects of the miotic pupil. Patients should be consistently dilated for subsequent fields if this strategy is employed. Changes in the refractive error secondary to pharmacological dilation are likely negligible in the largely non-presbyopic patient demographic that commonly undergo perimetric evaluation.

A standard background light intensity of 31.5 asb (apostilbs) is used for the HVF, to match the scotopic light conditions outlined by Goldmann perimetry standards. HVF targets come in sizes ranging from 0.25 $mm^2$ to 64.00 $mm^2$ represented by Roman numerals I through V (see Goldmann Visual Fields below). Typically, a size III stimulus (4 $mm^2$) is used in patients with good visual acuity (usually at least 20/200 or better). In these cases of decreased visual acuity, the use of larger size V (64 $mm^2$) test stimulus may be helpful, although many clinicians will opt for Goldmann Visual Fields for these low vision patients. Stimulus intensity, color, and duration can furthermore be varied by the operator based upon clinical needs.

Gaze tracking is possible with all HVF machines, and the reliability of an individual test can be further analyzed beyond the reliability indices calculated for each field. A real time fixation monitor is displayed at the bottom of each visual field printout. Upward deflections represent the moment a patient saccades away from a target, and downward deflections represent a tracking failure commonly secondary to blinking.

### 3.1.2 Testing algorithms – Swedish interactive testing algorithm (SITA)

SITA testing was designed to optimize visual field accuracy while reducing testing time. It is based on the concept of "threshold", which is a term that is defined as the intensity of light that a patient can detect 50% of the time. The threshold represents the minimal amount of light intensity that can be reliably detected. SITA testing determines this threshold by presenting points with varying intensities using a "bracketing" technique. Specifically, this technique involves measuring intensities above and below the threshold, as defined above. This technique is much more efficient than full threshold protocols, and generally is able to maintain a high degree of concordance in a much shorter time period. The SITA algorithm is dynamic, and the stimuli are timed based on an individual patient's response time. Algorithms are age-matched, so proper patient data entry is imperative. SITA-Fast and SITA standard algorithms remain options that can reduce test time by about 70% and 50%[23], respectively, when compared with full threshold tests. The differences between the protocols lies in the variability in response allowed when determining threshold values, with the SITA standard being more rigorous in repetition of points. In other words, the SITA-FAST strategy has a lower level of confidence needed to be achieved at each point relative to SITA-Standard. The SITA-fast protocol utilizes the expected thresholds based on normative population databases. The utilization of these normative assumptions increases the efficiency of the test, but is limited by the fact that it does not account for threshold variability at the individual level. The SITA fast protocol is generally more than adequate for screening examinations and for those patients who cannot perform SITA standard secondary to fatigue. Most glaucoma specialists rely on SITA standard testing to monitor for subtle changes indicating progression. This is particularly critical in the regions of the visual field surrounding an existing scotoma. A study by Budenz, et al demonstrated an overall sensitivity of 98% and 95% for SITA standard and SITA fast protocols when compared to full threshold testing. The same study demonstrated sensitivity in patients with mild glaucomatous damage as 92% and 85% respectively[24]. Specificity was determined to be 96% for both algorithms.

### 3.1.3 Short wavelength automated perimetry (SWAP) – Blue-on-yellow perimetry

SWAP testing is based upon the concept that glaucoma is characterized by damage to cells in the visual pathway that are more sensitive to blue light, with a peak activity at 440 nanometers. Blue cones in the photoreceptor layer of the retina eventually synapse in the koniocellular layers of the lateral geniculate body, via small bistratified retinal ganglion cells. The fact that SWAP testing isolates one type of ganglion cell should not imply that these cells are necessarily the first to be affected by glaucomatous injury. Moreover, SWAP testing avoids the masking effects of inherent redundancies within the visual pathways by isolating one particular system.[25,26]

SWAP testing is generally more fatiguing than SAP, and is also much more affected by lens opacification and drusen in patients with macular degeneration. Recent development of SITA-SWAP testing has helped reduce test duration while maintaining sensitivity. The stimulus size for the blue target in SWAP testing is larger than that of SAP (equivalent to Goldmann V vs. III sized targets, respectively). More light is needed to activate the blue cone system[27], and although the blue target is generally less bright, the larger test stimulus size partially compensates for it. The caveat is, that a larger test stimulus can over estimate fixation losses in patients with relatively small blind spots, even though fixation maybe maintained.

Many studies have demonstrated the ability of SWAP testing to detect visual field abnormalities earlier than SAP testing[28,29]. A recent publication demonstrated less persuasive results regarding the early predictive abilities of SWAP testing. However, methodological differences between Johnson's original data from the prior decade may help explain the varied results[30]. Other reports indicate that patients with visual field defects on SAP demonstrate dramatically larger defects when tested with SWAP[31-33]. As data is continually being collected regarding SWAP testing in glaucoma patients, a better understanding of the protocol's benefits and limitations will help elucidate the role of SWAP testing in functional assessment of the glaucoma patient. At the time of this publication, SWAP testing largely remains the test most commonly used in younger patients with high clinical suspicion for glaucoma. This is especially the case in patients with previous normal SAP testing.

### 3.1.4 Reliability indices

In order to make determinations about clinically significant functional progression, it is imperative that visual fields are as reliable and reproducible as possible. Assessment of a glaucomatous scotoma by *reliable* perimetry is expected to fluctuate given the natural history of the disease and the manner in which we quantify defects. Alternately stated, seemingly progressive visual field loss can often "reverse" with serial testing, indicating that the etiology of the deterioration may indeed be non-physiological. The establishment of a blind spot corresponding to the position of the optic nerve is accomplished by placing testing points within this region during reliable fixation. It is even more challenging to separate fluctuation from progression when analyzing visual fields that are considered "unreliable". The establishment of an adequate baseline is important clinically, and essential if progression analysis is desired (see GPA below).

Fixation losses are measured by introducing stimuli into the physiological blind spot, and monitoring whether patients are able to detect them. A fixation loss indicates that the blind spot has moved (i.e. the patient has refixated to an alternate location within the perimeter). False positives are defined as patient responses when no stimulus is present. False negative responses are defined as a lack of detection of a suprathreshold stimulus (i.e. not being able to detect a more intense stimulus after the threshold is determined).

Reliable fields generally are recommended to have false positive and negative rates fewer than 35%, and fixation losses less than 20%. In clinical practice, many patients are not able to adequately perform the testing regardless of algorithm, and alternate means of documenting functional progression are necessary. Birt, et al.,[33] demonstrated in a review of 768 visual field test from 106 glaucoma patients, that only 59.5% of test were considered reliable by the aforementioned criterion. Elevating the fixation loss threshold criterion from 20% to 33% increased the number of fields meeting reliability standards to over 75%. Newkirk[34], et al further demonstrated that artificially introducing false positives of 33% to a visual field improved the calculated mean deviation (MD) by 6dB; an amount that can easily mask progressive damage. Vingrys et al[35]demonstrated similar results, suggesting that the cutoffs for reliability of false positive results be reduced to 20% or less. Bengtsson, et al.[36], hve shown that false positive rates are the least variable in test-retest paradigms, and are likely to be the most reliable index of visual field accuracy based on the SITA algorithms.

### 3.1.5 Glaucoma Hemifield test/analysis (GHT)

The GHT was developed by Asman, et al in the early 1990s to measure asymmetries in threshold sensitivity around the horizontal meridian. It functionally analyzes five corresponding pairs of mirror image sectors in the superior and inferior horizontal fields, corresponding to the normal anatomy of the retinal nerve fiber layer. Outer edge, temporal, and blind spot points are excluded from the analysis, and can be used with either the 30- or 24-2 protocols. Abnormal GHT values indicate asymmetry around the horizontal meridian, and allows for rapid evaluation of zone defects that affect the superior or inferior hemifields in particular[37] The results are further stratified into 5 categories: "Outside Normal Limits", "Borderline", "Generalized Reduction of Sensitivity", "Abnormally High Sensitivity", and "Within Normal Limits". The definition of "Outside Normal Limits" is based upon defects between the respective upper and lower paired sectors greater than what would be expected in 1% of the normative database, or a sum difference at 0.5% normal population level. "Borderline" results indicate the same criterion at the 3% normal population level. Katz, et al analyzed the rate of incident field loss after one abnormal GHT, and found that GHT is not a consistent criterion for defining incident field loss. They further concluded that the use of two or three consecutive abnormal fields to define incident field loss makes it more likely that subsequent test results will be abnormal[38]. Susanna, et al. further analyzed the ability of the GHT to detect early glaucomatous changes, and found the sensitivity, specificity, and reproducibility of the GHT to be 100,100, and 83.3% respectively[39]. Johnson, et al more recently concluded that the GHT, GHT hemifield cluster, and Pattern Deviation plots provided the highest sensitivity and specificity of all the visual field metrics[40]

### 3.1.6 Glaucoma progression analysis (GPA)

Given the often large amounts of data provided by serial perimetry, the absolute need for automated detection of progressive visual field loss has lead to advancements in software that efficiently summarize function over time. This capability allows clinicians to rapidly detect areas of the visual field that have deteriorated from baseline threshold values. These are defined by the user as the first reliable field or fields (full threshold or SITA). The data output of GPA analysis summarizes the probability of the presence of glaucomatous progression. It factors in normal fluctuation from a large database, and subtracts out deficits secondary to media opacification as well. The data is summarized in probability plots, demonstrating the likelihood of functional progression with variably darkened triangular symbols. Triangles that are darker represent a portion of the visual field that has consistently worsened over multiple tests. A minimum of five examinations over at least three years must be included in GPA 2 for the linear regression results to be presented. The open triangles represent deterioration from baseline with a 0.5 confidence interval, the half-shaded triangles represent deterioration at the same point on 2 visual fields, and finally the darkened triangle represents deterioration at the same location on 3 visual fields. Deterioration is defined as greater than that of the normal fluctuation that occurs within a normative database. Again, the lack of a uniform definition of deterioration is a severe limitation when comparing progression analyses. Consensus regarding this definition continues to be the source of much debate. Furthermore, the clinical relevance of any defined progression must be evaluated on an individual case basis to avoid errors in treatment strategy. Regardless of the definition of progression, it is widely accepted that the accuracy of progression rates is vastly improved with additional data points. This functionally translates into establishing a reliable baseline, repeating visual fields often, and using a longitudinal analysis to determine the rate of progression. In this manner, the likelihood of clinically relevant deterioration can be most accurately assessed.

As the assessment of glaucoma progression involves some degree of subjectivity, there are often discrepancies in patients who demonstrate mild changes in function. A recent review of 510 Humphrey visual fields of 83 eyes by 3 examiners demonstrated that clinician agreement of progression on sequential fields was actually better without the GPA analysis[41]. Clinician agreement (inter-observer reliability) obviously may not be an appropriate reference standard for the determination of disease progression given the subjective nature of the analysis. Another review of 90 eyes with greater than 5 reliable visual fields demonstrated that the GPA performed better in the detection of progression, when compared to a pattern deviation based visual field index (VFI)[42]. Another retrospective review of 93 glaucoma patients with 5 reliable fields concluded that there is a strong correlation between GPA identification of glaucomatous progression and a thorough objective clinical assessment of the visual fields. They further concluded that GPA could be a useful test to aid clinicians in the detection of glaucomatous progression, with high specificity, strong positive likelihood ratio, good sensitivity and negative likelihood ratio[43]. Diaz-Aleman, et al[44] examined 56 eyes of 42 patients with at least 7 reliable fields, and compared threshold noiseless trend (TNT) to GPA, and showed that TNT had a higher specificity and concordance with clinical examiners than GPA.

It is important to note that no universal definition of glaucoma, whether via a statistical package or point-by-point analysis, has been universally accepted. The optimal characterization of glaucomatous progression is the source of much of the research on perimetry that is currently being performed. Furthermore, as the perimetric definitions of progression vary significantly amongst many of the major landmark glaucoma studies, comparisons of results between the major trials has been limited. Clinically relevant models derived from these studies lack reproducibility, and no one index has been shown to be superior at the time of this publication (Figures 3-8).

While a useful adjunctive tool, GPA has had variable success when compared to other methodologies. It is our opinion that GPA serves as a useful tool in conjunction with other standard examination techniques when compared to grossly comparing serial HVF examinations without point by point analysis. The software will unlikely replace careful clinical examination utilizing a gestalt technique in its current clinical application. Monitoring the rate of visual field deterioration by multiple metrics, while accurately predicting the onset of functional loss with particular regard to projected life expectancy, is likely the optimal strategy in determining optimal treatment.

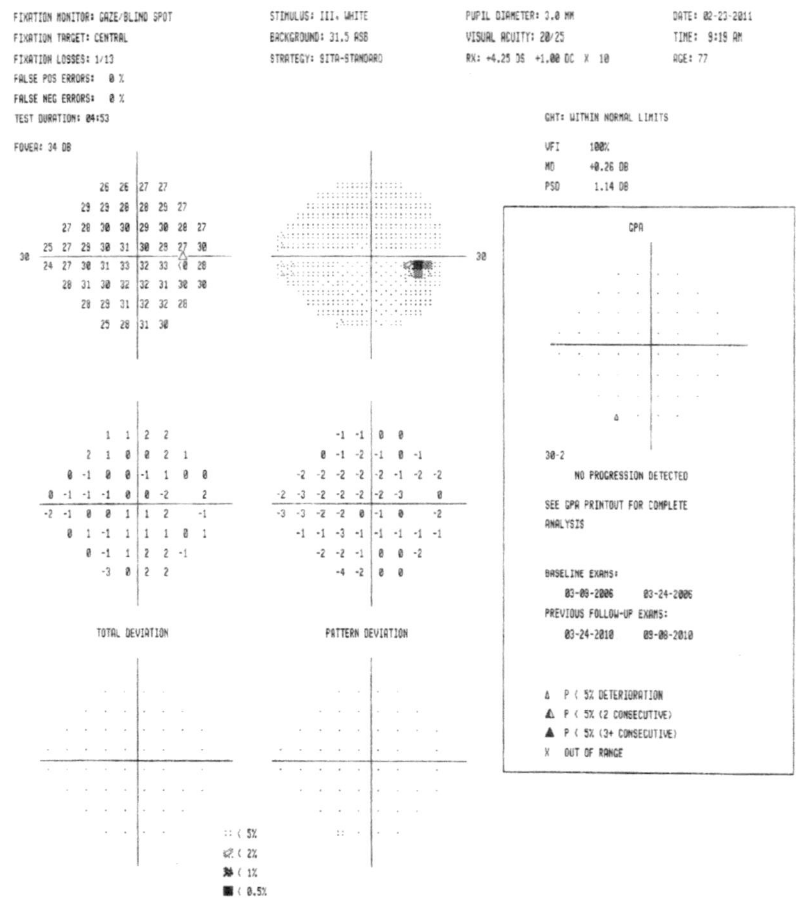

Fig. 3. HVF single field analysis with progression analysis summary: OD

This HVF is an example of the normal scan of the right eye of a patient being followed as a glaucoma suspect. Important demographic information is included at the top of the printout, including the date of birth. The type of visual field, in this case, Central 24-2 Threshold Test, is listed directly below. The type of Fixation Monitor (Gaze/Blind Spot), Stimulus Size (III) and Color (White stimulus on White Background), and the pupil diameter in mm (3.0 mm) is displayed in the next line, along with the date of the examination. The standard background intensity of 31.5 asb is used for this test, and the BCVA is further inputted from the chart. Reliability indices including Fixation Losses, False Positive and False Negative Errors, are displayed as a ratio and percentage respectively. The testing strategy is also displayed (SITA-Standard). Making clinical assessments of progression based upon serial analysis of fields utilizing different strategies should be avoided. The optimal refractive correction for the 30cm test distance is displayed, and it is one of the essential roles of the perimetrist to accurately correct the patient with large diameter loose lenses. The test duration is also recorded, and can give insight into a patient's performance. Longer test durations are likely to be prone to errors secondary to fatigue, and may have poorer reliability indices as well. Often the second eye tested will have lower test times, indicating the possibility of a learning curve effect during that perimetry session. Alternating the first eye tested for subsequent fields may "reverse" this phenomenon when unexplained asymmetry is found. The threshold sensitivities, along with mean and pattern deviations are plotted along with probability analysis for a given defect. Darker shaded boxes within the field indicate a higher probability that the defect is valid compared to age-matched controls (range from 0.5% - 5%). The glaucoma hemifield test (GHT) is displayed in the upper right hand corner of this scan, indicating in this case that no asymmetry was found between the upper and lower sectors analyzed. Finally, the GPA summary plot is found in the boxed results section. In this case, no progression was detected. Symbols are placed at any test point location that has changed from baseline by more than the variability you would see in 19 out of 20 stable glaucoma patients at the approximately the same stage of the disease. The dates of the baseline and previous fields, used by the software to determine the likelihood of progression, are further displayed. The accuracy of the progression analysis improves dramatically with both a reliable baseline, and a larger number of follow-up fields.

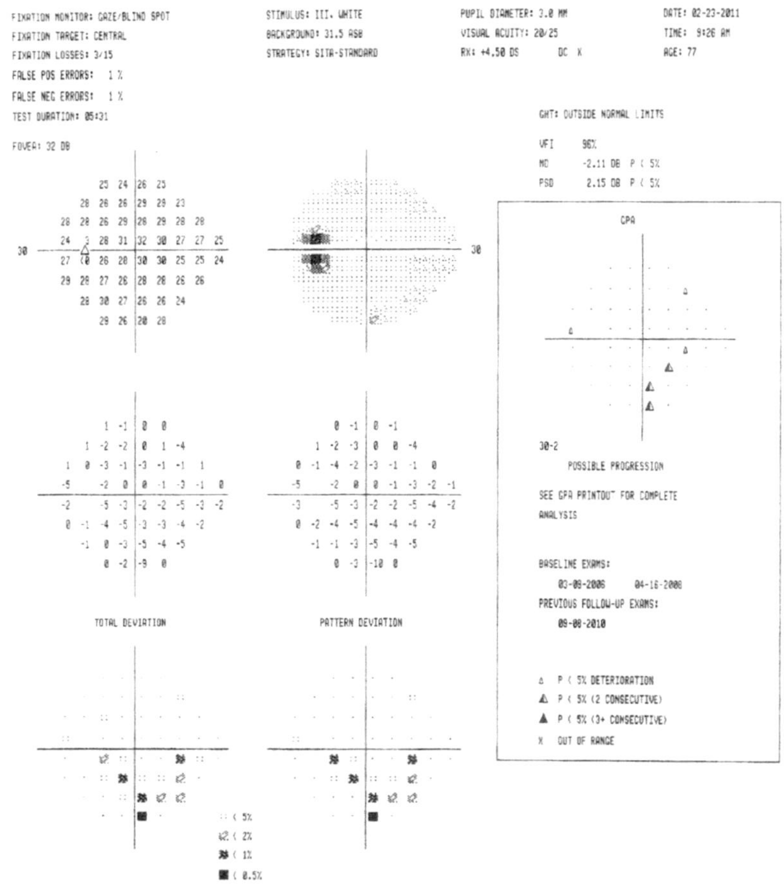


Fig. 4. Single field analysis: OS

In contrast to the right eye of the same patient, the left eye is demonstrating early changes in the pattern deviation of the inferior field (indicated by variably shaded boxes). The GHT is considered "Outside Normal Limits", and the GPA has determined the presence of "Possible Progression". The half-shaded triangles indicate p-values < 5% on 2 consecutive fields.

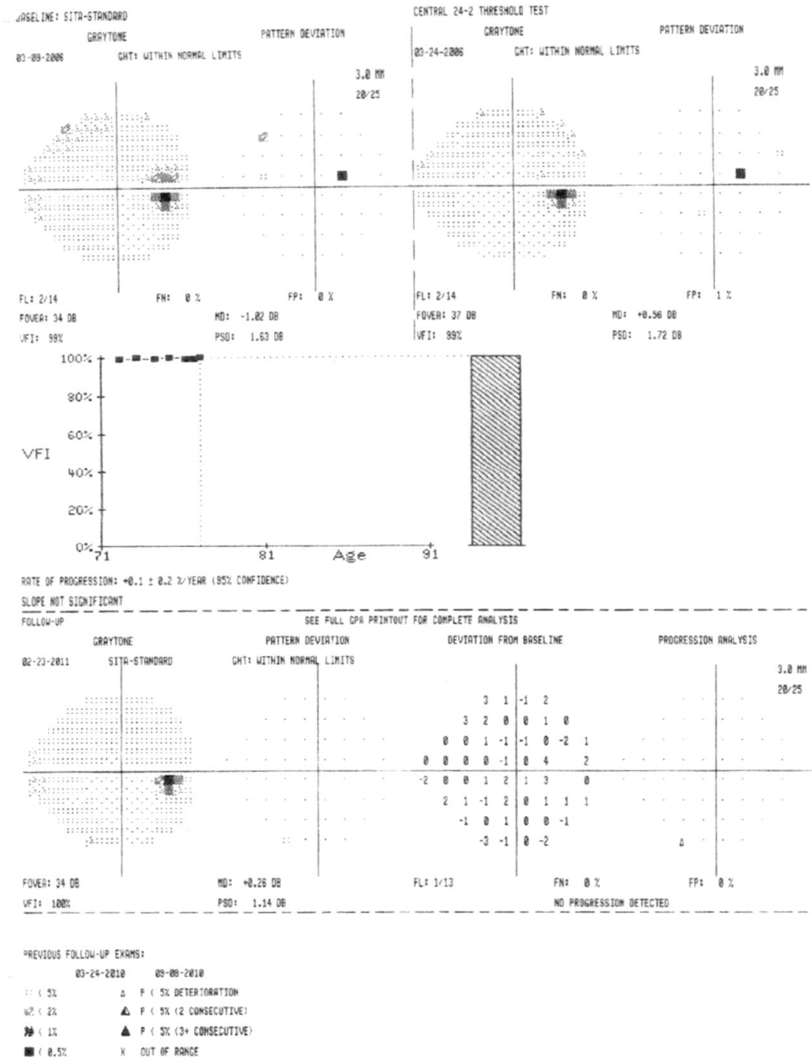


Fig. 5. GPA Summary OD

The GPA summary displays the grey scale for the baseline test, along with some of the indices for each of the tests displayed, including MD, PSD, GHT, Reliability Indices, Pupil size, and BCVA. The rate of change is also plotted over time (patient's age in years) against a visual field index (VFI). A VFI score of 100% represents a normal visual field, and 0% represents completely blackened perimetry. The VFI is calculated from pattern deviation plots, and was developed in response to the effects of media opacity on previous metrics. The rate of progression as a percentage is further displayed and analyzed. In this case, a +0.1 ± 0.2%/year was determined to be a normal slope. The shaded box at the far right of the plots is the extrapolated final VFI given a life expectancy of approximately 100 years old and the calculated rate of progression. The bottom half of the printout displays the results of the most recent exam, and provides probability plots for point-by-point likelihood of progression compared to baseline and prior follow-up examinations.

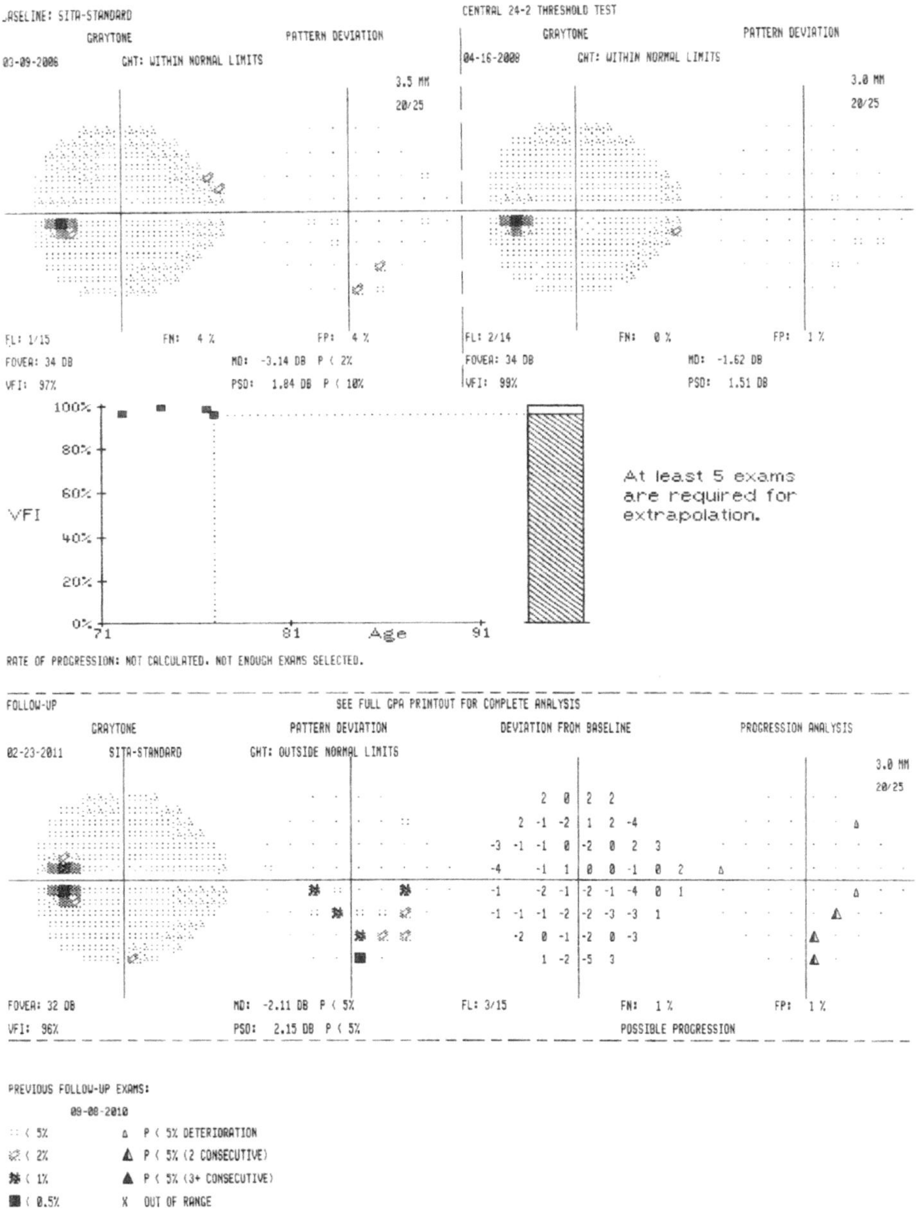


Fig. 6. GPA summary OS

In this case, it is demonstrated that the VFI extrapolation requires at least 5 consecutive tests to be considered reliable (only 4 visual fields are inputted), and a rate to be accurately calculated. The accuracy of this progression software significantly improves over time as additional fields are added to the analysis. The baseline visual fields in this patient are normal, in contrast to the defects noted in the most previous field detailed at the bottom of the printout. This patient is considered clinically to be at moderate risk of functional progression in this eye.

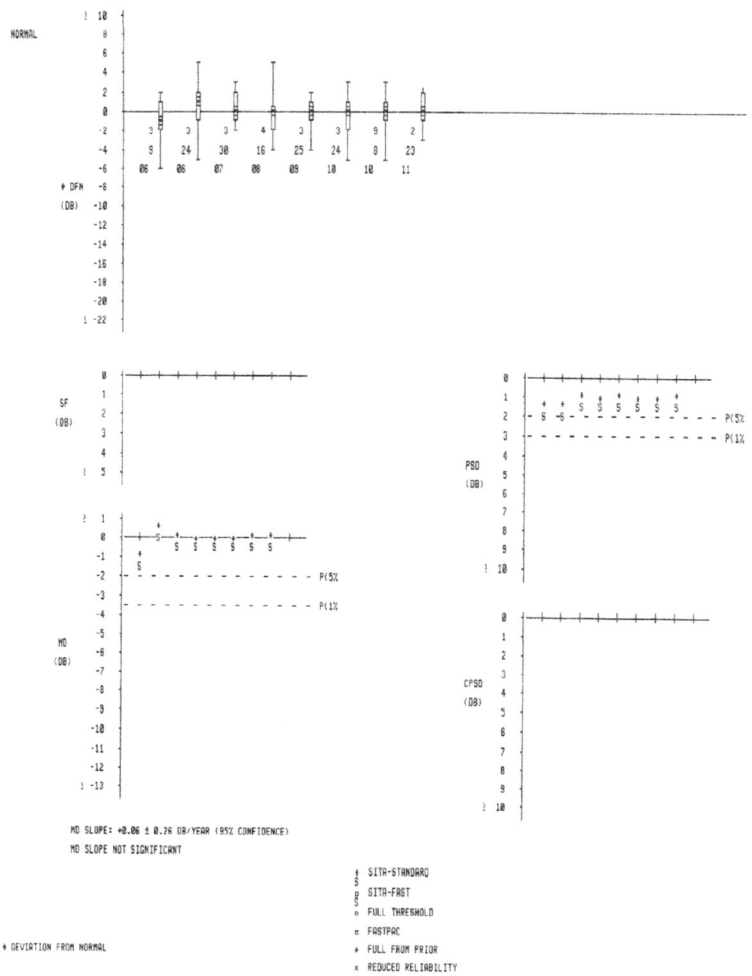


Fig. 7. Change analysis OD

The Change Analysis box plots display a variety of visual field metrics in the form of frequency distributions. The Y-axis is valued in Db, and represents the difference between the observed values relative to a normative database. The actual values observed are displayed in a chronological fashion centered on the 0 dB point (ie no deviation from normal). Positive deflections (above 0 db) indicate a "better than normal" threshold, and negative deflections indicate "worse than normal" threshold values. In this manner, the highest point (top of the "T") for each field represents the point with the highest threshold relative to normal. The shaded boxes for each data set indicate the percentile rank within each field. The highest value of the uppermost box for each data set is the 85th percentile, the middle represents the 50th percentile (ie half of the thresholds are above, and the other half below), and the bottom value represents the 15th percentile. The slope of the line for each visual field index is graphically displayed and then analyzed. In this example, the MD slope is calculated as +0.06 ± 0.26dB/year, indicating that no progression is noted during the testing interval. It is important to note that other diagnoses besides glaucoma can adversely affect the indices as well. Clinical correlation is always imperative.

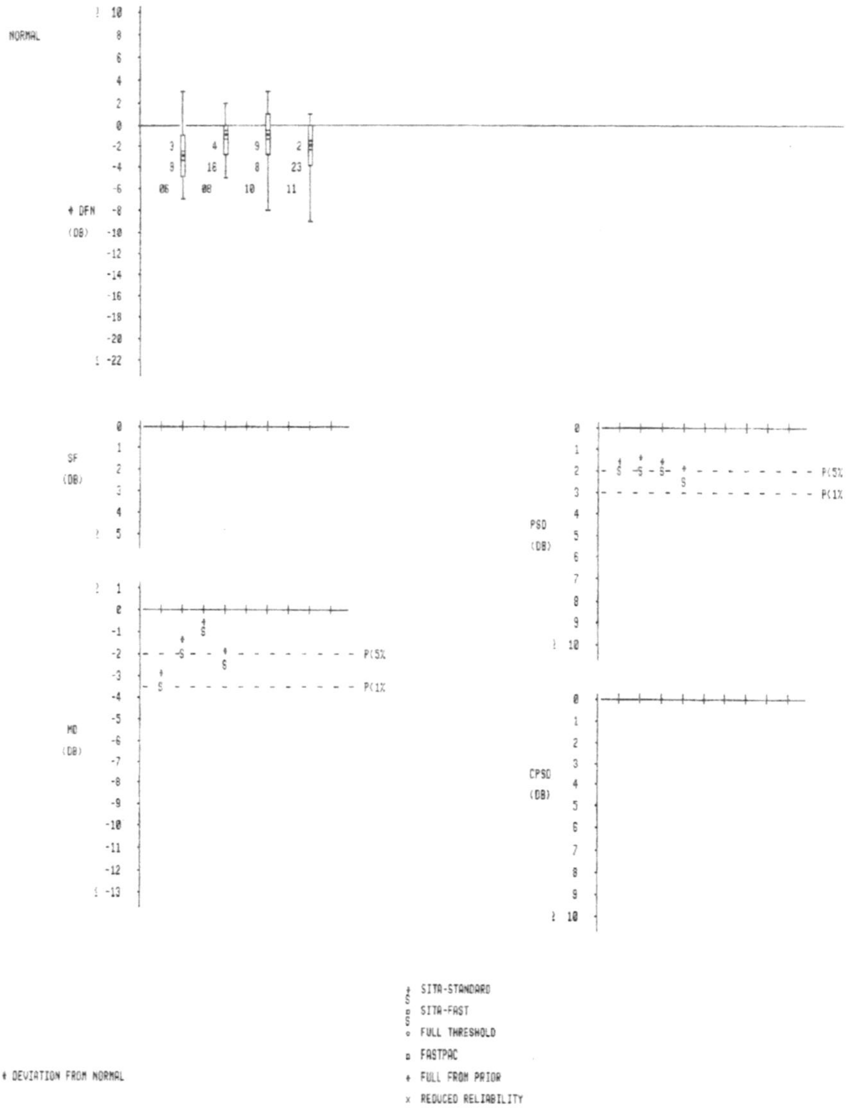


Fig. 8. Change analysis OS

In contrast to the right eye, the median values for the fields included are below the 0db line. The highest threshold points for each field (top of the "T") are above normal limits, however the range of percentile rankings tend to be below the 0 dB mark. The PSD plot further demonstrates possible worsening of the visual field, particularly in the latest examination.

### 3.2 Alternate functional assessment

When a patient is determined by multiple attempts and strategies to be a poor test taker by conventional SAP, alternate strategies may need to be employed to measure the visual field and establish an adequate baseline. As therapeutic algorithms are often advanced (ie topical therapy, laser, incisional surgery) based upon demonstration of functional progression of disease, it is optimal for the clinician to exhaust any and all options available to determine the functional status of a patient. The Octopus perimeter is an alternative to the HVF, and offers many advantages in these patients. The Goldmann kinetic perimeter is an also relatively commonly used option in these patients for multiple reasons. As fixation can be manually monitored, patients are able to take breaks during testing, and receive coaching and encouragement on a point by point basis. Frequency Doubling Technology (FDT), Matrix analyzers, while much faster than traditional SAP, may not necessarily be appropriate as an alternate testing protocol for many patients. Simple confrontational visual fields provide only a gross estimate of visual function, and are clearly not an appropriate way to follow patients with, or at risk for glaucoma.

### 3.2.1 Octopus visual field analyzer

The Octopus visual field analyzer (Haag-Streit International, Koeniz, Switzerland) has had major advancements over the past decade, which largely developed in response to many of the limitations of the HVF. One of the key advancements in the technology is an improved fixation/blink monitor which continually tracks and accounts for fixation losses and eye blinking, along with automatic adjustments based on head and eye positioning relative to the perimeter. This additional functionality can dramatically improve the accuracy of the test, and further limit lens/rim artifacts that may occur with traditional SAP. Furthermore, the Tendency Oriented Perimeter (TOP) strategy employed by the Octopus reduces test duration for threshold analysis to an average of 2.5 minutes per eye, significantly reducing patient fatigue. The Octopus' EyeSuite™ Progression software offers intuitive plots demonstrating both global and cluster progression, and has the ability to integrate structural assessment as well. The Octopus test stimuli and background intensities are matched to those of Humphrey and Goldmann perimeters (See HFA above and GVF below).

Studies comparing the Octopus and Humphrey visual field analyzers have demonstrated variable results. King, et al[45] demonstrated that the SITA Fast and TOP strategies were highly correlated in a study of 76 glaucoma patients. They did note that although the TOP strategy was faster than the SITA protocol, it tended to underestimate the focal visual field defects. A recent analysis by Lan, et al[46] demonstrated a similar finding when comparing the Octopus to FDT (see below). Often times, the establishment of newer baselines with an alternate protocol proves to be a major barrier to adaptation. As with many technologies, ease of integration into electronic medical records has proven to be a driving force for changes in clinical practice. The utility of testing patients with multiple functional assessments remains to be determined given the likelihood of discordance.

### 3.2.2 Goldmann visual field (GVF)

The major difference between SAP and Goldmann visual field testing is that the SAP is a static visual field, whereas Goldmann visual field testing is kinetic, defined as perimetry utilizing a moving stimulus (3-5 degrees/second)[47]. It is important to note that the GVF may be used as a manual static perimeter as well, and is generally reserved for improved isolation of an existing scotoma. In the case of kinetic Goldmann perimetry, the moving stimulus is controlled by a skilled operator. This subjectivity is a major drawback, as subtle changes in the visual field can easily be missed given the summative variability of both the patient and operator[48]. However, given that each patient response can be carefully monitored, the added reliability of GVF testing makes the test clinically useful in patients who are unable to perform SAP. This is especially true in patients with poor central visual acuity who are unable to reliably fixate for automated perimetry. This is indeed one of the most common reasons that GVF testing is ordered for glaucoma patients.

An additional advantage of the GVF is that it is it the only form of perimetry that is able to test the entire visual field. This encompasses 60 degrees superiorly and nasally, 75 degrees inferiorly, and 110 degrees temporally, although there are few clinical indications that demand testing far peripheral points. Neuro-ophthamic evaluation for functional visual loss and other central processes remains another common indication for GVF testing.

Definitions of stimuli and target sizes are summarized below.

| **Stimulus size** | **Stimulus Intensity** |
|---|---|
| 0 = 1/16 $mm^2$ | 1 - 4 : represent 5dB increments |
| I = 1/4 $mm^2$ | a - e : represent 1 dB increments |
| II = 1 $mm^2$ | |
| III = 4$mm^2$ | |
| IV= 16$mm^2$ | |
| V= 64 $mm^2$ | |

### 3.2.3 Frequency doubling technology (FDT) and the Matrix™ perimeter

FDT perimetry is based on a phenomenon that when an achromatic sinusoidal grating ,with low spatial frequency, flickers at a high temporal frequency, the apparent spatial frequency of the grating appears to be doubled[49]. Glaucoma is thought to preferentially effect cells in the magnocellular pathway, which have been demonstrated to be more sensitive to motion and flicker detection[50]. On the other hand, theories contend that the FDT illusion is based on higher cortical processing, and no retinal substrate exists to account for the phenomenon[51]. Regardless, the appeal of a technology that is theoretically able to preferentially detect damage to this visual pathway is obvious, and the clinical utility of FDT has advanced remarkably over the past decades. Current screening and full threshold strategies can be performed in minutes, reducing the inaccuracies of testing patients that are easily fatigued by the duration of SAP and similar strategies (Figures 9-10). Reproducibility of FDT results has further been demonstrated in multiple studies[52,53]. The reported sensitivity of FDT ranged from 0.51 to 1.00, and specificity from 0.58 to 1.00 determined by a meta-analysis of pooled data in 2006, with similar findings in more recent data.[54,55]

Nakagawa, et al.[56] recently examined 39 open angle glaucoma patients with low to moderate IOP, comparing FDT to SAP. With almost 5 years of follow-up, they determined that FDT was useful for monitoring defects detected in the SAP-normal hemifield in OAG eyes with low-to-normal IOP. A detailed study of 60 eyes with normal SAP ("pre-perimetric glaucoma") found that FDT testing was able to detect abnormalities in an astounding 65% of patients, of which 51% later developed defects by SAP over 4-27 months[57], a clear demonstration of the clinical utility of FDT in early detection of disease processes. Ferraras, et al[58] examined 278 subjects with pre-perimetric glaucoma by SAP, but with structural abnormalities by HRT, GDx-VCC, and OCT (see below). This study demonstrated that 20% of patients with structural loss had abnormalities on SWAP and FDT testing when SAP was found to be normal.

The Humphrey Matrix perimeter (Carl Zeiss Meditec, Dublin, Calif) was introduced in 2005, as a newer generation FDT perimetry option with the implementation of multiple efficiency measurements to reduce test taking duration. Fixation monitoring technology has been implemented, as have a wide variety of testing options ranging from screening to full threshold algorithms. The option of smaller stimuli able to resolve subtle maculopathies, etc. is a further advancement from older generation FDT perimeters.

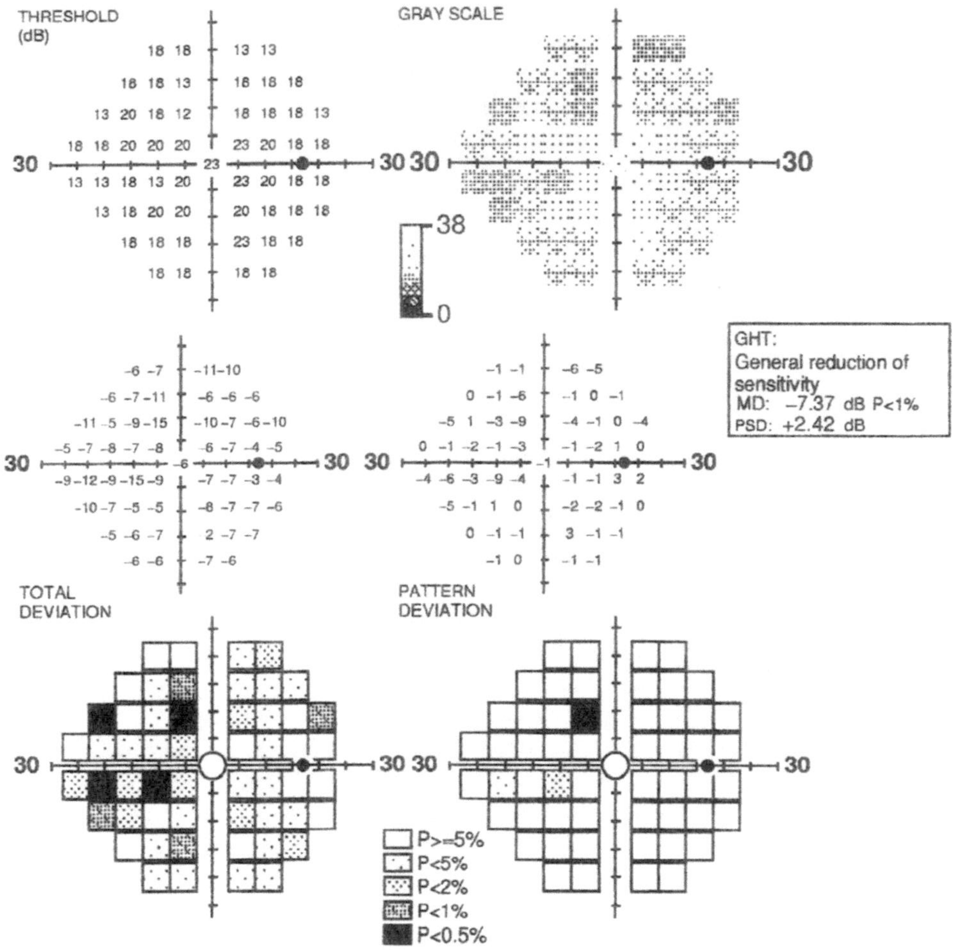


Fig. 9. Frequency doubling technology (FDT): Right eye of same patient on same day as HVF

The FDT plots of the right eye of the same patient show similar metrics to the HVF single field analysis (See Figure 1). The total deviation plot demonstrates more damage than the pattern deviation plot, likely indicating the presence of a media opacity in this patient. The pattern deviation plot demonstrates one point , in the superior field close to the vertical meridian, with a p<0.5 value not detected by the HVF. The significance of this point of visual field loss, as with any finding, needs to be correlated clinically with structural examination and careful ophthalmoscopy. This may indicate a false positive value, or possibly an early defect that the FDT was able to resolve prior to HVF change.

A recent prospective study of 115 glaucomatous eyes examined with the Humprey Matrix perimeterand SITA-SWAP demonstrated sensitivity of 87% for early glaucoma (pattern standard deviation was 94% and mean deviation was 91%); and nearly 100% sensitivity and specificity for moderate to advanced glaucoma when compared to SAP[59]. Another study comparing FDT to SAP in 50 patients with confirmed glaucoma by SAP demonstrated excellent sensitivities of greater than 90%, and demonstrated that FDT had greater specificity than SAP in detecting more severe defects.[60] These recent results certainly demonstrate that FDT is a technology that likely will play an increasing role in the functional assessment of glaucoma patients.

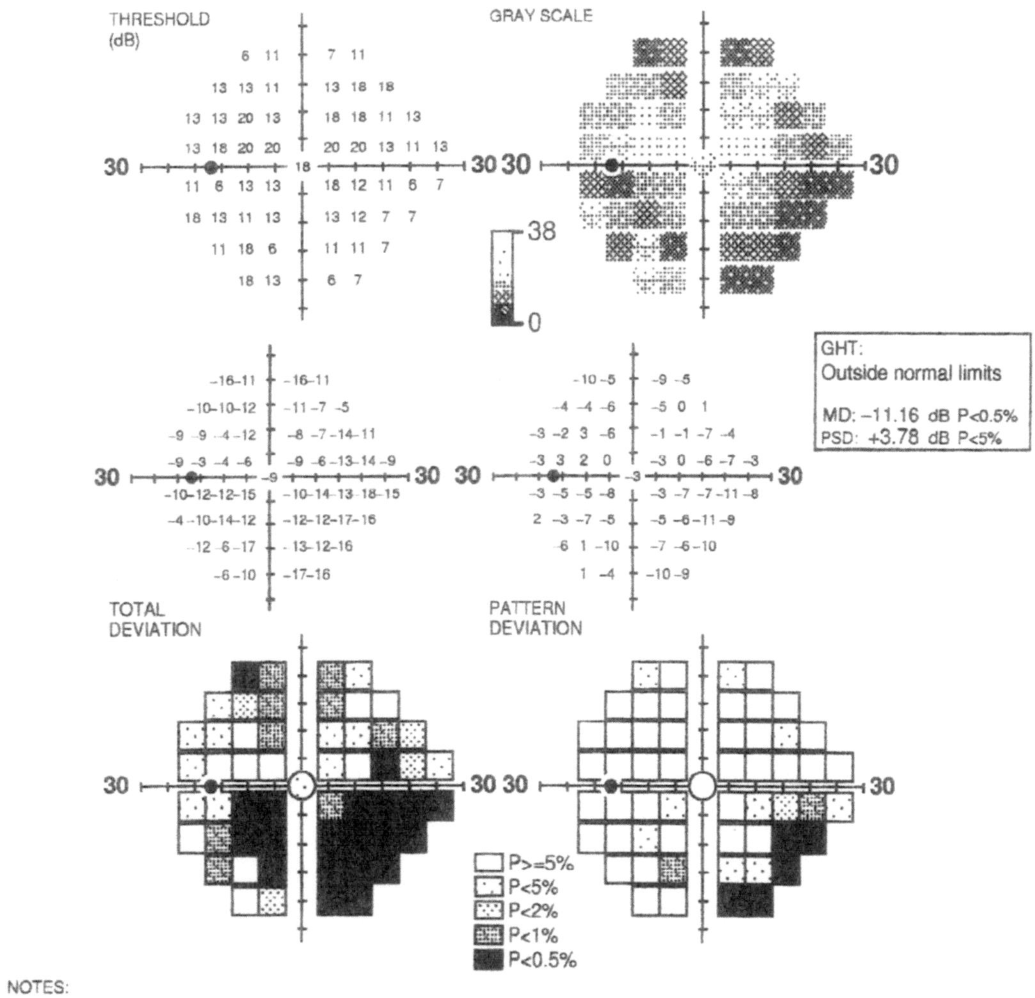


Fig. 10. Frequency doubling technology: Left eye of same patient on same day as HVF

The FDT plot clearly demonstrates a focal defect in the inferonasal field that corresponds to the HVF defects (See Figures 4-6). It is interesting to note that the MD is significantly lower (-11.16 dB) than that calculated from a HVF the same day (-2.11 dB). This large discrepancy may be indicative of the FDT's ability to detect disease at an earlier state. However, the rate of change demonstrated in subsequent FDT evaluations will provide more insight into the likelihood of clinical relevant progression.

## 4. Structural assessment of the glaucoma patient

The assessment of structural abnormalities of the anterior segment and the optic nerve can be performed utilizing a variety of technologies. Each of these diagnostic modalities offers a range of imaging resolutions, and the latest iterations offer extremely detailed images. Arguably, the largest advantage of adjunctive structural assessment is the fact that the measurements are purely objective (ie not subject to the inherent variability seen in all forms of subjective functional assessment). Another important ramification of these advancements is the ability to detect structural abnormalities prior to functional loss. In patients with documented functional loss, structural assessment further allows for quantification of the magnitude of defects. The detailed summary images rendered allow clinicians to actively engage patients in their diagnosis and treatment with simple color coded plots of the relevant anatomy. A great deal of research has been done utilizing these technologies, and it has clearly changed the manner in which clinicians diagnose, treat, and monitor disease progression. Furthermore, objective measurements are inherently less likely to be subject to test taking environments, and are therefore more translatable between practitioners. As structural assessments are not without limitations, it is the role of the clinician to reconcile discordant data, and make the most appropriate recommendations based on the totality of information available.

Prior to the modern imaging techniques further described below, clinicians relied on careful fundoscopic examination and red-free photography to visualize the retinal nerve fiber layer. A recent study by Suh, et al analyzed progressing normal tension glaucoma patients with red-free photography, visual fields, and stereo disc photography[61]. Four characteristic progression patterns were noted including: widening of the existing defect towards the macula, deepening of the defect without expansion, appearance of a new defect, and finally widening of a defect away from the macula. It was noted that almost 95% of these patients exhibited widening of the defect towards the macula, and deepening of the existing defect. Interestingly, no progression was clinically observed on the disc stereo photographs (n=65) or in the visual fields (n=55) in 64 eyes (98.5%) and 46 eyes (83.6%), respectively[61]. Although useful, reproducible high quality red-free images are often difficult and expensive to obtain. Serial red-free photography has largely been supplanted by the newer diagnostic modalities presented below for more routine cases.

### 4.1 Ocular coherence tomography (OCT)

OCT is one of the technologies that has absolutely revolutionized the field of ophthalmology. Clinicians are now able to resolve, at the micrometer level, exceptional three dimensional images of ocular tissues *in vivo*. These detailed images have allowed us to follow a variety of disease states with incredible accuracy, and help monitor the efficacy of therapeutic interventions. OCT is based upon the principle of interferometry, and provides a non-invasive "optical biopsy" of almost every aspect of the ocular anatomy. OCT is powered by low-coherence near infrared light (820nm), and renders images of microstructures based upon reflected signals. The light source at this wavelength offers excellent tissue penetration and has an exceptional safety profile. The super luminescent diode light source is split, simultaneously illuminating the ocular tissue specified,along with an internal reference mirror. The interference patterns of the backscattered light is detected by photo detectors, and then graphically interpreted into a standardized output format.

#### 4.1.1 Time-domain OCT

This technology is used by the Stratus® OCT (Carl Zeiss Meditec, Dublin, CA), allowing for approximately 10 micrometer resolution at an acquisition rate of approximately 400 scans/second. This technology has recently been somewhat supplanted by higher generation OCT scanners in many practices. (see Spectral Domain OCT below). The most commonly used protocol for glaucoma management is the Fast Retinal Nerve Fiber (RNFL) scan, with thinning of the RNFL serving as a surrogate for the measurement of ganglion cell loss. The optic nerve head can be further analyzed to determine rim volume, depth, and cup to disc ratio, amongst other parameters. The Fast RNFL protocol measures the thickness of the RNFL in a circumferential fashion around the optic nerve at around a 3.4mm diameter. The thicknesses of the RNFL from both eyes are then compared to an age-matched normative database. The results are displayed in graphical form with a color coding system designed to represent the severity of the thinning. The average RNFL thickness is calculated from the thicknesses of individually displayed measurements from all four quadrants of the optic nerve. Time-domain OCT has limitations with regards to resolution and data acquisition speeds. This is based on the fact that the technology is limited by the velocity of movement of-a mirror-interferometer Kanamori, et al.[62] compared the RNFL scans and mean deviation (MD) from SAP of 237 glaucomatous eyes versus 160 controls, and found a significant correlation between RNFL thinning and greater MD. Furthermore, the average RNFL thickness proved to be the most reliable parameter in monitoring glaucomatous progression. Gupta, et al.[63] in a recent review in the neuro-ophthalmic literature, demonstrated that patients with non-glaucomatous optic neuropathies had a thinner RNFL thickness than patients with glaucomatous optic neuropathy. Leung, et al.[64] conducted a large study of 137 eyes obtaining 1373 Fast RNFL scans, 1373 normal RFNL scans, and 1236 visual fields over a median period of 4 years, and determined that the Fast RNFL protocol was the most reliable Stratus OCT protocol to detect and follow progression in glaucomatous eyes.

Given the objective nature of OCT scans, there is a tendency amongst clinicians to rely on these examinations more than functional assessment with perimetry. While this may be deemed appropriate in patients unable to perform perimetric evaluation reliably, the limitations of OCT must be taken into account as well. Reliable OCTs are often impossible in patients with severe surface disease, miotic pupils, dense media opacification, high axial length with associated peripapillary atrophy, and vitreous disease. Correlations should routinely be performed between OCT results and the clinical appearance of the optic nerve, as the scans may underestimate cupping when there is glaucomatous undermining under the rim tissue.

Our group[65] recently published a study further demonstrating the confounding effects of vitreous traction on the retinal nerve fiber layer. Approximately 110 eyes of patients were examined with Stratus OCT. Those noted to have partial vitreous detachments at the optic nerve head were found to have artifactually elevated RNFL measurements when matched to controls. Given the relatively high incidence of partial posterior vitreous detachments in the glaucoma group, it was hypothesized that RNFL damage from glaucoma may be masked by the effects of the vitreo-retinal interface. It was concluded from these results that both structural and functional assessments are imperative to determine the presence of glaucomatous damage in these patients in particular. Further investigation of the natural history of PVD, along with changes in the measured retinal nerve fiber layer by OCT, is currently underway. A corollary analysis of the effects of aging on vitreous separation is furthermore being investigated The vitreoretinal interface has been extensively examined by

OCT, particularly in diabetics. Ophir et al, amongst others, have performed multiple analyses utilizing 3-D SD-OCT (see below) to demonstrate that the subtleties of the vitreoretinal interface can be resolved accurately[66,67].

### 4.1.2 Spectral domain (SD) OCT

SD-OCT, also known as Fourier Domain OCT or High Definition OCT (HD-OCT), is the latest commercially available iteration of the OCT technology at the time of this publication. The commercially available Cirrus® OCT (Carl Zeiss Meditec, Inc.) has tremendous advantages over the Stratus OCT in the evaluation and management of many eye conditions. SD-OCT measures the cross-spectral density, a Fourier transformation aimed to estimate the spectral density from a sequence of time samples. The measurements are performed at the detection arm of the interferometer[68]. This allows for much higher resolution and lower test times, as there are no "moving-part" limitations within the interferometer. Furthermore, the ability of the SD-OCT to capture approximately 20,000 axial scans per second, compared to 400 scans/sec for the Stratus OCT, allows for significantly more accurate imaging. This further translates into scans that are less subject to micro-saccadic eye movements during data acquisition. The resultant axial resolution of the scans can be less than 6 micrometers. The Cirrus OCT is furthermore able to match anatomical landmarks from prior scans, minimizing the errors associated with scan misalignment. Misalignment errors are indeed an important source of confounding data with previous versions of the OCT. This is especially the case when longitudinal progression analysis is performed. Lastly the ability to render 3-Dimensional imaging of complex ocular anatomy is yet another major advancement.

Many ophthalmic practices have updated the Stratus OCT to one of the SD-OCT modules in the recent past. It is important to note that the aforementioned differences do not easily allow clinicians to compare RNFL measurements between the two technologies, and accurate correction factors are currently lacking. The re-establishment of a new baseline RNFL thickness with the SD-OCT is quite commonly done in many of these cases. Knight, et al.[69] compared the Stratus OCT to the Cirrus OCT RNFL measurements of 130 eyes with glaucoma relative to normal controls. They demonstrated that the RNFL thickness measured by the Stratus OCT tended to be higher than that of the Cirrus OCT. Sung, et al[70], performed a similar comparative study of 60 normals, 48 glaucoma suspects, and 55 glaucoma patients, They demonstrated that the Cirrus OCT had better sensitivity and specificity for disease than the Stratus OCT, and classified a significantly higher proportion of patients as abnormal. Specifically, Cirrus OCT demonstrated higher sensitivity and specificity (63.6% and 100%) than the Stratus OCT (40.0% and 96.7%) Leung, et al.[64], in a study of 128 glaucomatous eyes over 2 years, similarly concluded that the Cirrus OCT detected glaucomatous changes earlier and more often that the Stratus OCT. A portion of this difference can be attributed to decreased measurement variability with the Cirrus OCT.

Newer versions being developed will likely offer even greater sensitivity and specificity, improved resolution, and clinical progression analysis. Incorporation and evaluation of perimetry in the analysis will likely help bridge the current gap that exists between structural damage and functional loss These advancements will likely be in part possible with the exponentially growing adoption of electronic medical record (EMR) systems. At the time of this publication, significant barriers exist with respect to the interface between EMR, and the variety of functional and structural assessment tools that were traditionally designed as stand-alone technologies.

### 4.2 Confocal scanning laser ophthalmoscopy (SLO)

Retinal imaging with a confocal scanning laser ophthalmoscope (cSLO) involves scanning a small laser beam over the retina, and constructing an image from the descanned reflected light. By applying the confocal principle, tomographic images can be produced[71]. The confocal principle involves measurement of reflected laser light which is concentrated through a pinhole. SLO is based upon acquiring point-by-point images from a series of depths, and then reconstructing them into three-dimensional topographic images.. The Heidelberg Retinal Tomography (HRT) unit scans the fundus with a 670-nm diode laser, creating a three-dimensional map of the fundus and optic nerve. This is accomplished by obtaining multiple optical sections at different depths using a confocal aperture[72] The commercially available (HRT) unit has undergone advancements since the advent of the technology, to its current form as the HRT-III. HRT is used clinically in a similar manner to OCT scans in the evaluation and management of glaucoma. Exceptional imaging quality and newer iterations of progression analysis have made the HRT one of the leading structural analysis tools in practice today. HRT scans further employ eye tracking technology to improve the validity and reproducibility of serial examination. The analysis of the optic nerve head further includes a variety of metrics designed to document morphological variants (Figure 11). The clinical and predictive utility of these parameters continues to be the subject of a great deal of research and subsequent debate. As with any testing modality, data from the HRT needs to be correlated to an individual patient's clinical picture to determine its validity.

Kalabhoukhava, et al.[72], analyzed 59 subjects with ocular hypertension and glaucoma over 50 months with HRT, perimetry, and stereo disk photography. After expert review of the patients at the 50 month time point, subjects were grouped as either progressive or non-progressive. HRT parameters (cup shape measurement, classification index, the third moment in contour, cup/disc ratio, cup area, rim area, and area below reference) showed statistically significant morphological changes in only the progressive group (ie no change from baseline in the "stable" group). These results effectively demonstrate the high diagnostic utility of HRT testing as an adjunctive assessment tool for glaucoma evaluation. Kilintizis, et al[73], demonstrated that changes in HRT parameters of "length of contour" (LC) and "standard deviation of contour" (SDC) were of particular significance when comparing almost 100 glaucoma patients to controls. Balasubramanian, et al.[74] compared HRT I and II parameters in 380 eyes, and concluded that the stereometric parameters were not significantly altered by the newer generation scans. Another study by this same group performed an observational cohort study of 246 eyes followed with HRT, topographic change analysis (TCA), SAP, and stereo photography. It was concluded from the variability in results that there is a great deal of discordance in the detection of longitudinal change[75] between these modalities. Somewhat conflicting assessments of the utility of the HRT, as with all of the aforementioned diagnostic modalities, reminds us that the clinical utility of any data collected greatly relies on the clinician's subjective correlations.

### 4.3 Scanning laser polarimetry (SLP)

The original GDx (Laser Diagnostic Technologies, San Diego, CA), and newer versions with variable corneal compensation GDx-VCC (Carl Zeiss Meditec, Dublin, CA), analyze RNFL thickness with a different method than the OCT and HRT. The RNFL is birifringent secondary to the highly ordered microtubule arrays of the axon microtubules. As the near infrared laser light (780 nm) is split by the birifringent tissue, a phase shift phenomenon

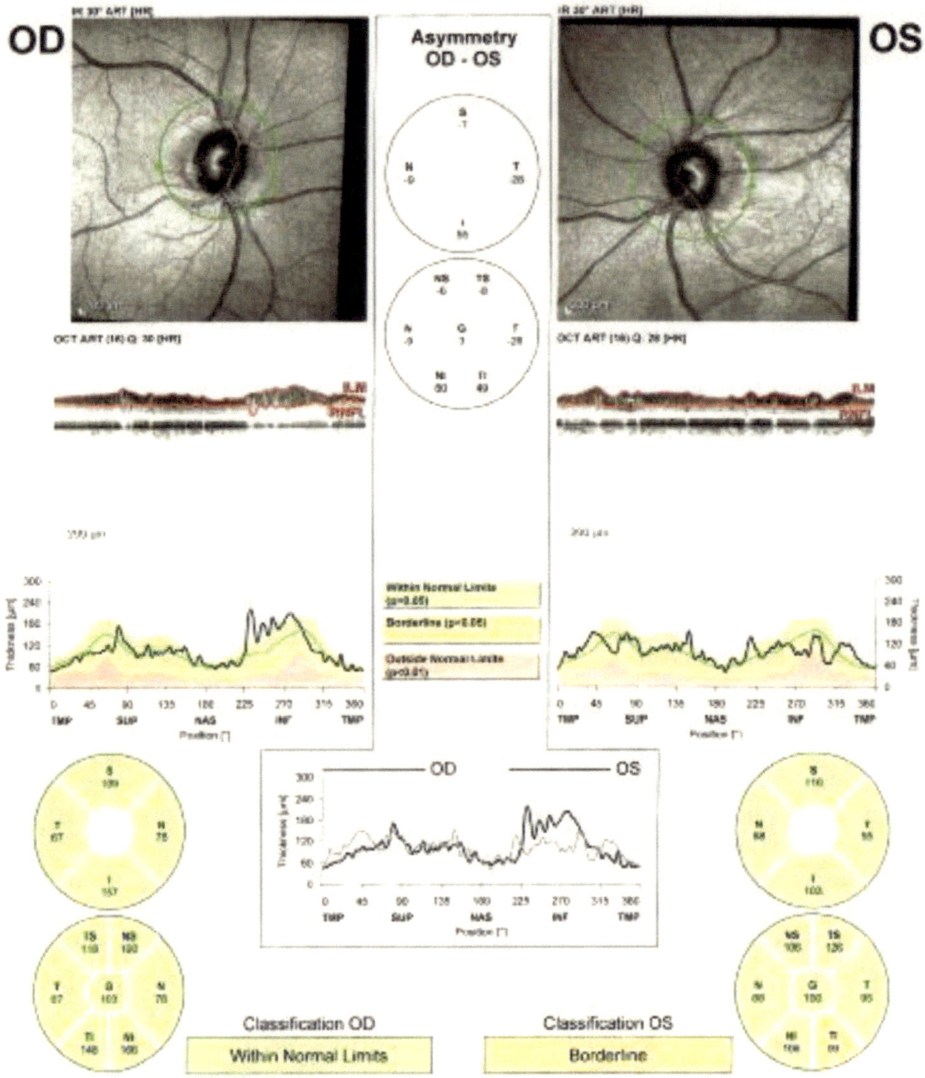


Fig. 11. Heidelberg retinal tomography (HRT) summary of RNFL of same patient on same day as HVF and FDT

Structural analysis may demonstrate an anatomical correlate to demonstrable visual field loss. The digital images are rendered at the top of the summary slide. The green circle demonstrates the limits of the area that is being examined. Centration is optimal in this case, and the newest generation HRT scanners are able to register and match previous scans to improve the reliability of progression analysis. The difference, or calculated asymmetry, between the two eyes is displayed in the top center of the summary printout. The difference in measure RNFL (OD - OS) is graphically displayed by location in the circumpapillary region with S= Superior, N= Nasal, I=Inferior, T=temporal, along with combinations in between the regions (ie TS = Temporal Superior, etc.). Negative values indicate that the left eye has a thicker RNFL, and positive values indicate the opposite. The circumpapillary RNFL.

occurs given the difference in velocity of the reflected light. RNFL thickness can be calculated based on the magnitude of this phase shift. As the anterior segment structures also demonstrate the property of biriferigence, it is necessary to subtract these effects, and newer versions with customized corneal compensation have proven to be much more accurate than prior versions utilizing a fixed compensation algorithm[76]. While the newest generation SLP is far more accurate than earlier versions, the technology is subject to some degree of variability in eyes that show so called "atypical birefringence patterns". Normal patterns of birefringence are generally characterized by the presence of high peripapillary retardation superiorly and inferiorly. This pattern corresponds histologically to the distribution of the superior and inferior arcuate nerve fiber bundles.[77] Abnormal patterns, that are considered normal variants, could therefore confound the data analysis and subsequent detection of disease.

Kim, et al.[78] measured the RNFL of 60 normal patients to 60 glaucoma patients with GDx VCCand Stratus OCT. The results demonstrated no significant differences between the instruments, with high correlations in the superior and inferior quadrants in particular. Pablo, et al[79]analyzed 181 eyes diagnosed with OHTN with GDx-VCC and Stratus OCT, and also found similar diagnostic accuracy between the two. Aptel, et al.[80], compared 120 eyes with Cirrus OCT and GDx-VCC (40 normals, 40 glaucoma suspects, 40 glaucoma) compared with visual field sensitivity, and found that the Cirrus OCT had a stronger correlation to function than the GDx-VCC. Lopez-Pena[81] performed a prospective study of 423 eyes 87 normal eyes, 192 ocular hypertensive eyes, 70 pre-perimetric glaucomas and 74 glaucomatous eyes) to compare SAP with GDx-VCC. The results of this large study showed only weak to moderate correlations with RNFL measurements and visual field defects in the glaucoma group. The relationship between HRT structural defects with functional visual field changes is clearly yet to be well defined.

## 5. Conclusions

The management of glaucoma in the modern era, despite the advent of a host of technologies, remains more of an art than a science in many respects. Improvements in tonometry will continue to improve the accuracy of IOP measurement, especially as the effects of corneal biomechanical properties continue to be elucidated. The potential for accurate home monitoring will allow for better assessment of diurnal and inter-visit IOP control. Similarly, improved imaging techniques will allow for earlier detection of disease with continually improving resolution and reproducibility. It is important to consider that early detection of glaucoma inherently carries the risk of over-diagnosis and subsequent overtreatment. Rates of progression, with all of the modalities described, need to be established prior to the initiation or advancement of therapy. Understanding the limitations of the testing is imperative when making assessments regarding both structure and function. A gestalt approach to glaucoma management allows the specialist to amalgamate a host of information, and effectively cater therapies based on the information available. The modern age of glaucoma care has had notable advancements, and the future of glaucoma management will allow for the optimal care of this globally disabling disease.

## 6. References

[1] Yeshigeta, G. et al. The Influence of Central Corneal Thickness on Intraocular Pressure Measured by Goldmann Applanation Tonometry Among Selected Ethiopian

Communities J Glaucoma: October/November 2010 - Volume 19 - Issue 8 - p 514–518

[2] Azuara-Blanco, T. Bhojani, A. Sarhan, C Pillai, H. Dua Tono-Pen determination of intraocular pressure in patients with band keratopathy or glued cornea *Br J Ophthalmol.* 1998 June; 82(6): 634–636.

[3] Broman AT, Congdon NG, Bandeen-Roche K, Quigley HA. Influence of corneal structure, corneal responsiveness, and other ocular parameters on tonometric measurement of intraocular pressure. *J Glaucoma.* 2007 Oct-Nov;16(7):581-8.3.

[4] Lester M, Mermoud A, Achache F, Roy S. New Tonopen XL: comparison with the Goldmann tonometer. *Eye* (Lond). 2001 Feb;15(Pt 1):52-8.

[5] Kirwan C, O'Keefe M. Corneal hysteresis using the Reichert ocular response analyser: findings pre- and post-LASIK and LASEK. *Acta* Ophthalmol. 2008 Mar;86(2):215-8.

[6] Ayala M. Corneal Hysteresis in Normal Subjects and in Patients with Primary Open-Angle Glaucoma and Pseudoexfoliation Glaucoma. *Ophthalmic Res.* 2011 Apr 6;46(4):187-191.

[7] Detry-Morel M, Jamart J, Pourjavan S. Evaluation of corneal biomechanical properties with the Reichert Ocular Response Analyzer. *Eur J Ophthalmol.* 2011 Mar-Apr;21(2):138-48.

[8] Anand A, De Moraes CG, Teng CC, Tello C, et al. Corneal hysteresis and visual field asymmetry in open angle glaucoma. *Invest Ophthalmol Vis Sci.* 2010 Dec;51(12):6514-8.

[9] Ang GS, Bochmann F, Townend J, Azuara-Blanco A. Corneal biomechanical properties in primary open angle glaucoma and normal tension glaucoma. *J Glaucoma.* 2008 Jun-Jul;17(4):259-62.

[10] Mollan SP, Wolffsohn JS, Nessim M, Laiquzzaman M, Sivakumar S, Hartley S, Shah S. Accuracy of Goldmann, ocular response analyser, Pascal and TonoPen XL tonometry in keratoconic and normal eyes. *Br J Ophthalmol* 2008;92:1661-1665.

[11] Knecht PB, Schmid U, Romppainen T, Hediger A, Funk J, Kanngiesser H, Kniestedt C. Hand-held dynamic contour tonometry. *Acta Ophthalmologica* Volume 89, Issue 2, pages 132–137, March 2011

[12] Gunvant P, Newcomb RD, Kirstein EM, Malinovsky VE, Madonna RJ Meetz RE Measuring accurate IOPs: Does correction factor help or hurt? 2010. *OPTH* 4:611-6

[13] Kotecha A, White E, Schlottmann PG, Garway-Heath DF. Intraocular pressure measurement precision with the Goldmann applanation, dynamic contour, and ocular response analyzer tonometers. *Ophthalmology.* 2010 Apr;117(4):730-7.

[14] Sullivan-Mee M, Gerhardt G, Halverson KD, Qualls C. Repeatability and reproducibility for intraocular pressure measurement by dynamic contour, ocular response analyzer, and goldmann applanation tonometry. *J Glaucoma.* 2009 Dec;18(9):666-73.

[15] Flemmons MS, Hsiao YC, Dzau J, Asrani S, Jones S, Freedman SF. Icare rebound tonometry in children with known and suspected glaucoma. *J AAPOS.* 2011 Apr;15(2):153-7.

[16] Scuderi GL, Cascone NC, Regine F, Perdicchi A, Cerulli A, Recupero SM. Validity and limits of the rebound tonometer (ICare®): clinical study. *Eur J Ophthalmol.* 2011 May-Jun;21(3):251-7.

[17] Munkwitz S, Elkarmouty A, Hoffmann EM, Pfeiffer N, Thieme H. Comparison of the iCare rebound tonometer and the Goldmann applanation tonometer over a wide IOP range. Graefes Arch Clin Exp Ophthalmol. 2008 Jun;246(6):875-9.

[18] Asrani S, Chatterjee A, Wallace DK, Santiago-Turla C, Stinnett S. Evaluation of the ICare rebound tonometer as a home intraocular pressure monitoring device. J Glaucoma. 2011 Feb;20(2):74-9.

[19] Kass MA, Heuer DK, Higginbotham EJ, et al. Ocular Hypertension Treatment Study Group. The Ocular Hypertension Treatment Study (OHTS): a randomized trial determines that topical ocular hypotensive medication delays or prevents the onset of primary open-angle glaucoma. *Arch Ophthalmol.* 2002;120:701–13

[20] The AGIS Investigators. The Advanced Glaucoma Intervention Study (AGIS):11. Risk factors for failure of trabeculectomy and argon laser trabeculoplasty in advanced glaucoma patients. *Am J Ophthalmol.* 2002;134:481–498

[21] Musch DC, Lichter PR, Guire KE, Standardi CL CIGTS Study Group. The Collaborative Initial Glaucoma Treatment Study: study design, methods, and baseline characteristics of enrolled patients. *Ophthalmology.* 1999;106:653–662

[22] Lindenmuth KA, Skuta GL, Rabbani R, Musch DC. Effects of pupillary constriction on automated perimetry in normal eyes. *Ophthalmology.* 1989 Sep;96(9):1298–1301.

[23] Nordmann JP, Brion F, Hamard P, Mouton-Chopin D. Evaluation of the Humphrey perimetry programs SITA Standard and SITA Fast in normal probands and patients with glaucoma. *J Fr Ophthalmol.* 1998 Oct;21(8):549-54

[24] Budenz DL, Rhee P, Feuer WJ, McSoley J, et al. Sensitivity and specificity of the Swedish interactive threshold algorithm for glaucomatous visual field defects. *Ophthalmology.* 2002 Jun;109(6):1052-8

[25] Martin PR, White AJ, Goodchild AK, et al. Evidence that blue-on cells are part of the third geniculocortical pathway in primates. *Eur J Neurosci.* 1997 Jul;9(7):1536-41.

[26] Dacey DM, Lee BB. The 'blue-on' opponent pathway in primate retina originates from a distinct bistratified ganglion cell type. *Nature.* 1994 Feb 24;367(6465):731-5.

[27] Tarek Shaarawy, Mark B. Sherwood, Roger A. Hitchings, Jonathan G. Crowston Glaucoma: Expert Consult Premium Edition Volume 2.

[28] Johnson CA, Adams AJ, Casson EJ, Brandt JD. Blue-on-yellow Perimetry can predict the development of glaucomatous visual field loss. *Arch Ophthalmol* 1993;111:645-50.

[29] Johnson CA, Adams AJ, Casson EJ, Brandt JD. Progression of early glaucomatous visual field loss as detected by blue-on-yellow and standard white-on-white automated Perimetry. *Arch Ophthalmol* 1993;111:651-6.

[30] Van Der Schoot J, Reus NJ, Colen TP, Lemij HG. The ability of short-wavelength automated perimetry to predict conversion to glaucoma. *Ophthalmology.* 2010; 117(1):30-34.

[31] Bengtsson B. A New Rapid Threshold Algorithm for Short-Wavelength Automated Perimetry Invest. *Ophthalmol.* Vis. Sci. March 2003 vol. 44 no. 3 1388-1394

[32] Bengtsson B, Heijl A. Diagnostic Sensitivity of Fast Blue-Yellow and Standard Automated Perimetry in Early Glaucoma:A Comparison between Different Test Programs. *Ophthalmology* July 2006; 113(7) 1092-1097

[33] Birt CM, Shin DH, Samudrala V, et al. Analysis of reliability indices from Humphrey visual field tests in an urban glaucoma population. *Ophthalmology.* 1997 Jul; 104(7):1126-30.

[34] Newkirk MR, Gardiner SK, Demirel S, Johnson CA. Assessment of False Positives with the Humphrey Field Analyzer II Perimeter with the SITA Algorithm. *Invest. Ophthalmol. Vis. Sci.* Oct 2006: 47(10) 4632-4637

[35] Vingrys AJ, Demirel S. False-response monitoring during automated perimetry. *Optom Vis Sci.* 1998 Jul;75(7):513-7.

[36] Bengtsson B, Olsson J, Heijl A, Rootze´n H. A new generation of algorithms for computerized threshold perimetry, SITA. *Acta Ophthalmol Scand.* 1997;75:368–375.

[37] Åsman P, Heijl A. Glaucoma Hemifield Test: Automated Visual Field Evaluation *Arch Ophthalmol.* 1992;110(6):812-819.

[38] Katz J, Quigley HA, Sommer A. Detection of incident field loss using the glaucoma hemifield test. *Ophthalmology.* 1996 Apr;103(4):657-63.

[39] Susanna R Jr, Nicolela MT, Soriano DS, Carvalho C. Automated perimetry: a study of the glaucoma hemifield test for the detection of early glaucomatous visual field loss. *J Glaucoma.* 1994 Spring;3(1):12-6.

[40] Johnson CA, Sample PA, Cioffi GA, et al. Structure and Function Evaluation (SAFE) (I. Criteria for glaucomatous visual field loss using standard automated perimetry (SAP) and short wavelength automated perimetry (SWAP). *Am J Ophthalmol.* 2002;134:177–185

[41] Lester M, Corallo G, Capris E, Capris P. Agreement in detecting glaucomatous visual field progression by using guided progression analysis and Humphrey overview printout. *Eur J Ophthalmol.* Feb 2011: 21(5): 6-6.

[42] Casas-Llera P, Rebolleda G, Muñoz-Negrete FJ, et al. Visual field index rate and event-based glaucoma progression analysis: comparison in a glaucoma population. *Br J Ophthalmol.* 2009 Dec;93(12):1576-9. Epub 2009 Jun 16.

[43] Arnalich-Montiel F, Casas-Llera P, Muñoz-Negrete FJ, Rebolleda G. Performance of glaucoma progression analysis software in a glaucoma population. *Graefes Arch Clin Exp Ophthalmo*l. 2009 Mar;247(3):391-7. Epub 2008 Nov 4.

[44] Diaz-Aleman VT, Anton A, de la Rosa MG, Johnson ZK, et al. Detection of visual-field deterioration by Glaucoma Progression Analysis and Threshold Noiseless Trend programs. *Br J Ophthalmol.* 2009 Mar;93(3):322-8. Epub 2008 Jul 11.

[45] King AJ, Taguri A, Wadood AC, Azuara-Blanco A. Comparison of two fast strategies, SITA Fast and TOP, for the assessment of visual fields in glaucoma patients. *Graefes Arch Clin Exp Ophthalmol.* 2002 Jun;240(6):481-7. Epub 2002 May 15.

[46] Lan YW, Hsieh JW, Sun FJ. Comparison of matrix perimetry with octopus perimetry for assessing glaucomatous visual field defects. *J Glaucoma.* 2011 Feb;20(2):126-32.

[47] Alward, W. Krachmer, J editor; Glaucoma the requisites in Ophthalmology. *Mosby,* St Louis; 2000; p57-61.

[48] Katz J, Tielsch JM, Quigley HA, Sommer A. Automated perimetry detects visual field loss before manual Goldmann perimetry. *Ophthalmology* 1995;102(1):21-6.

[49] Kelly DH. Frequency doubling in visual responses. J Opt Soc Am 1966;56:1628-33.

[50] Maddess T, Severt WL. Testing for glaucoma with the frequency-doubling illusion in the whole, macular and eccentric visual fields. *Aust N Z J Ophthalmol* 1999;27:194-6.43.

[51] White AJ, Sun H, Swanson WH, Lee BB. An examination of physiological mechanisms underlying the frequency-doubling illusion. *Invest Ophthalmol Vis Sci* 2002; 43:3590-9.

[52] Anderson AJ, Johnson CA. Frequency-doubling technology perimetry. *Ophthalmol Clin North Am.* 2003;16:213-25

[53] Spry PG, Johnson CA, McKendrick AM, Turpin A. Variability components of standard automated perimetry and frequency-doubling technology perimetry. *Invest Ophthalmol Vis Sci* 2001;42:1404-10.

[54] Paczka JA, Friedman DS, Quigley HA, et al. Diagnostic capabilities of frequency-doubling technology, scanning laser polarimetry, and nerve fiber layer photographs to distinguish glaucomatous damage. *Am J Ophthalmol* 2001;131:188-97.

[55] Cello KE, Nelson-Quigg JM, Johnson CA. Frequency doubling technology perimetry for detection of glaucomatous visual field loss. *Am J Ophthalmol* 2000;129:314-22.

[56] Nakagawa S, Murata H, Saito H, et al. Frequency Doubling Technology for Earlier Detection of Functional Damage in Standard Automated Perimetry-Normal Hemifield in Glaucoma With Low-to-Normal Pressure. *J Glaucoma.* 2011 May 3. [Epub ahead of print]

[57] Fan X, Wu LL, Ma ZZ, et al. Usefulness of frequency-doubling technology for perimetrically normal eyes of open-angle glaucoma patients with unilateral field loss. *Ophthalmology.* 2010 Aug;117(8):1530-7, 1537.

[58] Ferreras A, Polo V, Larrosa JM, Pablo LE, Pajarin AB, Pueyo V, Honrubia FM. Can frequency-doubling technology and short-wavelength automated perimetries detect visual field defects before standard automated perimetry in patients with preperimetric glaucoma? *J Glaucoma.* 2007 Jun-Jul;16(4):372-83.

[59] Clement CI, Goldberg I, Healey PR, Graham S. Humphrey matrix frequency doubling perimetry for detection of visual-field defects in open-angle glaucoma. *Br J Ophthalmol.* 2009 May;93(5):582-8.

[60] Leeprechanon N, Giangiacomo A, Fontana H, et al. Frequency-doubling perimetry: comparison with standard automated perimetry to detect glaucoma. *Am J Ophthalmol.* 2007 Feb;143(2):263-271.

[61] Suh MH, Kim DM, Kim YK, Kim TW, Park KH. Patterns of progression of localized retinal nerve fibre layer defect on red-free fundus photographs in normal-tension glaucoma. *Eye (Lond).* 2010 May;24(5):857-63.

[62] Kanamori A, Nakamura M, Escano MF, et al. Evaluation of the glaucomatous damage on retinal nerve fiber layer thickness measured by optical coherence tomography. *Am J Ophthalmol.* 2003 Apr;135(4):513-20.

[63] Gupta PK, Asrani S, Freedman SF, et al. Differentiating glaucomatous from non-glaucomatous optic nerve cupping by optical coherence tomography. *Open Neurol J.* 2011 Jan 26;5:1-7.

[64] Leung CK, Cheung CY, Weinreb RN, et al Evaluation of retinal nerve fiber layer progression in glaucoma: a comparison between the fast and the regular retinal nerve fiber layer scans. *Ophthalmology.* 2011 Apr;118(4):763-7

[65] Batta P, Engel HM, Shrivastava A, et al. Effect of partial posterior vitreous detachment on retinal nerve fiber layer thickness as measured by optical coherence tomography. *Arch Ophthalmol.* 2010 Jun;128(6):692-7.

[66] Ophir A, Martinez MR, Mosqueda P, Trevino A. Vitreous traction and epiretinal membranes in diabetic macular oedema using spectral-domain optical coherence tomography. *Eye (Lond).* 2010 Oct;24(10):1545-53.

[67] Mirza RG, Johnson MW, Jampol LM. Optical coherence tomography use in evaluation of the vitreoretinal interface: a review. *Surv Ophthalmol.* 2007 Jul-Aug;52(4):397-421.

[68] De Boer JF, Cense B, B. Park H, et al. Improved signal-to-noise ratio in spectral-do*main compared with time-domain optical coherence tomography. *Optics Letters.* November 1, 2003 / Vol. 28, 21.
[69] Knight OJ, Chang RT, Feuer WJ, Budenz DL. Comparison of retinal nerve fiber layer measurements using time domain and spectral domain optical coherent tomography. *Ophthalmology.* 2009 Jul;116(7):1271-7.
[70] Sung KR, Kim DY, Park SB, Kook MS. Comparison of retinal nerve fiber layer thickness measured by Cirrus HD and Stratus optical coherence tomography. *Ophthalmology.* 2009 Jul;116(7):1264-70.
[71] Vieira P, Manivannan A, Lim CS, Sharp P, Forrester JV. Tomographic reconstruction of the retina using a confocal scanning laser ophthalmoscope. *Physiol Meas.* 1999 Feb;20(1):1-19.
[72] Kalaboukhova L, Vanja Fridhammar V, Lindblom B. Glaucoma follow-up by the Heidelberg Retina Tomograph. *Graefe's Archive for Clinical and Experimental Ophthalmology* Volume 244, Number 6, 654-662.
[73] Kilintzis V, Pappas T, Chouvarda I, et al. Novel Heidelberg retina tomograph-based morphological parameters derived from optic disc cupping surface processing. *Invest Ophthalmol Vis Sci.* 2011 Feb 16;52(2):947-51.
[74] Balasubramanian M, Bowd C, Weinreb RN, Zangwill LM. Agreement between the Heidelberg Retina Tomograph (HRT) stereometric parameters estimated using HRT-I and HRT-II. *Optom Vis Sci.* 2011 Jan;88(1):140-9.
[75] Vizzeri G, Weinreb RN, Martinez de la Casa JM, Alencar LM, Bowd C, Balasubramanian M, Medeiros FA, Sample P, Zangwill LM. Clinicians agreement in establishing glaucomatous progression using the Heidelberg retina tomograph. *Ophthalmology.* 2009 Jan;116(1):14-24.
[76] Weinreb RN, Bowd C, Zangwill LM. Glaucoma detection using scanning laser polarimetry with variable corneal polarization compensation. *Arch Ophthalmol.* 2003 Feb;121(2):218-24.
[77] Bagga H, Greenfield MD, William DS, Feuer J, Quantitative assessment of atypical birefringence images using scanning laser polarimetry with variable corneal compensation *American Journal of Ophthalmology* Volume 139, Issue 3, March 2005, 437-446.
[78] Kim HG, Heo H, Park SW. Comparison of scanning laser polarimetry and optical coherence tomography in preperimetric glaucoma. *Optom Vis Sci.* 2011 Jan; 88(1):124-9.
[79] Pablo LE, Ferreras A, Schlottmann PG. Retinal nerve fibre layer evaluation in ocular hypertensive eyes using optical coherence tomography and scanning laser polarimetry in the diagnosis of early glaucomatous defects. *Br J Ophthalmol.* 2011 Jan;95(1):51-5.
[80] Aptel F, Sayous R, Fortoul V, Beccat S, Denis P. Structure-function relationships using spectral-domain optical coherence tomography: comparison with scanning laser polarimetry. *Am J Ophthalmol.* 2010 Dec;150(6):825-33.
[81] López-Peña MJ, Ferreras A, Polo V, Larrosa JM, Pablo LE, Honrubia FM. Relationship between standard automated perimetry and retinal nerve fiber layer parameters measured with laser polarimetry. *Arch Soc Esp Oftalmol.* 2010 Jan;85(1):22-31.

# 17

# Anterior Chamber Angle Assessment Techniques

Claudio Campa, Luisa Pierro, Paolo Bettin and Francesco Bandello
*Department of Ophthalmology, University Vita-Salute, Scientific Institute San Raffaele*
*Milan,*
*Italy*

## 1. Introduction

The anterior chamber angle is the actual anatomical angle created by the root of the iris and the peripheral corneal vault. Within it lie the structures involved in the outflow passage of the aqueous, namely the trabecular meshwork and the Schlemm's canal (figure 1).
The depth of the angle in a healthy eye is approximately 30°, with the superior part usually less deep than the inferior half. However the depth is influenced by gender, age and refractive error. Female gender has the greatest influence on iridocorneal angle reduction, followed by age and spherical equivalent (Rufer et al.).
The relationship of the iris plane to the cornea has a significant effect on the aqueous humor's accessibility to its outflow drainage system. In eyes where the iris and corneal endothelium are "closed"against one another, the aqueous will not be drained causing an increase of the intraocular pressure (angle closure glaucoma) (Lens, 2008).

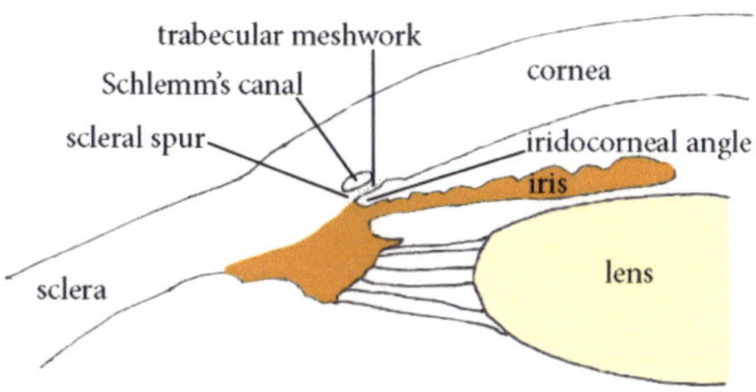


Fig. 1. Diagram of the anatomical structures forming the iridocorneal angle

Primary angle-closure glaucoma (PACG) is a leading cause of blindness worldwide (Quigley and Broman, 2006). Five overlapping conditions, not necessarily progressing in an orderly sequence, are usually described in this disease: angle closure suspect, intermittent (subacute) angle closure, acute angle closure, chronic angle closure and absolute angle closure (Kanski, 2007).
At the earliest stage (angle closure suspect), eyes have narrow or occludable angles without raised intraocular pressure (IOP) or glaucomatous optic neuropathy. It has been estimated that

22% of the eyes with angle closure suspect progress to acute angle closure (Thomas et al., 2003a) whereas 28.5% progress to chronic angle closure over 5-10 years (Thomas et al., 2003b). Prophylactic laser iridotomy performed in eyes with narrow angles may halt the progression of the angle closure process and prevent development of PACG (Nolan et al., 2003). Similarly peripheral iridoplasty, which may also be used to break an attack of acute angle-closure unresponsive to medical therapy or laser iridotomy, can be successfully employed in nonacute situations in patients with angle-closure when laser iridotomy fails to deepen the anterior chamber angle, i.e. particularly in case of plateau iris (Ritch et al., 2007, Ng et al., 2008).
Hence evaluation of anterior chamber angle (ACA) is of great importance to identify and treat those patients at risk for PACG.
It is well known that the depth and volume of the anterior chamber diminish with age and are related to the degree of ametropia. Male subjects have larger anterior chamber dimensions than female subjects. Although grading of limbal chamber depth using van Herick's technique (see below) is commonly used as a surrogate for measuring ACA, gonioscopy has represented for many years the only method able to adequately quantify ACA. However this technique has a subjective and semi-quantitative nature, is hardly reportable due to the difficulty of obtaining good images and requires a good training to be performed properly.
Moreover, in some circumstances such as plateau iris, the angle can be narrow despite a deep anterior chamber. For these reasons, with technology advancements, several new techniques have been proposed with the aim of providing a better imaging of the anterior segment. In this chapter we will show the clinical findings of each method reviewing the strengths and limitations of each approach.

## 2. van Herick test

Performed on the slit lamp without any additional aids, the van Herick test allows quick, not invasive assessment of anterior angle width. The technique was originally described by van Herich (Van Herick et al., 1969): a narrow slit of light is projected onto the peripheral nasal or temporal cornea at an angle of 60° as near as possible to the limbus. This results in a slit image on the surface of the cornea the width of which is compared with the peripheral anterior chamber depth ("black space") (figure 2). A four-point scale is then used, with each grade indicating the probability of angle closure. In grade 4 the anterior chamber depth (ACD) is ≥100% corneal thickness and the angle is wide open; in grade 3 it is > 25 to 50% and the angle is incapable of closure; in grade 2 it is 25% and the angle closure is possible; in grade 1 is < 25% and the angle closure is likely.
Studies have shown suboptimal results when using van Herick test to screen for primary angle closure (Alsbirk, 1986), (Congdon et al., 1997), (Thomas et al., 1996): particularly it has been found that measurements performed at the nasal limbus tend to overestimate the angle width. To improve precision in quantification of ACD, Foster (Foster et al., 2000a) proposed a modified scheme in which the original grade 1 was sub-divided into 0%, 5%, and 15% corneal thickness, and a grade of 75% corneal thickness was added to compensate for the gap between the original grades 3 and 4. This seven-point grading system resulted in 99% sensitivity compared to gonioscopic evaluation; the interobserver agreement for this augmented grading scheme was good (weighted kappa 0.76). However it is hardly reproducible in clinical practice.

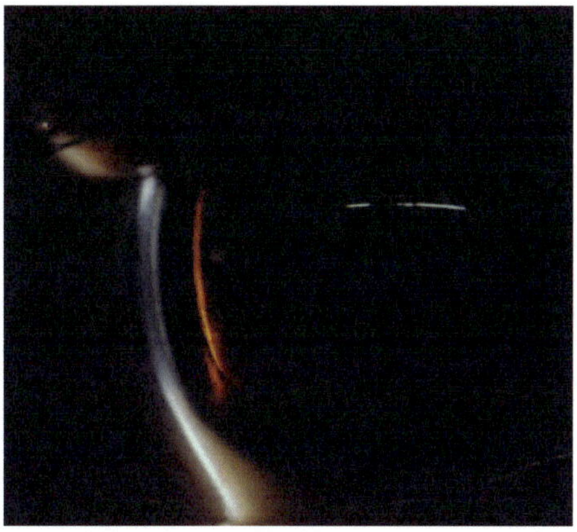

Fig. 2. An example of van Herick technique for assessing anterior chamber depth (a grade 4 is shown, see text)

## 3. Smith method

Another optical technique used to determine ACD is Smith's slit-length method (Smith, 1979). It is performed using a standard slit-lamp. The illumination system is located in the subject's temporal field at an angle of 60° and the slit-beam is projected horizontally. If measuring the patient's right eye the right ocular of the slit lamp is used and vice versa for the left eye. A beam of approximately 1.5 mm thickness, with its orientation horizontal, is placed across the cornea. The procedure involves focusing the slit-beam on the corneal surface while an out of focus image of the slit-beam is observed on the iris/lens surface. The length of the slit-beam when the two corneal and iris/lens images are just touching is multiplied by a constant to give the ACD in millimetres (figure 3). In the original description of the method by Smith the constant was 1.40, while others (Barrett et al., 1996) have proposed more recently 1.31. Both constants have been determined using an optical pachymetry.

The Smith method has been validated by a number of authors (Barrett et al., 1996) (Douthwaite and Spence, 1986). It allows the clinician to obtain reliable estimates of axial ACD, without any attachments to the slit-lamp biomicroscope. The axial ACD estimates are accurate to within ± 0.25 mm (Smith, 1979), ± 0.2 mm (Jacobs, 1979) and ± 0.33 mm (Barrett et al., 1996) as compared to pachymetry and to within ± 0.42 mm, as compared to ultrasonography. There is no effect of the central corneal thickness on the ACD estimate made using this method (Osuobeni et al., 2003), which has also a minimum inter and intra observer variation (Osuobeni et al., 2000).

From birth to the age of 13 years, the mean value of ACD increases from 2.37 to 3.70 mm for Northern European boys, and from 2.39 to 3.62 mm for girls (Larsen, 1971). There is very little change in the mean anterior chamber depth from the teenage years to about 30 years, while there is a decline in the mean anterior chamber depth from 30 to 60 years, probably because of the increase of lens thickness (Fontana and Brubaker, 1980). Between this age range the typical value is around 2.5 mm. The depth and volume of the anterior chamber are also related to the degree of ametropia. Male subjects usually have larger anterior chamber dimensions than female subjects. There is a direct association between narrow anterior chamber angle and shallow anterior chamber depth (Wishart and Batterbury, 1992).

Consequently, the ACD quantification represents an indirect means of assessing the anterior chamber angle and identifying patients who are more likely to develop PACG. Usually eyes with ACD <2 mm are considered at risk (Wishart and Batterbury, 1992).

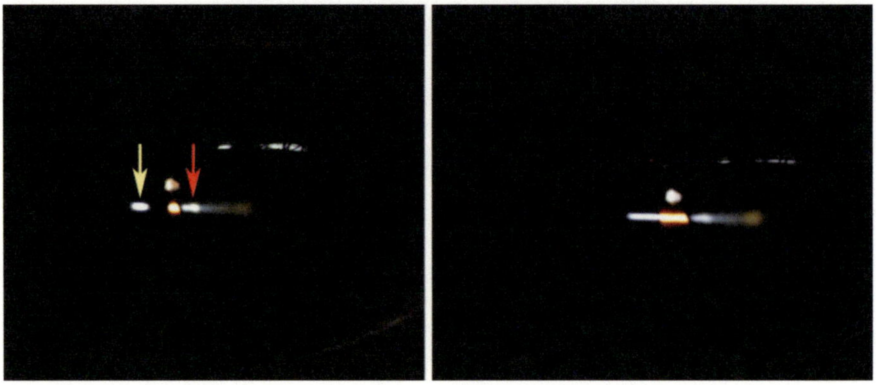

Fig. 3. Measurement of the anterior chamber depth using Smith's method. Yellow arrow indicates the focused horizontal corneal-imaged slit and red arrow the out-of-focus iris/lens-imaged slit (see text for details)

## 4. Gonioscopy

Gonioscopy still represents the gold standard for assessment of the angle. This technique was first developed by Trantas in the late 1800s and subsequently modified by Koeppe and Barkan to allow a direct visualization of the structure of the anterior chamber angle with a contact lens (Friedman and He, 2008). Nowadays however indirect gonioscopy (which relies on mirrors or prisms to reflect light from the angle to the viewer) is usually preferred because of several advantages over direct gonioscopy: the patient can be examined at the slit lamp using a variable magnification and there is no astigmatic aberration. Two lenses are commonly employed: the Zeiss-type and the Goldmann-type. The Zeiss-type lens has a 9-mm diameter corneal surface (radius of curvature 7.72 mm) and doesn't require a coupling agent. The Goldmann-type has larger base diameter (corneal surface 12 mm and radius of curvature 7.38 mm) and requires a coupling agent (thick artificial tears or hydroxypropyl methylcellulose) when placed on the cornea. Although use of Zeiss-type lens needs more training and expertise, it has undoubted advantages because leaves the anterior segment clear for later viewing of the posterior pole and compresses the cornea centrally, which in turns allows for greater dynamic assessment of the angle structures.

Moreover pressure on the larger base lenses can lead to compression over Schwalbe's line with a consequent alteration of angle's morphology.

Since illumination conditions and degree of pupil dilation may dramatically alter angle configuration, a strict assessment protocol should be followed: the patient should look straight ahead and should be examined in a dark room, using a 1-mm beam with adequate illumination to visualize angle structures (Weinreb and Friedman, as cited in (Friedman and He, 2008).

Three grading systems have been proposed for documenting angle findings seen in gonioscopy: Scheie (Scheie, 1957), Schaffer (Shaffer, 1960) and Spaeth (Spaeth, 1971) classification (table 1).

| **Scheie** | | **Schaffer** | | | **Spaeth** | | |
|---|---|---|---|---|---|---|---|
| *Classification* | *Findings* | *Classification* | *Findings* | *Angle width (deg.)* | *Classification* | | *Findings* |
| Wide open | All structures visible | Grade 4 | Ciliary body is visible | 35-45 | Iris insertion | A<br>B<br>C<br>D<br>E | Anterior<br>Behind<br>In sclera<br>Deep angle recess<br>Extremely deep recess |
| Grade I | Iris root not visible | Grade 3 | Scleral spur is visible | 20-35 | Width of angle recess | | 0, 10, 20, 30 and 40 degrees |
| Grade II | Ciliary body not visible | Grade 2 | Only trabecular meshwork is visible | 20 | Peripheral iris configuration | S<br>R<br>Q | Steep<br>Regular<br>Queer |
| Grade III | Posterior trabecular meshwork not visible | Grade 1 | Only Schwalbe's line is visible | ≤ 10 | 12 o'clock pigmentation | 0<br>1+<br>2+<br>3+<br>4+ | None<br>Just visible<br>Mild<br>Moderately dense<br>Dense |
| Grade IV | None of angle structures visible | Grade 0 | Angle is closed | 0 | | | |

Table 1. Angle grading systems

In the Scheie scheme grade zero represents a wide open angle. Grade 1 is a "slightly narrow" angle and the iris root is not visible; grade 2 means that the ciliary body is not visible while grade 3 means that the posterior (pigmented) trabecular meshwork is not visible. Grade 4 is a closed angle and therefore no angle structures are visible. Scheie believed that persons with grade 3 and grade 4 angles were at greatest risk of PACG.

The Shaffer system is currently the most popular grading system. It uses both angle width and angle structures to classify angle grade: this is confusing because sometimes width and structures seen may place an angle into different categories. In this grading system angles between 35 and 45 degrees are classified as grade 4, those between 20 and 35 as grade 3, those between 10 and 20 as grade 2 and those ≤10 as grade 1, with a closed angle (zero degrees) classified as grade 0. Angle width is often preferred to angle depth in the description of ACA, because the latter may differ in different locations. Taking into consideration the angle structures, Shaffer classification's grade 4 comprises all structures, grade 3 the structures up to the scleral spur, grade 2 up to the trabecular meshwork, in grade 1 only the Schwalbe's line is visible and in grade 0 none of the angle structures are visible.

Spaeth classification provides the most comprehensive approach to angle assessment. This classification includes three components: angular width of angle recess, configuration of the peripheral iris, insertion site of the iris root. The width of the angle recess is graded from 10 to 40 degrees. The iris configuration is reported as "r" (regular), "s" (steep, as in plateau iris configuration), or "q" (queer, or backward, bowing as may occur in pigment dispersion syndrome). The insertion of iris root ranges from A – anterior to the Schwalbe's line, B - behind Schwalbe's line, but anterior to scleral spur, C - posterior to scleral spur (i.e., scleral spur visible, but not ciliary body), D - ciliary body visible, and E - large amount of ciliary body visible. When the iris is appositional with the angle, the "apparent" iris insertion, seen without indentation, is noted as a letter placed in parenthesis, while the "actual" insertion is noted with a letter not placed in parenthesis. Finally the Spaeth system rates also the pigment of the posterior trabecular meshwork at 12 o'clock from 0 to 4+ (black pigmented meshwork) and the presence or absence of peripheral anterior synechiae (PAS). An example of wide open angle is given in figure 4.

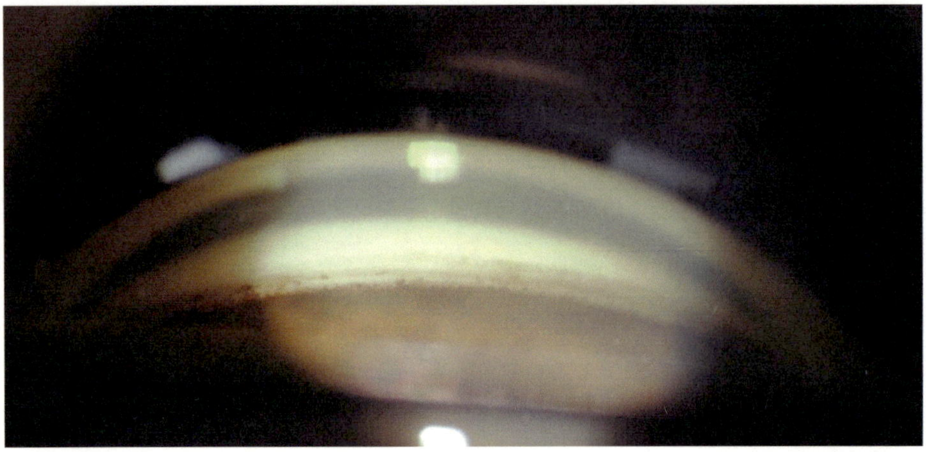

Fig. 4. Gonioscopy of a wide open angle. All angle structures are visible. From down to top: ciliary body band with some iris processes reaching the trabecular meshwork, scleral spur, pigmented (posterior) trabecular meshwork, nonpigmented (anterior) trabecular meshwork and Schwalbe's line delineated by some scattered pigment

Not many studies have been published on the reliability of the angle grading systems. Some authors have reported a weighted k values for inter-observer reproducibility of Shaffer classification in the ranges of 0.6 using a Goldmann-style lens (Foster et al., 2000b) (Aung et al., 2005). The Spaeth system has shown high reproducibility and comparability to UBM in 22 patients (Spaeth et al., 1995).

A quantitative grading of the angle has been proposed by some authors (Cockburn, 1980, Congdon et al., 1999), but has not gained popularity in clinical practice.

Once an angle is viewed and it is determined that there is iridotrabecular contact, it is necessary to determine whether the angle is appositionally closed or if there are permanent PAS. To pursue this task a gentle indentation with the goniolens is performed ("dynamic gonioscopy"). By indenting the central cornea (usually with a Zeiss-type lens) the aqueous is displaced into the peripheral anterior chamber where it bows the iris posteriorly and widens the chamber angle. This widening differentiates areas where the peripheral iris is permanently adherent to the peripheral cornea (i.e. PAS) from areas where the iris is merely reversibly apposed to the peripheral cornea.

Caution must be taken in distinguishing PAS from iris processes. Iris processes, either plastered across the surface of the angle or bridging from the peripheral iris to the angle structures, are pigmented strands continuous with and histologically identical to the iris. These are a normal variant and have no effect upon aqueous outflow. On the contrary PAS are abnormal adhesions of the peripheral iris to the angle structure that, if extensive enough, can eventually reduce trabecular outflow. Usually PAS tend to be wider (at least half of 1 clock hour in width) and are present to the level of the trabecular meshwork or higher.

Examples of PAS include the fibrovascular membrane formed in neovascular glaucoma, proliferating abnormal endothelial cells in the iridocorneal endothelial (ICE) syndromes, epithelialization of the angle due to epithelial ingrowth, or inflammatory trabecular and keratic precipitates in contact with an inflamed iris in uveitis.
The gonioscopic criteria for an occludable angle usually include: 1) trabecular meshwork invisible in 270° or more of the entire angle in the primary position of gaze without indentation and / or 2) angular width less than 20 degrees by the Shaffer grading (Kim and Jung, 1997). Often these criteria are used to identify angles that require treatment (i.e. iridotomy), although there is still no unanimous consensus (Friedman, 2001, Foster et al., 2002).

## 5. Pentacam

The Pentacam (Oculus, Inc., Lynnwood, WA, USA) is a rotating Scheimpflug camera with a short-wavelength slit light (475 nm, blue light-emitting diode laser) that is able to take 25 slit images of the anterior segment of the eye in 2 seconds with 500 true elevation points in each image. Any eye movement is detected (and the results corrected) by a second camera. A three-dimensional model of the anterior segment can therefore be built with the obtained data including the corneal thickness, corneal topographic parameters, central ACD, anterior chamber angle (ACA), anterior chamber volume (ACV) and other parameters. Interestingly the software doesn't require any manual initiation. Two chamber angles for each chosen meridian are provided. It is noteworthy to mention that ACA is calculated by lengthening the posterior cornea and the iris contour to compute the chamber angle using an interpolation method, because Pentacam cannot image the angle recess and scleral spur. Several studies have investigated the reliability of Pentacam (and other Scheimpflug cameras) in measuring ACA. Lam (Lam et al., 2002) found on 25 healthy subjects with open angles that the 95% limit of agreement on repeat measurements of angle width was 5°, and inter-observer agreement was 6°. Rabsilber showed good reliability of Pentacam in assessing ACA in 76 healthy volunteers (Rabsilber et al., 2006). Although measurement of the ACA obtained with the Pentacam seem to correlate significantly with Shaffer's grade determined by gonioscopy, a certain discrepancy has been reported between ACA and ACD measured by Pentacam and ultrasound biomicroscopy (UBM) or anterior-segment optical coherence tomography (AS-OCT) in eyes with a narrow angle (Liang et al.) (Kurita et al., 2009) (Mou et al.). This may be due to the inability of the Pentacam to visualize the most peripheral part of the iris. Alternatively the placement of an eye cup, which is necessary for UBM examination, may be responsible of a flattening of the cornea which in turns leads to an artificial reduction of the ACD. Hence ACV seems to be the most efficient parameter to screen patients with POAG or POAG suspect using the Pentacam (Kurita et al., 2009). However although Pentacam non-contact approach to angle assessment is highly appealing for screening purposes, it is limited to visualization of only the angle recess. Scheimpflug photography indeed does not display the retroiridal structures or the ciliary body, which are of great interest in glaucoma diagnosis.

## 6. Ultrasound Biomicroscopy (UBM)

Ultrasound-based diagnostic imaging uses a probe containing a piezoelectric transducer to emit a sound wave which propagates through tissues and is partially reflected –echoes-from anatomic structures differing in acoustic impedance (density × speed of sound). Some of the echoes return to the transducer and are converted back into voltages and amplified. The range of each echo is proportional to the time delay between sound wave emission and echo return, specifically, r = ct/2, where r is the range, c is the speed of sound (1532 m/s at 37°C in normal saline) and t is the time (Ursea and Silverman).

Each pulse/echo event thus provides information along one line of sight. By mechanically scanning the probe, information along an ordered series of lines is obtained. By converting echo amplitude into pixel intensity, a 2D cross-sectional B-scan image is then produced.

Ultrasonic imaging resolution improves by increasing the frequency of the transducer. However higher frequencies produce a correspondingly smaller wavelength which is less able to penetrate the tissues.

Ultrasound systems utilizing probes of approximately 35 MHz or more have come to be known as "ultrasound biomicroscopy" (UBM) or 'very high-frequency ultrasound systems'. Such systems have a tissue penetration of only 5 mm but provide lateral and axial resolutions approximately of 40 and 20 microns, respectively. They allow therefore for a more detailed assessment of the anterior ocular structures than was available using traditional B-scan ultrasound.

UBM systems are now produced by numerous companies, with probes ranging from 50 to 80 MHz. Handheld UBM probes are now often equipped with acoustically transparent, fluid-filled 'bubble tips' that can be placed directly onto the globe. These obviate the use of water-baths or scleral shells for acoustic coupling, greatly simplifying the examination and allowing the patient to be examined in a sitting position.

UBM provides both quantitative and qualitative information on the anterior segment of the eye. Pavlin and coworkers carried out the first clinical UBM study of the ocular structures in glaucomatous patients in the early 1990s (Pavlin et al., 1992). Subsequently many authors proposed different biometric parameters to characterize the angle and anterior segment. The most common include: angle-opening distance (AOD), trabecular-iris angle (TIA), trabecular–ciliary process distance (TCPD), iris thickness (ID), angle-recess area (ARA), iris ciliary process distance (ICPD), iris-lens contact distance (ILCD) (see Table 2 and figure 5 for details).

AOD and ARA can be measured at various distances from the sclera spur. Theoretically, 500 µm is the appropriate distance because it approximates the length of the trabecular meshwork. However, a longer measurement distance of 750 µm uses information from a large region of the image and may be more robust, especially for ARA, since it is less affected by local iris surface undulations. Henzan and coworkers studied the performance of the UBM parameters in differentiating primary angle closure/primary angle closure suspect from non-occludable angle eyes through the receiver operating characteristic (ROC) curve and the area under the curve (AUC). They found that $AOD_{500}$ and TIA under light conditions had the greatest AUC of 0.94. The ideal cutoff values for the $AOD_{500}$ and TIA under light conditions determined with the Youden index (=sensitivity - [1 - specificity]) were 0.17 mm (sensitivity, 0.82; specificity, 0.96) and 15.2 degrees (sensitivity, 0.83; specificity, 0.93), respectively (Henzan et al.).

A limitation of these findings is that UBM measurements of angle structures can be influenced by a number of variables including patient's age and gender (Friedman et al., 2008), direction of gaze, accommodation, room illumination, variation in image acquisition (position of the probe, meridians scanned) (Friedman and He, 2008).

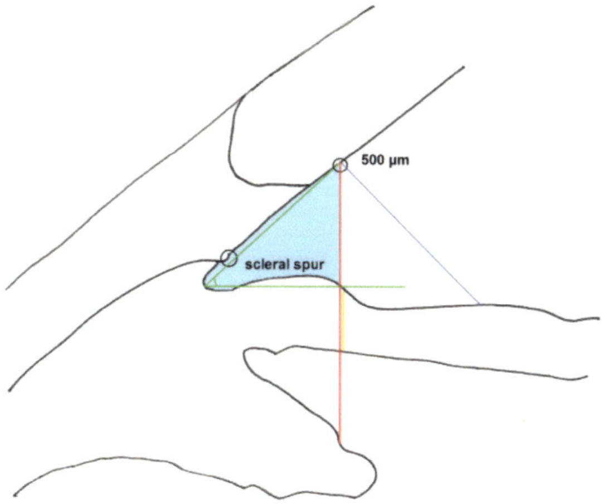


Fig. 5. Diagram illustrating several biometric descriptors of the angle, including angle-opening distance (blue line), iris thickness (yellow line), trabecular-iris angle (red line), trabecular-ciliary process distance (green line) and angle recess area (light blue area). In this example measurements are made 500 µm from the sclera spur

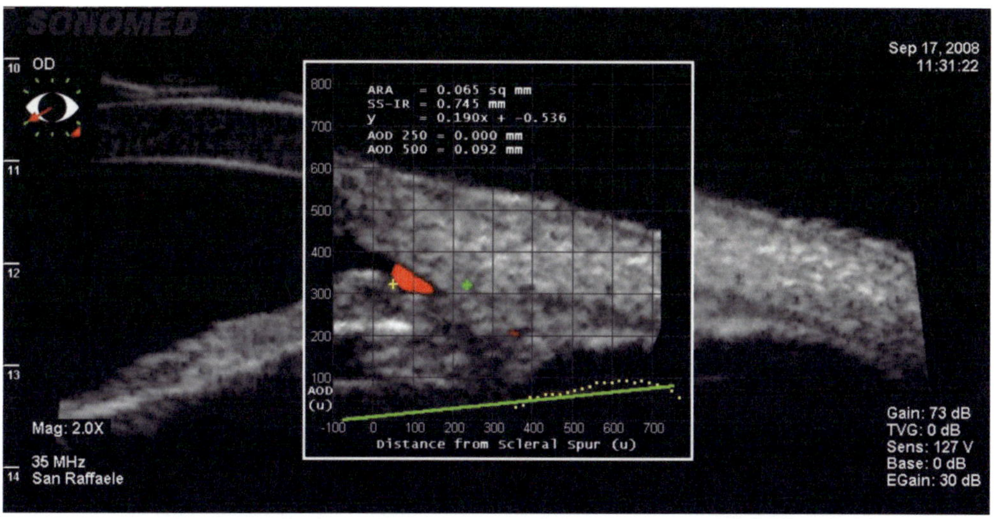


Fig. 6. Screen shot of the analysis software from the UBM Pro 2000 (UBM Pro 2000, Paradigm Medical Industries, Salt Lake City, UT, USA)

One would expect high variability in the measurements because of the partly subjective nature of the caliper placement on visualized anatomic landmarks. On the contrary the reported reproducibility of analyses on single UBM images seems to be pretty good.

Marchini showed high reproducibility in a paper comparing UBM parameters in angle closure patients (range of coefficient of variation 1.4 -16%) (Marchini et al., 1998).

Even better reproducibility was reported by Gohdo when measuring the ciliary body thickness (CBT) one and two millimeters posterior to the scleral spur (coefficient of variation < 2.5%) (Gohdo et al., 2000).

In any case image analysis using calipers to mark each structure takes a large amount of time due to the need to place a cursor at each point for any given measurement.
To overcome this issue, Ishikawa and colleagues created a semi-automated program (UBM Pro 2000, Paradigm Medical Industries, Salt Lake City, UT, USA) that provides several important parameters once the scleral spur is identified (figure 6) (Ishikawa et al., 2000).

| Parameter | Description | Range* | | References |
|---|---|---|---|---|
| | | Occludable angle (OA) | Nonoccludable angle (NOA) | |
| $AOD_{500}$ | Distance from cornea to iris at 500 µm from the scleral spur | 0.11± 0.04 | 0.29 ± 0.13 | (Henzan et al.) |
| TIA | Angle formed from angle recess to points 500 µm from scleral spur on corneal endothelium and perpendicular on surface of iris | 10.3±3.9 | 24.2± 9.3 | (Henzan et al.) |
| TCPD | Measured from point on endothelium 500 µm from scleral spur perpendicularly through iris to ciliary process | 0.62 ± 0.11 | 0.77±0.16 | (Henzan et al.) |
| ID | Measured from perpendicular 500 µm from scleral spur | 0.40 ±0.05 | 0.41±0.05 | (Henzan et al.) |
| $ARA_{750}$ | Area of triangle between angle recess, iris and cornea 750 µm from scleral spur | 0.10±0.08 | 0.13 ±0.01 | (Friedman et al., 2003) for NOA (Yoo et al., 2007) for OA |
| ICPD | Distance from the posterior iris surface to the ciliary process perpendicular 500 µm from scleral spur | 0.39± 0.21 | 0.40± 0.10 | (Sihota et al., 2005) |
| ILCD | Length of contact between surfaces of lens and iris | 0.79±0.22 | 0.98± 0.41 | (Sihota et al., 2005) |

*All values (mean±standard deviation) are in mm except TIA which is in degrees and $ARA_{500}$ which is in mm$^2$.
Abbreviations: AOD=angle-opening distance; TIA=trabecular-iris angle; TCPD=trabecular–ciliary process distance; ID:iris thickness; ARA=angle-recess area; ICPD=iris ciliary process distance; ILCD=iris-lens contact distance;

Table 2. Biometric parameters used in UBM for characterizing the angle and anterior segment in subjects with an occludable/nonoccludable angle

The software calculates $AOD_{250}$, $AOD_{500}$, $ARA_{750}$ and performs linear regression analysis of consecutive AODs, producing two figures: the acceleration and the y-intercept. Acceleration tells how rapidly the angle is getting deeper, using the tangent of the angle instead of degrees as the unit. The y-intercept refers to the distance between the scleral spur and the iris surface along the perpendicular to the trabecular meshwork plane.
Acceleration and the y-intercept can be negative numbers. A negative number for acceleration means that the angle has an almost normal configuration at its peripheral part and becomes very shallow or is attached to the cornea at its central part. A negative y-intercept means that the angle recess is very shallow or is attached to the cornea at its periphery, whereas it is relatively wide centrally. According to Ishikawa and colleagues this software dramatically improves the overall reproducibility, with a coefficient of variation ranging between 7.3 and 2.5 for the various parameters (Ishikawa et al., 2000).

UBM gives also valuable qualitative information which helps in the diagnosis and in the management of several ocular diseases. In plateau iris syndrome UBM well demonstrates the ciliary body anteriorly positioned compressing the iridocorneal angle and placing the peripheral iris in apposition to the trabecular meshwork (figure 7).

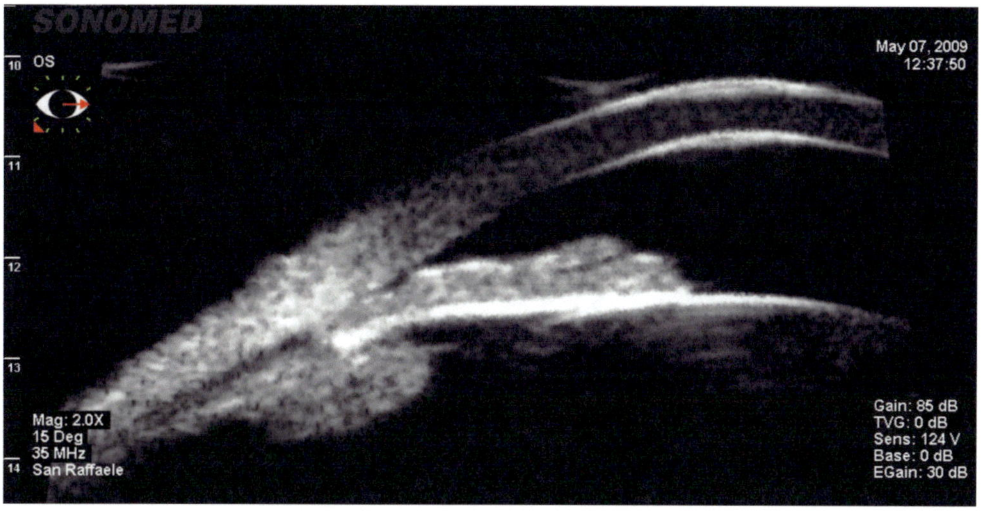


Fig. 7. Ultrasound biomicroscopy view of an eye with plateau iris syndrome

In pigment dispersion syndrome UBM shows an open angle, a characteristic concave iris and a ciliary body rotated posteriorly (figure 8).

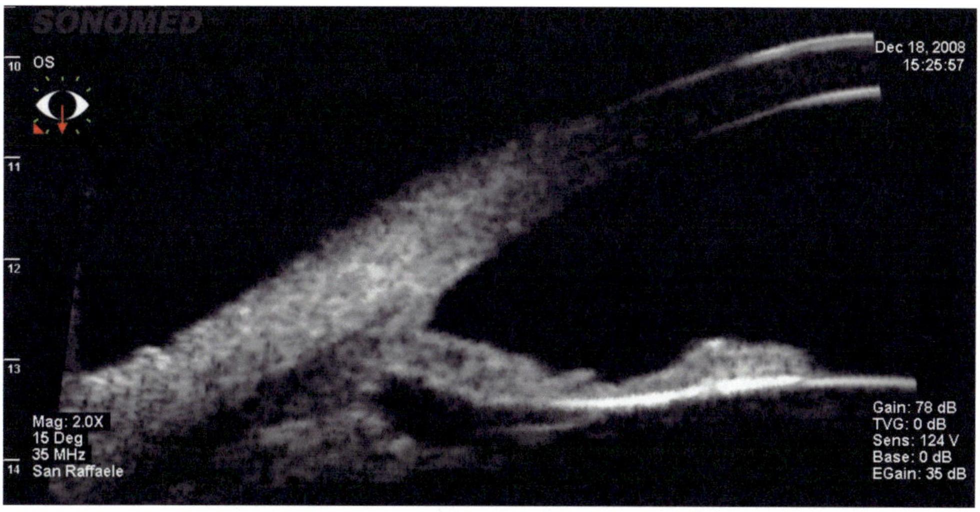


Fig. 8. Ultrasound biomicroscopy view of an eye with pigment dispersion syndrome

Angle recession, intraocular foreign bodies, ciliary body cysts are also easily detectable by UBM. Lastly UBM may represent a useful tool for the planning and guidance of glaucoma surgery, including the evaluation of filtering blebs, sclerectomy and canaloplasty, as well as the diagnosis and evaluation of postoperative complications.

## 7. Anterior segment optical coherence tomography (AS-OCT)

Optical coherence tomography (OCT) of the eye was first described by Huang and coworkers at the Massachusetts Institute of Technology (Boston, MA, USA) in 1991 (Huang et al., 1991). OCT uses a near-infrared light that is directed throughout ocular tissues. While most of the light is absorbed by the tissues or scattered, a small portion is reflected and collected by an interferometer in order to produce an image. In time-domain OCT, the reference mirror is mechanically scanned in the range axis, and this allows determination of the range to optical reflections along the tissue path, which are represented by interference fringes in the OCT signal.

OCT was initially developed only for retinal imaging; in 1994 Izatt et al. (Izatt et al., 1994) for the first time used it also for imaging the anterior chamber (anterior segment OCT, AS-OCT). Since then, AS-OCT has rapidly become popular for ACA assessment.

Originally anterior and posterior segment imaging used the same wavelength (830 nm). Subsequently a longer wavelength of 1310 nm was preferred for AS-OCT. This increases the depth of penetration by reducing the amount of light scattered by the sclera and limbus, allowing for visualization of the ACA morphology in greater detail. In addition, the 1310 nm light incident on the cornea is strongly absorbed by water in the ocular media, with only 10% reaching the retina. This enables the AS-OCT to utilize higher power, enhancing imaging speed and eliminating motion artifacts (Quek et al.). The Visante™ OCT (Carl Zeiss Meditec, Dublin, CA, USA) and the SL-OCT (Heidelberg Engineering, GmbH, Dossenheim, Germany) are 2 commercially available devices which use this wavelength providing an axial and transverse resolution of 18 μm and 60 μm, respectively, for the Visante and <25 μm and 20–100 μm for the SL-OCT (Quek et al.). SL-OCT incorporates OCT technology into a modified slit-lamp biomicroscopy system: this requires slower image acquisition speed and more operator skills.

More recently the new frequency (Fourier) domain OCTs have been developed, where the broadband signal is broken into a spectrum using a grating or linear detector array (i.e. sensitive detectors arranged in grating or single row), and depth is determined from the Fourier transform of the spectrum without motion along the reference arm (Ursea and Silverman). The fast readout speed of the detectors (typically tens of kilohertz) allows acquisition at video frame rates (30 fps) while the multiplexed scheme provides a signal-to-noise ratio (SNR) advantage over time domain OCT (TD-OCT). Fourier (also called Spectral) domain OCTs (SD-OCTs) allows scans at a rate of 26,000 A-scans per second and more images to be taken in a single pass. These devices produce therefore detailed cross-sectional images of structures at an axial resolution of 5 μm and a transverse resolution of 15 μm.

The RTVue (Optovue Inc.,Fremont, CA, USA), the Cirrus high-definition OCT (HD-OCT) 4.0 (Cirrus; Carl Zeiss Meditec Inc.) and the OPKO Spectral OCT SLO (OPKO Health, Inc.) are all SD-OCT systems that can be used for either retinal or anterior segment imaging (when used with a corneal adaptor module).

AS-OCTs provide same type of ACA measurements of UBM, with the same advantages and limitations (i.e. they are influenced by patient's age and gender, direction of gaze, accommodation, room illumination, meridians scanned). Furthermore, likewise UBM, some AS-OCTS have a built-in semi-automated software which offers the most common biometric parameters of ACA after the manual localization of the scleral spur (figure 9) (table 3). Contradictory results are present in literature on the agreement between UBM and AS-OCT in quantitative ACA measurement and detection of narrow angles. Some authors have found the two methods to be quite similar (Radhakrishnan et al., 2005, Dada et al., 2007); others have shown poor agreement (Mansouri et al.). In a study including 32 patients Wang et al. have reported that low-resolution OCT is similar to UBM for most of the studied angle measurements, while high-resolution OCT tends to give higher measurements than both low-resolution OCT and UBM. Furthermore AS-OCT measurements seem more reproducible than those from UBM (Wang et al., 2009). Likewise UBM, AS-OCT may be used for qualitative evaluation of ACA in a variety of ocular diseases (plateau iris syndrome, pigment dispersion syndrome, etc.) and it is undoubtedly safer than UBM in the evaluation of filtering blebs because AS-OCT is non-contact technique.

| Parameter | Description | Range* | | References |
|---|---|---|---|---|
| | | Occludable angle (OA) | Nonoccludable angle (NOA) | |
| **$AOD_{500\ nasal}$** | Distance from cornea to iris at 500 µm from the scleral spur | 0.33±0.14 | 0.50±0.21 | (Grewal et al.) |
| **$AOD_{500\ temporal}$** | See above | 0.30±0.11 | 0.51±0.22 | (Grewal et al.) |
| **$TISA_{500nasal}$** | Trapezoidal area with the following boundaries: anteriorly, AOD500; posteriorly, a line drawn from the scleral spur perpendicular to the plane of the inner scleral wall to the opposing iris; superiorly, the inner corneo-scleral wall; and inferiorly, the iris surface. | 0.23±0.14 | 0.34±0.11 | (Grewal et al.) |
| **$TISA_{500temporal}$** | See above | 0.23 ±0.14 | 0.33±0.12 | (Grewal et al.) |
| **$ARA_{750\ nasal}$** | Area of triangle between angle recess, iris and cornea 750 µm from scleral spur | 0.08 | 0.29 | (Pekmezci et al., 2009) |
| **$ARA_{750temporal}$** | See above | 0.09 | 0.28 | (Pekmezci et al., 2009) |

*All values (mean±standard deviation) are in mm except ARA and TISA which are in $mm^2$.
Abbreviations: AOD=angle-opening distance; TISA=trabecular-iris space area; ARA=angle recess area;

Table 3. Most common biometric parameters used in AS-OCT for characterizing the angle and anterior segment in subjects with an occludable/non-occludable angle

Compared to UBM, AS-OCT is a technique more rapid, more easily practiced by a technician, better tolerated because requires no contact. A limitation of AS-OCT is that it doesn't allow visualizing the ciliary body and the supra-choroidal space. Using gonioscopy as reference standard several authors have shown sensitivities of AS-OCT in detecting narrow angles up to 98%, although often the specificity was significantly lower (between 55 and 85%) (Nolan et al., 2007, See et al., 2007) (Pekmezci et al., 2009). AS-OCT tends indeed to detect more closed ACAs than gonioscopy, particularly in the superior and inferior quadrants (Nolan et al., 2007, Sakata et al., 2008a).

Angle recess area at 750 µm from scleral spur ($ARA_{750}$) and angle-opening distance at 500 µm from the scleral spur ($AOD_{500}$) seem to have the highest correlation with gonioscopy (Pekmezci et al., 2009).

Radhakrishnan indicated an AOD 500 cutoff of 190 µm for detecting occludable angles (Radhakrishnan et al., 2005).

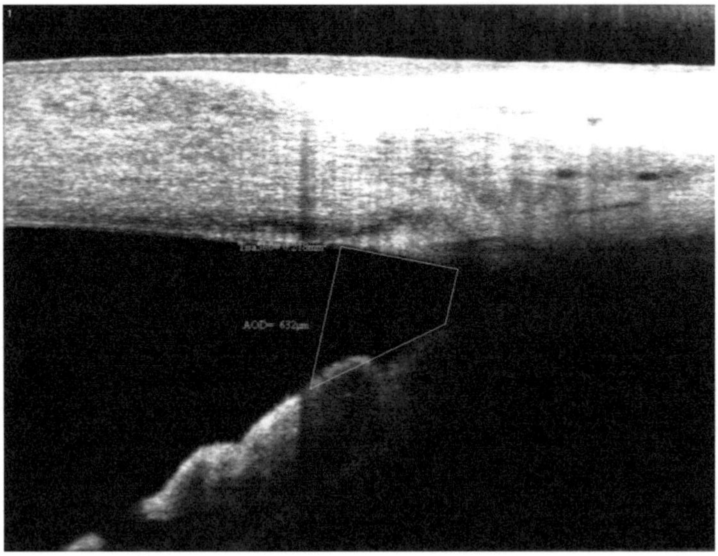

Fig. 9. Screen shot of the ACA measurements (angle-opening distance and trabecular-iris space area at 500) provided by the analysis software of RTVue OCT (Optovue Inc., Fremont, CA, USA)

As for UBM, also for AS-OCT angle classification hinges on accurate localization of the scleral spur, as it is used as the reference point for all the other quantitative measurements. However, this localization is not always easy to be found possibly generating non-negligible intra- and inter-observer variance.

The sclera spur can be defined as the point where there is a change in curvature of the inner surface of the angle wall, often appearing as an inward protrusion of the sclera.

Studies investigating the visibility of the sclera spur with AS-OCT showed a visualization between 70% and 78.9% of analyzed images (Sakata et al., 2008b) (Wong et al., 2009). Most of the cases in which the scleral spur could not be detected occurred in images in which the internal surface of the sclera formed a smooth continuous line (with no inward protrusion of the sclera or change in its curvature) or in images with suboptimal quality. Less frequently, the scleral spur was difficult to identify owing to an atypical contour of the inner corneoscleral wall.

Despite the possible difficulty in localization of sclera spur, several studies have shown low intra- and inter-observer variability of AS-OCT ACA measurements, which tends to increase only when AS-OCT image acquisitions are performed by less-experienced operators (Khor et al., Tan et al., Muller et al., 2006, Li et al., 2007) In a recent study the range of intra-observer variability in image analysis was from 9.4% to 12.5% in the experts and from 4.2% to 17.4% in the non-experts. Inter-observer variability was 10.7% in the experts and 10.2% in the non-experts. The reproducibility was high, 0.875 and 0.942 in the experts and 0.906 in the non-experts (Tan et al.).

## 8. Conclusions

Several new technologies are becoming more and more popular for the assessment of the angle and anterior segment. They can provide useful additional qualitative information to those obtained with the traditional tools (slit-lamp and gonioscopy). Furthermore they can offer also precise ACA measurements which however are often not comparable each other. Hence we believe that one should build its normative data - using gonioscopy as reference standard- to use them for screening for angle closure purposes.

However, as technologies evolve, it is likely that the diagnostic performance of different techniques/instruments may soon reach acceptable specificity and sensitivity levels for mass screening for angle closure.

## 9. References


Alsbirk, P.H. (1986). Limbal and axial chamber depth variations. A population study in Eskimos. *Acta Ophthalmol (Copenh),* Vol. 64, No. 6, (Dec 1986) pp. (593-600), 0001-639X (Print)

Aung, T., Lim, M.C., Chan, Y.H., Rojanapongpun, P. & Chew, P.T. (2005). Configuration of the drainage angle, intraocular pressure, and optic disc cupping in subjects with chronic angle-closure glaucoma. *Ophthalmology,* Vol. 112, No. 1, (Jan 2005) pp. (28-32), 1549-4713 (Electronic)

Barrett, B.T., McGraw, P.V., Murray, L.A. & Murgatroyd, P. (1996). Anterior chamber depth measurement in clinical practice. *Optom Vis Sci,* Vol. 73, No. 7, (Jul 1996) pp. (482-486), 1040-5488 (Print)

Cockburn, D.M. (1980). A new method for gonioscopic grading of the anterior chamber angle. *Am J Optom Physiol Opt,* Vol. 57, No. 4, (Apr 1980) pp. (258-261), 0093-7002 (Print)

Congdon, N.G., Spaeth, G.L., Augsburger, J., Klancnik, J., Jr., Patel, K. & Hunter, D.G. (1999). proposed simple method for measurement in the anterior chamber angle: biometric gonioscopy. *Ophthalmology,* Vol. 106, No. 11, (Nov 1999) pp. (2161-2167), 0161-6420 (Print)

Congdon, N.G., Youlin, Q., Quigley, H., Hung, P.T., Wang, T.H., Ho, T.C. & Tielsch, J.M. (1997). Biometry and primary angle-closure glaucoma among Chinese, white, and black populations. *Ophthalmology,* Vol. 104, No. 9, (Sep 1997) pp. (1489-1495), 0161-6420 (Print)

Dada, T., Sihota, R., Gadia, R., Aggarwal, A., Mandal, S. & Gupta, V. (2007). Comparison of anterior segment optical coherence tomography and ultrasound biomicroscopy for assessment of the anterior segment. *J Cataract Refract Surg,* Vol. 33, No. 5, (May 2007) pp. (837-840), 0886-3350 (Print)

Douthwaite, W.A. & Spence, D. (1986). Slit-lamp measurement of the anterior chamber depth. *Br J Ophthalmol,* Vol. 70, No. 3, (Mar 1986) pp. (205-208), 0007-1161 (Print)

Fontana, S.T. & Brubaker, R.F. (1980). Volume and depth of the anterior chamber in the normal aging human eye. *Arch Ophthalmol,* Vol. 98, No. 10, (Oct 1980) pp. (1803-1808), 0003-9950 (Print)

Foster, P.J., Buhrmann, R., Quigley, H.A. & Johnson, G.J. (2002). The definition and classification of glaucoma in prevalence surveys. *Br J Ophthalmol,* Vol. 86, No. 2, (Feb 2002) pp. (238-242), 0007-1161 (Print)

Foster, P.J., Devereux, J.G., Alsbirk, P.H., Lee, P.S., Uranchimeg, D., Machin, D., Johnson, G.J. & Baasanhu, J. (2000a). Detection of gonioscopically occludable angles and primary angle closure glaucoma by estimation of limbal chamber depth in Asians: modified grading scheme. *Br J Ophthalmol,* Vol. 84, No. 2, (Feb 2000a) pp. (186-192), 0007-1161 (Print)

Foster, P.J., Oen, F.T., Machin, D., Ng, T.P., Devereux, J.G., Johnson, G.J., Khaw, P.T. & Seah, S.K. (2000b). The prevalence of glaucoma in Chinese residents of Singapore: a cross-sectional population survey of the Tanjong Pagar district. *Arch Ophthalmol,* Vol. 118, No. 8, (Aug 2000b) pp. (1105-1111), 0003-9950 (Print)

Friedman, D.S. (2001). Who needs an iridotomy? *Br J Ophthalmol,* Vol. 85, No. 9, (Sep 2001) pp. (1019-1021), 0007-1161 (Print)

Friedman, D.S., Gazzard, G., Foster, P., Devereux, J., Broman, A., Quigley, H., Tielsch, J. & Seah, S. (2003). Ultrasonographic biomicroscopy, Scheimpflug photography, and novel provocative tests in contralateral eyes of Chinese patients initially seen with acute angle closure. *Arch Ophthalmol,* Vol. 121, No. 5, (May 2003) pp. (633-642), 0003-9950 (Print)

Friedman, D.S., Gazzard, G., Min, C.B., Broman, A.T., Quigley, H., Tielsch, J., Seah, S. & Foster, P.J. (2008). Age and sex variation in angle findings among normal Chinese subjects: a comparison of UBM, Scheimpflug, and gonioscopic assessment of the anterior chamber angle. *J Glaucoma,* Vol. 17, No. 1, (Jan-Feb 2008) pp. (5-10), 1057-0829 (Print)

Friedman, D.S. & He, M. (2008). Anterior chamber angle assessment techniques. *Surv Ophthalmol,* Vol. 53, No. 3, (May-Jun 2008) pp. (250-273), 0039-6257 (Print)

Gohdo, T., Tsumura, T., Iijima, H., Kashiwagi, K. & Tsukahara, S. (2000). Ultrasound biomicroscopic study of ciliary body thickness in eyes with narrow angles. *Am J Ophthalmol,* Vol. 129, No. 3, (Mar 2000) pp. (342-346), 0002-9394 (Print)

Grewal, D.S., Brar, G.S., Jain, R. & Grewal, S.P. Comparison of scheimpflug imaging and spectral domain anterior segment optical coherence tomography for detection of narrow anterior chamber angles. *Eye (Lond),* (Feb 18, 1476-5454 (Electronic)

Henzan, I.M., Tomidokoro, A., Uejo, C., Sakai, H., Sawaguchi, S., Iwase, A. & Araie, M. Comparison of Ultrasound Biomicroscopic Configurations Among Primary Angle Closure, Its Suspects, and Nonoccludable Angles: The Kumejima Study. *Am J Ophthalmol,* (Mar 28, 1879-1891 (Electronic)

Huang, D., Swanson, E.A., Lin, C.P., Schuman, J.S., Stinson, W.G., Chang, W., Hee, M.R., Flotte, T., Gregory, K., Puliafito, C.A. & et al. (1991). Optical coherence tomography. *Science,* Vol. 254, No. 5035, (Nov 22 1991) pp. (1178-1181), 0036-8075 (Print)

Ishikawa, H., Liebmann, J.M. & Ritch, R. (2000). Quantitative assessment of the anterior segment using ultrasound biomicroscopy. *Curr Opin Ophthalmol,* Vol. 11, No. 2, (Apr 2000) pp. (133-139), 1040-8738 (Print)

Izatt, J.A., Hee, M.R., Swanson, E.A., Lin, C.P., Huang, D., Schuman, J.S., Puliafito, C.A. & Fujimoto, J.G. (1994). Micrometer-scale resolution imaging of the anterior eye in vivo with optical coherence tomography. *Arch Ophthalmol,* Vol. 112, No. 12, (Dec 1994) pp. (1584-1589), 0003-9950 (Print)

Jacobs, I.H. (1979). Anterior chamber depth measurement using the split-lamp microscope. *Am J Ophthalmol,* Vol. 88, No. 2, (Aug 1979) pp. (236-238), 0002-9394 (Print)

Kanski, J.J. (2007). *Clinical ophthalmology: a systematic approach,* (6th), Butterworth Heinemann Elsevier, 9780080449692 (hbk.)

Khor, W.B., Sakata, L.M., Friedman, D.S., Narayanaswamy, A., Lavanya, R., Perera, S.A. & Aung, T. Evaluation of scanning protocols for imaging the anterior chamber angle with anterior segment-optical coherence tomography. *J Glaucoma,* Vol. 19, No. 6, (Aug 365-368), 1536-481X (Electronic)

Kim, Y.Y. & Jung, H.R. (1997). Clarifying the nomenclature for primary angle-closure glaucoma. *Surv Ophthalmol,* Vol. 42, No. 2, (Sep-Oct 1997) pp. (125-136), 0039-6257 (Print)

Kurita, N., Mayama, C., Tomidokoro, A., Aihara, M. & Araie, M. (2009). Potential of the pentacam in screening for primary angle closure and primary angle closure suspect. *J Glaucoma,* Vol. 18, No. 7, (Sep 2009) pp. (506-512), 1536-481X (Electronic)

Lam, A.K., Chan, R., Woo, G.C., Pang, P.C. & Chiu, R. (2002). Intra-observer and inter-observer repeatability of anterior eye segment analysis system (EAS-1000) in anterior chamber configuration. *Ophthalmic Physiol Opt,* Vol. 22, No. 6, (Nov 2002) pp. (552-559), 0275-5408 (Print)

Larsen, J.S. (1971). The sagittal growth of the eye. 1. Ultrasonic measurement of the depth of the anterior chamber from birth to puberty. *Acta Ophthalmol (Copenh),* Vol. 49, No. 2, 1971) pp. (239-262), 0001-639X (Print)

Lens, A., Nemeth, S.C., Ledford, J.K. (2008). *Ocular Anatomy and Physiology,* (Second Edition), Slack Incorporated, 978-1-55642-792-3,

Li, H., Leung, C.K., Cheung, C.Y., Wong, L., Pang, C.P., Weinreb, R.N. & Lam, D.S. (2007). Repeatability and reproducibility of anterior chamber angle measurement with anterior segment optical coherence tomography. *Br J Ophthalmol,* Vol. 91, No. 11, (Nov 2007) pp. (1490-1492), 0007-1161 (Print)

Liang, J., Liu, W., Xing, X., Liu, H., Zhao, S. & Ji, J. Evaluation of the agreement between Pentacam and ultrasound biomicroscopy measurements of anterior chamber depth in Chinese patients with primary angle-closure glaucoma. *Jpn J Ophthalmol,* Vol. 54, No. 4, (Jul 361-362), 1613-2246 (Electronic)

Mansouri, K., Sommerhalder, J. & Shaarawy, T. Prospective comparison of ultrasound biomicroscopy and anterior segment optical coherence tomography for evaluation of anterior chamber dimensions in European eyes with primary angle closure. *Eye (Lond),* Vol. 24, No. 2, (Feb 233-239), 1476-5454 (Electronic)

Marchini, G., Pagliarusco, A., Toscano, A., Tosi, R., Brunelli, C. & Bonomi, L. (1998). Ultrasound biomicroscopic and conventional ultrasonographic study of ocular dimensions in primary angle-closure glaucoma. *Ophthalmology,* Vol. 105, No. 11, (Nov 1998) pp. (2091-2098), 0161-6420 (Print)

Mou, D., Fu, J., Li, S., Wang, L., Wang, X., Wu, G., Qing, G., Peng, Y. & Wang, N. Narrow- and open-angle measurements with anterior-segment optical coherence tomography and Pentacam. *Ophthalmic Surg Lasers Imaging,* Vol. 41, No. 6, (Nov 1 622-628), 1938-2375 (Electronic)

Muller, M., Dahmen, G., Porksen, E., Geerling, G., Laqua, H., Ziegler, A. & Hoerauf, H. (2006). Anterior chamber angle measurement with optical coherence tomography: intraobserver and interobserver variability. *J Cataract Refract Surg,* Vol. 32, No. 11, (Nov 2006) pp. (1803-1808), 0886-3350 (Print)

Ng, W.S., Ang, G.S. & Azuara-Blanco, A. (2008). Laser peripheral iridoplasty for angle-closure. *Cochrane Database Syst Rev,* No. 3, 2008) pp. (CD006746), 1469-493X (Electronic)

Nolan, W.P., Baasanhu, J., Undraa, A., Uranchimeg, D., Ganzorig, S. & Johnson, G.J. (2003). Screening for primary angle closure in Mongolia: a randomised controlled trial to determine whether screening and prophylactic treatment will reduce the incidence of primary angle closure glaucoma in an east Asian population. *Br J Ophthalmol,* Vol. 87, No. 3, (Mar 2003) pp. (271-274), 0007-1161 (Print)

Nolan, W.P., See, J.L., Chew, P.T., Friedman, D.S., Smith, S.D., Radhakrishnan, S., Zheng, C., Foster, P.J. & Aung, T. (2007). Detection of primary angle closure using anterior segment optical coherence tomography in Asian eyes. *Ophthalmology,* Vol. 114, No. 1, (Jan 2007) pp. (33-39), 1549-4713 (Electronic)

Osuobeni, E.P., Hegarty, C. & Gunvant, P. (2003). The effect of central corneal thickness on estimates of the anterior chamber depth. *Clin Exp Optom,* Vol. 86, No. 6, (Nov 2003) pp. (371-375), 0816-4622 (Print)

Osuobeni, E.P., Oduwaiye, K.A. & Ogbuehi, K.C. (2000). Intra-observer repeatability and inter-observer agreement of the Smith method of measuring the anterior chamber depth. *Ophthalmic Physiol Opt,* Vol. 20, No. 2, (Mar 2000) pp. (153-159), 0275-5408 (Print)

Pavlin, C.J., Harasiewicz, K. & Foster, F.S. (1992). Ultrasound biomicroscopy of anterior segment structures in normal and glaucomatous eyes. *Am J Ophthalmol,* Vol. 113, No. 4, (Apr 15 1992) pp. (381-389), 0002-9394 (Print)

Pekmezci, M., Porco, T.C. & Lin, S.C. (2009). Anterior segment optical coherence tomography as a screening tool for the assessment of the anterior segment angle. *Ophthalmic Surg Lasers Imaging,* Vol. 40, No. 4, (Jul-Aug 2009) pp. (389-398), 1542-8877 (Print)

Quek, D.T., Nongpiur, M.E., Perera, S.A. & Aung, T. Angle imaging: advances and challenges. *Indian J Ophthalmol,* Vol. 59 Suppl, (Jan S69-75), 1998-3689 (Electronic)

Quigley, H.A. & Broman, A.T. (2006). The number of people with glaucoma worldwide in 2010 and 2020. *Br J Ophthalmol,* Vol. 90, No. 3, (Mar 2006) pp. (262-267), 0007-1161 (Print)

Rabsilber, T.M., Khoramnia, R. & Auffarth, G.U. (2006). Anterior chamber measurements using Pentacam rotating Scheimpflug camera. *J Cataract Refract Surg,* Vol. 32, No. 3, (Mar 2006) pp. (456-459), 0886-3350 (Print)

Radhakrishnan, S., Goldsmith, J., Huang, D., Westphal, V., Dueker, D.K., Rollins, A.M., Izatt, J.A. & Smith, S.D. (2005). Comparison of optical coherence tomography and ultrasound biomicroscopy for detection of narrow anterior chamber angles. *Arch Ophthalmol,* Vol. 123, No. 8, (Aug 2005) pp. (1053-1059), 0003-9950 (Print)

Ritch, R., Tham, C.C. & Lam, D.S. (2007). Argon laser peripheral iridoplasty (ALPI): an update. *Surv Ophthalmol,* Vol. 52, No. 3, (May-Jun 2007) pp. (279-288), 0039-6257 (Print)

Rufer, F., Schroder, A., Klettner, A., Frimpong-Boateng, A., Roider, J.B. & Erb, C. Anterior chamber depth and iridocorneal angle in healthy White subjects: effects of age, gender and refraction. *Acta Ophthalmol,* Vol. 88, No. 8, (Dec 885-890), 1755-3768 (Electronic)

Sakata, L.M., Lavanya, R., Friedman, D.S., Aung, H.T., Gao, H., Kumar, R.S., Foster, P.J. & Aung, T. (2008a). Comparison of gonioscopy and anterior segment ocular coherence tomography in detecting angle closure in different quadrants of the anterior chamber angle. *Ophthalmology,* Vol. 115, No. 5, (May 2008a) pp. (769-774), 1549-4713 (Electronic)

Sakata, L.M., Lavanya, R., Friedman, D.S., Aung, H.T., Seah, S.K., Foster, P.J. & Aung, T. (2008b). Assessment of the scleral spur in anterior segment optical coherence tomography images. *Arch Ophthalmol,* Vol. 126, No. 2, (Feb 2008b) pp. (181-185), 0003-9950 (Print)

Scheie, H.G. (1957). Width and pigmentation of the angle of the anterior chamber; a system of grading by gonioscopy. *AMA Arch Ophthalmol,* Vol. 58, No. 4, (Oct 1957) pp. (510-512), 0096-6339 (Print)

See, J.L., Chew, P.T., Smith, S.D., Nolan, W.P., Chan, Y.H., Huang, D., Zheng, C., Foster, P.J., Aung, T. & Friedman, D.S. (2007). Changes in anterior segment morphology in response to illumination and after laser iridotomy in Asian eyes: an anterior segment OCT study. *Br J Ophthalmol,* Vol. 91, No. 11, (Nov 2007) pp. (1485-1489), 0007-1161 (Print)

Shaffer, R.N. (1960). Primary glaucomas. Gonioscopy, ophthalmoscopy and perimetry. *Trans Am Acad Ophthalmol Otolaryngol,* Vol. 64, (Mar-Apr 1960) pp. (112-127), 0002-7154 (Print)

Sihota, R., Dada, T., Gupta, R., Lakshminarayan, P. & Pandey, R.M. (2005). Ultrasound biomicroscopy in the subtypes of primary angle closure glaucoma. *J Glaucoma,* Vol. 14, No. 5, (Oct 2005) pp. (387-391), 1057-0829 (Print)

Smith, R.J. (1979). A new method of estimating the depth of the anterior chamber. *Br J Ophthalmol,* Vol. 63, No. 4, (Apr 1979) pp. (215-220), 0007-1161 (Print)

Spaeth, G.L. (1971). The normal development of the human anterior chamber angle: a new system of descriptive grading. *Trans Ophthalmol Soc U K,* Vol. 91, 1971) pp. (709-739), 0078-5334 (Print)

Spaeth, G.L., Aruajo, S. & Azuara, A. (1995). Comparison of the configuration of the human anterior chamber angle, as determined by the Spaeth gonioscopic grading system and ultrasound biomicroscopy. *Trans Am Ophthalmol Soc,* Vol. 93, 1995) pp. (337-347; discussion 347-351), 0065-9533 (Print)

Tan, A.N., Sauren, L.D., de Brabander, J., Berendschot, T.T., Passos, V.L., Webers, C.A., Nuijts, R.M. & Beckers, H.J. Reproducibility of anterior chamber angle measurements with anterior segment optical coherence tomography. *Invest Ophthalmol Vis Sci,* Vol. 52, No. 5, 2095-2099), 1552-5783 (Electronic)

Thomas, R., George, R., Parikh, R., Muliyil, J. & Jacob, A. (2003a). Five year risk of progression of primary angle closure suspects to primary angle closure: a population based study. *Br J Ophthalmol,* Vol. 87, No. 4, (Apr 2003a) pp. (450-454), 0007-1161 (Print)

Thomas, R., George, T., Braganza, A. & Muliyil, J. (1996). The flashlight test and van Herick's test are poor predictors for occludable angles. *Aust N Z J Ophthalmol,* Vol. 24, No. 3, (Aug 1996) pp. (251-256), 0814-9763 (Print)

Thomas, R., Parikh, R., Muliyil, J. & Kumar, R.S. (2003b). Five-year risk of progression of primary angle closure to primary angle closure glaucoma: a population-based study. *Acta Ophthalmol Scand,* Vol. 81, No. 5, (Oct 2003b) pp. (480-485), 1395-3907 (Print)

Ursea, R. & Silverman, R.H. Anterior-segment imaging for assessment of glaucoma. *Expert Rev Ophthalmol,* Vol. 5, No. 1, (Feb 1 59-74), 1746-9899 (Electronic)

Van Herick, W., Shaffer, R.N. & Schwartz, A. (1969). Estimation of width of angle of anterior chamber. Incidence and significance of the narrow angle. *Am J Ophthalmol,* Vol. 68, No. 4, (Oct 1969) pp. (626-629), 0002-9394 (Print)

Wang, D., Pekmezci, M., Basham, R.P., He, M., Seider, M.I. & Lin, S.C. (2009). Comparison of different modes in optical coherence tomography and ultrasound biomicroscopy in anterior chamber angle assessment. *J Glaucoma,* Vol. 18, No. 6, (Aug 2009) pp. (472-478), 1536-481X (Electronic)

Wishart, P.K. & Batterbury, M. (1992). Ocular hypertension: correlation of anterior chamber angle width and risk of progression to glaucoma. *Eye (Lond),* Vol. 6 ( Pt 3), 1992) pp. (248-256), 0950-222X (Print)

Wong, H.T., Lim, M.C., Sakata, L.M., Aung, H.T., Amerasinghe, N., Friedman, D.S. & Aung, T. (2009). High-definition optical coherence tomography imaging of the iridocorneal angle of the eye. *Arch Ophthalmol,* Vol. 127, No. 3, (Mar 2009) pp. (256-260), 1538-3601 (Electronic)

Yoo, C., Oh, J.H., Kim, Y.Y. & Jung, H.R. (2007). Peripheral anterior synechiae and ultrasound biomicroscopic parameters in angle-closure glaucoma suspects. *Korean J Ophthalmol,* Vol. 21, No. 2, (Jun 2007) pp. (106-110), 1011-8942 (Print)

# 18

# End Stage Glaucoma

Tharwat H. Mokbel
*Mansoura University Mansoura, Egypt*

## 1. Introduction

Glaucoma is the second leading cause of blindness in the general population. The definition of end-stage glaucoma may be based on a very constricted visual field, or a markedly severed visual acuity (Gillies& Brooks et al., 2000). Many factors have been postulated to put the patient at a high risk. Achieving an individually fashioned target IOP is supposed to minimize the risk of glaucoma progression (Nouri-Mahdavi & Hoffman et al., 2004). Medical regimens may induce significant short and long term IOP fluctuations. Surgery should be considered in end stage glaucoma. Trabeculectomy has been reported to be associated with less diurnal IOP fluctuation compared to maximum medical therapy. Wipe-out phenomenon is a rare complication and may be considered as a blast from the past. Meanwhile, Trabeculectomy has many surgical difficulties. Emphasis on guidelines for a successful trabeculectomy without toil is presented, besides the new modalities to achieve a favorable outcome.

## 2. What is end stage glaucoma?

There is no universally accepted definition of end-stage glaucoma. It may be based on a very constricted visual field, less than 10 or a visual acuity of 20/200 or worse that is attributable to glaucoma (Gillies & Brooks et al., 2000).

### 2.1 Importance

Glaucoma is the second leading cause of irreversible blindness in the general population, and the leading cause of blindness in black patients. Besides, patients with end-stage glaucoma have a high risk of further disease progression. Although peripheral vision is seriously affected, these patients may maintain good central vision sufficient enough to perform simple daily tasks.

### 2.2 Diagnostic challenge

End stage glaucoma carries a diagnostic challenge. Visual field examination is either unreliable or impossible. Only when a central island of vision remains, visual field tests of the central degrees should be chosen. Small changes in the visual field may be deleterious to central vision but it can be difficult to differentiate them from inter-test fluctuation. Small neuroretinal rim changes may correspond to significant changes in the visual acuity. On the other hand, OCT may be useful in the detection of glaucomatous progression. In advanced or progressive glaucoma, imaging can be justified every 3–4 months to look for change (Bartz-Schmidt & Thumann G et al., 1999).

### 2.3 Risk factors for progression

Many factors have been proved to increase the risk of glaucoma progression in end stage glaucoma, The most important are elevated intraocular pressure (IOP), IOP fluctuations, male gender, less formal education, severity of disease, pseudoexfoliation syndrome, worsening visual fields during follow up, optic disc hemorrhage, advanced stage of disease, migraine, patient's expected longevity, and the possibility of systemic diseases e.g hypertension, diabetes, and myopia (Law & Nguyen et al., 2007).

## 3. Target IOP in end stage glaucoma

Target IOP is the IOP that minimizes the risk of glaucoma progression with minimum impact on the quality of life. Although the concept of a target IOP is debated, it is recommended that every patient should have an individualized target IOP and re-estimated according to the follow up. Target IOP may be a percent reduction from a baseline IOP or may be an absolute IOP reduction. It is generally assumed that aiming to achieve a target IOP of at least a 20% reduction from the initial pressure at which damage occurred is a useful starting point. For moderate and advanced damage, a 30 and 40% decrease of IOP from baseline, respectively, is proposed. In each individual, the efficacy of any treatment lowering the IOP less than 15% should be questioned. The range of IOP fluctuations should also be considered and when in doubt a diurnal curve is indicated. Besides, the greater the pre-existing glaucoma damage, the lower the target IOP should be. It is clinically relevant that in eyes with severe pre-existing damage, any further damage may be functionally important. Thus, IOP should be set low in end-stage glaucoma. Target pressures seem to drop to lower and lower levels each decade. Even a more lower target IOP may be needed if other risk factors are present specially diabetes mellitus and hypertension. Severe pre-existing damage in the fellow eye is another possible risk factor, as well as a positive family history of visual handicap caused by primary open-angle glaucoma (POAG). A further 3% IOP lowering for each risk factor or for each decade of life expectancy is advised. Periodical re-evaluation and adjustments are necessary if the visual field continues to worsen at a rate that is clinically significant, it may be necessary to aim for a lower target IOP after other causes have been excluded (Miglior & Bertuzzi , 2010)..

### 3.1 Medical versus interventional strategy

The target IOP may not be achieved despite maximum medical therapy. Even if end stage glaucoma could be controlled medically, the lack of adherence and persistence with medication regimens may induce significant short and long term IOP fluctuations. These fluctuations have a deleterious effect on the visual outcomes. Medication may be inappropriate in some clinical situations. Extremely high IOP may be unlikely to be sufficiently reduced by medications. In this case medical treatment may be initiated briefly in order to operate at lower IOP.Some patients may have secondary conditions that interfere with the ability to administer medication such as dementia, mental illness, or arthritis.Economic problems are also challenges for patients in many locations. This may limit or effectively exclude access to medical treatment for glaucoma. Limited access to medical resources may be based on other factors such as distance from medical care and limited availability of practitioners and medications.On the other hand, glaucoma procedures are associated with more tight IOP control and minimal IOP fluctuations. There is a growing evidence that glaucoma procedures are more helpful in prevention of visual field loss when further IOP reduction is needed despite maximum medical therapy. There are no clearly defined and accepted rules to decide when surgery is the appropriate therapeutic choice, but there are principles that seem to guide this decision. Several assumptions underlie the recommendation of surgery for the treatment of glaucoma. Among these are the observation that surgical IOP lowering stops or slows progressive glaucoma damage. Even more, greater IOP lowering can be achieved with surgery than with medication in many patients, while surgery has greater risk than medical treatment of glaucoma. Intra-operative risks such as suprachoroidal haemorrhage, and post-operative risks such as hypotony and bleb related infection can result in rapid and profound visual loss.For example, trabeculectomy has been reported to be associated with less diurnal IOP fluctuation compared with maximum medical therapy in patients with end stage glaucoma . On the contrary, if the central fixation has already been lost, glaucoma procedures add no more beneficial effect and it is suggested to consider withholding surgery.

## 4. Surgical intervention in end stage glaucoma

### 4.1 Surgical options of end stage glaucoma

The surgical options for end stage glaucoma are generally the same as those of earlier stages of glaucoma. Many trabeculectomy modalities are suitable for end stage glaucoma. While trabeculectomy is the treatment of choice in primary open angle glaucoma, consider lens removal (combined surgery) in patients with end-stage chronic angle closure glaucoma. This offers the best chance to deepen the anterior chamber and widen the angle. Trabeculectomy with antimetabolites reduces IOP more compared with trabeculectomy alone. Ologen collagen matrix is a new promising modality that carries a superior advantage over conventional trabeculectomies and antimetabolites. Glaucoma drainage implants are indicated after glaucoma filtration surgery failure, on the other hand cycloablation in the form of cyclophotocoagulation or cyclocryotherapy are indicated for eyes with poor vision.

### 4.2 Preoperative preparation

A proper preoperative preparation is essential for a successful glaucoma surgery outcome. Adequate management of blood pressure, coagulation profile by the physician is crucial .Preoperative Visual field is important for medical and medico-legal reasons. Topical corticosteroids such as fluoromethelone may be used to calm down any claimed inflammation. Glaucoma lowering agents should be stopped several days in advance.

### 4.3 Anaesthetic precautions

Ophthalmic anaesthesia planning is of great help in end stage glaucoma surgery. General anaethesia is considered for one-eyed patients as possible. Certain precautions are mandatory during local anesthesia particularly reduction of the volume, addition of hyaluronidase and avoidance of orbital compression. Facial block is important to produce enough facial akinesia. Subtenon or peribulbar anaethesia do worth consideration particularly for myopia.

### 4.4 Difficulties of surgical intervention in end stage glaucoma

It has been well noticed that procedures in end stage glaucoma carries more surgical difficulties. This is because of the possibility of previous operations (glaucoma or cataract) and the long term use of topical glaucoma drugs. These co-morbidities have negative effects on the conjunctiva, and on the outcome of a new operation.

## 5. Conventional trabeculectomy in end stage glaucoma

Trabeculectomy should be fashioned properly and with extreme caution in end stage glaucoma to achieve the best favorable outcomes. Fornix-based flaps are preferred for better exposure of the sclera and less chance of a posterior scar formation. A corneal traction suture is suggested to avoid formation of a superior rectus haematoma.An anterior segment infusion system through the paracentesis is helpful in stabilizing the IOP during surgery, decrease the risk of serious complications, and enable more accurate suturing of the scleral flap. Bleb is fashioned under the upper lid to minimize discomfort and bleb-related complications, such as leak or infection. The scleral flap must be sufficiently large and of adequate thickness to provide resistance to aqueous outflow, especially if antimetabolites are used. Besides, the side incisions are left incomplete (1–2 mm from limbus) to encourage posterior flow and achieve a diffuse bleb. Scleral flap sutures can be pre-placed while the eye is still firm. Adjustment of sutures of the scleral flap should be based on intraoperative evaluation of flow.

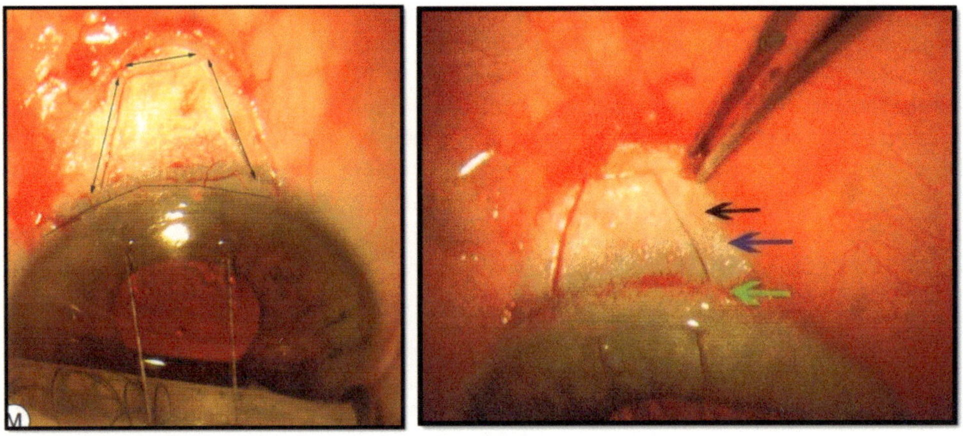

Fig. 1. (RT) Fornix-based flaps for better exposure of the sclera and less chances of a posterior scar. A corneal traction suture avoids the formation of a superior rectus haematoma, (LT) The scleral flap must be sufficiently large and of adequate thickness to provide resistance to aqueous outflow. (Fellman, 2009)

Many modalities of scleral flap sutures are of great help. Among those are fixed interrupted sutures that can be lasered later, releasable sutures that can be pulled out postoperatively and adjustable sutures that can be loosened transconjunctivally. Meticulous conjunctival closure is a priority to avoid hazardous postoperative bleb leakage and hypotony. Careful postoperative IOP measurement is indicated to detect early IOP spikes which could result in optic nerve damage. Bleb leakage and signs of inflammation should always be examined.

## 6. Trabeculectomy with antimetabolites

Tissue healing can be modulated with antimetabolites to improve outcomes of trabeculectomy. Antimetabolites are not very often used for the first trabeculectomies, but are mandatory after previous trabeculectomy or cataract surgery and for combined cataract-trabeculectomy surgery. Also they are indicated with trabeculectomy failure in the other eye and for dark skin and young patients. Antimetabolites are applied with a low dose, short duration, and on the largest possible area. While preoperative subconjunctival mitomycin-C (MMC) has less cytotoxic effect on the ciliary body compared with intraoperative episcleral application, both preoperative and intraoperative applications of MMC are effective in controlling IOP with a safer course and less postoperative complications in preoperative subconjunctival injection. Argon laser trabeculoplasty as an adjuvant therapy before or after trabeculectomy is an issue of controverse. Black and white patients with advanced glaucoma respond differently. Blacks with end stage glaucoma benefit more from a regimen that begins with laser surgery, and whites benefit more from one that begins with trabeculectomy.

## 7. Glaucoma filtering surgery with amniotic membrane transplantation

### 7.1 Principle

Antimetabolites may influence the integrity of the conjunctival barrier, resulting in a thin-walled avascular bleb (Hutchinson & Grossniklaus et al., 1997). The end result is often poor epithelialization and increased susceptibility to leakage and hypotony or infection, sometimes months after surgery (Parrish & Minckler, 1996). On the other hand, amniotic membrane exhibits a number of characteristics that might be of benefit in glaucoma surgery, that is good epithelization, good integration with the surrounding tissue, a low healing response, suppression of TGF-B activity and poor immunogenicity (Willoch & Nicolaissen, 2003). These features of amniotic membrane make it an attractive tissue for use in glaucoma surgery. It has been used in filtration surgery as an adjunct to reduce scarring, for repair of leaking blebs and as a cover for valve implant (Fujishima & Shimazaki et al., 1998).

### 7.2 Operative technique

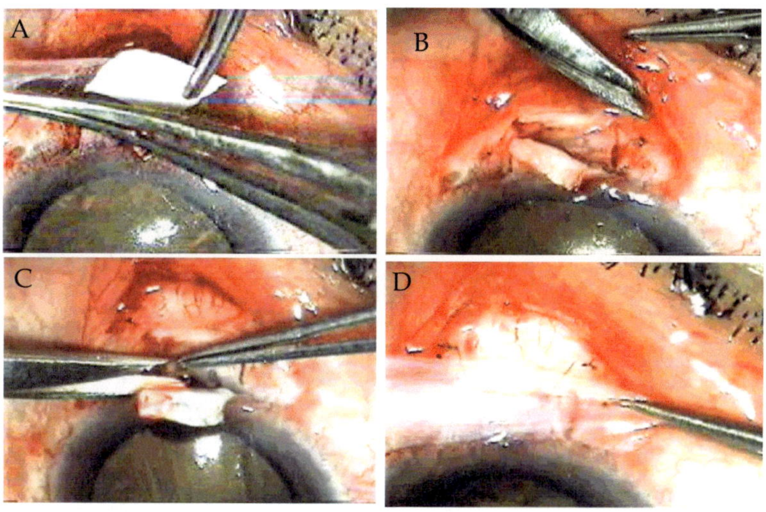


Fig. 2. (A) Peeling of aminiotic membrane from Nitro celluose paper, (B) Amniotic membrane graft is placed under the scleral flap and suturing of the graft to the sclera, (C) Trabeculectomy measuring 2X3 mm is done (D) Second graft over the scleral flap ( Mokbel & El-hefny et al., 2005)

Fornix based conjunctival flap, care was taken to ensure haemostasis during the whole surgical procedure. Scleral flap was done measuring 4x5 mm. Previously prepared amniotic membrane which is preserved in Dulbeccos Modified Eagles Media (DME) at -80ºC and was known to be free from HIV, HCV, HBV and syphilis was used Fig. 2(A). Amniotic membrane graft measuring 3x8 mm with its epithelial side up was placed between the scleral flap and deep sclera and attached to the scleral with four 10-0 nylon sutures at the corners Fig. 2(B). The amniotic membrane was then retracted and trabeculectomy measuring 2x3 mm was done Fig. 2(C). The scleral flap was then closed by two 10/0 nylon sutures. A second graft of amniotic membrane measuring 1.5x1.5 cm was placed over the sclera and attached near the limbus by two 10-0 nylon sutures and posteriorly by other two sutures Fig. 2(D). The conjunctiva was then closed using two 8/0 virgin sutures at the corners. Postoperatively each patient recieved a subconjunctival injection of Dexamethazone and garamycin followed by topical application of 5 times daily tobramycin & Dexamethazone drops for 4 weeks. All antiglaucoma medications were stopped ( Mokbel & El-hefny et al., 2005).

## 8. Ologen collagen matrix

Ologen is porcine extracellular matrix made of atelocollagen cross-linked with glycosaminoglycan. Ologen is a biodegradable scaffolding matrix that induces a regenerative wound healing process without the need for antifibrotic agents. It is well known that episcleral fibrosis and sub-conjunctival scarring are the major causes of failure in glaucoma filtering surgery. Ologen collagen matrix can creat the sub-conjunctival bleb and modulate the wound healing for the surgery. Ologen collagen matrix is a 3-D scaffold porous structure that can guide fibroblast to grow randomly, instead of linear alignment. This can reduce sub-conjuctival and trabdoor scars. Thus, Ologen collagen matrix carries the

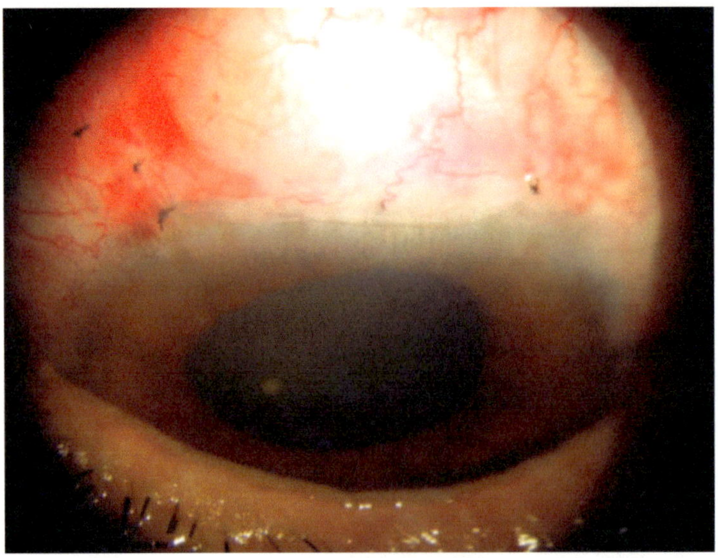

Fig. 3. Ologen implant,diffuse bleb and a well formed anterior chamber (photo of the author)

advantage of lowering IOP more safely and efficiently than standard trabeculectomy with MMC, with the merit of less possibility of bleb leaks and endophthalmitis compared with antimetabolites (Sarkisian, 2010).

The collagen matrix helps to limit hypotony through a tamponading effect over the scleral flap. On the other hand Ologen collagen matrix carry the disadvantage of increased cost, besides the difficulty of laser suture lysis.

### 8.1 Technique

According to the surgeon preference, limbal - or a fornix-based conjunctival flap are accepted. A loose stitch sclera flap is done in order to encourage aqueous flow for the filtering surgery. Ologen collagen matrix disc is implanted over the scleral flap. No suture is required to secure the implant, and as soon as it touches the sclera, it absorbs aqueous and molds to cover the scleral tissue. Collagen matrix therefore need not be presoaked or prepared in any way. After the collagen matrix's placement, the surgeon closes the conjunctiva in his or her usual meticulous fashion to ensure that the wound is watertight.

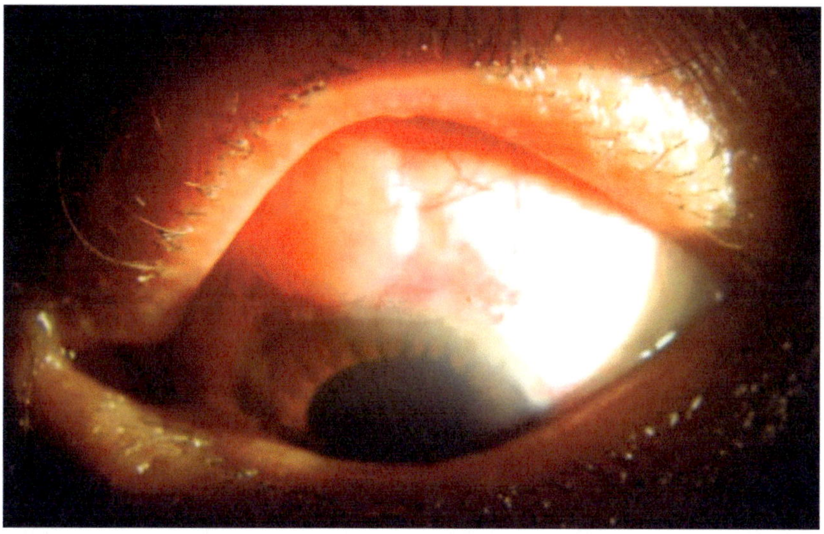

Fig. 4. Ologen implant, next day after surgery (photo of the author)

Ologen currently comes in two sizes for glaucoma filtering surgery: 6 X 2 mm and 12 X 1 mm. The numbers 6 and 12 stands for the diameter of the round implant, and the numbers 2 and 1 refer to its thickness. Ologen is biodegradable in 90 to 180 days. Ologen has been approved by the FDA in August 2009 (Sarkisian, 2010).

## 9. Aqueous shunting procedures with glaucoma drainage devices

Glaucoma drainage devices (GGDs) are indicated when trabeculectomy is unlikely to be successful. Besides, GDDs should be considered for socioeconomic or logistical issues relating to safety, follow-up care, etc. GDDs that do not have mechanisms to restrict aqueous flow require a suture ligature or internal stent or other flow restricting mechanism because the restriction of flow of aqueous humor from the eye is important in the prevention of postoperative hypotony. There are several type of devices; however, they can be divided into two categories:anterior drainage devices and posterior drainage devices. Most posterior drainage devices are composed of a silicone or Silastic tube that is placed into the eye (through the limbus or pars plana) and through which aqueous humor passes into the episcleral-subconjunctival space near the globe's equator. In this area there is an episcleral plate that is designed to maintain an aqueous reservoir. There are three design features which distinguish different implants; the presence of a valve or mechanism to restrict the flow of aqueous humor from the eye, the surface area and configuration of the episcleral plate, and the the material used.Drainage devices without a built in flow restriction mechanism, such as the Molteno, Baerveldt, and Schocket band implants, may be inserted in a one-stage procedure, where the flow of aqueous is restricted by a suture ligature around the tube or an internal stent. On the other hand krupin Valve implant and Ahmed Glaucoma Valve implant have pressure-sensitive valves or mechanisms which restrict the flow of aqueous from the eye (Mokbel, 2005).

## 10. Cyclodestruction

Cyclodestructive procedures aim to decrease aqueous humor secretion by damaging the ciliary processes, thereby reducing intraocular pressure (IOP). Modalities for cyclodestruction include cyclocryotherapy, and cyclophotocoagulation, using the Nd:YAG or diode laser. Endoscopic, non-contact and contact modes of cyclophotocoagulation are available, with the contact diode mode most widely used, laser diode cyclophotocoagulation is the procedure of choice for end stage glaucoma when trabeculectomy and drainage implants have a high probability for failure or have high risk of surgical complications. Less intense laser therapy on a repeated basis rather than a single high dose treatment is suggested to minimize complications of treatment. The effectiveness of treatment should be assessed after 3-4 weeks, at which time re-treatment may be considered.

## 11. Risk of losing vision

The patient should be informed about the relative risk of losing vision from a surgical procedure in end-stage glaucoma eyes. Visually devastating complications include chronic hypotony (leading to hypotony maculopathy), retinal detachment, malignant glaucoma, corneal decompensation, endophthalmitis, and phthisis bulbi. A detailed clearly written patient consent is important.It should entail all the potential hazards from suggested surgical procedure.

### 11.1 Wipe-out phenomenon

The wipe-out phenomenon is unexplained vision loss following glaucoma surgery. Wipe-out phenomenon data comes from older retrospective reports using older surgical techniques. Newer data does not report the occurrence of the wipe-out phenomenon.

## 12. Conclusion

In end stage glaucoma there is a higher incidence of visual loss than early glaucoma. So, frequent patient monitoring and quick decision making should be done.The target IOP in end stage glaucoma is lower than in early stage. Surgery should be considered in end stage glaucoma. Wipe-out phenomenon is a rare complication and may be considered as a blast from the past.

## 13. References


Bartz-Schmidt K. U., Thumann G., Jonescu-Cuypers C. P., et al. (1999) Quantitative morphologic and functional evaluation of the optic nerve head in chronic open-angle glaucoma. *Surv Ophthalmol* 44; 1, pp.541-553.

Fellman R. (2009). Trabeculectomy, In: *Glaucoma volume two surgical management*, Shaarawy T. & Sherwood M. & Hitchings R. and Crowston J. pp.(111-150), Saunders, 978-0-7020-2978-3,China.

Fujishima H., Shimazaki J., Shinozaki N., Tsubota K. (1998) Trabeculectomy with the use of amniotic membrane for uncontrollabe glaucoma. Ophthalmic Surg. 29; pp.928-943.

Gillies W. E., Brooks A. M., Strang N. T. (2000). Management and prognosis of end stage glaucoma. *Clin Experiment Ophthalmol,* 28, PP.(405-408).

Hutchinson A. K., Grossniklaus H. E., Brown R. H., McManus P. E. and Bradley G. K. (1997) Clinicopathologic features of excised mitomycin filtering bleb. Arch Ophthalmol 112, pp. 74-79.

Law S. K., Nguyen A. M., Coleman A. L., et al. (2007) Severe loss of central vision in patients with advanced glaucoma undergoing trabeculectomy. *Arch Ophthalmol,* 125, pp.1044-1050.

Miglior S. and Bertuzzi F. (2010). IOP: Target Pressures, In: *Pearls of Glaucoma Management,* Giaconi, J. & Law, S. & Coleman A. and Caprioli J. pp.(99-104), Springer-Verlag Berlin Heidelberg, 978-3-540-68238-7, New York.

Mokbel T., (2005) Long term clinical experience with Ahmed valve in refractory glaucoma. *Bull. Ophthalmol. Soc . Egypt, 98(3); pp 479-484.*

Mokbel T., El-hefny E., El-bendary A. (2005) Glaucoma filtering surgery with amniotic membrane transplantation. *Bull. Ophthalmol. Soc. Egypt, 98(3); pp 419-423.*

Nouri-Mahdavi K., Hoffman D., Coleman A. L., et al. (2004) Predictive factors for glaucomatous visual field progression in the Advanced Glaucoma Intervention Study. *Ophthalmology* 111; pp1627-1635.

Palmberg, P. (2005).outcome measures for Studies of glaucoma surgery, In: Glaucoma urgery Open Angle Glaucoma, Weinreb,R and Crowston,J.pp(1-7), Kugler, ISBN 90 6299 203 X, Netherlands.

Parrish R. K. II and Minckler D. (1996) "Late endophthalmitis" filtering surgery time bomb? Ophthalmology. 103, pp. 1167-1168.

Sarkisian, S. (2010). A Replacement for Antimetabolites? Ologen is a new product that modulates wound healing in glaucoma surgery. *Glaucoma Today.*winter2010,pp.22-24 .

Topouzis, F. (2010). Procedural Treatments:Surgery in End-Stage Glaucoma, In: *Pearls of Glaucoma Management,* Giaconi J & Law S. & Coleman A. and Caprioli J. pp.(323-330), Springer-Verlag Berlin Heidelberg, ISNB 978-3-540-68238-7, New York.

Willoch C. M., Nicolaissen B. (2003). Amnion sheilded trabeculectomy. Acta Ophthalmologica Scand. pp.658-659.

19

# Update on Modulating Wound Healing in Trabeculectomy

Hosam Sheha
*Ocular Surface Center & Tissue Tech Inc., Miami, Florida*
*United States*

## 1. Introduction

Trabeculectomy is the most commonly used surgical procedure for managing medically uncontrolled glaucoma. It reduces intraocular pressure (IOP) by creating an artificial drainage pathway of the aqueous humor from the anterior chamber to the subconjunctival space, forming a filtering bleb. Aqueous humor in the subconjunctival space may then exit by multiple pathways including transconjunctival filtration and absorption through the episcleral veins (Fig. 1).

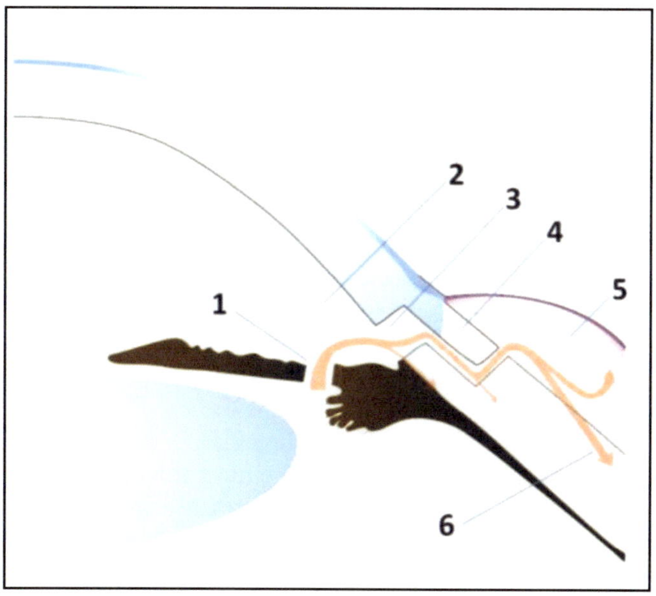


Fig. 1. Aqueous pathway after trabeculectomy through peripheral iridectomy (1) to the anterior chamber (2), the internal ostium (3), the route under the scleral flap (4), and the edge of the scleral flap to be absorbed via the bleb wall (5), and the episcleral venous plexus (6)

The success of trabeculectomy has been limited by postoperative fibrosis at the surgery site, leading to bleb failure months or years after surgery. High risk factors that lead to the failure in trabeculectomy include previous ocular surgery, specific types of glaucoma e.g. secondary

glaucoma such as neovascular, uveitic, post-traumatic, and lens-induced glaucoma, and to a lesser extent, young age and black race (Sturmer et al, 1993; Broadway and Chang, 2001).
Several surgical and pharmacologic techniques have been introduced to enhance the success in eyes with poor surgical prognoses. Until now, no effective and safe agent has been identified that can inhibit fibrosis, without complications, in the glaucoma filtering wound created by trabeculectomy. Although antimetabolites have revolutionized glaucoma surgery, the use of these agents is still associated with substantial risk (Chen, 1983). The common clinical practice of using mitomycin C (MMC) in trabeculectomy as an anti-fibrotic and anti-metabolic agent has achieved only limited success in cases with high-risk glaucoma while raising notable sight-threatening complications such as hypotony, bleb leaks, and infection (Lama and Fechtner, 2003).
To circumvent complications caused by MMC, there is a great need to improve the outcome of trabeculectomy by identifying a physiological modulator that may suppress pathological fibrosis without compromising the normal reparative wound healing process.
Our recent clinical research suggests that amniotic membrane (AM) could be a physiological modulator of wound healing that prevents scar formation in the subconjunctival space. We have demonstrated that AM not only prevents scar formation via its anti-inflammatory and anti-scarring actions but also serves as a spacer integrated into the intra-bleb structure to avert early over-filtration complications associated with trabeculectomy, and to stabilize the patency of the filtering fistula for prolonged maintenance of the bleb function (Sheha et al, 2008). This chapter reviews recent advances in the use of amniotic membrane as a biological modulator of wound healing that suppresses pathological fibrosis in trabeculectomy.

## 2. Wound healing process following trabeculectomy

Wound healing is triggered by activating the body's innate immunity and is characterized by inflammation in the acute phase, granulation tissue formation in the intermediate phase, and scarring in the chronic phase. This wound healing process is mediated by a number of cell types and is orchestrated by complex arrays of growth factors, cytokines, chemokines, and non-protein mediators. Trabeculectomy differs from most surgical procedures in that inhibition of wound healing is desirable to achieve surgical success (Dvorak, 1986).
Experimental and human studies have outlined a sequence of events that occurs in early bleb failure (Summarized in Fig. 2) (Skuta and Parrish, 1987). After surgical trauma, plasma proteins, including fibrinogen, fibronectin, and plasminogen, form a gel-like fibrin-fibronectin matrix, into which inflammatory cells (including monocytes and macrophages), new capillaries, and fibroblasts migrate. Macrophages from monocytes appear in about 12 hours, reaching peak numbers around day 3. These macrophages activate an inflammatory response, including the activation of lymphocytes and fibroblasts. T-cells appear on day 5, and after reaching a peak in numbers by the end of two weeks, they are activated into specific T-cells, which release various cytokines to control the activity and proliferation of fibroblasts. The fibrin-fibronectin matrix is eventually degraded by inflammatory cells, and fibroblasts subsequently synthesize fibronectin, interstitial collagens, and glycosaminoglycans to form fibrovascular granulation tissue (Desjardins et al, 1986; Grierson et al, 1988; Reichel et al, 1998; Miller et al, 1989; Chang et al, 2000).
The proliferated fibroblasts gradually begin to differentiate; this process is suspected to be mediated by various factors: transforming growth factor (TGF)-beta (Wipff et al, 2007), connective-tissue growth factor (CTGF) (Sherwood, 2006), Rho-associated serine-threonine

kinase (ROCK1) (Meyer-ter-Vehn et al, 2006), and the matrix-metalloproteinases (MMPs) (Chintala et al, 2005). Unlike undifferentiated fibroblasts, the newly-differentiated myofibroblasts transform the secreted extracellular matrix into an actin-based component which creates stronger scar tissue (Desmouliere et al, 1993). Blood vessels retract over time and fibroblasts largely disappear as the tissue is remodeled to form a dense collagenous subconjunctival scar.

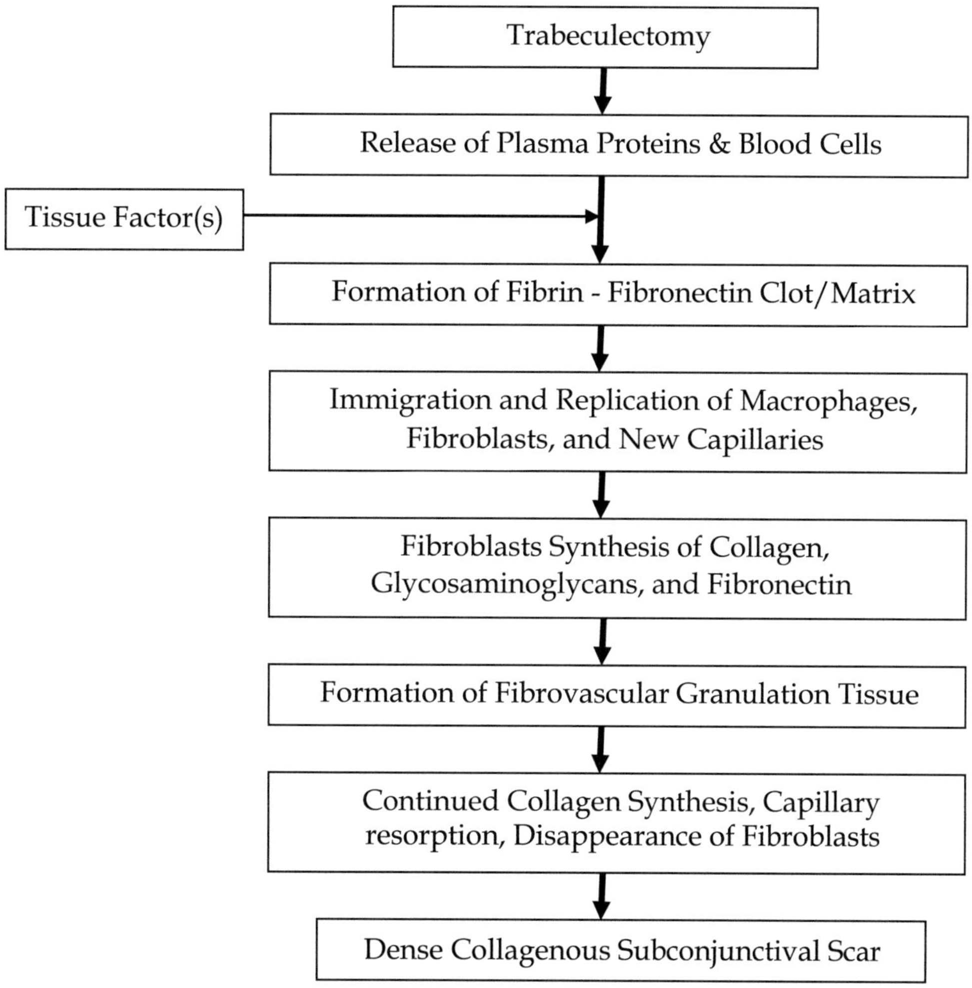


Fig. 2. Events of wound healing in trabeculectomy failure

## 3. Risk factors and potential causes of trabeculectomy failure

### 3.1 External factors

External factors at the episceral-conjunctival interface are responsible for most cases of trabeculectomy failure. Fibroblast proliferation, synthesis of the extracellular matrix, and subsequent development of subconjunctival fibrosis play prominent roles in external failure. Chemotactic factors for fibroblasts include lymphokines, complement, native collagens of types I to V, fibronectin, some proteolytic digestion fragments of collagen and fibronectin, and platelet-derived growth factor (Ross et al, 1986).

Intense preoperative and postoperative inflammation induces a cellular response that accelerates wound healing. The presence of blood beneath the conjunctiva may also increase the probability of bleb failure. As noted above, serum derivatives including fibronectin and platelet-derived growth factor may stimulate fibroblast migration and proliferation. In addition, macrophages, which may be activated by blood, appear to play a key role in inducing the fibroproliferative response in wound repair (Leibovich and Ross, 1975). Extrapolation of these observations to trabeculectomy wound healing is consistent with the clinical impression that the presence of blood increases the likelihood of postoperative fibrosis.

### 3.2 Intraocular factors

In the absence of scar formation, an inadequate opening into the anterior chamber due to scleral remnants or Descemet's membrane in the fistula may lead to primary failure. Blockage of the filtration site by prolapsed iris, vitreous, or ciliary body may also lead to early postoperative failure (Maumenee, 1960). Many of these potential causes of bleb failure can be avoided by careful surgical technique. A spacer during surgery can enhance the likelihood of a patent fistula.

## 4. Measures to improve the trabeculectomy outcome

Trabeculectomy success relies on the continued patency of the fistula and the continued ability of the filtering bleb created out of the conjunctiva to absorb aqueous humor. Thus, the success of the procedure lies not only on the surgical technique but also the intraoperative and postoperative measures to minimize scar formation.

Preoperative inflammation should be treated with anti-inflammatory agents, usually corticosteroids. Miotics, which break down the blood-aqueous barrier, should be discontinued at least two weeks before trabeculectomy. Treatment of postoperative inflammation is also important. Cycloplegic agents help restore the blood-aqueous barrier and may reduce the release of plasma proteins, which may contribute to the postoperative healing response.

With respect to surgical technique, tissue trauma should be minimized by avoiding unnecessary manipulation of the conjunctiva, Tenon and iris. Hemostasis should be performed to decrease bleeding. Removal of the inner sclerectomy block should establish a patent channel without remnants of Descemet's membrane. A basal iridectomy prevents postoperative iris incarceration at the filtering site.

Although a fornix-based conjunctival flap might prevent scarring of the posterior conjunctiva and Tenon's capsule, randomized studies of limbus versus fornix-based conjunctival flaps in primary trabeculectomies failed to document significant differences in surgical success between the two techniques (Shuster et al, 1984; Traverso et al, 1987). The effect of the excision of Tenon's capsule on trabeculectomy success is also controversial.

## 5. Pharmacologic modulation of wound healing

Unlike most surgical procedures, success of glaucoma filtering surgery is achieved through the inhibition of wound healing. The use of pharmacologic agents is based on suppression of proliferation of cells, mainly fibroblasts, which would limit the healing at the site of the fistulizing surgery and consequently limit postoperative scarring.

### 5.1 Corticosteroids

As stated above, the initial steps in wound healing are inflammation and coagulation, leading to a cascade of biological events including cellular, hormonal, and growth factor release. These events finally lead to scar tissue formation (Skuta and Parrish, 1987). Corticosteroids regulate wound healing through the inhibition of macrophage functions, such as phagocytosis and the release of enzymes like collagenase, plasminogen activator, and growth factors, and thus suppress inflammation. Specific anti-inflammatory effects include suppression of fibrin deposition, capillary permeability, migration of leukocytes and macrophages, and phagocytic activity (Starita et al, 1985). Corticosteroids also inhibit vascular permeability and fibroblast proliferation (Lama and Fechtner, 2003). Tissue culture studies of human Tenon capsule fibroblasts have shown that corticosteroids inhibit cell attachment and proliferation (Nguyen and Lee, 1992).

Postoperative topical corticosteroids have been reported to significantly increase the success of trabeculectomy (Araujo 1995). Sub-Tenon injection of triamcinolone acetonide (TA) appears to be a more effective mean of high-dose corticosteroid delivery and may increase the success rate of trabeculectomy (Hosseini 2007). Tham and associates reported that the use of TA (1.2 mg) injection into filtration blebs at the conclusion of trabeculectomy was associated with good intraocular pressure (IOP) control for 3 months (Tham 2006). However, Yuki et al reported no significant differences between the success rates of trabeculectomy with or without intraoperative sub-Tenon injection of 20 mg TA within the 12-month follow-up period (Yuki, 2009).

Besides intra- and post-operative administration, some studies have highlighted the beneficial effect of preoperative use of corticosteroids and non steroidal anti-inflammatory agents in improving the success rate of filtration surgery. Baudouin demonstrated that fluorometholone drops one month before filtering surgery has effectively reduced inflammation, as indicated by the expression of human leukocyte antigen (HLA)-DR after impression cytological analysis (Baudouin 2002). Breusegem compared preoperative topical anti-inflammatory medications to placebo before trabeculectomy. Significantly fewer postoperative needling procedures were needed in the steroid-treated group (5%) than in the placebo group (41%). Furthermore, none of the patients in the steroid group required topical IOP-lowering medication to maintain a subtarget IOP, compared with 24% of patients in the placebo group. However, there was no significant overall difference in absolute IOP values or in relative IOP reduction between two groups at any point (Breusegem 2010). Despite the aforementioned advantages, topical steroids pose a risk for steroid-induced IOP elevation and cataract.

### 5.2 Antimetabolites

Anti-mitotic agents such as MMC and 5-fluorouracil (5-FU) help suppress post-surgical scarring by causing widespread non-selective cell death and apoptosis. The intraoperative application of MMC in trabeculectomy was introduced by Chen (Chen, 1983), while Heuer was the first to report the use 5-FU postoperatively as subconjunctival injections (Heuer et al, 1984).

While 5-FU can be used both for intraoperative application and postoperative injection (Parrish et al, 2001), the use of MMC as a postoperative injection is not as widely accepted as

5-FU (Apostolov and Siarov, 1996). The concentration of 5-FU used intraoperatively is 50 mg/mL applied for up to 5 minutes. The concentration of MMC used intraoperatively ranges from 0.1-0.5 mg/mL applied for 2-5 minutes, depending on the risk of failure. The antifibrotic agent can be applied to the scleral bed before or after the scleral flap is made, using cellulose sponges. The antifibrotic-soaked sponges should be applied to the area where aqueous flow is desired and should not be placed too close to the limbus or in contact with the wound edges. After all the sponges have been removed, the site is irrigated with copious amounts of saline solution to remove residual antifibrotic agents.

Although anti-mitotic agents improved the success rate of trabeculectomy (Chen et al, 1990;Kitazawa et al, 1991), there is an increased risk of early postoperative complications such as hypotony, bleb rupture, and infectious endophthalmitis (Shields et al, 1993; Greenfield and Parrish, 1996; Singh et al, 2000; WuDunn et al, 2002; Palanca-Capistrano et al, 2009). Another common late complication is bleb leakage, which may cause other serious complications such as infection, hypotony related maculopathy, and corneal endothelial decompensation (Greenfield et al, 1996; Nuyts et al, 1994). Thus, understanding, mechanisms of wound healing following MMC treatment is important to reduce bleb-related complications of leakage.

As a mechanism of MMC action, it is commonly accepted that inhibiting fibroblast proliferation leads to decreased conjunctival adhesion and maintaining the bleb (Lama and Fechtner, 2003). In terms of the pharmacokinetics of MMC, the t1/2 in blood doses of 30, 20, and 10 (mg/body) is 50, 43, and 10 minutes, respectively (Fujita, 1982). This suggests that the half-life of MMC is very short. Because we use MMC at a dosage of less than 1% on the sclera for several minutes in trabeculectomy, its effective lifespan seems to be less than several hours. As stated above, fibroblasts appear and are activated at 12 hours after surgery by macrophages and various cytokines that are released from T-cells. Therefore, it seems unreasonable that MMC directly suppresses fibroblasts' proliferation.

It is more likely that MMC initially suppresses the proliferation of mast cells, including chymase-positive cells which may promote inflammatory response. As a result of this, fibroblast proliferation is then restrained (Okada et al, 2009). In fact, topical instillation of an anti-mast-cell agent, tranilast, was useful for filtering bleb formation and IOP
reduction (Chihara et al, 2002). Therefore, suppression of mast cells might be related to formation of the filtering bleb. In addition, chymase inhibition might play a role in maintaining filtering blebs for an extended period of time. It has been reported that a chymase inhibitor prevents adhesion for up to three months in an abdomen adhesion model (Okamoto et al, 2004), so bleb formation may be maintained for a long period if MMC inhibits chymase function after tissue injury. Further investigation is needed to verify that chymase inhibitors are appropriate for glaucoma surgeries.

### 5.3 Anti-vascular endothelial growth factor (VEGF) antibodies

Pathologic angiogenesis is frequently associated with massive inflammation and migration of fibroblasts. It was shown that cultured conjunctival fibroblasts could be stimulated to produce VEGF by pro inflammatory cytokines (sano-Kato et al, 2005), and Tenon's capsule fibroblasts were inhibited by angiogenesis inhibitors (Wong et al, 1994). Based on these findings, it is imaginable that a selective inhibition of growth factors such as VEGF could be an approach to prevent or treat extensive wound healing. To further elucidate the direct effect of anti-VEGF agents on fibroblasts, Guerriero et al. illustrated in vitro effects of bevacizumab on human corneal and conjunctival fibroblast cell lines. Their research concluded that when corneal stromal fibroblasts are exposed to bevacizumab, loss of cell-to-cell adhesions and morphological changes are seen. They further stated that these changes are dose-dependent (Guerriero et al. 2006).

Currently, two therapeutic anti-VEGF antibodies exist; bevacizumab and ranibizumab. The use of subconjunctival bevacizumab 1mg in 0.04ml to treat a failing filtering bleb in addition to a needling procedure has been described in one patient (Kahook et al, 2006b). This patient showed an immediate decrease in IOP and was symptomatically improved as well. Bevacizumab has also been used in neovascular glaucoma (Kahook et al, 2006a; Michels et al, 2005). Kapetansky et al. studied the utility of subconjunctival bevacizumab injections administered proximal to blebs after trabeculectomy at the earliest sign of vascularization (Kapetansky et al, 2007). They noted that nearly two thirds of the blebs had an observable reduction in vascularity while decreasing IOP from a mean of 17.8 to 14mmHg 1 month after injection. Improved results were noted when the injections were given earlier in the postoperative phase. Coote et al presented a case of subconjunctival injection of bevacizumab that resulted in a dramatic reduction of bleb vascularity for 6 weeks. In their case, even 6 months after injection, a healthy bleb with minimal scar tissue was seen (Coote et al., 2008).

Ranibizumab is a fully humanized monoclonal antibody-fragment and therefore has a low molecular weight, which results in good tissue penetration. The antibody deactivates all isoforms of VEGF-A. Although intraocular injection of the drug showed no toxic side effects in an animal model (Manzano et al, 2006), the disadvantage of this form of application in trabeculectomy is the short half life of the drug. Although ranibizumab has a longer intravitreal half-life (6 days), this form of application does not cover the main peak of scarring reaction that is occurring around 2-3 weeks after surgery (Choi et al, 2010). For example, Purcell et al. noted decreased IOP and bleb vascularization after bleb needle revision using ranibizumab. But, this effect was short-lived, as increased vascularization was noted after 1 month of follow-up (Purcell, et al. 2008).

Further studies are needed to better understand how anti-VEGF agents might benefit patients undergoing glaucoma filtration surgery. There are ongoing safety studies to better analyze the importance of route of administration - intracameral, sub-Tenon and intravitreal - and to determine whether unknown side effects co-exist. It is important to delineate duration of action when anti-VEGF agents are injected in the intra or sub-Tenon's space and how this might influence efficacy.

## 6. Amniotic membrane as a modulator of trabeculectomy wound healing

### 6.1 Fetal strategy of wound healing

The amniotic membrane shares the same cell origin as the fetus. The majority of the studies testify the clinical efficacy of amniotic membrane transplantation (AMT) in gearing adult wound healing toward regeneration with minimal inflammation and scarring, suggesting that amniotic membrane (AM), like the fetal tissue, carries similar features that may not only facilitate regeneration but also inhibit scar formation (Mast et al, 1992; Adzick and Lorenz, 1994)

A number of mechanisms have been put forth to explain the AM's biological actions in modulating adult wound healing toward the fetal direction with anti-inflammation, anti-scarring and anti-angiogenesis. (Tseng et al, 2004).

It remains unclear whether such therapeutic actions are directly or indirectly linked to modulate healing and differentiation. AM has been shown to down-regulate transforming growth factor-β signaling in cultured normal conjunctival fibroblasts (Tseng et al., 1999; Lee et al., 2000) and to inhibit the cellular migration triggered by vascular endothelial growth factor (VEGF) (Shey et al., 2011). Furthermore, AM can exert potent anti-inflammatory effects by facilitating macrophage apoptosis (Li et al, 2006).

### 6.2 Preliminary studies

Several investigators have explored the clinical efficacy of deploying AM as an adjunctive therapy to improve the surgical outcome of various glaucoma procedures, including trabeculectomy (Sheha et al, 2010). They have shown that transplantation of a single (Fujishima et al, 1998; Lu and Mai, 2003; Yue et al, 2003; Drolsum et al, 2006) or folded (Bruno et al, 2006; Eliezer et al, 2006) sheet of AM under the scleral flap (Fujishima et al, 1998; Yue et al, 2003; Drolsum et al, 2006; Bruno et al, 2006), and/or under the conjunctiva (Yue et al, 2003; Drolsum et al, 2006; Bruno et al, 2006; Eliezer et al, 2006), with additional MMC (Fujishima et al, 1998; Drolsum et al, 2006; Bruno et al, 2006), reduces IOP in eyes with refractory glaucoma. Experimental rabbit studies demonstrated that the AM, inserted under the scleral flap, achieves the same reduction of subconjunctival fibroblasts and macrophages around the trabeculectomy sites as that achieved by MMC (Demir et al, 2002; Wang et al, 2005), as well as reduces the number of fibroblasts at trabeculectomy sites when inserted under the scleral flap even without MMC (Zhong et al, 2000; Barton et al, 2001).

### 6.3 Potential advantages of AM

We have conducted the first prospective randomized trial to demonstrate the clinical efficacy of transplanting a single layer of cryopreserved AM under and around the scleral flap (Fig. 3), in conjunction with application of MMC in refractory glaucoma. In this study of 37 eyes, 18 received 0.2 mg/ml MMC under the flap for 2 min while 19 received additional implantation of cryopreserved AM under and around the scleral flap (Sheha et al, 2008).

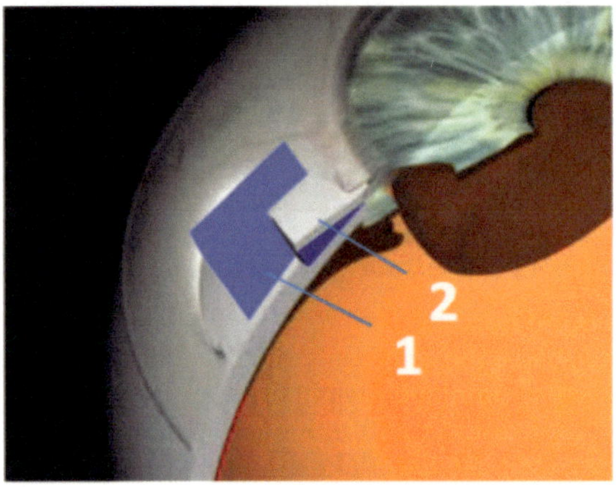


Fig. 3. AMT in trabeculectomy. AM (1) inserted under and around the scleral flap (2)

In the control MMC only group, IOP continuously rose between 3 and 12 months postoperatively. The incidence of encapsulated blebs, which are caused by collagen-producing fibroblasts (Ophir, 1992), was greater in the control group (38.9% vs. 5.3%) at 12 months postoperatively. This indicates that the effect of MMC was not sufficient to suppress scar formation, potentially due to its short half-life.

At 12 months postoperatively, the group with AM transplantation achieved significantly higher rates of complete (IOP ≤ 21 mmHg without medications) and qualified success (IOP ≤ 21 mmHg with or without additional medications). Furthermore, the resultant blebs were diffuse and translucent, but still retained normal vascularity (Fig. 4A). This bleb morphology was notably different from a MMC-induced ischemic bleb, which is prone to develop late complications such as bleb leak and infection (Fig. 4B). There were significantly fewer early postoperative complications such as shallow anterior chamber and choroidal effusion. These beneficial effects may be attributed to the fact that AM inserted under the scleral flap effectively halts rapid drainage of aqueous humor from the trabeculectomy site to reduce immediate hypotony from overfiltration and reduces scarring in the filtration site in the long run.

Hence, it is plausible that AM implanted in subconjunctival and subscleral spaces might reduce the adverse side effects intrinsically associated with MMC and with over-filtration, making AM a unique natural biological modulator that may exert a similar anti-scarring action to MMC while eliminating the potential sight-threatening complications known to MMC.

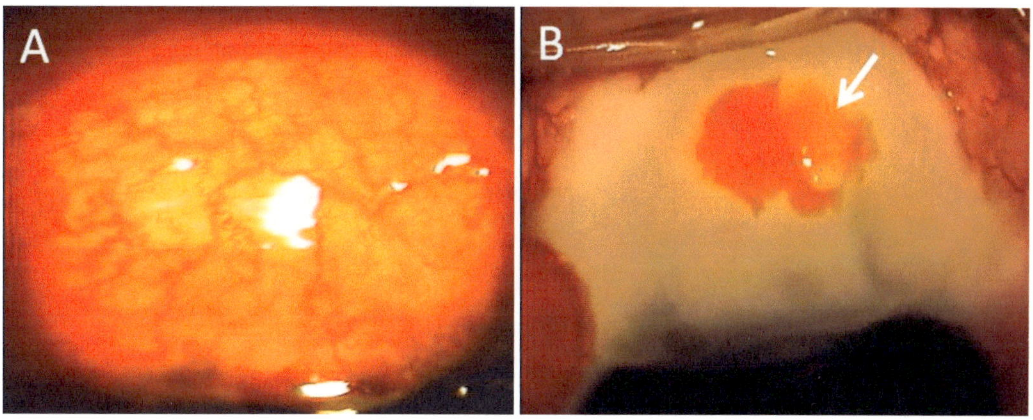


Fig. 4. Comparison between functioning bleb with normal vascularity after AMT (A) and ischemic leaking bleb after MMC (B); arrow indicates the bleb leak revealed by fluorescein staining (B)

The aforementioned favorable results could be attributed to a synergistic beneficial effect of MMC and AM on controlling fibrosis at the trabeculectomy site. It remains unclear whether the AM can substitute MMC completely in trabeculectomy. Furthermore, the mechanism through which the AM exerts its effects as well as its fate in the subscleral space over time remains largely unknown. The AM may not only prevent scar formation via its known anti-inflammatory and anti-scarring actions but may also serve as a spacer integrated into the internal bleb structure to stabilize the patency of the filtering fistula and maintain a functioning bleb.

Currently we are studying the fate of AM and internal bleb morphology. Although histological studies showed that human AM dissolves at 1 month postoperatively in rabbits (Wang et al, 2005), we do not know whether similar AM dissolution also occurred in human patients. We have gathered preliminary data supporting the feasibility of using anterior segment optic coherence tomography (OCT) to detect the presence of AM and the evidence of host cell integration into the AM after being transplanted in the subconjunctival space to cover the glaucoma shunt tube. Our results showed that implanted AM maintained its thickness over a period of 12 months (Anand et al, 2011).

### 6.4 Evidence of AM anti-angiogenic action

Pathologic angiogenesis that is frequently associated with uncontrolled inflammation may lead to fibrosis. While reducing fibrosis in subconjunctival and subscleral spaces as shown above, AM was found to deliver anti-angiogenic actions to resolve rubeosis iridis that is known to occur in neovascular glaucoma. In our study, there were 7 eyes with neovascular glaucoma in each group, which was accompanied by circumcorneal congestion, neovascularization at the angle and the iris in the form of rubeosis iridis (Fig. 5A), and hyphema (Fig. 6A). Interestingly, 2 weeks following implantation of AM, we observed rapid resolution of the circumcorneal congestion and dramatic regression of the anterior chamber neovascularization (Fig. 5B) and hyphema (Fig. 6B). The effect was persistent through 12 months of follow-up.

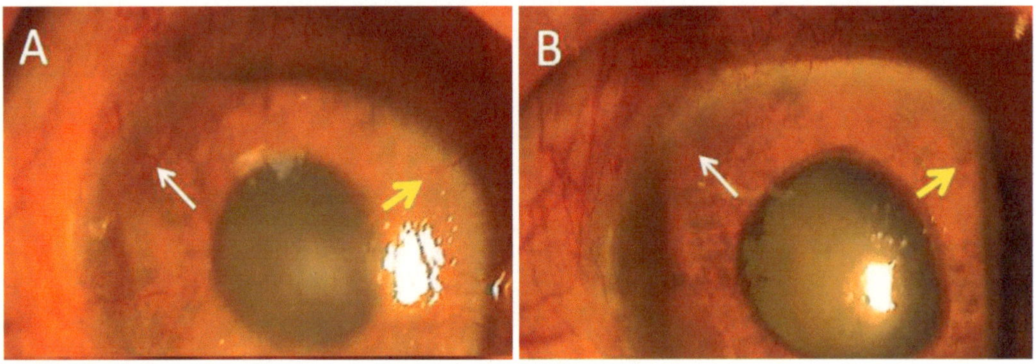


Fig. 5. Resolution of rubeosis iridis (arrows) in neovascular glaucoma

Hence, our study was the first showing AM's anti-angiogenic clinical efficacy. Because such an action was not associated with reduction of the normal vascularity of the bleb (Fig.4A), we speculate that AM's anti-angiogenic action is preferentially directed toward abnormal neovascularization. This novel therapeutic action against neovascularization may add an extra benefit in the management of high-risk neovascular glaucoma.

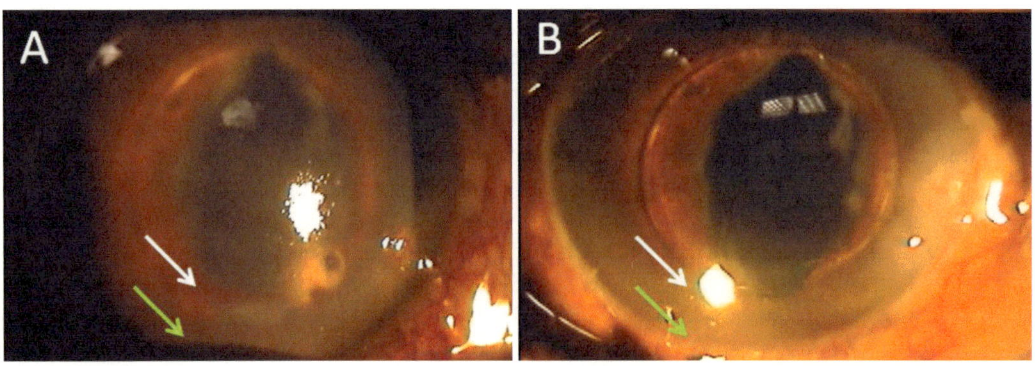


Fig. 6. Rapid resolution of rubeosis iridis (white arrow) and hyphema (green arrow) in neovascular glaucoma

## 7. Future research

Our preliminary studies designate that the implantation of AM to lower IOP in trabeculectomy represents a significant advance in treating glaucoma by eliminating complications associated with MMC and over-filtration. Further understanding of the fate of AM via imaging studies will not only confirm its anti-inflammatory and anti-scarring effects but will also teach us how intrableb wound healing can be modulated by the AM regarding integration into the surrounding operated tissue. Such knowledge will further strengthen our belief that AM can be a natural biological matrix derived from the fetus that may modulate adult wound healing toward regeneration through the reduction of inflammation, scarring, and unwanted new blood vessel formation. Further proof of the anti-angiogenic action of AM in reverting neovascularization in cases of neovascular glaucoma will generate a direct impact on using AM to treat ocular diseases where angiogenesis threatens vision. We expect that such a treatment will be more effective than the conventional approach based on an antibody blockade against VEGF, because AM not only suppresses angiogenesis mediated by VEGF and other growth factors, but also curtails inflammation and scarring. This innovative concept can then be applied to other parts of the body where pathological fibrosis or angiogenesis is considered detrimental and undesirable.

## 8. Financial disclosure and acknowledgement

The clinical research mentioned in this article was supported in part by grant #EY019785 from the National Eye Institute via TissueTech, Inc., which owns US patents on the method of preparation and clinical uses of human amniotic membrane. The content is solely the responsibility of the author and does not necessarily represent the official views of the National Eye Institute or the National Institutes of Health. The author thanks Lingyi Liang, MD, PhD and Shunsuke R. Sakurai for assistance in editing the text.

## 9. References

Adzick NS, Lorenz HP. (1994). Cells, matrix, growth factors, and the surgeon. The biology of scarless fetal wound repair. *Ann Surg,* Vol.220, pp.10-18.

Anand A, Sheha H, Teng C, Liebmann JM, Ritch R, Tello C. (2011). Use of Amniotic Membrane Graft in Glaucoma Shunt Surgery. *Ophthalmic Surg Lasers Imaging.*

Apostolov VI, Siarov NP. (1996). Subconjunctival injection of low-dose Mitomycin-C for treatment of failing human trabeculectomies. *Int Ophthalmol,* Vol.20, No.1-3, pp.101-105.

Araujo SV, Spaeth GL, Roth SM, Starita RJ. A ten-year follow-up on a prospective, randomized trial of postoperative corticosteroids after trabeculectomy. Ophthalmology 1995; 102:1753–1759.

Barton K, Budenz D, Khaw PT, Tseng SCG. (2001). Glaucoma filtration surgery using amniotic membrane transplantation. *Invest Ophthalmol Vis Sci,* Vol.42, pp.1762-1768.

Baudouin C, Nordmann JP, Denis P, et al. Efficacy of indomethacin 0.1% and fluorometholone 0.1% on conjunctival inflammation following chronic application of antiglaucomatous drugs. Graefes Arch Clin Exp Ophthalmol 2002;240:929–35.

Breusegem C, Spielberg L, Van Ginderdeuren R, Vandewalle E, Renier C, Van de Veire S, Fieuws S, Zeyen T, Stalmans I. Preoperative Nonsteroidal Anti-inflammatory Drug or Steroid and Outcomes after Trabeculectomy. Ophthalmology 2010;117:1324–1330

Broadway DC, Chang LP. (2001). Trabeculectomy, risk factors for failure and the preoperative state of the conjunctiva. *J Glaucoma,* Vol.10, No.3, pp.237-249.

Bruno CA, Eisengart JA, Radenbaugh PA, Moroi SE. (2006). Subconjunctival placement of human amniotic membrane during high risk glaucoma filtration surgery. *Ophthalmic Surg Lasers Imaging,* Vol.37, No.3, pp.190-197.

Chang L, Crowston JG, Cordeiro MF, Akbar AN, Khaw PT. (2000). The role of the immune system in conjunctival wound healing after glaucoma surgery. *Surv Ophthalmol,* Vol.45, No.1, pp.49-68.

Chen CW, Huang HT, Bair JS, Lee CC. (1990). Trabeculectomy with simultaneous topical application of mitomycin-C in refractory glaucoma. *J Ocul Pharmacol,* Vol.6, No.3, pp.175-182.

Chen C. (1983). Enhanced intraocular pressure controlling effectiveness of trabeculectomy by local application of mitomycin C. *Trans Asia Pac Acad Ophthalmol,* Vol.9, pp.172-177.

Chihara E, Dong J, Ochiai H, Hamada S. (2002). Effects of tranilast on filtering blebs: a pilot study. *J Glaucoma,* Vol.11, No.2, pp.127-133.

Chintala SK, Wang N, Diskin S, Mattox C, Kagemann L, Fini ME, Schuman JS. (2005). Matrix metalloproteinase gelatinase B (MMP-9) is associated with leaking glaucoma filtering blebs. *Exp Eye Res,* Vol.81, No.4, pp.429-436.

Choi JY, Choi J, Kim YD. (2010). Subconjunctival bevacizumab as an adjunct to trabeculectomy in eyes with refractory glaucoma: a case series. *Korean J Ophthalmol,* Vol.24, No.1, pp.47-52.

Coote MA, Ruddle JB, Qin Q, Crowston JG (2008). Vascular changes after intra-bleb injection of bevacizumab. *J Glaucoma* Vol.17, No., pp.517–518.

Demir T, Turgut B, Akyol N, Ozercan I, Ulas F, Celiker U. (2002). Effects of amniotic membrane transplantation and mitomycin C on wound healing in experimental glaucoma surgery. *Ophthalmologica,* Vol.216, No.6, pp.438-442.

Desjardins DC, Parrish RK, Folberg R, Nevarez J, Heuer DK, Gressel MG. (1986). Wound healing after filtering surgery in owl monkeys. *Arch Ophthalmol,* Vol.104, No.12, pp.1835-1839.

Desmouliere A, Geinoz A, Gabbiani F, Gabbiani G. (1993). Transforming growth factor-beta 1 induces alpha-smooth muscle actin expression in granulation tissue myofibroblasts and in quiescent and growing cultured fibroblasts. *J Cell Biol,* Vol.122, No.1, pp.103-111.

Drolsum L, Willoch C, Nicolaissen B. (2006). Use of amniotic membrane as an adjuvant in refractory glaucoma. *Acta Ophthalmol Scand,* Vol.84, No.6, pp.786-789.

Dvorak HF. (1986). Tumors: wounds that do not heal. Similarities between tumor stroma generation and wound healing. *N Engl J Med,* Vol.315, No.26, pp.1650-1659.

Eliezer RN, Kasahara N, Caixeta-Umbelino C, Pinheiro RK, Mandia C, Jr., Malta RF. (2006). Use of amniotic membrane in trabeculectomy for the treatment of glaucoma: a pilot study. *Arq Bras Oftalmol,* Vol.69, No.3, pp.309-312.

Fujishima H, Shimazaki J, Shinozaki N, Tsubota K. (1998). Trabeculectomy with the use of amniotic membrane for uncontrolled glaucoma. *Ophthalmic Surg Lasers,* Vol.29, pp.428-431.

Fujita H. (1982). [Pharmacokinetics of mitomycin C and its derivative (KW-2083)]. *Gan To Kagaku Ryoho,* Vol.9, No.8, pp.1362-1373.

Greenfield DS, Parrish RK. (1996). Bleb rupture following filtering surgery with mitomycin-C: clinicopathologic correlations. Ophthalmic Surg Lasers, Vol.27, No.10, pp.876-877.

Greenfield DS, Suner IJ, Miller MP, Kangas TA, Palmberg PF, Flynn HW, Jr. (1996). Endophthalmitis after filtering surgery with mitomycin. *Arch Ophthalmol,* Vol.114, No.8, pp.943-949.

Guerriero E, Yu JU, Kahook MY. (2006) Morphologic evaluation of bevacizumab (Avastin) treated corneal stromal fibroblasts. *Invest Ophthalmol Vis Sci, Vol*47, E-Abstract 1642.

Grierson I, Joseph J, Miller M, Day JE. (1988). Wound repair: the fibroblast and the inhibition of scar formation. *Eye (Lond),* Vol.2 ( Pt 2), pp.135-148.

Heuer DK, Parrish RK, Gressel MG, Hodapp E, Palmberg PF, Anderson DR. (1984). 5-fluorouracil and glaucoma filtering surgery. II. A pilot study. *Ophthalmology,* Vol.91, No.4, pp.384-394.

Hosseini H, Mehryar M, Farvardin M. Focus on triamcinolone acetonide as an adjunct to glaucoma filtration surgery. Med Hypotheses 2007;68:401- 403

Kahook MY, Schuman JS, Noecker RJ. (2006a). Intravitreal bevacizumab in a patient with neovascular glaucoma. *Ophthalmic Surg Lasers Imaging,* Vol.37, No.2, pp.144-146.

Kahook MY, Schuman JS, Noecker RJ. (2006b). Needle bleb revision of encapsulated filtering bleb with bevacizumab. Ophthalmic Surg Lasers Imaging, Vol.37, No.2, pp.148-150.

Kapetansky FM, Pappa KS, Krasnow MA, et al (2007). Subconjunctival injection(s) of bevacizumab for failing filtering blebs. *Invest Ophthalmol Vis Sci* 2007 [E-Abstract 837

Kitazawa Y, Kawase K, Matsushita H, Minobe M. (1991). Trabeculectomy with mitomycin. A comparative study with fluorouracil. *Arch Ophthalmol,* Vol.109, No.12, pp.1693-1698.

Lama PJ, Fechtner RD. (2003). Antifibrotics and wound healing in glaucoma surgery. *Surv Ophthalmol,* Vol.48, No.3, pp.314-346.

Lee S-B, Li D-Q, Tan DTH, Meller D, Tseng SCG. (2000). Suppression of TGF-b signaling in both normal conjunctival fibroblasts and pterygial body fibroblasts by amniotic membrane. *Curr Eye Res,* Vol.20, pp.325-334.

Leibovich SJ, Ross R. (1975). The role of the macrophage in wound repair. A study with hydrocortisone and antimacrophage serum. *Am J Pathol,* Vol.78, No.1, pp.71-100.

Li W, He H, Kawakita T, Espana EM, Tseng SCG. (2006). Amniotic membrane induces apoptosis of interferon-gamma activited macrophages in vitro. *Exp Eye Res,* Vol.82, No.2, pp.282-292.

Lu H, Mai D. (2003). [Trabeculectomy combined amniotic membrane transplantation for refractory glaucoma]. *Yan Ke Xue Bao,* Vol.19, No.2, pp.89-91.

Manzano RP, Peyman GA, Khan P, Kivilcim M. (2006). Testing intravitreal toxicity of bevacizumab (Avastin). *Retina,* Vol.26, No.3, pp.257-261.

Mast BA, Diegelmann RF, Krummel TM, Cohen IK. (1992). Scarless wound healing in mammalian fetus. *Surgery,* Vol.174, pp.441-451.

Maumenee AE. (1960). External filtering operations for glaucoma: the mechanism of function and failure. *Trans Am Ophthalmol Soc,* Vol.58, pp.319-328.

Meyer-ter-Vehn T, Sieprath S, Katzenberger B, Gebhardt S, Grehn F, Schlunck G. (2006). Contractility as a prerequisite for TGF-beta-induced myofibroblast transdifferentiation in human tenon fibroblasts. *Invest Ophthalmol Vis Sci,* Vol.47, No.11, pp.4895-4904.

Michels S, Rosenfeld PJ, Puliafito CA, Marcus EN, Venkatraman AS. (2005). Systemic bevacizumab (Avastin) therapy for neovascular age-related macular degeneration twelve-week results of an uncontrolled open-label clinical study. *Ophthalmology,* Vol.112, No.6, pp.1035-1047.

Miller MH, Grierson I, Unger WI, Hitchings RA. (1989). Wound healing in an animal model of glaucoma fistulizing surgery in the rabbit. Ophthalmic Surg, Vol.20, No.5, pp.350-357.

Nguyen KD, Lee DA. Effect of steroids and nonsteroidal anti-inflammatory agents on human ocular fibroblast. Invest Ophthalmol Vis Sci 1992;33:2693–2701

Nuyts RM, Felten PC, Pels E, Langerhorst CT, Geijssen HC, Grossniklaus HE, Greve EL. (1994). Histopathologic effects of mitomycin C after trabeculectomy in human glaucomatous eyes with persistent hypotony. *Am J Ophthalmol,* Vol.118, No.2, pp.225-237.

Okada K, Sugiyama T, Takai S, Jin D, Ishida O, Fukmoto M, Oku H, Miyazaki M, Ikeda T. (2009). Effects of mitomycin C on the expression of chymase and mast cells in the conjunctival scar of a monkey trabeculectomy model. *Mol Vis,* Vol.15, pp.2029-2036.

Okamoto Y, Takai S, Miyazaki M. (2004). Significance of chymase inhibition for prevention of adhesion formation. *Eur J Pharmacol,* Vol.484, No.2-3, pp.357-359.

Ophir A. (1992). Encapsulated filtering bleb. A selective review--new deductions. *Eye,* Vol.6 ( Pt 4), pp.348-352.

Palanca-Capistrano AM, Hall J, Cantor LB, Morgan L, Hoop J, WuDunn D. (2009). Long-term outcomes of intraoperative 5-fluorouracil versus intraoperative mitomycin C in primary trabeculectomy surgery. *Ophthalmology,* Vol.116, No.2, pp.185-190.

Parrish RK, Schiffman JC, Feuer WJ, Heuer DK. (2001). Prognosis and risk factors for early postoperative wound leaks after trabeculectomy with and without 5-fluorouracil. *Am J Ophthalmol,* Vol.132, No.5, pp.633-640.

Purcell JM, Teng CC, Tello C, et al (2008). Effect of needle bleb revision with ranibizumab as a primary intervention in a failing bleb following trabeculectomy. *Invest Ophthalmol Vis Sci* 2008. [E-Abstract 4165]

Reichel MB, Cordeiro MF, Alexander RA, Cree IA, Bhattacharya SS, Khaw PT. (1998). New model of conjunctival scarring in the mouse eye. *Br J Ophthalmol,* Vol.82, No.9, pp.1072-1077.

Ross R, Rainee EW, Bowen-Pope DF. (1986). The biology of platelet-derived growth factor. Cell, Vol.46, pp.155-169.

Sano-Kato N, Fukagawa K, Okada N, Kawakita T, Takano Y, Dogru M, Tsubota K, Fujishima H. (2005). TGF-beta1, IL-1beta, and Th2 cytokines stimulate vascular endothelial growth factor production from conjunctival fibroblasts. *Exp Eye Res,* Vol.80, No.4, pp.555-560.

Sheha H, Liang L, Tseng SCG (2010). Amniotic Membrane Grafts for Glaucoma Surgery. In: Paul N.Schacknow, John R.Samples, editors. *The Glaucoma Book;* A Practical, Evidence-Based Approach to Patient Care.New York:Springer. p. 861-869.

Sheha H, Kheirkhah A, Taha H. (2008). Amniotic membrane transplantation in trabeculectomy with mitomycin C for refractory glaucoma. *J Glaucoma,* Vol.17, No.4, pp.303-307.

Sherwood MB. (2006). A sequential, multiple-treatment, targeted approach to reduce wound healing and failure of glaucoma filtration surgery in a rabbit model (an American Ophthalmological Society thesis). *Trans Am Ophthalmol Soc,* Vol.104, pp.478-492.

Shey E, He H, Sakurai S, Tseng SC. (2011) Inhibition of Angiogenesis by HC{middle dot}HA, a Complex of Hyaluronan and the Heavy Chain of Inter-{alpha}-Inhibitor, Purified from Human Amniotic Membrane. Invest Ophthalmol Vis Sci. [Epub ahead of print]

Shields MB, Scroggs MW, Sloop CM, Simmons RB. (1993). Clinical and histopathologic observations concerning hypotony after trabeculectomy *with* adjunctive mitomycin C. *Am J Ophthalmol,* Vol.116, pp.673-683.

Shuster JN, Krupin T, Kolker AE, Becker B. (1984). Limbus- v fornix-based conjunctival flap in trabeculectomy. A long-term randomized study. Arch Ophthalmol, Vol.102, No.3, pp.361-362.

Singh K, Mehta K, Shaikh NM, Tsai JC, Moster MR, Budenz DL, Greenfield DS, Chen PP, Cohen JS, Baerveldt GS, Shaikh S. (2000). Trabeculectomy with intraoperative mitomycin C versus 5-fluorouracil. Prospective randomized clinical trial. *Ophthalmology,* Vol.107, No.12, pp.2305-2309.

Skuta GL, Parrish RK. (1987). Wound healing in glaucoma filtering surgery. *Surv Ophthalmol,* Vol.32, No.3, pp.149-170.

Starita RJ, Fellman RL, Spaeth GL, Poryzees EM, Greenidge KC, Traverso CE. (1985). Short- and long-term effects of postoperative corticosteroids on trabeculectomy. *Ophthalmology,* Vol.92, No.7, pp.938-946.

Sturmer J, Broadway DC, Hitchings RA. (1993). Young patient trabeculectomy. Assessment of risk factors for failure. *Ophthalmology,* Vol.100, No.6, pp.928-939.

Tham CC, Li FC, Leung DY. Intrableb triamcinolone acetonide injection after bleb-forming filtration surgery (trabeculectomy, phacotrabeculectomy, and trabeculectomy revision by needling): a pilot study. Eye 2006;20:1484 –1486.

Traverso CE, Tomey KF, Antonios S. (1987). Limbal- vs fornix-based conjunctival trabeculectomy flaps. *Am J Ophthalmol,* Vol.104, No.1, pp.28-32.

Tseng SCG, Espana EM, Kawakita T, Di Pascuale MA, Wei Z-G, He H, Liu TS, Cho TH, Gao YY, Yeh LK, Liu C-Y. (2004). How does amniotic membrane work? *The Ocular Surface,* Vol.2, No.3, pp.177-187.

Tseng SCG, Li D-Q, Ma X. (1999). Suppression of Transforming Growth Factor isoforms, TGF-b receptor II, and myofibroblast differentiation in cultured human corneal and limbal fibroblasts by amniotic membrane matrix. *J Cell Physiol,* Vol.179, pp.325-335.

Wang L, Liu X, Zhang P, Lin J. (2005). [An experimental trial of glaucoma filtering surgery with amniotic membrane]. *Yan Ke Xue Bao,* Vol.21, No.2, pp.126-131.

Wipff PJ, Rifkin DB, Meister JJ, Hinz B. (2007). Myofibroblast contraction activates latent TGF-beta1 from the extracellular matrix. *J Cell Biol,* Vol.179, No.6, pp.1311-1323.

Wong J, Wang N, Miller JW, Schuman JS. (1994). Modulation of human fibroblast activity by selected angiogenesis inhibitors. *Exp Eye Res,* Vol.58, No.4, pp.439-451.

WuDunn D, Cantor LB, Palanca-Capistrano AM, Hoop J, Alvi NP, Finley C, Lakhani V, Burnstein A, Knotts SL. (2002). A prospective randomized trial comparing intraoperative 5-fluorouracil vs mitomycin C in primary trabeculectomy. *Am J Ophthalmol,* Vol.134, No.4, pp.521-528.

Yue J, Hu CQ, Lei XM, Qin GH, Zhang Y. (2003). Trabeculectomy with amniotic membrane transplantation and combining suture lysis of scleral flap in complicated glaucoma. *Zhonghua Yan Ke Za Zhi,* Vol.39, No.8, *pp.476-480.*

Yuki K, Shiba D, Kimura I, Ohtakey Y, Tsubota K. Trabeculectomy With or Without Intraoperative Sub-Tenon Injection of Triamcinolone Acetonide in Treating Secondary Glaucoma Am J Ophthalmol 2009;147:1055–1060

Zhong Y, Zhou Y, Wang K. (2000). Effect of amniotic membrane on filtering bleb after trabeculectomy in rabbit eyes. *Yan Ke Xue Bao,* Vol.16, No.2, pp.73-6, 83.

20

# Novel Glaucoma Surgical Devices

Parul Ichhpujani[1] and Marlene R. Moster[2]
[1]*Glaucoma Facility, Department of Ophthalmology, Government Medical College and Hospital, Chandigarh,*
[2]*Anne and William Goldberg Glaucoma Service, Wills Eye Institute, Philadelphia, PA,*
[1]*India*
[2]*USA*

## 1. Introduction

An ideal glaucoma procedure is the one that is easy to perform, reproducible, with a low incidence of early postoperative hypotony, and long-term adequate IOP control. Furthermore, it should be minimally cataractogenic, allow rapid visual recovery and have the potential to be combined with phacoemulsification without one procedure potentially affecting the outcome of the other. Unfortunately, the quest for an ideal glaucoma procedure is on. The Landmarks in the course of surgical innovations for glaucoma management highlight the fact that we have come a long way.

**Landmarks in the history of surgical innovations for glaucoma**

- 1857 - Albrecht von Graefe: Surgical iridectomy "to reduce aqueous production" in glaucoma. Iridectomy helped many cases of angle closure, but not by the mechanism proposed.
- 1859 - Coccius: Iridectomy with iris inclusion
- 1876 - Argyll-Robertson: Scleral trephination
- 1878 - Louis De Wecker: Anterior sclerectomy
- 1903 - Bader and Lagrange: Iridosclerectomy
- 1905 - Heine: Cyclodialysis
- 1906 - Soren Holth: Iridenclesis
- 1909 - Elliot: Corneoscleral trephination
- 1924 - Preziozi: Electrocautery to create a full thickness fistula between the anterior chamber and the subconjunctival space.
- 1936 - Otto Barkan: Goniotomy for chronic glaucoma in adults.
- 1956 - Meyer-Schwickerath: Laser iridotomy with a xenon arc photocoagulator.
- 1958 - Harold Scheie: Modified Preziozi's procedure. Entered the eye with a knife and then used cautery to extend the scleral wound.
- 1968 - Cairns: Trabeculectomy. Removed a rectangular section of trabecular meshwork and deep cornea. He aimed to remove a block of the canal of Schlemm to get aqueous to flow freely into its cut ends.

- 1968 – Anthony Molteno: Glaucoma drainage device that directly shunted aqueous from the anterior chamber into a episcleral reservoir.
- 1976 – Theodore Krupin: First valved glaucoma drainage tube, at first without a reservoir.
- 1979 – James B. Wise and Stanton L. Witter: Argon laser "trabeculoplasty."
- 1982 – Robert Ritch: Iridoplasty for acute angle closure crisis unresponsive to medication.
- 1983 – Chen Wu Chen: Mitomycin C as an adjunctive in trabeculectomy.
- 1984 – 5-Fluorouracil was first reported in an animal model and in a pilot study in glaucoma filtering surgery.
- 2002 - ExPRESS miniature glaucoma shunt
- 2003 - Reay Brown and Mary Lynch: EYEPASS glaucoma shunt
- 2004 - George Baerveldt and Don Minckler: FDA approved, Trabectome microelectrocautery device
- 2004 - Richard Hill and Mory Ghareb: Trabecular micro-bypass stent, iStent. Undergoing FDA review
- 2005 – Deep light Gold shunt
- 2009 - Bruce Shields: Aquashunt
- 2009 - Transcend CyPass glaucoma implant

## 2. Trabeculectomy

Despite several available options, trabeculectomy—arguably is the most-performed glaucoma surgery till today. Although improved techniques and the adjunctive use of antimetabolites has enhanced long-term success as measured by intraocular pressure (IOP) control, trabeculectomy has a sizeable risk profile to glaucoma patients, over both the short and long term.

Blebitis, bleb related endophthalmitis, hypotony, overfiltration, bleb leaks, bleb fibrosis and encapsulation, bleb overhang, corneal endothelial cell loss, dellen, and aqueous misdirection are among the many risks associated post trabeculectomy. (Borisuth et al, 1999)

## 3. Drainage devices

Glaucoma drainage devices (GDD) were initially developed for use in complex glaucoma patients, many of whom had failed medical, laser, and prior surgical treatments. (Molteno, 1969; Krupin et al., 1976; Lloyd et al., 1994 & Coleman et al., 1995) Typically, these devices consist of a tube placed into the anterior chamber to allow for aqueous humor to flow posteriorly into an encapsulated filtration area typically 10–12 mm posterior to the limbus, into a reservoir sutured to the sclera.

Though complications associated with anterior bleb formation were avoided, GDD resulted in a high risk of hypotony and overfiltration, sometimes leading to suprachoroidal hemorrhage. As a result several measures for flow restriction and regulation were adopted, but despite all efforts complication profile of GDD is significant. Overfiltration, fibrosis, tube exposure, tube occlusion, tube retraction and diplopia to list a few potential complications. (Kupin et al., 1995; Ticho and Ophir, 1993 & Gedde et al., 2007)

Since neither trabeculectomy nor GDDs are without their fair share of complications, the quest for the development and advancement of glaucoma surgery to provide alternative means of shunting aqueous humor out of the anterior chamber is on.

Surgical procedures augmenting either conventional outflow pathway or uveoscleral outflow pathway have been developed. For conventional outflow enhancement, goniosurgical procedures (Epstein et al., 1985) and surgeries involving schlemm canal (both ab interno and ab externo) have recently emerged as successful surgical options.
Surgical approaches to augment suprachoroidal outflow have also been explored with cyclodialysis, suprachoroidal implants, seton devices, and most recently, an ab externo gold shunt placed in the suprachoroidal space. (Pinnas and Boniuk, 1969; Krejci, 1972; Ozdamar et al., 2003; Jordan et al., 2006)

| Type | Glaucoma surgery |
|---|---|
| Non penetrating | Viscocanalostomy<br>Deep sclerectomy<br>Canaloplasty |
| Minimally penetrating | Ex-PRESS glaucoma filtration device<br>Trabecular micro-bypass iStent<br>Trabectome microelectrocautery<br>Gold microshunt (GMS) device<br>Eyepass implant |
| Penetrating | Trabeculectomy |

Table 1. Types of glaucoma surgeries

This chapter, addresses the available knowledge for the novel drainage devices; devices which attempt to assist with flow regulation such as the Ex-PRESS mini-glaucoma shunt (Alcon Laboratories, Inc., Fort Worth, TX) (Wamsley et al., 2004), Schlemm's canal surgical procedures, including nonpenetrating canaloplasty surgery ( Lewis et al., 2007), the Glaukos trabecular micro-bypass iStent (Nichamin, 2009) the Trabectome microelectrocautery device (Nguyen, 2008) and the suprachoroidal outflow gold microshunt device (GMS) (Melamed et al., 2009) (Table 1).Published data is limited as many of these devices are currently in investigation and undergoing clinical trials.

## 4. Minimally penetrating procedures

### 4.1 Ex-PRESS glaucoma filtration device

Ophthalmic surgery has evolved over the last several decades into sophisticated microsurgery involving continually smaller incisions. The Ex-PRESS shunt is on the forefront of this evolution toward smaller incision glaucoma filtration surgery. Since there is an added cost to using the Ex-PRESS rather than trabeculectomy, its place in the surgical management of glaucoma has not been clear so far.

**Device**

Ex-PRESS stands for "excessive pressure regulating shunt system".
The Ex-PRESS implant is a miniature unvalved glaucoma implant. It was originally developed by Optonol, Ltd. (Neve Ilan, Israel), as an alternative procedure to trabeculectomy

and to the other types of glaucoma filtering surgery for patients with open angle glaucoma (Nyska et al., 2003). Now, it is available as EX-PRESS Glaucoma Filtration Device (Alcon Laboratories, Inc., Fort Worth, TX).

The device is approximately 3 mm long, stainless steel tube (outer diameter 400 µm (27 gauge)) with a beveled, sharpened, rounded tip, a disc-like flange (<1 $mm^2$) at the device proximal end, and a spur-like projection that prevents its extrusion. (Nyska et al., 2003; Geffen et al., 2010) The external flange and inner spur are angled to conform to the anatomy of the sclera, and the distance between them corresponds to the scleral thickness at the site of implantation.

The EX-PRESS® Glaucoma Filtration Device is preloaded on a specially designed disposable introducer, the EX-PRESS® Delivery System (EDS). The EDS is an inserter designed to maintain the correct orientation of the EX-PRESS® Glaucoma Filtration Device throughout the implantation procedure. The commercially available versions are: R-50, P-50 and P-200. (Table 2; Figure 1)

| Characteristic | Ex PRESS R50 | Ex PRESS P50 | Ex PRESS P200 |
|---|---|---|---|
| External body device | Round | Round | Round |
| Device length | 2.96 | 2.64 | 2.64 |
| Internal lumen size | 50 | 50 | 200 |
| Tip shape | Pointed | Pointed | Pointed |
| Backplate shape | Uniform | Vertical split | Vertical split |
| Preincision needle gauge | 27G | 25G | 25G |

Table 2. Comparative characteristics of the available models of Ex- PRESS implant

**Indications**

- Open Angle Glaucoma refractory to medical and laser treatment
- Open Angle Glaucoma with a failed filtration procedure
- Combined glaucoma and cataract procedure (Ex-PRESS may have the advantage of faster visual recovery compared with trabeculectomy)
- Aphakic glaucoma (As no iridectomy is required with the Ex-PRESS implantation, there is less risk of vitreous moving forward through a new iridectomy)
- Sturge-Weber syndrome and other situations as high hyperopia and nanophthalmos (Since chances of choroidal effusions following trabeculectomy are high in these subset of patients; Ex-PRESS implantation may offer a safer alternative because of its lower rate of prolonged postoperative hypotony)

**Contraindications**

The implantation of the EX-PRESS® Glaucoma Filtration Device is contraindicated if one or more of the following conditions exist:

- Presence of ocular disease such as uveitis, ocular infection, severe dry eye or severe blepharitis.
- Pre-existing ocular or systemic pathology that, in the opinion of the surgeon, is likely to cause postoperative complications following implantation of the device.
- Patient diagnosed with angle closure glaucoma.

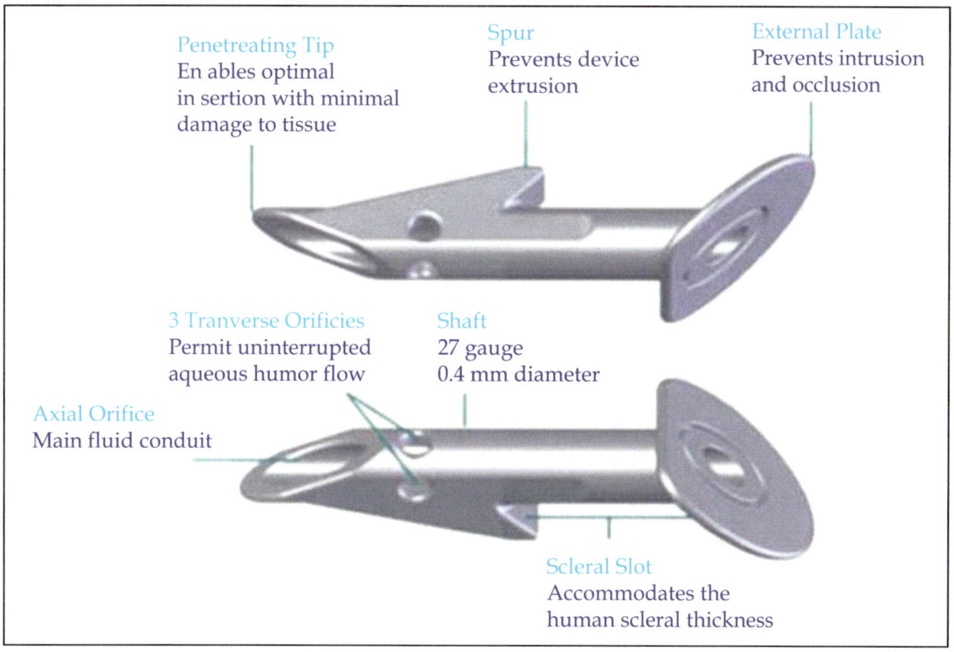


Fig. 1. R 50 Ex-PRESS device

**Surgical procedure**

Originally, the device was designed to be inserted at the limbus directly under the conjunctiva with formation of a subconjunctival bleb which served as a flow modulator. Poor conjunctival covering of the device, conjunctival erosions over the external flange and conjunctival scarring with subsequent decreased aqueous humour filtration, were some of the complications that were encountered because of direct subconjunctival implantation. (Kaplan Messa et al., 2002; Gandolfi et al., 2002; Traverso et al., 2005; Wamsley et al., 2004; Stewart et al., 2005; Rivier et al., 2007; Tavolato et al., 2006; Garg et al., 2005) Conjunctivoplasty or tube removal had to be performed to avoid secondary infection.

To overcome these complications, Dahan and Carmichael suggested implanting the device under a limbus based 50% deep scleral flap extending into clear cornea. (Dahan and Carmichael, 2005) This operation is similar to standard trabeculectomy without the need of an iridectomy or scleral removal.

This implant may also be used in deep sclerectomy to simplify the difficult dissection of Schlemm's canal and Trabeculo-Descemet's membrane.

### 4.2 Placement of device under a scleral flap

To place the Ex-PRESS filtration device, a conjunctival peritomy, limbal or fornix-based, is first created as in conventional trabeculectomy. Gentle cautery is applied to the sclera prior to creation of a scleral flap. The dimensions of the scleral flap may need to be slightly larger than the trabeculectomy flap and it should be initiated more posteriorly in order to ensure full coverage of the shunt plate.

Scleral spur is identified by a white, glistening band of fibers that crosses the bed of this section. The blue zone is a transition zone to the clear cornea. The surgeon should make sure that they implant the EX-PRESS device in the anterior chamber, just at the level of the scleral spur, but not too far posteriorly. It is important for the device to enter the eye exactly at the anterior aspect of the scleral spur and for it to remain at the iris plane so that it does not point downward towards the iris.

Once the scleral spur has been visualized, the anterior chamber should be filled with viscoelastic or air in the area of anticipated shunt entry. Rather than an ostium created by a punch, trephine, or scissors, a 25- or 27-gauge needle or a 400 µm wide blade is used to enter the anterior chamber at the level of the scleral spur, parallel to the iris, and the Ex-PRESS device is injected into this needle tract.

**Complications**

The Ex-PRESS device relies on nonphysiologic subconjunctival flow as its mechanism of IOP lowering. As a result, all of the issues that limit trabeculectomy and the complication profile associated with blebs accompany the Ex-PRESS shunt too, but to a much lesser extent.

Recently, external blockade of the tube has been reported as a possible device-related complication of Ex-PRESS implants, which can be visualized on a systematic gonioscopic examination. (Bagnis et al., 2011) It should be considered whenever IOP increases and a flat bleb is observed. Neodymium: Yttrium Argon Garnet (Nd:YAG) laser at the tip of the device is a viable therapeutic option to treat the external occlusion of Ex-PRESS devices, regardless the nature of the obstruction. Obstruction may also occur inside the lumen of the device where it may not be visualized by gonioscopy, at the point where the diameter constricts to 50 mm. Since this constriction point is close to the opening into the anterior chamber, Nd:YAG laser works in this scenario as well (Netland, 2011).

Corneal dislocation of the Ex-PRESS implant may occur and when associated with ocular hypertension, needs surgical treatment. (Vetrugno et al., 2011) Before considering a trabeculectomy, it could be valuable to attempt an implant reposition. Reopening of the conjunctiva and the scleral flap, excision of the corneal tissue covering the flange, and stitching the implant to the sclera with polyprolene suture has been tried with success.

The Magnetic Resonance Imaging (MRI) systems in clinical use today operate with magnetic fields ranging from 0.2 to 3.0 Tesla. To ascertain MRI compatibility, the Ex-PRESS glaucoma drainage device (316L stainless steel) has been examined for magnetic field interactions under standard 1.5, 3.0, and 4.7 T MRI scanning protocols. (Seibold et al., 2011) During induced torque testing, no displacement was noted under 1.5 and 3.0 T conditions, although a significant amount of displacement occurred in the 4.7 T environment. Increasing amounts of angular deflection were demonstrated at all three field strengths. So, it should be remembered that Ex-PRESS moves in the presence of high magnetic fields.

### 4.3 Scientific evidence so far

**Ex-PRESS versus trabeculectomy**

Maris et al in a retrospective comparative case series analysed data of 49 eyes with the Ex-PRESS and 47 eyes with a standard trabeculectomy. (Maris et al., 2007) The authors noted that although the mean IOP was significantly higher in the early postoperative period in the Ex-PRESS group compared with the trabeculectomy group, the reduction of IOP was similar in both groups after 3 months. The number of postoperative glaucoma medications in both groups was not significantly different. Kaplan-Meier survival curve analysis showed no significant difference in success between the two groups ($P = 0.594$). The success rate at an average of 11 months was 90% for the Ex-PRESS shunt compared with 92% for trabeculectomies at last follow up. Early postoperative hypotony and choroidal effusion were significantly more frequent after trabeculectomy than after Ex-PRESS implants under a scleral flap ($P < 0.001$). There was no difference between a limbal based or a fornix based approach with either procedure (trabeculectomy vs. Ex-PRESS shunt). After 3 months, the percentage decrease in IOP was similar for the groups, Ex-PRESS group (39.9 to 46.6%) and the trabeculectomy group (28.6 to 45.4%). For IOP control during the postoperative period, a significantly greater number of laser suture lysis procedures were performed in the Ex-PRESS group compared with the control group. The authors concluded that the Ex-PRESS implant under a scleral flap had similar IOP-lowering efficacy with a lower rate of early hypotony compared with trabeculectomy.

**Ex-PRESS in previously operated eyes**

Moster and co workers reported intermediate-term results of the Ex-PRESS implant (R-50 and T-50), under a scleral flap in previously operated eyes (cataract or failed glaucoma surgeries). (Lankaranian et al., 2010) To compare the outcome between patients who had previous trabeculectomy or cataract surgery the definition of success was IOP of 5-15mmHg. One hundred eyes of 100 patients were studied. The mean follow-up period was $27 \pm 13.2$ months (range: 12-66). Success was defined as complete if IOP was 5-21 mmHg without medication or surgical intervention, and qualified if IOP was within the same range with glaucoma medication. Success was complete in 60 (60%) and qualified in 24 (24%) eyes. The mean preoperative IOP of $27.7 \pm 9.2$ mm Hg (range, 14-52 mmHg) with $2.73 \pm 1.1$ drugs declined to $14.02 \pm 5.1$ mm Hg with $0.72 \pm 1.06$ drugs at the last follow up ($P < 0.0001$). The causes of failure were uncontrolled IOP (11%), bleb needling (4%), and persistent hypotony (1%). Bleb needling may induce an erratic wound healing response in some cases and lead to failure. The probability of success in the patients with previous cataract surgery and trabeculectomy at 3 years was 60.6% and 50.9%, respectively. Figure 2 shows Ex-PRESS implant in a case with previously failed trabeculectomy.

Ates and coworkers studied 15 eyes with postpenetrating keratoplasty glaucoma unresponsive to medical antiglaucomatous therapy in which Ex-PRESS mini glaucoma shunt implantation was done. (Ates et al., 2010)

IOP decreased from 41.46 mm Hg to 12.06 mm Hg over a mean follow-up of 12.2 months ($P<0.001$).

IOP was below 21 mm Hg in 14 of 15 eyes (93.3%) with or without antiglaucomatous drugs. Complete success (IOP<21 mm Hg without medication) rate was 86.6%. Average number of antiglaucomatous drug usage decreased from 3.20 (range: 2 to 4) preoperatively to 0.26 postoperatively (range: 0 to 3) ($P<0.001$). In 93.3% of the cases, the decrease in IOP was 30%

or above postoperatively. After Ex-PRESS implantation, clear grafts remained clear while edematous grafts became clearer due to IOP decrease. Neither biomicroscopy nor pachymetry showed worsening of preoperatively opaque grafts.
Similarly, Vetrugno and colleagues also reported good results in vitrectomized patients who required glaucoma surgery for persistent ocular hypertension (Vetrugno et al., 2010).

**Ex-PRESS with deep sclerectomy**

Bissig and colleagues did a prospective, nonrandomized trial to study Deep Sclerectomy with the Ex-PRESS X-200 implant in 26 eyes. (Bissig et al., 2010) A posterior deep sclerectomy was dissected without opening the Schlemm's canal and an Ex-PRESS X-200 device was inserted under the scleral flap into the anterior chamber to drain aqueous humour into the intrascleral space. Eighty-five percent of patients achieved an IOP < 18 mmHg with or without medication and 69% without medication. Post-operative complications were hyphaema (15%), wound leak (15%), encysted blebs (54%) and bleb fibrosis in 8% of patients.

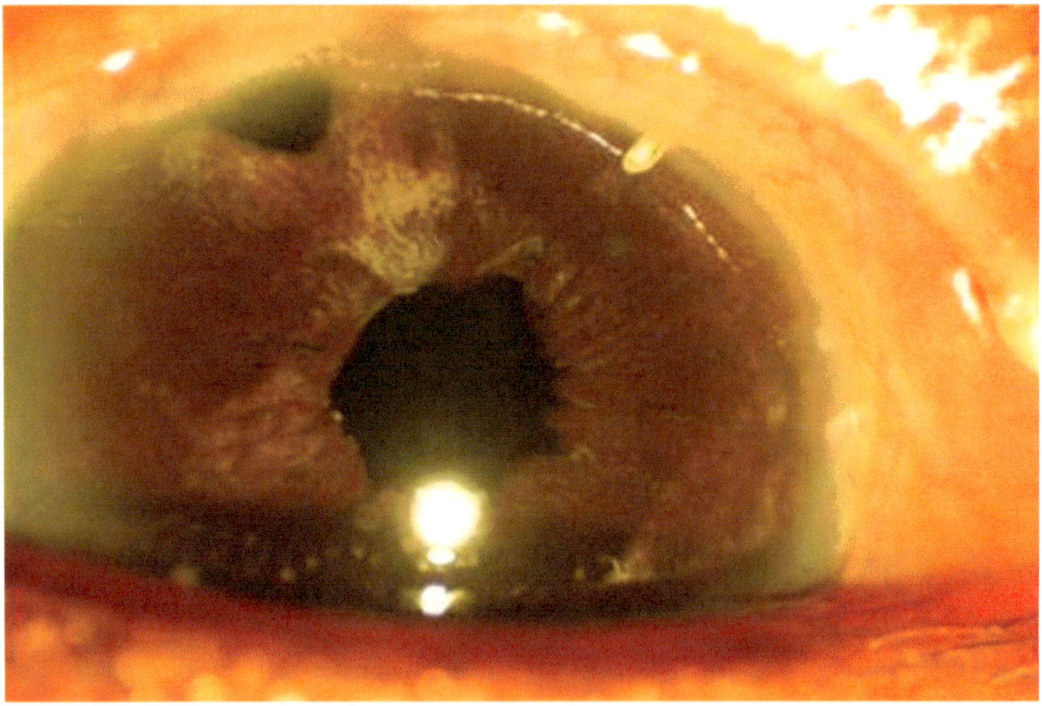

Fig. 2. Ex-PRESS in a previously failed glaucoma surgery

Gindroz and coworkers conducted a prospective study reporting on modified deep sclerectomy using the Ex-PRESS LR-50 in combined cataract and glaucoma surgery in 24 eyes. (Gindroz et al., 2011) Preoperative data had, IOP: 18.1±5.3 mmHg, best-corrected visual acuity (BCVA): 0.6±0.3, and number of medications: 2.3±1.1. The IOP decreased by 25.4% at 24 months and by 27.0% at 48 months. At 24 months, 19 patients (86.3%) achieved a BCVA of 0.5 or better, and at 48 months the mean BCVA was 0.7±0.3. At the last visit, the mean number of medications reduced to 0.6±0.8 (P<0.05). The complete and qualified success rates were 45.6% and 85.2%. No conjunctival erosions over the Ex-PRESS LR-50 were noted.

**Ex-PRESS with phacoemulsification**

Kanner and co workers implanted Ex-PRESS device under a scleral flap either as a single procedure in 231 eyes of 200 patients or combined with cataract surgery in 114 eyes of 100 patients, for a total of 345 eyes in 300 patients who received the implant. (Kanner et al., 2009) They found that the Ex-PRESS implant under a scleral flap could lower IOP alone or in combination with cataract surgery. The most common device-related complication was blockage of the lumen of the implant, which was effectively treated with Nd:YAG laser treatment of the tube tip in the anterior chamber.

### 4.4 Place in surgical armamentarium

The advantages of this device as an adjunct to filtration surgery may be a lowered incidence of early postoperative hypotony and elimination of the need for a surgical iridectomy. The device is easily placed either temporally or nasally in an eye with prior scarring, as long as there are 2 to 3 clock hours of mobile conjunctiva available. There is often enough conjunctivae available between the side port vitrectomy scars to form a posterior bleb following a pars plana vitrectomy. Ex-PRESS requires less healthy tissue than for placement of a traditional drainage implant.

Since the resulting blebs are usually low and diffuse, there is little risk of developing delle or bleb dysethesias, even when the surgery is located off to one side.

In eyes with prior failed trabeculectomies, Ex-PRESS can help to reestablish the aqueous flow without having to repeat the original procedure. The Ex-PRESS fits easily in the middle ground between a repeat trabeculectomy and a larger glaucoma drainage device like a Baerveldt, Molteno, or an Ahmed tube shunt.

Additionally, because of the technical familiarity of trabeculectomy, the learning curve for the incorporation of this device into filtering surgery is not a steep one, and it has shown to be effective when combined with phacoemulsification.

Initial doubts about the Ex-PRESS filtration device are decreasing with recent advances offering possibly a wider spectrum of indications while diminishing the potential complications.

## 5. Trabecular bypass devices

The site of abnormal outflow resistance within the meshwork is probably the juxtacanalicular tissue adjacent to Schlemm's canal, a layer of the meshwork approximately 10 μm thick. Removal or bypassing this thin layer of tissue should decrease the elevated IOP, without the need for creating a hole in the sclera and a filtration bleb.

Recent work has focused on using small tubes to bypass the meshwork, creating a direct route from the anterior chamber into Schlemms' canal. (Razeghinejad and Spaeth, 2011)

### 5.1 Trabecular micro-bypass iStent

**Device**

The iStent® trabecular micro-bypass stent (Glaukos Corp, Laguna Hills, California) is the first *ab-interno* micro bypass stent. It is a heparin-coated with Duraflo (Edwards Lifesciences, Irvine, CA), nonferromagnetic, surgical grade titanium (Ti6Al4V ELI) stent less than one mm in length and approximately 0.3 mm in height, with a snorkel length of 0.25 mm and a nominal snorkel bore diameter of 120 μm. It is about 1/5000 of the size of the Baerveldt implant. (Samuelson et al., 2011) The iStent® is inserted through a small temporal clear corneal incision, bypassing the trabecular meshwork, and placed in Schlemm's canal at the lower nasal quadrant. The dimensions of the stent are customized for a natural fit and retention within the 270μ canal space, with three retention arches to ensure secure placement.

**Indications**

- Mild-to-moderate primary open angle glaucoma
- Pigmentary glaucoma
- Pseudoexfoliative glaucoma, stand alone or in combination with cataract surgery.

**Contraindications**

- Presence of ocular disease such as uveitis, ocular infection
- Patients diagnosed with angle closure glaucoma

**Surgical technique**

The iStent® is preloaded in a single-use, light release force, sterile applicator (Figure 3) with a secure, rotatable grip to facilitate manipulation and placement into Schlemm's canal. Separate orientations of the stent are available for the right and left eye. iStent® implantation can be performed under topical anesthesia. Prior to implanting the iStent®, the angle anatomy and targeted stent site must be in clear view. The Swan-Jacob gonioprism is used to inspect the angle to ensure a good view at the nasal implant location. The iStent® is implanted through the same small, temporal, clear corneal incision used for phacoemulsification or a 1.5 mm incision when the stent is implanted as a stand-alone procedure. iStent in inserted in trabecular meshwork with "*Penetrate, lift and slide*" insertion technique.

For best possible angle visualization; iStent® insertion should be performed from the temporal side with the microscope magnified 12X and tilted towards the surgeon. The patient's head is tilted away from the surgeon.

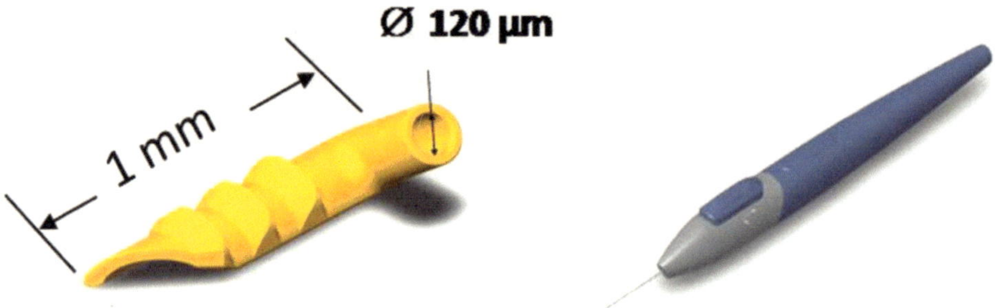


Fig. 3. Snorkel shaped iStent; iStent Applicator

Implantation is performed in the nasal position (3 to 4 o'clock for the right eye; 8 to 9 o'clock for the left eye) with the tip of the implant directed inferiorly. The tip of the stent should approach the trabecular meshwork at 15° angle to facilitate penetration of the tissue (Figure 4). Excessive resistance indicates that the approach is too perpendicular to the trabeculum. Once the stent is covered with meshwork it is released by pressing the applicator button. Only the proximal end of the stent remains visible in the anterior chamber. The iStent® is seated into position by gently tapping the side of the snorkel with the applicator tip. A small reflux of blood from the Schlemm's canal reflects correct positioning of the stent. Extraction of the viscoelastic material and hydration of the corneal incision conclude the procedure.

Proper stent placement is confirmed by flushing the anterior chamber of any refluxed blood, performing a high-magnification examination to confirm that the base of the implant is parallel with the circumferential axis of the Schlemm canal, and gently nudging the snorkel to confirm that the snorkel axis is parallel with the iris plane and that the base is well seated and fully through the trabecular meshwork.

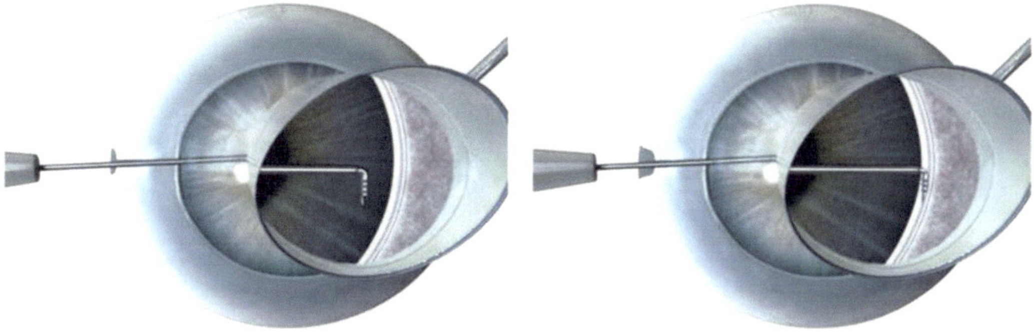

Fig. 4. Technique of iStent implantation

**Complications**

The stent is small (1 mm) and hence it may sometimes be difficult to verify exact placement of the implant via gonioscopy, particularly in cases of corneal edema, peripheral anterior synechiae, or an uncooperative or anxious patient. In such cases there is a possibility of accidentally misplacing the iStent. Ichhpujani and coworkers carried out an in vitro study, in which they used a human cadaver eye, unsuitable for transplantation, as a model to visualize the position of the stent. (Ichhpujani et al., 2010) They reported that in cases where gonioscopy is not successful, UBM can aid in localization of the iStent, in both the anterior and posterior chambers, provided the probe is moved to provide a favorable signal, whereas AS-OCT is limited to detection of stents in the anterior chamber alone and B-scan is of no value.

A theoretical problem with bypass of the meshwork is blood reflux from Schlemm's canal into the anterior chamber via the tube, creating a microhyphema. Any activity that raises episcleral venous pressure higher than IOP, such as prolonged bending with the head down or vigorous Valsalva maneuver, would be most likely to cause this problem. Since such maneuvers also increase IOP by increasing the choroidal blood volume, this would counter the elevated episcleral venous pressure. This may explain why microhyphemas have not been reported till date with an iStent.

### 5.2 Scientific evidence so far

US iStent Study group assessed the safety and efficacy of the iStent in combination with cataract surgery in subjects with mild to moderate open-angle glaucoma. (Samuelson et al., 2011) A total of 240 eyes with mild to moderate open-angle glaucoma with IOP ≤ 24 mmHg controlled on 1 to 3 medications were randomized to undergo cataract surgery with iStent implantation (treatment group) or cataract surgery only (control). The primary efficacy measure was unmedicated IOP≤ 21 mmHg at 1 year. The study met the primary outcome, with 72% of treatment eyes versus 50% of control eyes achieving the criterion ($P< 0.001$). At 1 year, IOP in both treatment groups was statistically significantly lower from baseline values. Sixty-six percent of treatment eyes versus 48% of control eyes achieved ≥20% IOP

reduction without medication ($P< 0.003$). The overall incidence of adverse events was similar between groups with no unanticipated adverse device effects.
The ocular hypotensive efficacy seen with the stent in this study was found to be consistent with the trabecular bypass mechanism of action and results described in literature. (Fea, 2010; Spiegel et al., 2008 & 2009)
Compared with cataract surgery alone, implantation of the iStent concomitant with cataract extraction significantly increases trabecular outflow facility, reduces IOP and the number of medications. (Fernandez- Barrientos et al., 2010)
A study in cultured human anterior segments has shown that a single stent created the largest change in IOP, resulting in a mean of 12.4 ± 4.2 mm Hg, corresponding to an 84% increase in facility of outflow. Interestingly, IOP seemed to reach a baseline level of approximately 12 mm Hg, even with multiple stents. (Bahler et al., 2004)
The probable explanation is that only one is enough to bypass the barrier of the Schlemm's canal and the lumen of the iStent is large enough to drain the aqueous as if the Schlemm's wall is well functioning.

### 5.3 Place in the surgical armamentarium

The iStent is believed to reestablish natural trabecular outflow, and it leaves the conjunctiva untouched, and avoids the lifelong risk of complications associated with filtering blebs. Thus, iStent implantation in patients with mild to moderate open-angle glaucoma undergoing cataract surgery represents a novel therapeutic approach that provides clinically significant reductions in IOP and medication use.

### 5.4 Trabectome electrocautery device

**Device**

The Trabectome surgical device was cleared by the US Food and Drug Administration in January 2004 for the treatment of adult and juvenile open-angle glaucoma. The concept is similar in principle to *ab interno* trabeculotomy, the key difference being that a microelectrocautery device is used to ablate a strip of the trabecular meshwork and inner wall of Schlemm's canal, thus allowing direct access of aqueous to the collector channels. This theoretically bypasses the main site of resistance to aqueous outflow and reestablishes the natural drainage passageway out of the eye.
The Trabectome consists of a disposable footpedal activated handpiece and a console to adjust infusion, aspiration and electrosurgical energy. The handpiece consists of a 19-gauge infusion sleeve, a 25-gauge aspiration port, and a bipolar electrocautery unit 150 µm away from an insulated footplate (Figure 5). The footplate is 800 µm in length from the heel to the tip, has a maximum width of 230 µm, and maximum thickness of 110 µm.

**Indications**

Trabectome may be an excellent surgical option for patients who require postoperative IOPs in the mid-to-high teens. It can be combined with cataract surgery.

- Early to moderate Primary open-angle glaucoma
- Pigmentary and pseudoexfoliative glaucoma.
- Patients with elevated IOP despite previous glaucoma surgery (trabeculectomy or a drainage tube)

**Contraindications**

Angle closure with or without peripheral anterior synechiae is the only contraindication. Trabecular meshowork without pigment may pose difficulty for proper gonioscopic identification of structures.

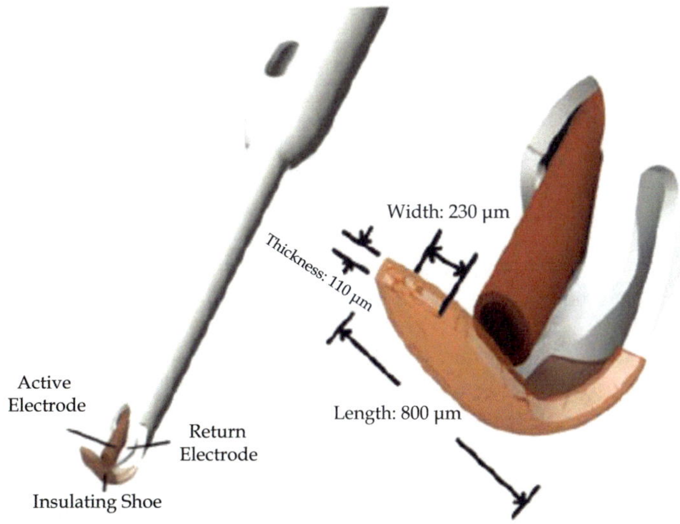


Fig. 5. Trabectome hand piece

**Surgical procedure**

Surgery is carried out with a temporal approach through a clear corneal incision of 1.6-1.8 mm to accommodate the electrocautery unit. Alternatively, when combined with clear cornea coaxial phacoemulsification, the main incision may be used for the Trabectome handpiece. Ophthalmic visco-devices are used to inflate and stabilize the anterior chamber and a gonioprism is used for direct visualization of the angle. Once the instrument has been inserted into Schlemm's canal, the foot pedal is depressed to begin electrocautery. The surgeon's hand simultaneously moves in one direction to ablate the tissue until the tip of the handpiece has reached the limit of visibility. The handpiece may then be turned to achieve ablation in the opposite direction again, to the limits of view. Total arc length amenable to treatment through a single incision is 60–90°. Tissue debris released during electrocautery can obscure the view hence aspiration and continuous irrigation are carried out. A clear corneal suture is applied and intracameral air is injected at the conclusion of Trabectome ablation to prevent postoperative hyphema.

When combined Trabectome and cataract surgery are done then the ab interno trabeculotomy is completed before starting the phacoemulsification. This order of operation prevents the formation of phacoemulsification-related corneal edema that could impair visualization of the angle structures.

Too low power settings and rapid movement of the handpiece should be avoided as it may lead to inadvertent tear of the trabecular meshwork and cause tissue from the inner wall of Schlemm's canal to accumulate in the gap of the footplate. In addition, the surgeon should make sure that the eye does not rotate during the treatment, as this indicates excessive pressure on the posterior wall of Schlemm's canal.

Many surgeons advocate the use of pilocarpine 1% 1 to 2 hours prior to Trabectome-only surgery to improve surgical visualization of the angle and to protect the crystalline lens in phakic patients. Postoperatively, pilocarpine can enhance aqueous outflow and prevent the development of peripheral anterior synechiae. The tapering of glaucoma medications is generally undertaken approximately 1 month after surgery.
The procedure has a learning curve, especially for surgeons not familiar with operating temporally or with various patient head positions.

**Complications**

Transient hyphemas are the typical complication, clearing within a few days. Other complications are rare in this procedure, but can include iridodialysis, cyclodialysis, and IOP spike. Sustained hyphema, wound leak, infection, choroidal effusion, and hemorrhage are not typically seen after this procedure.

### 5.5 Scientific evidence so far

Minckler et al reported a retrospective case series of 1127 Trabectome surgeries, with 738 Trabectome-only and 366 Trabectome-cataract surgeries. (Minckler et al., 2008) Overall, IOP reduced to 39% at 24 months (n=50), and with Trabectome only cases (n=46) the reduction was 40%. Surgery combined with cataract removal (n=45) showed an 18% decrease in IOP at 12 months. Medications were decreased by at least half in each cohort.
Francis et al for the Trabectome study group reported the short-term results of combined phacoemulsification and trabeculotomy by the internal approach with a follow-up to 21 months. (Francis et al., 2008) This prospective interventional case series comprised of 304 consecutive eyes with open-angle glaucoma and cataract having combined phacoemulsification and trabeculotomy with a Trabectome. The mean IOP was 20.0 mm Hg ±6.3 (SD) preoperatively, 14.8±3.5 mm Hg at 6 months, and 15.5±2.9 mm Hg at 1 year. There was a corresponding drop in glaucoma medications from 2.65±1.13 at baseline to 1.76±1.25 at 6 months and 1.44±1.29 at 1 year. Subsequent secondary glaucoma procedures were performed in 9 patients. The only frequent complication, blood reflux in 239 patients (78.4%), resolved within a few days.
Previous laser trabeculoplasty does not appear to significantly impact IOP, but may increase the need for glaucoma medication in patients undergoing Trabectome surgery (Vold and Dustin, 2010).

### 5.6 Place in surgical armamentarium

Early clinical experience with this technology has shown that patient selection, surgical technique, and postoperative medical management affect patients' outcomes. Though it is efficacious in IOP lowering, we still do not know what is the maximal amount of IOP lowering that can be attained, and whether this relates to other factors such as episcleral venous pressure.

### 5.7 Canaloplasty

Canaloplasty is an *ab externo* procedure which entails 360° intubation of Schlemm's canal, along with suture-assisted distension of the canal in order to restore physiologic outflow via the conventional pathway without the formation of a fistula or bleb (Khaimi, 2009). The iTrack 250 flexible microcatheter (iScience Interventional, Menlo Park, CA) for canaloplasty received FDA approval in 2008.

**Device**

The iScience device has a 45-mm working length flexible polymer microcatheter of 200-mm shaft diameter with a rounded 250-mm tip diameter (Figure 6).The catheter consists of a central support wire designed to provide a backbone for guidance during advancement and to add resistance to potential kinking of the microcatheter. The optical fibers in the microcatheter allow for transmission of a red blinking light from a laser-based micro-illumination system to the tip to assist in visualization and localization of the tip during passage. The microcatheter possesses a true lumen for the delivery of substances such as viscoelastic to expand the canal during passage or retraction. The proximal end of the device connects to the nonsterile laser-based micro-illumination light source on a mayo stand from one arm, with another arm connected to a sterile screw-mechanism syringe designed to assist in controlled injection of viscoelastic into Schlemm's canal.

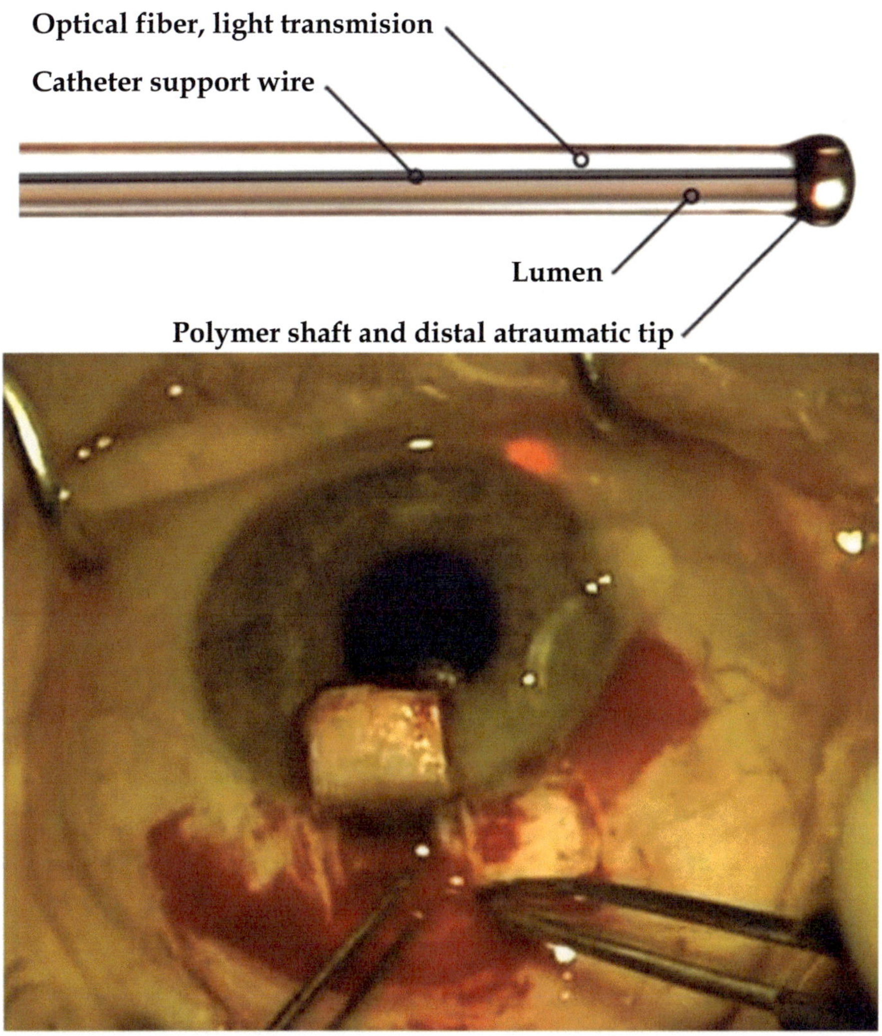


Fig. 6. iTrack250A canaloplasty microcatheter

**Indications**

- Mild-to-moderate open angle glaucoma
- Pigmentary glaucoma (Ichhpujani et al., 2011)
- Pseudoexfoliative glaucoma

**Contraindications**

- Scarring from prior trabeculectomy
- Patients with obvious scarring in Schlemm's canal due to prior medication use, laser, surgery or corneoscleral trauma at the limbus
- Anomalies in the anterior chamber angle

**Surgical procedure**

The chosen surgical site is the superior sclera and hence a traction suture is needed for maintaining a downgaze position. For a corneal traction a careful site selection is required so as to ensure the suture is placed several clock hours away from the intended surgical site.

A fornix based conjunctival peritomy is done leaving an anterior skirt of conjunctiva attached to the limbus with blunt dissection carried out posteriorly. Light wet field cautery is applied to the sclera, being careful to avoid aqueous and ciliary veins. A superficial parabolic scleral flap of approximately 5 mm anterior–posterior length by 5 mm width and one-third scleral thickness is fashioned with the help of a crescent knife, forward into clear cornea. A deep inner scleral flap is then created approximately 1 mm inside from the edge of the superficial scleral flap. An approximately 100 mm thick layer of sclera should be left covering the choroid at the base of the deep dissection. Once the white limbus-parallel fibers of the scleral spur are visible at the deep dissection, fibers of the outer wall of Schlemm's canal should be visible by lifting of the deep flap with a toothed forceps. A paracentesis incision should be made in the clear cornea to lower the IOP to prevent outward bulging of Descemet's membrane and the inner wall of Schlemm's canal, reducing the likelihood of penetration into the anterior chamber during the ensuing delicate dissection. The deep flap is now advanced forward approximately another 1 mm to expose Descemet's membrane. Mermoud forceps can be used to delicately strip the inner wall of Schlemm's canal away. The corneal stroma should be separated from Descemet's window with surgical sponges such as Merocel. Once the window has been fashioned, the underside of the deep flap is scored with a sharp tip blade at the very anterior aspect and cut off with Vannas scissors. Each cut end of Schlemm's canal is then intubated with a 150-mm outer bore viscocanalostomy cannula, and a miniscule amount of high viscosity sodium hyaluronate is injected into each end to dilate the ostia and facilitate entrance of the iScience device into the canal.

With the help of nontoothed forceps, the microcatheter is introduced into one of the cut ends of Schlemm's canal and advanced 360° until the tip emerges from the other cut end of the canal. In a minority of patients successful catheterisation through the entirety of the canal fails. At times the microcatheter may pass into the suprachoroidal space posterior to Schlemm's canal. In such cases, the catheter should be immediately retracted and passage attempted in the opposite direction. Once the microcatheter has been passed 360° and the tip has emerged, a 10–0 Prolene suture with the needles cut off is tied around the shaft of the device near the tip with the two loose ends tied to the loop. The device is then withdrawn slowly from the opposite direction with controlled injection of viscoelastic every 2-3 clock hours, taking care not to cause Descemet's detachment.

Once the catheter has been removed, the 10–0 Prolene is cut from the tip, leaving two single 10–0 Prolene sutures in the canal with two loose ends emerging from each cut end of

Schlemm's canal. Each suture is tied to itself in a slipknot fashion with some back and forth movement in the canal, known as "flossing, " to ensure that the suture sits anteriorly in Schlemm's canal. Suture tension is then assessed by pulling the suture knot posteriorly, until it is only barely able to reach the scleral spur. Suture tension is felt to play an important role in canaloplasty, where a greater suture tension results in more distension of Schlemm's canal with resultant greater IOP reduction and increased flow. The superficial scleral flap is then placed back into position and sutured in a watertight fashion with interrupted 10–0 nylon sutures. Conjunctiva is also closed in a water tight fashion with 10-0 vicryl sutures.

**Complications**

In trabeculectomy the natural anterior chamber fluid outflow is by-passed via an artificial fistula. Unlike trabeculectomy, canaloplasty attempts to re-establish the physiological anterior chamber fluid draining system by means of dilation of Schlemm's canal and its collector channels. If the anterior chamber pressure temporarily lowers the level of the venous capillary pressure, it is consistent with a patent piping system when a reverse flow with blood reflux into the anterior chamber can be observed as long as a minimal physiological pressure gradient from the anterior chamber in the direction of channel Schlemm's canal has been restored. Thus, an anterior chamber haemorrhage shows the desired consistency of the draining system and hence it should logically be expected after each successful procedure where hypotony in the postoperative period occurs. (Koch et al., 2010)

The surgery is technically challenging and hence there is a learning curve. Microhyphema (7.9%), early and late IOP elevations (7.9% and 2.4%, respectively), wound hemorrhage (2.4%), suture extrusion (1.6%), Descemet membrane detachment (DMD) (1.6%), and hypotony (0.8%) have been reported. (Grieshaber et al., 2010; Palmiero et al., 2010) Trabeculo-Descemet window fibrosis may occur in postoperative course.

### 5.8 Scientific evidence so far

Lewis and coworkers reported 3-year results of the safety and efficacy of canaloplasty either as a standalone procedure or in combination with cataract surgery in adult open angle glaucoma subjects. (Lewis et al., 2011) Three years postoperatively, all study eyes (n = 157) had a mean IOP of 15.2 mm Hg ± 3.5 (SD) and mean glaucoma medication use of 0.8 ± 0.9 compared with a baseline IOP of 23.8 ± 5.0 mm Hg on 1.8 ± 0.9 medications. Eyes with combined cataract-canaloplasty surgery had a mean IOP of 13.6 ± 3.6 mm Hg on 0.3 ± 0.5 medications compared with a baseline IOP of 23.5 ± 5.2 mm Hg on 1.5 ± 1.0 medications. Intraocular pressure and number of medication, in all eyes were significantly decreased from baseline at every time point ($P<0.001$). Late postoperative complications included cataract (12.7%), transient IOP elevation (6.4%), and partial suture extrusion through the trabecular meshwork (0.6%).

Koerber reported a comparative case series of 30 eyes of 15 adult patients with bilateral primary open-angle glaucoma who underwent canaloplasty in one eye and viscocanalostomy in the contralateral eye. (Koerber, 2011) With a follow-up period of 18 months, both the canaloplasty and viscocanalostomy groups showed statistically significant reductions in mean IOP ($P<0.01$) and number of supplemental medications ($P<0.01$) as compared with preoperative values. In the canaloplasty cohort, eyes had a mean IOP of 14.5±2.6 mm Hg on 0.3±0.5 medications at 18 months postoperatively as compared with preoperative levels of 26.5±2.7 mm Hg on 2.1±1.0 medications. In the viscocanalostomy cohort, eyes had a mean IOP of 16.1±3.9 mm Hg on 0.4±0.5 medications at 18 months as compared with preoperative levels of 24.3±2.8 mm Hg on 1.9±0.8 medications ($P=0.02$). No patient in either cohort

experienced significant complications. The author concluded that canaloplasty showed slightly better efficacy to viscocanalostomy in the reduction of IOP (P=0.02).
Grieshaber and coworkers have shown that Canaloplasty produced a sustained long-term reduction of IOP in 60 eyes of black Africans with POAG independent of preoperative IOP. (Grieshaber et al., 2010)

### 5.9 Place in surgical armamentarium

The analogy of cardiac surgery is most appropriate to educate patients. In some patients, cardiac surgeons can stent or dilate the obstructed vessel with a less invasive angioplasty, while in others with more serious disease, surgeons may have to open the chest and perform a more complex procedure." For glaucoma patients, this means transitioning from canaloplasty to trabeculectomy.

## 6. Deeplight gold micro shunt

**Device**

The GMS (SOLX Ltd, Boston, Massachusetts) is a nonvalved flat-plate drainage device made from 24-K medical-grade (99.95%) gold. The device is composed of two leaflets fused together vertically concealing nine channels within the body that connect the anterior openings to the posterior ones (Figure 7). Two different models of the device exist, the GMS (XGS-5) and the GMS Plus (XGS-10), both measuring 5.2 mm long, 2.4 mm wide anteriorly and 3.2 mm wide posteriorly, but differing in weight and channel size. The XGS-5 model weighs 6.2 mg and is 60mm in thickness with the channels measuring 25mm in width and 44mm in height while the XGS-10 model weighs 9.2 mg and the channels measure 25mm in width by 68mm in height. Aqueous humor from the anterior chamber exiting through the uveoscleral pathway to the suprachoroidal space is enhanced by this device by allowing fluid to travel both through the channels in the shunt and also around the body of the shunt. (Melamed et al., 2009)

**Indications**

The suprachoroidal space appears to be an excellent pathway option for those patients who have had failed trabeculectomy or Schlemm's canal procedures.

**Contraindications**

- Recent angle closure glaucoma episode
- Uveitic glaucoma, iridocorneal endothelial syndrome, traumatic glaucoma, or neovascular glaucoma
- Other significant ocular disease, except cataract
- Active ocular infection
- Expected ocular surgery in next 12 months
- No suitable quadrant for implant

**Surgical procedure**

After a 4 mm fornix-based conjunctival peritomy, an approximately 3.5 mm scleral incision is created 2 mm posterior to the limbus or slightly further posteriorly in high myopes (can be inserted in any quadrant but easier in superotemporal quadrant). The dissection is carried out to near full thickness depth, where the choroid is visible through a thin layer of sclera. A scleral pocket at 95% depth is then created by tunneling anteriorly towards the scleral spur. At this point, a vertical incision is made into the choroidal space and a small amount of suprachoroidal anesthesia and viscoelastic are administered with a blunt cannula. Via a sideport incision viscoelastic is filled in the anterior chamber at the anticipated site of entry of the gold shunt. Alternatively, an AC maintainer can be used and an entry is made into the anterior chamber at the level of the scleral spur through the previously constructed scleral tunnel.

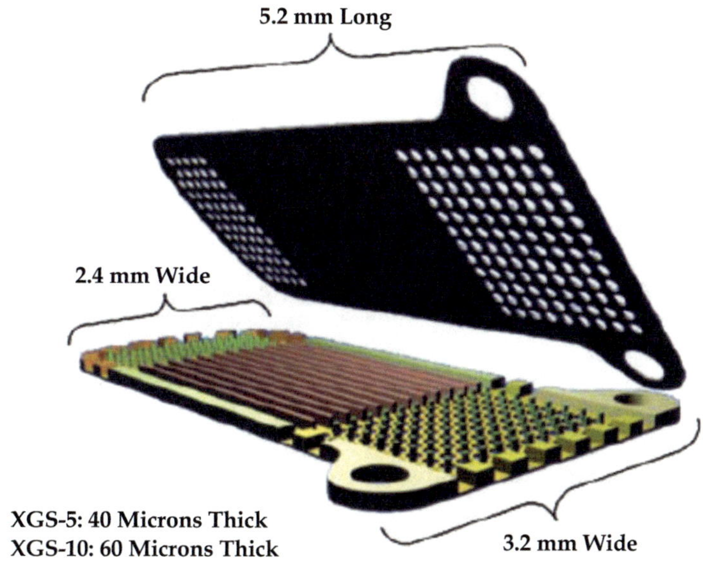


Fig. 7. Gold microshunt

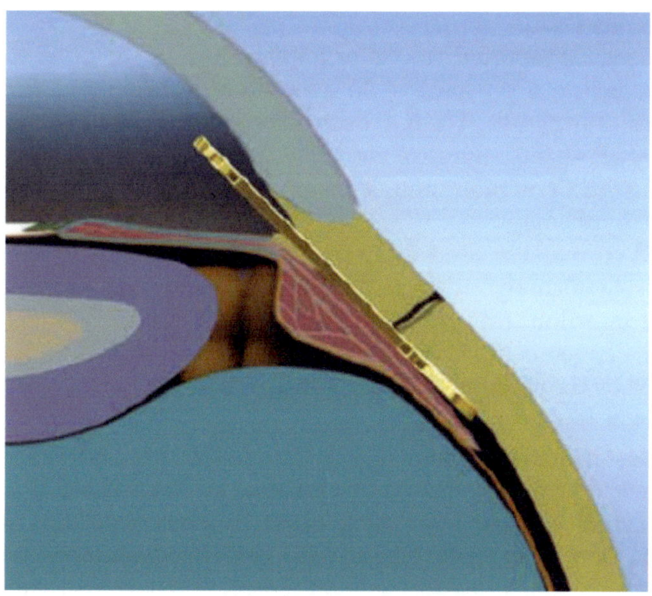

Fig. 8. Cross-section of eye showing correct GMS position

The shunt is placed through the scleral incision, ensuring the head of the device is in the anterior chamber (Figure 8). Positioning of the shunt is achieved posteriorly in the suprachoroidal space using a sharp 27-gauge needle against the shunt to gently encourage it into the suprachoroidal pocket expanded previously by viscoelastic while grasping the wound with a toothed forceps. A "Push then pull" approach works well while inserting the shunt through scleral incision in the anterior chamber.
Alternatively, an instrument such as a Sinskey hook can be utilized on the lateral positioning holes. All of the shunt openings on the posterior aspect should be concealed under the posterior scleral lip of the wound. The anterior aspect of the wound can also be manipulated through the anterior chamber to aid in positioning of the shunt. Intraoperative gonioscopy can help to confirm the proper and intended positioning of the gold shunt in the anterior chamber.
The overlying scleral wound is tightly sutured with 4–5 interrupted 10-0 nylon sutures to ensure watertight closure, as subconjunctival reservoir is not the intended mode of filtration in this surgical procedure. Finally, a 10-0 vicryl horizontal mattress suture is placed to reappose conjunctiva. The crescent-shaped anterior aspect of the shunt consists of a positioning hole, which can be used to adjust shunt positioning with an instrument such as a Sinskey hook. The posterior aspect of the shunt likewise possesses two lateral wings for shunt manipulation. Flow is directed through and around the shunt via the natural pressure gradient from the anterior chamber to the suprachoroidal space.
Placement of GMS in anterior chamber allows future access with 790nm Ti: sapphire laser and goniolens to selectively open specific windows.

**Complications**

Mild hyphema, hypotony, choroidal effusion, haemorrhage or detachment and shunt migration have been noted in few cases, in decreasing order of their occurrence.

### 6.1 Surgical evidence so far

Melamed and colleagues reported results of implantation of the GMS in 38 patients with uncontrolled glaucoma in a prospective 2-center study. (Melamed et al., 2009) The mean follow-up time was 11.7 months. The IOP decreased a mean (SD) of 9 mmHg from 27.6 (4.7) to 18.2 (4.6) mmHg (P <0.001). Surgical success was achieved in 30 patients (79%) (IOP >5 and <22 mm Hg, with or without antiglaucoma medication). Eight patients had mild to moderate transient hyphema.
Mastropasqua and co workers used in vivo confocal microscopy to show that successful GMS implantation significantly increased conjunctival microcysts density and surface at the site of the device insertion. (Mastropasqua et al., 2010) These findings suggest that the enhancement of the aqueous filtration across the sclera may be one of the possible outflow pathways exploited by the shunt.

### 6.2 Place in surgical armamentarium

The European Agency for the Evaluation of Medicinal Products (EMEA) gave this shunt CE approval in October 2005. It is undergoing Phase III trials in USA. The results till date appear promising. One of the advantages with gold micro-shunt is that in addition to working as an implantable microscopic shunt, the level of IOP control can be titrated by the laser. Additional micro channels can be opened with the laser in the clinicians' office.

### 6.3 EYEPASS Bi-Directional glaucoma implant

**Device**

The Eyepass Bi-Directional glaucoma implant (GMP Vision Solutions, Inc.) consists of a dual 6.0 mm long silicone tube bonded at 1 end for less than 1.0 mm, creating a Y-shape (Figure 9). (Dietlein et al., 2008) The inner diameter of the silicone tube is 125 μm and the outer diameter is 250 μm, making the tube narrow enough to fit the lumen of the Schlemm canal. The implant is sterilized by gamma radiation and is a single-use device that should be stored at a temperature between 15°C and 30°C.

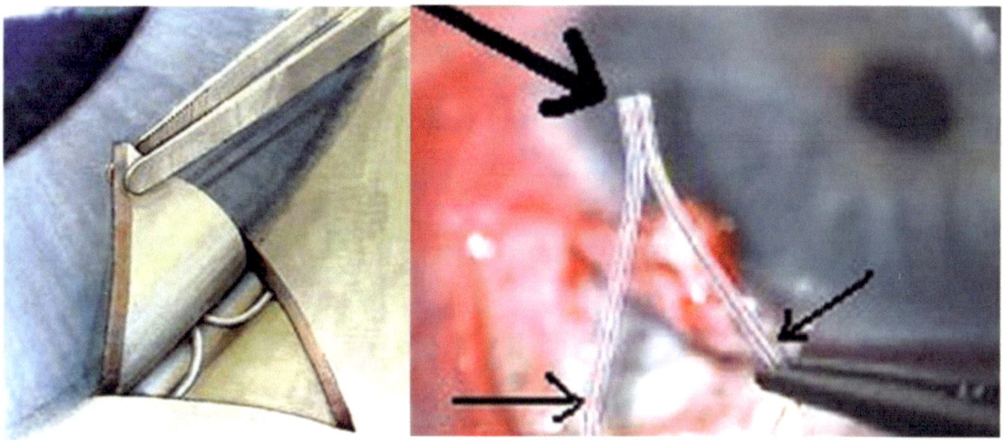

Fig. 9. Eyepass bidirectional implant

**Surgical procedure**

It can be used as a standalone procedure or in combination with cataract surgery. After a fornix-based superomedial conjunctival dissection and a mild wet field cautery, a two-third thickness triangular scleral flap with a 4 mm basis is dissected. Before the Schlemm canal is unroofed, clear corneal cataract surgery is performed. This is followed by the Schlemm canal unroofing by dissecting a second scleral flap or by opening the canal with small Vannas scissors. Before the Eyepass device is implanted in both lumina of the Schlemm canal, the openings on both sides of the canal are dilated by gentle injection of an OVD such as sodium hyaluronate 1.0% [Healon] through a viscocanalostomy cannula. Thereafter, the arms of the "Y" are inserted into the lumina of the Schlemm canal without exerting pressure in the direction of the anterior chamber. After both ends are buried in the Schlemm canal, the bonded end is inserted into the anterior chamber via a paracentesis almost 1.0 mm from the trabecular meshwork, toward the center of the anterior chamber and under the scleral flap. The implant does not need to be secured by sutures. The scleral flap is sutured to a watertight fit using interrupted 10-0 nylon sutures. The conjunctiva is closed with 8-0 polyglactin (Vicryl) sutures at the limbus.

**Complications**

The implant actually acts as a wick underneath the scleral flap, encouraging transscleral filtration in the early days after surgery; hence early postoperative hypotony may occur. Intraoperative perforation of the trabecular meshwork may also occur. Since this procedure entails conjunctival dissection, it may compromise other future ab-externo glaucoma surgery.

### 6.4 Surgical evidence so far

Dietlein et al conducted a small study to evaluate the safety and pressure-reducing efficacy of the Y-shaped Eyepass glaucoma implant in 12 glaucoma and cataract patients and found that combined cataract surgery with Eyepass shunt implantation was safe and appeared to be beneficial in glaucomatous eyes with cataract not requiring a low target IOP. (Dietlein et al., 2008) Perforation of the trabecular meshwork during Eyepass implantation occurred in 2 eyes requiring explantation and conversion to trabeculectomy. In the remaining 10 eyes, the mean maximum IOP was 30.4 mm Hg preoperatively, 12.0 mm 1 day postoperatively, 17.2 mm Hg at 4 weeks, and 18.3 mm at the end of the preliminary follow-up.
In case of trabecular meshwork perforation while inserting an arm of Eyepass, whether opening just 1 arm of the canal could achieve sufficient degree of surgical success is yet to be ascertained. Over the long term, the transscleral filtration seems to play a minor role in the IOP reducing effect of the Eyepass implant because of scarring and no antimetabolite induced favourable wound modulation. Role of antimetabolites to improve transscleral filtration is questionable at present.

### 6.5 Place in surgical armamentarium

The implant is currently undergoing Phase III trials.

## 7. Cypass micro stent

**Device**

Cypass (Transcend) is made from a biocompatible material (polyimide) and features a unique delivery system. The CyPass is a micro-implantable device, 6 mm in length, with a small lumen of 300 ìm (Figure 10). It allows for an *ab interno* surgical approach, which spares the conjunctiva, does not penetrate the sclera and leaves the trabecular meshwork intact.

**Surgical procedure**

It is implanted in the suprachoroidal space through a clear corneal incision, which coincides with the phacoemulsification incision in combined procedures. A special inserter is used to make the distal end of the device penetrate into the suprachoroidal space, while the proximal collar remains in the anterior chamber. Three rings on the collar keep the device in place, preventing movement.

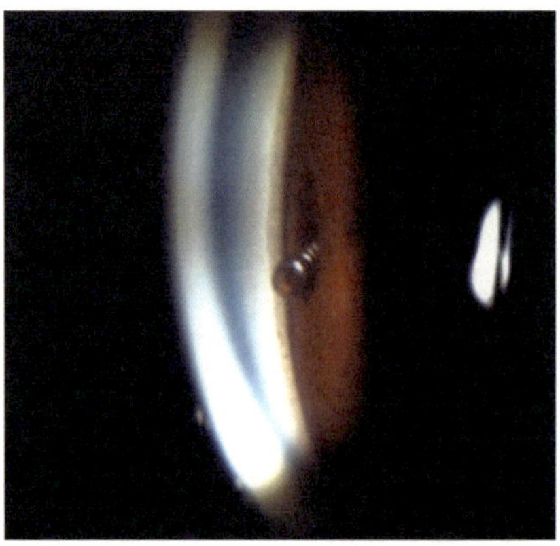

Fig. 10. Cypass microstent

### 7.1 Scientific evidence so far

Early clinical results, with the Cypass being placed in combination with cataract surgery (study by Transcend; unpublished data), showed promising results, with a 42% IOP decrease and a 60% decrease in medication use at six months.

**Ongoing clinical trials**

**Combination cypass and cataract surgery trial (COMPASS):** Transcend's 480 patient domestic pivotal clinical trial, combines the Cypass and cataract surgery. Enrollment began in the second half of 2009 and the company hopes to complete it by the end of 2011 or in early 2012.
**Cypass clinical evaluation trial (CYCLE):** This is a European prospective, non-randomized multi-center trial that includes "all-comers" with a goal to assess the Cypass in a broad variety of glaucoma patients.
**DUETTE:** This is another European trial. Evaluating two different versions of the Cypass in a prospective and randomized study.

**Place in surgical aramamentarium**

Cypass has been found to have few and minor complications compared with filtering procedures. In addition, it is a repeatable procedure, which leaves an intact superior conjunctiva, allowing filtering procedures to be performed at a later stage in case of failure. Preliminary findings need to be confirmed in prospective trials with larger series, evaluating long-term results.

## 8. Conclusion

The current gold standard, trabeculectectomy, has done well for many medically refractory glaucoma patients in the past 40 years. Despite its efficacy in lowering IOP, relatively easy learning curve, it is fraught with not only short time but lifetime potential sight threatening issues. Glaucomatologists and bioengineers are leaving no stone unturned to find a better alternative which addresses the flaws of trabeculectomy. Ex-PRESS glaucoma filtration implant, Trabectome electrocautery device, iStent, Canaloplasty, Gold microshunt and Eyepass bidirectional valve are few milestones along the path of finding an ideal glaucoma device. Although for most devices, the studies are ongoing and the verdict on long term safety and efficacy is awaited, the future definitely seems promising. One size does not fit all in glaucoma. Much remains to be resolved about all these new innovative procedures in glaucoma. It is not wise to abandon time-tested trabeculectomy but it's time to be more selective in choosing surgical procedures.

## 9. References

Ates, H, Palamar, M, Yagci, A, Egrilmez, S. (2010) Evaluation of Ex-PRESS mini glaucoma shunt implantation in refractory postpenetrating keratoplasty glaucoma. *J Glaucoma.*; 19:556-60.

Bagnis, A, Papadia, M, Scotto, R, Traverso, CE. (2011) Obstruction of the Ex-PRESS Miniature Glaucoma Device: Nd: YAG Laser as a Therapeutic Option. *J Glaucoma.* 2011 Mar 21. (Epub ahead of print).

Bahler, CK, Smedley, GT, Zhou, J, Johnson, DH (2004). Trabecular bypass stents decrease intraocular pressure in cultured human anterior segments. *Am J Ophthalmol.*; 138:988–94.

Bissig, A, Feusier, M, Mermoud, A, Roy, S. (2010) Deep sclerectomy with the Ex-PRESS X-200 implant for the surgical treatment of glaucoma. *Int Ophthalmol.*; 30:661-8.

Borisuth, NS, Phillips, B, Krupin T. (1999). The risk profile of glaucoma filtration surgery. *Curr Opin Ophthalmol*, 10, 2:112–116.

Coleman, AL, Hill, R, Wilson, MR, et al (1995). Initial clinical experience with the Ahmed glaucoma valve implant. *Am J Ophthalmol*, 120:23–31.

Dahan, E, Carmichael, TR. (2005) Implantation of a miniature glaucoma device under a scleral flap. *J Glaucoma*; 14:98-102.

Dietlein, TS, Jordan, JF, Schild, A, et al. (2008) Combined cataract-glaucoma surgery using the intracanalicular Eyepass glaucoma implant: first clinical results of a prospective pilot study. *J Cataract Refract Surg.*; 34:247-52.

Epstein, DL, Melamed, S, Puliatio, CA, Steinert, RF. (1985). Neodymium: YAG laser trabeculopuncture in open-angle glaucoma. *Ophthalmology*, 92:931–937.

Fea, AM (2010). Phacoemulsification versus phacoemulsification with micro-bypass stent implantation in primary open-angle glaucoma: randomized double-masked clinical trial. *J Cataract Refract Surg.*, 36:407-12.

Fernández-Barrientos, Y, García-Feijoó, J, Martínez-de-la-Casa JM, Pablo LE, Fernández-Pérez C, García Sánchez J. (2010). Fluorophotometric study of the effect of the glaukos trabecular microbypass stent on aqueous humor dynamics. *Invest Ophthalmol Vis Sci.*, 51:3327-32.

Francis, BA, See, RF, Rao, NA, et al (2006). Ab interno trabeculectomy: development of a novel device (Trabectome) and surgery for open-angle glaucoma. *J Glaucoma.*15:68-73.

Francis, BA, Minckler, D, Dustin, L, Kawji, S, Yeh, J, Sit, A, Mosaed S, Johnstone M; (2008) Trabectome Study Group. Combined cataract extraction and trabeculotomy by the internal approach for coexisting cataract and open-angle glaucoma: initial results. *J Cataract Refract Surg.*; 34:1096-103.

Gandolfi S, Traverso CF, Bron A, Sellem E, Kaplan-Messas A, Belkin M. (2002) Short-term results of a miniature drainage implant for glaucoma in combined surgery with phacoemulsification. *Acta Ophthalmol Scand Suppl*; 236:66.

Garg, SJ, Kanitkar, K, Weichel, E, Fischer, D. Trauma-induced extrusion of an Ex-PRESS glaucoma shunt presenting as an intraocular foreign body. *Arch Ophthalmol* 2005; 123:1270-2.

Gedde, SJ, Schiffman, JC, Feuer, WJ, Herndon, LW, Brandt, JD, Budenz DL (2007). Treatment outcomes in the tube versus trabeculectomy study after one year of follow-up. *Am J Ophthalmol*, 143:9–22.

Geffen, N, Trope, GE, Alasbali, T, et al (2010). Is the EX-PRESS glaucoma device magnetic resonance imaging safe? *J Glaucoma*, 19:116-118.

Gindroz, F, Roy, S, Mermoud, A, Schnyder, CC (2011).Combined Ex-PRESS LR-50/IOL implantation in modified deep sclerectomy plus phacoemulsification for glaucoma associated with cataract. *Eur J Ophthalmol.*, 21:12-9.

Grieshaber, MC, Pienaar, A, Olivier, J, Stegmann, R. (2010) Canaloplasty for primary open-angle glaucoma: long-term outcome. *Br J Ophthalmol.*, 94:1478-82.

Ichhpujani, P, Katz, LJ, Gille, R, Affel, E (2010). Imaging modalities for localization of an iStent (®). *Ophthalmic Surg Lasers Imaging*, 41:660-3.

Ichhpujani, P, Barahimi, B, Shields, CL, Eagle, RC Jr, Katz LJ (2011). Canaloplasty for pigmentary glaucoma with coexisting conjunctival lymphoma. *Ophthalmic Surg Lasers Imaging*. Feb 10; 42 Online:e10-1. doi: 10.3928/15428877-20110203-01.

Jordan, JF, Engels, BF, Dinslage, S, et al (2006). A novel approach to suprachoroidal drainage for the surgical treatment of intractable glaucoma. *J Glaucoma*, 15:200–205.

Kaplan-Messas, A, Traverso, CF, Sellem, E, Zbigniew, Z, Belkin, M. (2002) The Ex-PRESS ™ miniature glaucoma implant in combined surgery with cataract extraction: prospective study. *Invest Ophthalmol Vis Sci*; 43:3348A

Kanner, EM, Netland, PA, Sarkisian, SR, et al (2009). Ex-PRESS miniature glaucoma device implanted under a sclera flap alone or combined with phacoemulsification cataract surgery. *J Glaucoma.*; 18:488–491.

Koch, JM, Heiligenhaus, A, Heinz, C. (2010) Canaloplasty and Transient Anterior Chamber Haemorrhage: a Prognostic Factor? *Klin Monbl Augenheilkd.* Nov 16. [Epub ahead of print]

Koerber, NJ (2011). Canaloplasty in One Eye Compared With Viscocanalostomy in the Contralateral Eye in Patients With Bilateral Open-angle Glaucoma. *J Glaucoma.* Jan 26. [Epub ahead of print]

Khaimi, MA. (2009) Canaloplasty using iTrack 250 Microcatheter with Suture Tensioning on Schlemm's Canal. *Middle East Afr J Ophthalmol.*; 16:127-9.

Krejci, L. (1972) Cyclodialysis with hydroxyethyl methacrylate capillary strip. *Ophthalmologica*; 164:113–121.

Krupin, T, Podos, SM, Becker, B, Newkirk, JB. (1976). Valve implants in filtering surgery. *Am J Ophthalmol*, 81:232–235.

Kupin, TH, Juzych, MS, Shin, DH, Khatana, AK, Olivier, MM (1995).Adjunctive mitomycin C in primary trabeculectomy in phakic eyes. *Am J Ophthalmol*, 119:30–39.

Lankaranian, D, Razeghinejad, MR, Prasad, A, et al (2010). Intermediate-term results of the Ex-PRESS miniature glaucoma implant under a scleral flap in previously operated eyes. *Clin Experiment Ophthalmol.* Dec 22. doi: 10.1111/j.1442-9071.2010.02481.x. [Epub ahead of print].

Lewis, RA, von Wolff, K, Tetz, M, et al (2007). Canaloplasty: circumferential viscodilation and tensioning of Schlemm's canal using a flexible microcatheter for the treatment of open-angle glaucoma in adults: interim clinical study analysis. *J Cataract Refract Surg*; 33:1217–1226.

Lewis, RA, von Wolff, K, Tetz, M, et al. (2011) Canaloplasty: Three-year results of circumferential viscodilation and tensioning of Schlemm canal using a microcatheter to treat open-angle glaucoma. *J Cataract Refract Surg.*; 37:682-90.

Lloyd, MA, Baerveldt, G, Heuer, DK, et al. (1994). Initial clinical experience with the Baerveldt implant in complicated glaucomas. *Ophthalmology*, 101:640–650.

Maris, PJ, Jr, Ishida, K, Netland, PA. (2007) Comparison of trabeculectomy with Ex-PRESS miniature glaucoma device implanted under scleral flap. *J Glaucoma* 16: 14 - 19.

Mastropasqua, L, Agnifili, L, Ciancaglini, M, et al (2010). In vivo analysis of conjunctiva in gold micro shunt implantation for glaucoma. *Br J Ophthalmol.*; 94:1592-6.

Melamed, S, Ben Simon, GJ, Goldenfeld, M, Simon, G (2009).Efficacy and safety of gold micro shunt implantation to the supraciliary space in patients with glaucoma: a pilot study. *Arch Ophthalmol*; 127:264-9.

Minckler, DS, Mosaed, S, Dustin, L, Francis, BA. (2008) Trabectome (trabeculectomy-internal approach): additional experience and extended follow-up. *Trans Am Ophthalmol Soc.*106:1-12.

Molteno, ACB. (1969) New implant for drainage in glaucoma: clinical trial. *Br J Ophthalmol*, 53:606–615.

Netland, PA. Obstruction (Also Known as Occlusion or Blockage) of the Ex-PRESS Miniature Glaucoma Device. *J Glaucoma.* Mar 21. [Epub ahead of print]

Nichamin, LD. (2009) Glaukos iStent Trabecular Micro-Bypass. *Middle East Afr J Ophthalmol.*, 16 (3):138-40.

Nguyen, QH. Trabectome: a novel approach to angle surgery in the treatment of glaucoma. *Int Ophthalmol Clin*. Fall; 48:65-72.

Nyska, A, Glovinsky Y, Belkin M, Epstein Y. (2003) Biocompatibility of the Ex-PRESS miniature glaucoma drainage implant. *J Glaucoma*; 12:275-80.

Ozdamar, A, Aras, C, Karacorlu, M (2003). Suprachoroidal seton implantation in refractory glaucoma: a novel surgical technique. *J Glaucoma*; 12:354–359.

Palmiero, PM, Aktas, Z, Lee, O, Tello, C, Sbeity, Z (2010). Bilateral Descemet membrane detachment after canaloplasty. *J Cataract Refract Surg*.; 36:508-11.

Pinnas, G, Boniuk, M. (1969) Cyclodialysis with teflon tube implants. *Am J Ophthalmol*; 68:879–883.

Razeghinejad, MR, Spaeth, GL. (2011). A history of the surgical management of glaucoma. *Optom Vis Sci*., 88:E39-47.

Rivier, D, Roy, S, Mermoud, A. (2007). Ex-PRESS R-50 miniature glaucoma implant insertion under the conjunctiva combined with cataract extraction. *J Cataract Refract Surg*, 33:1946-52.

Samuelson, TW, Katz, LJ, Wells, JM, Duh, YJ, Giamporcaro JE (2010); US iStent Study Group. Randomized evaluation of the trabecular micro-bypass stent with phacoemulsification in patients with glaucoma and cataract. *Ophthalmology*.; 118:459-67.

Seibold, LK, Rorrer, RA, Kahook, MY. (2011). MRI of the Ex-PRESS stainless steel glaucoma drainage device. *Br J Ophthalmol*., 95:251-4.

Spiegel, D, Wetzel, W, Neuhann, T, et al. (2009).Coexistent primary open-angle glaucoma and cataract: interim analysis of a trabecular micro-bypass stent and concurrent cataract surgery. *Eur J Ophthalmol*., 19:393-9.

Spiegel, D, García-Feijoó, J, García-Sánchez, J, Lamielle, H. (2008). Coexistent primary open-angle glaucoma and cataract: preliminary analysis of treatment by cataract surgery and the iStent trabecular micro-bypass stent. *Adv Ther*.; 25:453-64.

Stewart, RM, Diamond, JG, Ashmore, ED, Ayyala, RS. (2005). Complications following Ex-PRESS glaucoma shunt implantation. *Am J Ophthalmol*, 140:340-1.

Tavolato, M, Babighian, S, Galan, A (2006). Spontaneous extrusion of a stainless steel glaucoma drainage implant (Ex-PRESS). *Eur J Ophthalmol*; 16:753-5.

Ticho, U, Ophir, A. (1993). Late complications after glaucoma filtering surgery with adjunctive 5-fluorouracil. *Am J Ophthalmol*, 115:506–510.

Traverso, CE, De Feo, F, Messas-Kaplan, A, Denis, P, Levartovsky, S, Sellem, E, *et al*. (2005) Long term effect on IOP of a stainless steel glaucoma drainage implant (Ex-PRESS) in combined surgery with phacoemulsification. *Br J Ophthalmol*; 89:425-9.

Wamsley, S, Moster, MR, Rai, S, Alvim, HS, Fontanarosa, J. (2004) Results of the use of the Ex-PRESS miniature glaucoma implant in technically challenging, advanced glaucoma cases: a clinical pilot study. *Am J Ophthalmol*; 138:1049-51.

Wamsley, S, Moster, MR, Rai, S, Alvim, H, Fontanarosa, J, Steinmann, WC. (2004). Optonol Ex-PRESS miniature tube shunt in advanced glaucoma. *Invest Ophthalmol Vis Sci*; 45:994A.

Vetrugno, M, Ferreri, P, Sborgia, C (2010). Ex-PRESS miniature glaucoma device in vitrectomized eyes. *Eur J Ophthalmol*.; 20:945-7.

Vetrugno, M, Ferreri, P, Cardascia, N, Sborgia, C. (2011)Surgical reposition of a dislocated Ex-PRESS miniature device. *Eur J Ophthalmol*.; 21:212-4.

Vold, SD, Dustin, L. Impact of laser trabeculoplasty on trabectome ((r)) outcomes. *Ophthalmic Surg Lasers Imaging*. 2010; 41:443-51.

# 21

# Cyclodestructive Procedures

Sima Sayyahmelli and Rakhshandeh Alipanahi
*From the Glaucoma Division, Tabriz Medical Sciences University, Tabriz, Iran*

## 1. Introduction

Several method used when an initial filtering procedure is not adequate to control the refractory glaucoma and when resumption of medical therapy,revision of original surgery, repeat filtering surgery at a new site, or aqueous shunt implantation is not successful; finally all cyclodestructive procedures reduce aqueous secretion by destroying part of the secretory ciliary epithelium portion of the ciliary body including cyclocryotherapy, contact and non-contact trans-scleral thermal lasers such as continuous-wave with the 1064-nm Nd:YAG, argon, and portable 810-nm semiconductor Diode laser.[1-4] Cryotherapy, the original technique, is increasingly being supplanted by laser photocoagulation, originally with the 1064-nm Nd:YAG laser and lately with the portable 810-nm semiconductor Diode laser.[2-3] An endoscopic laser delivery system has been advocated for use with cataract surgery or in pediatric, pseudophakic, or aphakic eyes. Use of the argon laser aimed at the ciliary processes through a goniolens is possible in a small percentage of patients. Transcleral diod laser cyclophotocoagulation (CPC ) reducing aqueous secretion by destroying, is generally considered to be better tolerated and perhaps more effective than cyclocryotherapy, and it has a lower incidence of complications such as postoperative pain, inflammation, phthisis bulbi and retinal detachment, possibly because of better absorption of this wave length by the pigmented tissues of the ciliary body. Diode laser cyclophotocoagulation (CPC) is often the choice treatment of lOP-lowering in painful blind eyes or in eyes unlikely to respond to other modes of therapy. Interventions methods such as retrobulbar alcohol injection, retrobulbar chlorpromazine injection, or enucleation are rarely performed now because of improved CPC techniques. Treatment of glaucoma in the pediatric population is frequently challenging and may require multiple surgical interventions. In the past it was used mainly in uncontrolled end-stage secondary glaucoma with minimal visual potential mainly to control pain. However it is now apparent that it can also be used in eyes with reasonably good vision which may be retained provided control of IOP is adequate. This section studies the indications, success rate and long term efficacy and complications of the cyclodestructive procedures in refractory glaucoma. Laser cycloablation is generally considered to be better tolerated and perhaps more effective than cyclocryotherapy.[3,4] The most commonly used technique for cyclodestructive surgery is the transscleral approach, in which the destructive element must pass through conjunctiva, sclera, and ciliary musculature, before reaching and destroying the ciliary processes. These procedures have the advantages of being noninvasive and relatively quick and easy because of variable success in adults (34-92%) and significant postoperative pain and complications including phthisis and retinal detachment, transscleral neodymium:YAG (Nd:YAG) and Diode lasers are replacing cyclocryotherapy as the preferred form of cyclodestruction in these eyes.[5-7] The cyclophotocoagulation has a lower incidence of complications such as pain, postoperative inflammation and phthisis bulbi, possibly because of better absorption of this wave length by the pigmented tissues of the ciliary body.[7-9] Several methods of Diode laser photocyclocoagulation have been reported to lower IOP and reduce pain in the eyes of refractory glaucoma Diode cyclophotocoagulation and sequential tube shunt following primary tube shunt failure in childhood glaucoma showed similar efficacy and complication rates. Ten to fifty percent of patients with primary congenital glaucoma fail goniotomy surgery and require further surgical intervention, Childhood glaucoma associated with systemic or ocular anomalies and secondary glaucoma such as that associated with congenital aphakia or pseudophakia have a worse surgical prognosis compared to primary congenital glaucoma. Trabeculectomy surgery with adjunctive mitomycin has a lower chance of successful control of children less than two years of age and in children who have had congenital cataract surgery. Additionally, compared to adults, the adjunctive use of anti-fibrotic agents with trabeculectomy in children may be associated with greater risk of late bleb-related infections. When a tube shunt fails to adequately control the intraocular pressure, limited treatment options remain. These options include a sequential tube shunt in another quadrant of the eye revision or replacement of the existing tube shunt, or a cyclodestructive procedure (usually transscleral or endoscopic Diode cyclophotocoagulation or cyclocryotherapy). Both tube shunts and transscleral Diode cyclophotocoagulation have been examined for treatment of refractory pediatric glaucoma. Compare the results of Contact Diod Laser Cyclophotocoagulation Versus Cyclocryotherapy in Refractory Glaucoma.[10-15]

Ciliary ablation is indicated to lower lOP in eyes that have glaucoma resistant to conventional medical and surgical therapies (refractory glaucoma, neovascular glaucoma, congenital glaucoma, secondary glaucoma, Post-surgical glaucoma, poor visual potential or that are poor candidates for incisional surgery(because of the small risk of sympathetic ophthalmia), painful blind eyes or in eyes unlikely to respond to other modes of therapy were treated with transscleral Diode laser Cyclophotocoagulation (CPC).

Ciliary ablation is relatively contraindicated in eyes with good vision because of the risk of loss of visual acuity.

Preoperative evaluation is the same as for incisional glaucoma surgery.

## 2. Methods and considerations

All patients signed an informed consent for the Ciliary body ablation procedures, after an explanation of the risks and benefits. Cyclophotocoagulation was performed under local anaesthesia (A sub-Tenon or peri bulbar ) with the Laser settings arc 1.5-2 sec and 1500-2000 mW with semiconductor Diode laser system (810 nm laser wavelength) with a spherical polished tip oriented by a handpiece, "G-Probe.". Figures 1 and 2. Duration was set at 2000 ms (2 seconds), and the initial power setting was 1750 MW. After the edge of the probe is aligned with the limbus, approximately 17-19 applications are placed 270° around the limbus, with a power of 1.5-2 Wand a duration of approximately 2 seconds The power was increased in 250 MW increments to a maximum of 2000 MW until an audible 'popping' sound is heard, and then the power was reduced by 250 MW to just below that level. Approximately 2-40 burns arc (typically five per quadrant for 270 degrees of treatment) placed 1.2 mm posteriorly to the limbus over 180 °but avoiding the posterior ciliary nerves at 3 and 9 o'clock. In all cases, the probe tips were carefully examined. The Diode laser handpiece attachment from one manufacturer is shown in figure 2. A strong topical steroid is prescribed hourly on the day of treatment and then q.i.d. for 2 weeks. Oral non-steroidal anti-inIlammatory agents are prescribed for 2 days. Figure 1 showed cyclodestructive procedures to relieve pain. Figure 2 showed Semiconductor Diode laser. Figure 3 showed "G probe" handpiece for contact Diode TCP.

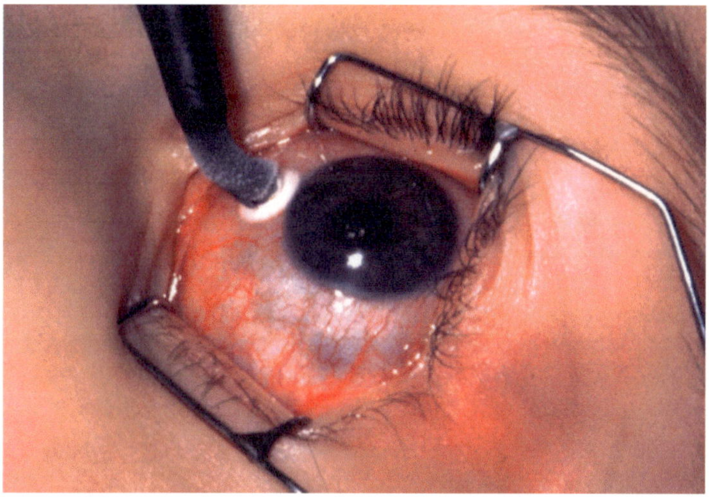

Fig. 1. Cyclodestructive procedures to relieve pain

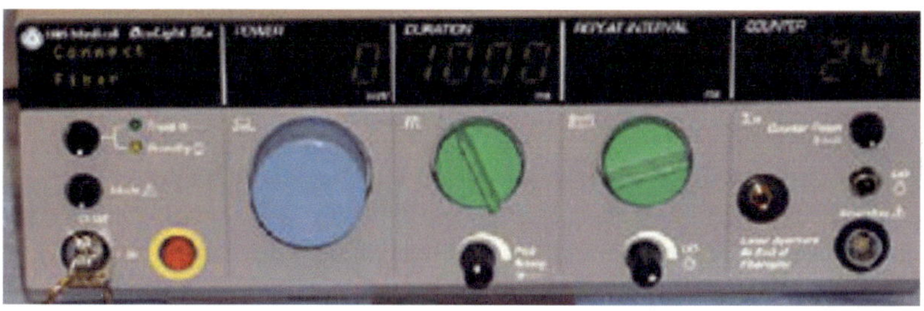

Fig. 2. Semiconductor Diode laser (IRIS Oculight SLx, Iris Medical Inc) for Diode contact TCP

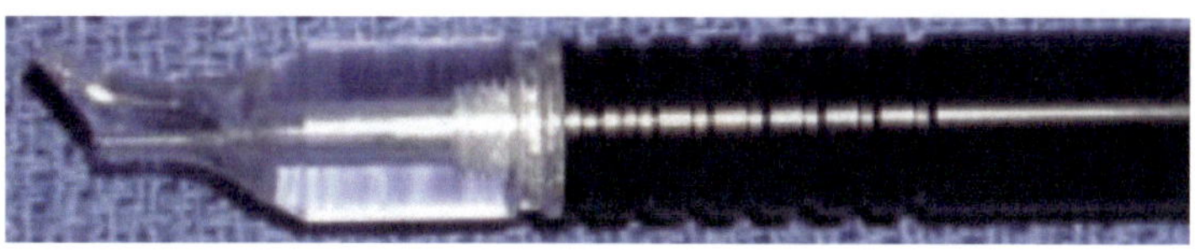

Fig. 3. Showed "G probe" handpiece for contact Diode TCP

Frequently more than one treatment session is required for adequate pressure control. The outcome of cycloDiode therapy was determined in terms of:

1. Success rate: defined as the percentage of eyes achieving and IOP between 5 and 21mm Hg with or without topical medication with cessation of oral carbonic anhydrase inhibitor use in all eyes after cycloDiode therapy at their final follow-up visit.

2. Response rate: defined as the percentage of patients achieving >30% drop from baseline IOP with cessation of oral carbonic anhydrase inhibitor use. This included eyes that developed hypotony (IOP<5mm Hg).
3. Failure rate: defined as percentage of patients who developed hypotony (IOP<5mm Hg) or phthisis, or those whose IOP drop was <30% from baseline.

The success rate is dependent on the type of glaucoma, frequently more than one treatment session is required for adequate pressure control and the procedure has to be repeated. Pain relief is generally good. After surgery intra ocular pressure and mean number of antiglaucoma medications would be dropped.

Criteria for success included intraocular pressure (IOP) of 21 mmHg or less with no devastating complications or need for further glaucoma surgery.

Pain following these procedures may be substantial, and patients should be provided with adequate analgesics, including narcotics, during the immediate postoperative period.

Cyclophotocoagulation may be associated with vision loss, prolonged hypotony, pain, inflammation, cystoid macular edema, hemorrhage, and even phthisis bulbi. Sympathetic ophthalmia is a rare but serious complication. Mildpostoperative pain and anterior segment innammation are common. Serious complications are rare and include conjunctival burns, prolonged uveitis, hyphema, chronic hypotony, phthisis bulbi, scleral thinning, corneal decompensation and retinal or choroidal detachment. However, since the aim of the procedure is usually to relieve pain. Vision-threatening complications do not have the same significance as those following conventional filtering procedures.

Transscleral Diode laser cycloablation is a recognized therapeutic approach to refractory glaucoma that involves photocoagulation of the pars plicata of the ciliary body with consequent reduction of aqueous secretion.[7,11] Diode laser cyclophotocoagulation appeared to be an effective and safe primary surgical treatment of medically uncontrolled chronic angle closure glaucoma, with intraocular pressure lowering effect persisting for up to two years.[16]

TSCPC has a significant ocular hypotensive effect on glaucoma refractory to both tube shunt and medical therapy.[17]

An unqualified success after cycloablation would be the attainment of a target IOP without the need for further medication, coupled with preservation of visual function. CycloDiode therapy appears to be effective in lowering IOP, in both the short and long term. Endoscopic cyclophotocoagulation (ECP) was introduced as an alternative to trans-scleral cyclophotocoagulation for treating refractory glaucomas in order to minimise complications such as phthisis and hypotony by providing direct visualisation of the ciliary processes. Glaucoma following penetrating keratoplasty, which has an incidence ranging from 10–52%, often proves refractory to medical treatment.1–3 We introduce a case of refractory post-PKP glaucoma in order to demonstrate the efficacy of ECP in treating post-PKP glaucoma and to describe its potential delayed effect in achieving intraocular pressure control Diode Laser Transscleral Cyclophotocoagulation as Primary Surgical Treatment for Medically Uncontrolled Chronic Angle Closure Glaucoma Long-Term Clinical Outcomes.[17] Endoscopic cyclophotocoagulation (ECP) was introduced as an alternative to trans-scleral cyclophotocoagulation for treating refractory glaucomas in order to minimise complications such as phthisis and hypotony by providing direct visualisation of the ciliary processes. Glaucoma following penetrating keratoplasty, which has an incidence ranging from 10–52%, often proves refractory to medical treatment.[1-3] We introduce a case of refractory post-PKP glaucoma in order to demonstrate the efficacy of ECP in treating post-PKP glaucoma and to describe its potential delayed effect in achieving intraocular pressure control Diode Laser Transscleral Cyclophotocoagulation as Primary Surgical Treatment for Medically Uncontrolled Chronic Angle Closure Glaucoma Long-Term Clinical Outcomes Diode Laser Transscleral Cyclophotocoagulation for Refractory Glaucoma.[18]

Contact Diode laser transscleral cyclophotocoagulation is useful in eyes with refractory glaucoma in which the risks of outflow surgery are deemed unacceptable, Diode laser transscleral cyclophotocoagulation (DCPC) is one of the most widely used methods of ciliary body ablation, with reported success rates ranging from 40% to 80% cyclodestructive procedures are generally reserved for eyes with glaucoma refractory to other forms of medical or surgical intervention. In the past 10 years, cyclocryotherapy has been replaced by other techniques, especially laser cyclophotocoagulation with Nd:YAG or Diode laser systems,[5-10] that achieve good results with a lower complication rate.[19-24] Diode laser transscleral cyclophotocoagulation is effective in lowering the intraocular pressure in chronic angle-closure glaucoma and its effect lasts for at least 1 year.[20] Transscleral Diode laser cyclophotocoagulation is an effective and safe method for the treatment of advanced, refractory glaucoma. However, repeated treatments are often necessary. Success of treatment depends on the age of patients, previous surgery, and the type of glaucoma.[21] Types of glaucoma that are often difficult to treat include neovascular glaucoma, posttraumatic glaucoma, glaucoma associated with aphakia severe congenital/developmental glaucoma, postretinal surgery glaucoma, glaucoma associated with penetrating keratoplasties, and glaucoma in eyes with scarred conjunctiva from surgery or disease processes.[22] Delgado et al. (2003) reported that use of noncontact transscleral neodymium:yttrium-aluminum-garnet cyclophotocoagulation for NVG in 115 eyes, while providing long-term IOP reduction, was associated with complications that included inflammation, visual loss, and hypotony, and that repeat treatments may be necessary to main good control of IOP.[27] Table 1showed demographics and treatment results of Transscleral diode laser cyclophotocoagulation at the different studies.

| | No. of eyes (%) | Age (yrs) (range) | Follow-up (mos) | Successfully treated eyes (%) | Reference number |
|---|---|---|---|---|---|
| A. Mistlberger et al | 93 | 9–92 | 12 | 74.2% | 19 |
| Mr J P Diamond et al | 263 | 4–99 | 17 | 89% | 15 |
| Ness et al | 32 | 22-92 | 17.1 | 28.6 | 17 |
| Bloom et al | 34 | | 34.1 | 34.1 | 9 |
| Sood and Beck | 9 | 1-15 | 12 | 66.7% | 13 |
| Jimmy et al | 14 | 48- 76 | 12 | 92.3% | 16 |
| T. Schlote et al. | 93 | 9–92 | 12 | 74.2% | 21 |
| F. A. Hauber and W. J. Scherer | 47 | 38–100 | 12 | 94.4%) | 24 |
| Ataullah, Biswas, Artes, et al | 53 | 6–90 | 23.1 | 84% | 25 |
| Iliev, Gerber | 131 | 69-84 | 30.1 | 69.5% | 26 |

Table 1. Demographics and treatment results of Transscleral diode laser cyclophotocoagulation at the different studies

Previous studies have demonstrated this, with ocular hypotensive responses.[7-9] Our study showed that in 50.6 % of patients the IOP was below 21 mmHg.
Complications of transscleral Diode CPC include conjunctival surface burns that may occur if tissue debris becomes coagulated on the tip and chars. We inspected all tips for this and found no debris. In addition, increased perilimbal conjunctival pigmentation may occur. One of patients had hypotony and phthisis after treatment 21 months after treatment. The risks of hypotony and phthisis are directly proportional to the dosage of laser energy delivered in a treatment session,[7] although, a clear relationship between treatment energy and IOP response, which is essential to accurate prediction of desirable effect, remains to be demonstrated. The published literature suggests that this type of treatment is usually reserved for eyes with end stage disease and poor visual potential. In conclusion, this study showed an increase of visual acuity after transscleral Diode laser cyclophotocoagulation therapy. Diode laser cyclophotocoagulation produces very characteristic injury to pars plicata, which frequently extends into pars plana, but with only mild persisting inflammation. Ciliary processes are, however, frequently spared within the treatment zone and may account for early or late treatment failure.[22-24]
Histopathological studies of enucleation specimens following laser cyclophotocoagulation (Diode and Nd:YAG laser) and cyclocryotherapy have been performed in humans [25-29] and animals.[12, 30-35] We have previously reported histopathology of two cases of clinical failure following Diode laser cyclophotocoagulation.[36] This study examines histological outcomes in nine cases in humans, and correlates this with the clinical c course in each eye.[28] Repeated use of the G-probe in transscleral cyclophotocoagulation, with ethylene oxide sterilization in between, resulted in an average decrease of 3% in laser energy delivered per repeated cycle of use up to the fourth cycle. No signs of physical damage were found.[25-28]
Laser G-probes remain functional after repeated use and ethylene oxide resterilization for up to four cycles. No visible physical damage to the probes was identified. It is safe and cost-effective to reuse G-probe for transscleral cyclophotocoagulation with ethylene oxide sterilization, provided the surgeon stays alert for signs of probe damage. This alertness should be retained regardless of whether new or old G-probes are used.[29-30] We noticed microscopic contamination of the G-probe by the tear film fluid in all the probes examined by us. The review of literature indicates that repeated use of the G-probe is not uncommon. The types of techniques used for making it suitable for repeated use indicate that it is not universally recognized that the lumen of the G-probe can accumulate fluid during the procedure, which makes it potentially hazardous when used for other patients.
Treatment with cyclophotocoagulation in patients with refractory glaucoma leads to increase in acuity and lower intraocular pressure. In our opinion the G-probe should not be reused as inadequately reprocessed G-probe can lead to risk of nosocomial infections, serious iatrogenic complications, and medico-legal problems.[30] Underlying diagnosis of neovascular glaucoma is a significant risk factor for hypotony post TCP. Hypotony was defined as IOP <5 at the end of 1-year follow-up period. Factors, such as underlying diagnosis, total energy used, age, earlier operations, and retreatment rates, which may influence the development of hypotony were analyzed using univariate analysis.[31-32]
CycloDiode therapy is highly effective but there is a significant risk of hypotony, which may be reduced by applying lower energy in cases of very high pretreatment IOP and in neovascular glaucoma.The dose-response association remains unpredictable, although a linear relation was found for neovascular glaucoma. Cyclophotocoagulation is necessary in some intractable cases but should be avoided whenever possible because of its potential

adverse effects on the lens and the retina. retrobulbar alcohol injection, retrobulbar chlorpromazine injection, or enucleation are rarely performed now because of improved CPC techniques.

## 3. References


[1] The Eye M,D, Association. Glaucoma In: Basic and Clinical Science Course; The American Academy of Ophthalmology: Copyright @2008. San Francisco LEO 2009; pp: 214-15.

[2] Kanski J. Glaucoma In Clinical Ophthalmology. 6th ed. Butherworth Heinmann Elsevier London, 2007. 429-431

[2] Youn J, Cox T, Herndon L, Allingham R, Shields M. (1998). A Clinical Comparison of Transscleral Cyclophotocoagulation with Neodymium: YAG and Semiconductor Diode Lasers. *Am J Ophthalmol, Vol.* 126, pp. 640-47.

[3] Kirwan J, Shah P, Khaw P. (2002) Diode Laser Cyclophotocoagulation: Role in the Management of Refractory Pediatric Glaucomas. *Ophthalmology, Vol.* 109, pp. 316-23.

[4] Semchyshyn T, Tsai J, Joos K. (2002) Supplemental Transscleral Diode Laser Cyclophotocoagulation after Aqueous Shunt Placement in Refractory Glaucoma *Ophthalmology,* Vol. 109, pp. 1078-84.

[5] Lai J, Tham C, Chan J, Lam D. (2005) Diode laser transscleral cyclophotocoagulation as primary surgical treatment for medically uncontrolled chronic angle closure glaucoma: long-term clinical outcomes. *Glaucoma,* Vol. 14, pp. 114-19.

[6] Waggle N, Freedman S, Buckley E, Davis J, Biglan A. (1998) Long-term outcome of Cyclocryotherapy for Refractory Pediatric Glaucoma. *Ophthalmology, Vol.* 105, pp. 1921- 27

[7] Vernon S, Koppens J, Menon J, Negi A. (2006) Diode laser cycloablation in adult a results of standard protocol and review of current literature. *Clinical and Experimental Ophthalmology, Vol.* 34, pp. 411-20.

[8] Agarwal H, Gupta V, Sihota R. (2004) Evaluation of contact versus non-contact Diode laser cyclophotocoagulation for refractory glaucomas using similar energy *Clin Exp Ophthalmol, Vol.* 32, pp. 33-38

[9] Bloom P, Tsai J, Sham K. Miller M. Rice N, Hitchings R. (1997) "Cycloid"Trans-scleral Diode laser cyclophotocoagulation in the treatment of advanced refractory glaucoma. *Ophthalmology, Vol.* 104, pp. 1519-29.

[10] Wong E, Chew P, Chee C, Wong J. (1997) Diode laser contact transscleral cyclophotocoagulation for refractory glaucoma in Asian patients. *Am J Ophthalmol, Vol.* 124, pp. 797-04.

[11] Goldenberg-Cohen N, Bahar I, Ostashinski M, Lusky M, Weinberger D, Gaton DD. (2005) Cyclocryotherapy versus transscleral Diode laser cyclophotocoagulation for uncontrolled intraocular pressure. *Ophthalmic Surg Lasers Imaging, Vol.* 36, pp. 272-9.

[12] Pastor S, Singh K, Lee D, Juzych M, Lin S, Netland P, et al. (2001) Cyclophotocoagulation A Report by the American Academy of Ophthalmology. *Ophthalmology,* Vol. 108, pp. 2130-36.

[13] Shalini Sood, MDa,b and Allen D. (2009) Cyclophotocoagulation versus sequential tube shunt as a secondary intervention following primary tube shunt failure in pediatric glaucoma, *J AAPOS.* Vol. 13, pp. 379–383.

[14] Cioffi G, Durcan J, Girkin C, Gross R, Netland P, Samples J, Samuelson T. (2009-2010) Surgical Therapy for Glaucoma, *American Academy of Ophthalmology*

[15] Murphy C, Spry P, Burnett C, Broadway C, Diamond D. (2003) Two centre study of the dose-response relation for transscleral Diode laser cyclophotocoagulation in refractory glaucoma. *Br J Ophthalmol, Vol.* 87, pp. 1252–1257

[16] Jimmy S. M. Lai, FRCS, FRCOphth,*† Clement C. Y. Tham, FRCS*§ Jonathan C. H. Chan, MRCSEd,*† and Dennis S. C. Lam, FRCS, FRCOphth*‡ (J Glaucoma 2005;14:114–119)

[17] Ness P, Khaimi M, Feldman R, Tabet R, Sarkisian S, Skuta G, Chuang A, and Mankiewicz K. Intermediate Term Safety and Efficacy of Transscleral Cyclophotocoagulation After Tube Shunt Failure. J Glaucoma 2011;00:000–000

[18] Hollander D, Lin S. Delayed therapeutic success with endoscopic cyclophotocoagulation in treating refractory post-penetrating keratoplasty glaucoma. Br J Ophthalmol 2003;87:791–803

[19] Mistlberger A, Liebmann J, Tschiderer H, Ritch R, Ruckhofer J, and Grabner G.Contact Diode laser transscleral cyclophotocoagulation is useful in eyes with refractory glaucoma in which the risks of outflow surgery are deemed, Journal of Glaucoma 10:288–293

[20] Lai J, Tham C, Chan J, and Lam D. Diode Laser Transscleral Cyclophotocoagulation in the Treatment of Chronic Angle-Closure Glaucoma: A Preliminary Study. *Journal of Glaucoma* 12:360–364

[21] Schlote T, Derse M, Rassmann K Nicaeus T, Dietz K, and Thiel H. Efficacy and Safety of Contact Transscleral Diode Laser Cyclophotocoagulation for Advanced Glaucoma.*Journal of Glaucoma* 10:294–301

[22] Lin S. Endoscopic and Transscleral Cyclophotocoagulation for the Treatment of Refractory Glaucoma. J Glaucoma 2008;17: 238–247

[23] S Lin.Endoscopic cyclophotocoagulation.Br J Ophthalmol 2002;86:1434–1438

[24] Hauber A, Scherer W. Influence of Total Energy Delivery on Success Rate after Contact Diode Laser Transscleral Cyclophotocoagulation: A Retrospective Case Review and Meta-analysis.*Journal of Glaucoma* 11:329–333

[25] S Ataullah, S Biswas, P H Artes, E O'Donoghue, A E A Ridgway, A F Spencer. Long term results of Diode laser cycloablation in complex glaucoma using the Zeiss Visulas II system Br J Ophthalmol 2002;86:39–42

[26] M E Iliev, S Gerber. Long-term outcome of trans-scleral Diode laser cyclophotocoagulation in refractory glaucoma. Br J Ophthalmol 2007;91:1631–1635.

[27] Hayreh S. Neovascular glaucoma.*Prog Retin Eye Res.* 2007 September; 26(5): 470–485 NVG is a severely blinding,

[28] McKelvie P, Walland M. Pathology of cycloDiode laser: a series of nine enucleated eyes. Br J Ophthalmol 2002;86:381–386

[29] Tham C, Lai J, Fung P, Chua J, Poon A, and Lam D. Physical Effects of Reuse and Repeated Ethylene Oxide Sterilization on Transscleral clophotocoagulation Laser G-Probes *Journal of Glaucoma* 11:21–25

[30] Bansal A, and Ramanathan.Potential Contamination of the G-probe Used for Transscleral CycloDiode(J Glaucoma 2008;17:157–158)

[31] Hla Myint Htoon, PhD,z Ching Lin Ho, MMed (Ophth), MMed(Paed), FRCS (Ed),*Tin Aung, MMed (Ophth), FRCS(Ed), PhD,*zy and Shamira Perera, MBBS, BSc, FRCOphth Ramli N,.Risk Factors for Hypotony After Transscleral Diode Cyclophotocoagulation., (J Glaucoma 2010;00:000–000)

[32] Alipanahi R. (2008) Long-Term Outcome of Transscleral Diode Laser Cyclophotocoagulation for Refractory Glaucoma. *Rawal Med J,* Vol. 33, pp. 173-175.

# 22

# Another Look on Cyclodestructive Procedures

Antonio Fea, Dario Damato,
Umberto Lorenzi and Federico M. Grignolo
*Dipartimento di Fisiopatologia Clinica- Clinica Oculistica*
*University of Torino*
*Italy*

## 1. Introduction

Cycloablation is a destructive procedure used to decrease the intra-ocular pressure (IOP) trough the ablation of the ciliary body that produces aqueous humour. Many destructive techniques, including diathermy, cryotherapy, ultrasounds, beta irradiation, and laser photocoagulation have been employed with a wide range of results and side effects. Although all above techniques can effectively destroy the ciliary body, only few of them have been used widely enough to convincingly demonstate their clinical usefulness and gain general acceptance. The ideal method of cyclodestruction should produce clinically useful and predictable reduction of intraocular pressure (IOP), with minimal complications and side effects. (Bartamian & Higginbotham, 2001). Ideally it should have a wide therapeutic window between insufficient and too aggressive treatment intensity, that can result in either insufficient IOP reduction or hypotony/phtisis. Cyclodestructive procedures are usually reserved for cases of glaucoma in eyes with little or no visual potential that proved refractory to medical treatment and outflow surgeries. (Lin, 2008) As an exception to this long established indication, cyclodestructive procedures performed with the 810 nm infrared diode laser transscleral cyclophotocoagulation have been successfully applied also in eyes with refractory glaucoma and good visual potential (Rotchford et al., 2010; Wilensky & Kammer, 2004) supporting an emerging notion that the indications for transscleral laser cyclophotocoagulation should not be limited to eyes with poor visual acuity or potential.

## 2. Background

Coagulation or destruction of the ciliary body to reduce aqueous production has been advocated in the treatment of glaucoma since the 1930s with the introduction of penetrating cyclodiathermy (Voght et al., 1936). In the 1950s, cyclocryotherapy was proven reasonably safe and effective to reduce IOP with less tissue destruction and better predictability compared to cyclodiathermy (Bietti, 1950). Problems still existed, however, including intense postoperative pain, intraocular pressure (IOP) rise, marked inflammation, hemorrhage, and a significant incidence of hypotony and visual loss. Ciliary ablation with ultrasounds was also briefly utilized, but it was eventually abandoned because of marked scleral thinning and ectasia at the treatment site (Coleman at al., 1985).

### 2.1 Laser cyclophotocoagulation

Laser cyclophotocoagulation has become the principal surgical method for reducing aqueous production. The first laser transscleral cyclophotocoagulation (TSCPC) was described by Beckam and Sugar in the early 1970s. Initially, they used the 694 nm ruby laser, but later reported that the 1064 nm infrared Neodymium : Yttrium-Aluminium-Garnet laser (Nd : YAG) was more effective due to its superior transmission through the sclera and absorption by the ciliary epithelium. The delivery of laser energy to the ciliary processes through the sclera may be performed either with an indenting contact probe or a noncontact projected beam. The development of the compact, portable 810 nm I.R. ophthalmic diode laser has made it more convenient to perform contact TSCPC. The same 810 nm I.R. diode laser beam can also be delivered inside the eye through an endoscope to directly photocoagulate the ciliary body under endoscopic guidance. This technique, named endoscopic cyclophotocoagulation (ECP), has become an increasingly important weapon in the glaucoma surgeon's armamentarium for the treatment of refractory glaucoma at the time of ocular surgery and may have some distinct advantages over the transscleral approach in eyes with visual potential. In 1976, Merritt described his method of transpupillary cyclophotocoagulation of the ciliary processes under indirect visualization via a gonioscopic laser lens. This interesting approach, potentially safer than the more invasive ECP, did not become popular because of the difficulty in visualizing and treating the ciliary processes through the gonio-lens, but it may still represent a good option for aniridic eyes.

Laser cyclo-destructive procedures can be divided as follows:

- Transpupillary CPC
- Transvitreal endophotocoagulation
- Transscleral CPC
    - Noncontact and contact 1064 nm Nd:YAG laser
    - Contact 810 nm diode laser
- Endoscopic 810 nm diode laser CPC

In the United States, CPC is used predominantly for refractory glaucoma difficult to control with conventional glaucoma filtration, such as neovascular glaucoma, traumatic glaucoma, glaucoma in aphakic eyes, advanced developmental glaucoma, inflammatory glaucoma, glaucoma associated with corneal transplantation, silicone oil-induced glaucoma, and glaucoma in eyes with conjunctival scarring from previous surgery. Cyclophotocoagulation is also used in eyes with limited visual potential, in urgent situations with dangerously elevated IOP, or for pain relief in eyes with no visual potential. It has uncommonly been used in patients who are not candidates for conventional glaucoma therapy due to poor compliance with care or poor postoperative follow-up. Cyclophotocoagulation has also been evaluated for use as primary surgical treatment in developing countries where conventional glaucoma therapy is not available (Egbert 2001).

## 3. Description of the various CPC procedures

### 3.1 Transpupillary cyclophotocoagulation

Direct transpupillary treatment of the ciliary processes with the argon laser (488/514 nm) is rarely used, because a clear visual axis and a well-dilated pupil are required to enable photocoagulation of the entire length of the ciliary processes. Clinical results have been poor when treatment was limited to the anterior most portions of the ciliary processes. Transpupillary CPC of the ciliary processes, exposed through peripheral iridectomy or a widely dilated pupil, can be effective. The mechanism may be related to a laser-induced retraction of the ciliary body.

### 3.2 Transvitreal endophotocoagulation

Transvitreal endophotocoagulation using a visible or infrared laser beam (514 nm argon, 532 nm solid-state or 810 nm diode) delivered through a vitreo-retinal endoprobe has been used with some success when performed in conjunction with a vitrectomy in the operating room. It requires clear media, aphakia or pseudophakia to directly treat the ciliary processes visible in the field of the operating microscope with scleral indentation. The laser power is titrated to produce a visible burn using continuous wave exposure durations that favour some thermal spread in the deeper layers of the ciliary processes.

### 3.3 Transscleral cyclophotocoagulation (TSCPC)

Due to the optical properties of the human sclera, TSCPC is performed with infrared emitting lasers, most commonly with the 810 nm Diode Laser delivered via a contact probe or with the 1064 nm Nd:YAG laser, delivered either with a non-contact projected beam or with a contact probe.

### 3.4 1064 nm Nd:Yag Laser Non-Contact TSCPC

Transscleral ciliary body ablation utilizing the Nd:YAG laser at 1064 nm wavelength has the theoretical advantage of better transmission through the scleral with less back scatter than shorter wavelengths, such as 514 nm argon and 810 nm diode lasers. Non-contact TSCPC was performed using the Nd:YAG laser in the free-running thermal mode (Microruptor III Lasag, Thun, Switzerland, no longer commercially available) for a duration of 20 msec, and the defocus setting number, which offsets the focal point of the 1064 nm infrared treating beam 3.6 mm posteriorly to the focal point of the red aiming beam. In this way, when the red aiming beam is focused on the conjunctiva, the infrared treatment beam is focused 3.6 mm below, supposedly within the ciliary processes. The laser energy is adjusted from 5 to 8 Joules (J) per application. Retrobulbar or peribulbar anaesthesia is given, and the patient is seated at the laser slit lamp. The treatment is directed parallel to the visual axis, focusing the aiming beam on the sclera, 1.5 mm posterior to the limbus, superiorly and inferiorly, and 1.0 mm posterior to the limbus nasally and temporally. A contact lens with 1.0 mm markings parallel to the limbus can be used to facilitate the placing of the applications, to hold the eyelids open and to bleach the conjunctiva. Alternatively, a lid speculum can be used to open the eyelids, and the red aiming beam can be focused on the centre of a 3 mm slit beam. Approximately eight to ten applications per quadrant are placed from 270 to 360 degrees. Treatment may be reduced to 180 degrees in patients judged to be clinically at risk for hypotony (Pastor et al., 2001).

### 3.5 1064 nm Nd:Yag Laser Contact TSCPC

Retrobulbar or peribulbar anaesthesia is given, the patient lies supine, and a eyelid speculum is placed. The anterior edge of the 2.2 mm sapphire tip of the delivery fibre optic handpiece (Surgical Laser Technologies, Inc., Malvern, PA) is placed 0.5 to 1.0 mm posterior to the limbus (the probe is centred 1.5 to 2.0 mm posterior to the limbus). Gentle pressure is applied with the probe, which is oriented perpendicular to the sclera. The laser energy setting is 5 to 9 Joules, for a duration of 0.7 seconds, with approximately eight spots per quadrant placed from 270 to 360 degrees. After the procedure, atropine and dexamethasone ointments are applied and the eye is patched. The patch may be removed in the evening and anti-glaucoma drops should be reinstituted. Prostaglandin analogues may be excluded in the short term if cystoid macular edema (CME) is a concern, and cholinergics should be temporarily discontinued to avoid increased anterior segment inflammation. Postoperative prednisolone acetate 1% is applied 4 times daily for 10 to 14 days and tapered according to inflammation (Lin, 2008).

### 3.6 810 nm Diode Laser Contact TSCPC

It is performed using a semiconductor diode laser system (IRIS Oculight SLx, IRIDEX Corp., Mountain View, CA), its 810 nm wavelength exhibits lower scleral transmission (35%) but considerably greater absorption by melanin than the 1064 nm wavelength. The laser energy is transmitted through a 600 μm diameter quartz fiber with a spherical protruding tip oriented by the footplate of the hand-piece called "G-Probe". Positioning the G-Probe parallel to the optical visual axis with the shorter edge of the footplate next to the anterior border of the limbus will centre the fibre optic tip 1.0-1.2 mm posterior to the corneoscleral limbus and direct the energy toward the ciliary processes. The tip protrudes 0.7 mm beyond the footplate contact surface, which indents the conjunctiva and sclera to enhance the transmission of the laser energy. The probe footplate is curved spherically to match the scleral curvature. Maximum settings from the system are 3.0 watts power and 9.9 seconds duration. Retrobulbar or peribulbar anesthesia is given and a lid speculum is placed. Duration is set at 2000 ms (2 seconds), and the initial power setting is 1750 mW. The power is increased in 250 mW increments to a maximum of 2500mW until an audible "pop" (caused by tissue explosion of the ciliary process, the iris root anteriorly or the retina posteriorly) is heard, then the power is reduced by 250 mW and treatment is completed at this power. Some surgeons recommend lower power and longer burn duration, for example 1250 mW at 4 seconds (5.0 Joules) in heavily pigmented eyes and 1500 mW at 3.5 seconds in lightly pigmented eyes (5.25 Joules). Six applications per quadrant are typically placed over 270 degrees involving the inferior, nasal and superior quadrants for a total of 18 applications per treatment. This is based on burns spaced half the width of the G-Probe footplate (2 mm), but various reports have used from 18 to 40 spots, with 180 to 360 degrees for the initial treatment (Pastor et al., 2001). Generally, the incidence of retreatment increases when a lower energy and/or a lower number of spots are applied. With all non-contact or contact TSCPC procedures, the outcome predictability is limited by the inability to visualize treated tissue. In lieu of direct visualization, trans-illumination may be used to identify the location of the ciliary body, especially in eyes with abnormal anatomy or in enlarged eyes (congenital glaucoma). An ocular trans-illuminator is placed against the posterior globe and directed towards the ciliary sulcus. In a darkened room, the diffuse illumination will demarcate the ciliary body, which can be marked externally (Sharkey & Murray, 1994).

### 3.7 810 nm diode laser endoscopic cyclophotocoagulation (ECP)

The laser unit for ECP (Endo Optiks, Little Silver, NJ) incorporates 1) a diode laser that emits 810 nm continuous-wave energy, 2) a 175W Xenon light source, 3) a Helium-Neon laser aiming beam, and 4) a video imaging and recording camera. All 4 optical elements are transmitted through a 18-gauge or 20-gauge fibre-optic probe, which is inserted into the eye. The optimal focus for the laser is 0.75 mm from the probe tip, and the endoscope provides a 70-degree field of view. The main unit is compact and portable with a maximum power output of 2.0 W. The laser power and the exposure duration (up to 9.99 seconds) are adjustable with the controls in the console. The foot pedal controls the laser firing, with the actual duration of each application determined by the exposure duration setting or by the pedal depression, whichever ends first. The 2 main approaches to reach the ciliary processes are via a limbal or a pars plana entry. The limbal approach is preferred to avoid the anterior vitrectomy and the associated risks for choroidal and retinal detachment. However, certain cases are more safely treated through the pars plana, for example, aphakic eyes with posterior synechiae limiting the access to the ciliary sulcus. In both situations, a retrobulbar block with lidocaine and bupivicaine is performed or general anaesthesia can be considered in selective cases. In the limbal approach, after dilation of the pupil with cyclopentolate 1% and phenylephrine 2.5%, a paracentesis is created and the anterior chamber is filled with viscoelastic agent, which is further used to expand the nasal posterior sulcus. This viscoelastic expansion of the posterior chamber allows for easier approach to the pars plicata with the ECP probe. A 2.2-mm keratome is then used to enter into the anterior chamber at the temporal limbus. After orientation of the probe image outside of the eye, the 18-gauge or 20-gauge endoprobe is inserted through the incision into the posterior sulcus. At this time, the ciliary processes are viewed on the monitor and treatment can begin. The laser is set at continuous-wave and power settings are 300 to 900 mW. Approximately a 180-degree span of ciliary processes is photocoagulated (more area can be treated if a curved probe is used). Laser energy is applied to each process until shrinkage and whitening occur. The ciliary processes are treated individually or in a "painting" fashion across multiple processes. If excessive energy is used, the process explodes with a "pop" sound due to bubble formation, leading to excessive inflammation and breakdown of the blood-aqueous barrier. After the nasal 180 degrees of ciliary processes are treated, a separate incision is created at the nasal limbus in a similar fashion as above. The temporal processes are then photocoagulated for a total of up to 360 degrees, if desired. Typically, 180 to 360 degrees are treated. Before closure of the wounds, the viscoelastic material is removed from the anterior chamber with irrigation and aspiration. In the pars plana approach, an infusion port is inserted through the inferior pars plana and 2 superior entries are created for vitrectomy and illumination. Only a limited anterior vitrectomy is performed to allow adequate and safe access to all of the ciliary processes. The ECP probe can be inserted through each superior entry for treatment of the opposite 180 degrees of processes. There may be a few superior processes that cannot be accessed because the entry ports are not exactly 180 degrees opposite to each other. Laser CPC is carried out with the same parameters and end points as described for the limbal approach. If the anterior segment surgeon has not had extensive experience in posterior segment surgery, assistance from a retinal surgeon should be sought for the establishment of the pars plana entry ports and the limited anterior vitrectomy. Risk of inadvertent choroidal and/or retinal detachment is a serious concern and should be minimized. In all patients, whether under local or general anaesthesia, retrobulbar bupivicaine is administered before or at end of the surgery to minimize postoperative pain. Sub-Tenon's injection of 1mL of triamcinolone (40 mg/mL) is also given for inflammation. On postoperative day 1, patients are placed on a regimen of topical antibiotics, steroids, nonsteroidal anti-inflammatory agents, cycloplegics, and their preoperative glaucoma medications except for miotics and prostaglandin analogues because these may exacerbate intraocular inflammation or its sequelae. Antibiotics are discontinued after 1 week, and the steroids, nonsteroidal anti-inflammatory agents, and cycloplegics are tapered as inflammation subsides. Glaucoma medications are removed according to the intraocular pressure (IOP) requirements. Administration of acetazolamide during the evening of surgery may be used to prevent a spike in IOP from underlying glaucoma, inflammation, or possible retained viscoelastic (Lin, 2008).

## 4. Published results

It is difficult if not impossible to compare studies that have different entry criteria and definitions of success. In fact, "success" in cyclophotocoagulation procedures has been defined as achieving IOP < 21 or 22 mmHg, and/or an IOP reduction of 20% or 30%; some study considered IOP < 5 mmHg as hypotony and, thus, a failure. Most studies allow the postoperative use of medications to achieve this definition of success.

### 4.1 Transscleral cyclophotocoagulation

#### 4.1.1 1064 nm Nd:Yag Laser Non-Contact TSCPC

In a retrospective study, Youn et al. (Youn et al., 1996) reviewed 479 patients in a follow-up period of 3-75 months (mean 22 months). The range of laser energy settings was 4 to 8 J. Postoperative IOP was between 5 and 20 mmHg in 52% of the patients. Forty percent of the patients lost two or more Snellen visual acuity lines. Visual deterioration was significantly associated with neovascular glaucoma, African descent, post-treatment hypotony, and more than 6 months of follow-up. Phthisis was encountred in 14% of treated patients. Noncontact Nd:YAG cyclophotocoagulation enhances the risk of graft failure in patients with previous penetrating keratoplasty. In a prospective, unmasked randomized trial, Shields et al. (Shields et al., 1993) assigned two groups of 89 patients to two energy settings, 4 J (range 3.7 to 4.5 J) for the Group A and 8 J (range 7 to 8.5 J) for the Group B, with 30 applications utilizing a contact lens. Among the patients who did not require further surgery, better success (75% versus 60%) and fewer retreatments (25% versus 40%) were observed in the higher energy. Among those patients who received no further surgery, vision loss was 56% of patients in Group A (4 J) versus 42% of patients in group B (8 J). There was no significant difference between the two groups. Mean follow-up was 12.6 months, ranging from 5 to 20 months. Delgado et al. (2003) studied the results of Nd:YAG laser non-contact TSCPC on neovascular glaucoma. Mean follow-up was 27 months (range 1 - 148), 115 eyes were evaluated using 7.8 J energy setting (20 to 40 application over 270 degrees) and the success rate was 65%, 49.8% and 34.8% after 1, 3 and 6 years respectively. There were 11.5% phtisis and 39.1% eyes had a loss of two or more Snellen visual acuity lines. An interesting retrospective study (Ayyala et al., 1998) attempted to compare mitomycin C trabeculectomy, glaucoma drainage device (GDD) and Nd:YAG non-contact TSCPC in the glaucoma management after penetrating keratoplasty. This was a non-comparative case series with fewer than 20 patients in each group. Mean follow-up was 12.9 months. There was no statistically significant difference in successful IOP control between mitomycin C trabeculectomy (77% success), GDD (80% success), or non-contact TSCPC (63%). There was no significant difference in the rate of failure of the corneal graft following trabeculectomy (15%), GDD (0%), or TSCPC (17%) that compared fairly with the 11% to 65% failure rate of the corneal graft following glaucoma surgery reported in the literature. (Pastor et al., 2001). As the criteria for success varied in the different studies, it is not surprising that the rate of success spanned from 35% to 83%. The most common complications included the loss of two or more Snellen visual acuity lines in up to 40% of patients, phthisis in 0 to 14%, hyphema in 0 to 4%, and corneal oedema in 0 to 6% of patients. Sympathetic ophthalmia has also been reported as an extremely rare complication. (Bechrakis et al., 1994).

| STUDY | LASER TYPE | GLAUCOMA | F -UP (mo) | N (eyes) | VA LOSS (%) | N. TREAT | POWER | DEGREES | N. SPOTS | SUCCESS (%) | SUCCESS CRITERIA |
|---|---|---|---|---|---|---|---|---|---|---|---|
| Delgado et al., 2003 | nc YAG | neovascular | 27 | 115 | 39 | 1,4 | 7,8 (J) | 270 | 20-40 | 50 | IOP<22; no pthysis; no further surgery |
| Youn et al., 1998 | nc YAG | all | 10,4 | 46 | 0 | 1,13 | 5,21 to 7,5 (J) | 360 | 32 | 83 | 5<IOP<21 |
| Shields et al., 1993 | nc YAG | all | 12 | 45 | 26 | 1 | 4 (J) | 360 | 30 | 60 | no additional glaucoma surgery |
| Shields et al., 1993 | nc YAG | all | 12 | 44 | 36 | 1 | 8 (J) | 360 | 30 | 75 | no additional glaucoma surgery |
| Youn et al., 1996 | nc YAG | all | 22 | 479 | 40 | 1 | 6 (J) | N/A | 25 | 52 | 5<IOP<20 |
| Lin et al., 2004 | c YAG | all | 67 | 68 | 16 | 1,4 | 7 to 9 (W) | 360 | 32 - 40 | 60,3(1 yr.); 48,5 (10 yrs.) | 3<IOP<25; no other TCP |
| Schuman et al., 1992 | c YAG | all | 19 | 116 | 31 | 1,27 | 7 to 9 (W) | N/A | 32 - 40 | 65 | 3<IOP<22 |

Table 1. Nd: YAG Laser

#### 4.1.2 1064 nm Nd:Yag laser contact TSCPC

There are fewer studies (see Table 1) reporting the use of Nd:YAG laser contact TSCPC than there are reporting non-contact TSCPC. Schuman et al. (Schuman et al., 1992) reported retrospectively on a series of 116 eyes of 114 patients with a mean follow-up of 1 year (range 6-19 months). Treatment consisted of 32 to 40 applications, for a total of 7 to 9 W of power delivered for 0.7 seconds. IOP control of 3 to 22 mmHg was achieved in 65% of eyes. Twenty-seven percent were retreated. Hypotony with less than 3 mmHg occurred in nine eyes, six of which were phthisical. Nineteen eyes (16%) lost light perception, and 47% of eyes with V.A. of 20/200 or better lost two or more Snellen visual acuity lines (17 of 36 eyes). Lin et al (Lin et al., 2004) in 2004 reported similar results about a series of 68 eyes with a mean follow-up of 5.58 years (range 0.1 - 10 years). Treatment consisted of 32 to 40 applications, for a total of 7 to 9 watts of power delivered for 0.7 seconds. Intraocular pressure control of 3 to 25 mmHg was achieved in 60 % of eyes after one year and in 48% after ten years with only one treatment. 40% of patient where retreated, and this has been considered a failure. Hypotony less than 3 mmHg was seen in 3 eyes, none of which were phthisical. Eleven eyes worsened their visual acuity.

#### 4.1.3 810 Nm diode laser contact TSCPC

For a variety of reasons, mainly clinical effectiveness and practicality, 810 nm diode laser contact TSCPC has been universally adopted to the point to become the standard of care for specific conditions. As a result, there are more publications in the literature on 810nm diode TSCPC (see Table 2) than on any other CPC modality, although many of them are only retrospective. As indicated in Table 2, the mean number of eyes reported in the studies was 55.82 (SD =+/- 58.26) (Standard Deviation) eyes with a variety of diagnoses and of laser treatment parameters. Laser power ranged from 1.25 to 3 watts (mean 1.94 W) for a mean exposure time of 2.16 seconds, for a mean number of applications of 22.10 (SD=+/- 7.02) over 180 to 360 degrees, sometimes adjusting the power for pops and sometimes not. Mean follow-up was 19.86 months (SD=+/- 12.71). Mean success rate was 67.26% (SD=+/- 15.70), but this cannot be a good indicator, because the definition of success was heterogeneous (see Table 2). Mean number of medication was 2.52 (SD=+/- 0.63) pre-operatively and 1.62 (SD=+/- 0.71) post-operatively. Mean loss of visual acuity was 24.74% (SD=+/- 16.78). Retreatment rate was 1.48 (SD=+/- 0.45). Complications were, hypotony (0 to 25%), phthisis (0 to 11%), AS inflammation (0 to 27%), choroidal detachment (0 to 10%), cataract progression (0 to 40%), atonic pupil (0 to 70%) and hyphema (0 to 13%). Rarely reported complications were endophthalmitis, failure of corneal graft, CMO, bullous keratopathy, band keratopathy, persistent ocular pain. Rarely reported complications included necrotizing scleritis (Ganesh et al., 2006), scleral perforation (Kwong at al., 2005), iris retraction and retroflexion (Sony et al., 2003) and malignant glaucoma (Azuara-Blanco et al., 1999). Table 2 stratifies the outcomes among various types of glaucoma. In Neovascular Glaucoma success rate ranges from 40% to 64% with a mean follow up from 9 to 60 months; in Silicon Oil Glaucoma success rate ranges from 44% to 82% with a mean follow up from 4 to 22 months; in Pediatric Glaucoma success rate ranges from 67% to 72% with a mean follow up from 20 to 21 months; in Chronic Angle Closure Glaucoma (CACG) success rate ranges from 86% to 92% with a mean follow up from 12 to 26 months; and in Keratoprosthesis Glaucoma success rate is 66% with a mean follow up of 26.6 months. 810 nm Diode Laser Contact TSCPC has also been used in 49 eyes with a good visual acuity (20/60 or better).

| STUDY | GLAUCOMA | F-UP (mo) | N (eyes) | N. TREAT | POWER (W) | TIME (s) | DEGREES | N. SPOTS | SUCCESS CRITERIA | SUCCESS (%) | VA LOSS (%) |
|---|---|---|---|---|---|---|---|---|---|---|---|
| Spencer et al., 1999 | all | 21,5 | 58 | 1,6 | 2,00 | 2 | 270 | 14 | IOP <= 22 | 81 | 20,7 |
| Yildirim et al., 2009 | nv | 24 | 33 | 1 | 1,50 | 2 | 270 | 17 | 5<IOP<21 | 61 | 18,2 |
| Ghosh et al., 2010 | nv | 9 | 14 | 1 | 2,00 | 2 | 180-270 | 25 | 30% IOP reduction | 64 | 21,4 |
| Preussner et al., 2010 | africans | 6 | 75 | N/A | 5,00 | 0,2 | 360 | 20 | N/A | N/A | N/A |
| Malik et al., 2006 | all | 35 | 28 | 2 | 2,12 | 2 | 360 | 24 | 6<IOP<21 | 64 | 46,4 |
| Semchyshyn et al., 2002 | all | 26,9 | 21 | 1,38 | 2,00 | 2 | 270 | 21,9 | 5<IOP<=21 | 66 | 52,4 |
| Schlote et al., 2000 | inflammatory | 12 | 22 | 2 | 2,00 | 2 | 270 | 12,5 | 5<IOP<21 in va>0,02 or IOP<30% in va<0,02 | 77,3 | 36,4 |
| Rotchford et al., 2010 | good vision | 60 | 49 | 1,73 | 2,00 | 2 | N/A | 14,4 | IOP<=21 | 89,8 | 61,2 |
| Sood et al., 2009 | pediatric | 19,8 | 9 | 1 | 1,25 | 3,5 | 180-270 | 17,4 | IOP<22;no complications; no further surgery | 66,7 | 20,0 |
| Kirwan et al., 2009 | pediatric | 21 | 77 | 2,3 | 1,50 | 1,5 | 300 | 40 | IOP<22 or 30% IOP reduction | 72 | 7,5 |
| Lai et al., 2002 | CACG | 12 | 14 | 1,14 | 2,00 | 2 | 270 | 16,3 | IOP < 21 | 85,7 | 0,0 |
| Lai et al., 2005 | CACG | 26,5 | 13 | 1,15 | 2,00 | 2 | 270 | 17,5 | IOP < 21 | 92,3 | 38,5 |
| Han et al., 1999 | silicon oil | 12 | 11 | 1,18 | 2,00 | 2 | 360 | 23,5 | IOP < =21 | 81,8 | 18,2 |
| Agarwal et al., 2004 | all types | 15,8 | 30 | 1,2 | 1,50 | 2 | 360 | 40 | IOP < 22 | 94 | 6,7 |
| Rivier et al., 2009 | keratoprotesis | 26,6 | 18 | 1,3 | 1,87 | 2 | 270 | 17,5 | lowering digital pressure | 66 | 38,9 |
| Noureddin et al., 2006 | all | 13,69 | 36 | 1,25 | 2,25 | 2 | 360 | 28 | IOP<=21 | 72,2 | 22,2 |
| Sivagnanavel et al., 2005 | silicone oil glaucoma | 21,8 | 18 | 1,5 | 2,00 | 1,5 | 180 | 25 | IOP < 22 | 44 | 55,6 |
| Egbert et al., 2001 | all | 13,2 | 40 | 1,22 | 1,50 | 1,5 | 360 | 20 | IOP <=22 | 48 | 25,0 |
| Egbert et al., 2001 | all | 13,2 | 39 | 1,22 | 1,25 | 2,5 | 360 | 20 | 20% IOP reduction | 46 | 20,5 |

Table 2. (continues on next page) 810 nm diode laser contact TSCPC

| STUDY | GLAUCOMA | F-UP (mo) | N (eyes) | N. TREAT | POWER (W) | TIME (s) | DEGREES | N. SPOTS | SUCCESS CRITERIA | SUCCESS (%) | VA LOSS (%) |
|---|---|---|---|---|---|---|---|---|---|---|---|
| Ansari et al., 2007 | all | 12,5 | 74 | 1,01 | 2,00 | 2 | 360 | 30 | 30% IOP reduction | 82 | 13,0 |
| Kaushik et al., 2008 | all | 14,3 | 66 | 1,16 | 2,00 | 2 | 270 | 18 | 5<IOP<22 | 78,8 | 4,5 |
| Nabili et al., 2004 | diabetic neovascular glaucoma | N/A | 20 | 1,45 | 2,00 | 2 | 270 | 15 | 5<IOP<22 | 40 | 40,0 |
| Kramp et al., 2002 | all | 13,9 | 193 | 1,3 | 1,60 | 2 | 360 | 27 | 10<IOP<22 | 76,4 | N/A |
| Grueb et al., 2006 | all | 24 | 90 | 1,3 | 2,00 | 2 | 180 | 17,5 | 4<IOP<18; 20% IOP reduction | 36,7 | 11,1 |
| Iliev et al., 2007 | all | 30,1 | 131 | 1,54 | 2,00 | 2 | 270 | 22 | 6<IOP<21 or IOP reduction >30% | 69,5 | 26,0 |
| Schlote et al., 2007 | aphakic and posttraumatic | 42 | 46 | 2,58 | 2,00 | 2 | 180 | 20 | 5<IOP<21 | 43,8 | 63,0 |
| Heinz et al., 2006 | juvenile idiopathic arthritis | 10,1 | 21 | 2,15 | 2,00 | 2 | 180 | 25 | IOP<=21 | 32 | 14,3 |
| Ocakoglu et al., 2005 | all | 11,4 | 32 | 1,68 | 2,50 | 2 | 270-300 | 22 | IOP<=22 | 72 | 0,0 |
| Murphy et al,. 2003 | all | 17 | 263 | 1,5 | N/A | N/A | N/A | N/A | 5<IOP<22 or 30% IOP reduction | 79,5 | 19,4 |
| Walland, 1998 | all | 10,1 | 22 | 1 | 1,50 | 1,5 | 360 | 40 | IOP<22 | 54,5 | 31,8 |
| Walland, 1998 | all | 11,4 | 8 | 1 | 1,50 | 1,5 | 180 | 20 | IOP<22 | 62,5 | 31,8 |
| Frezzotti et al., 2010 | all | 17 | 124 | 1,26 | 2,00 | 2 | 180-270 | 15 | 5<IOP<21 or pain relief | 67,3 | 12,9 |
| Leszcynski et al., 2009 | neovascular | 60 | 30 | 2,4 | 1,75 | N/A | 270 | 17,5 | N/A | N/A | 10,0 |
| Raivio et al., 2008 | all | 26 | 60 | 1,4 | 0,43 | 10 | 180 | 20 | 8<IOP<21 | 80 | 30,0 |
| Gangwani et al., 2010 | silicon oil | 4 | 9 | 2,34 | 1,87 | 2 | 270 | 30 | IOP<21 | 66,7 | 11,1 |
| Youn et al., 1998 | all | 10,4 | 49 | 1,2 | 2,37 | 2 | 360 | 24,63 | 5<IOP<22 | 71 | 8,2 |
| Brancato et al., 1995 | all | 20,7 | 68 | N/A | 2,60 | 2 | 360 | 18 | 2<IOP<=21 | 70,8 | N/A |

Table 2. (continued) 810 nm diode laser contact TSCPC

The success rate on pressure reduction (IOP <21) was 90%, but 60% of eyes lost 1 Snellen visual acuity line and 30% of the eyes lost more than 2 Snellen visual acuity lines. 810 nm Diode Laser Contact TSCPC has been compared to Ahmed Valve implantation by Yildirim et al. (Yildirim et al., 2009) who found a success rate of 61% for TSCPC vs. 59% for Ahmed Valve with a mean follow up of 24 months. In a similar study Sood et al (Sood et al., 2009) compared 810 nm Diode TSCPC to Ahmed Valve implantation in Pediatric Glaucoma and found a success rate of 66.7% for TSCPC vs 62.5% for Ahmed Valve with a mean follow up of 19.8 and 26.3 months respectively. Malik et al (Malik et al., 2006) compared 810 nm Diode TSCPC to Molteno tube shunt and found a success rate of 64% for TSCPC vs 81% for Molteno tube shunt with a mean follow up of 35 months. Youn et al (Youn et al., 1998) compared non-contact TSCPC with 1064 nm Nd:YAG and 810 nm diode lasers in a prospective, randomized, unmasked trial. Mean follow-up was 10.4 months. Success was 83% and 71% of the YAG and diode patients, respectively, (no statistically significant difference). Retreatment in the YAG group was lower (8.7%; 4/46) than the diode group (18%; 6/49). Although not statistically significant, the Nd:YAG group had a slightly higher success. In clinical practice the 1064 nm Nd:YAG laser in the free-running thermal mode is not commercially available anymore and most clinicians have elected to use the more compact and user-friendly 810 nm diode laser with the contact G-Probe. Agarwal et al (Agarwal et al., 2004) compared the 830 nm Diode Laser contact TSCPC to the 830 nm Diode Laser non-contact TSCPC 830 and found a success rate of 94% for Contact vs. 90% for Non-Contact after a mean follow up of 15.8 months. Although there is not a general agreement, most studies have found that the amount of energy used for 810 nm diode laser contact TSCPC seems to correlate with treatment success rate, without implying a higher complication or vision loss rate.

### 4.2 Endoscopic cyclophotocoagulation

#### 4.2.1 810 Nm diode laser endoscopic cyclophotocoagulation (ECP)

810 nm diode laser ECP is a relatively new method for CPC, and this is reflected in the relatively smaller number of publications (see Table 3). It's very difficult to compare such studies because laser parameters are different or not well specified. In Table 3 we summarized six studies that evaluated a 33.3 mean number of patients (SD=+/- 18.3) range 12 - 68, with various types of glaucoma, including pediatric glaucoma, for a mean follow-up of 11.9 months (SD=+/- 5.5) range 4.5-21.3 and with different definition of success. Mean success rate was 59.1% (SD=+/- 23.7) range 17-82.9%. Mean pre- and post-operative number of medication was 2.2 (SD=+/- 0.5) and 1.5 (SD=+/- 0.5) respectively. Mean visual acuity loss of two or more Snellen lines was 9% (SD=+/- 8) range 0-22% and retreatment rate was 1.16 (SD=+/- 0.2). Complications were hypotony (0 to 8%), phthisis (0 to 3%), anterior segment inflammation (0 to 6%), hyphema (0 to 9%), and RD (0 to 8%). In pediatric glaucoma (refractory glaucoma with corneal opacities) the success rate (IOP <21mmHg without complication and further surgery) was 17% at 13 months of follow up. (Al-Haddad et al., 2007). The authors attributed the poor results to the surgical difficulties of refractory pediatric glaucoma. Lima et al (Lima et al., 2004) compared ECP to Ahmed Valve implantation in 6\8 patients and found a success rate of 73.5% vs 70.6% (p = 0.7) respectively (mean follow up of 21.3 and 19.8 months respectively). Complications were different: ECP reported more cases of hypotony, phthisis, anterior segment inflammation, while Ahmed valve reported more cases of endophthalmitis, choroidal detachment and

| STUDY | GLAUCOMA | F-UP (mo) | N (eyes) | VA LOSS (%) | N. TREAT | DEGREES | SUCCESS (%) | SUCCESS CRITERIA |
|---|---|---|---|---|---|---|---|---|
| Lima et al., 2004 | all | 21,3 | 68 | 9 | 1 | 210 | 73,5 | 6<IOP<21 |
| Yip et al., 2009 | all | 15,9 | 29 | 17 | 1 | 270 | 48,3 | IOP<20%, no medications added |
| Kahook et al., 2007 (1 site) | all | 4,5 | 15 | 0 | 1 | 240-300 | 47 | IOP reduction of 3 mmHg at least; 1 medication reduction |
| Kahook et al., 2007 (2 sites) | all | 4,5 | 25 | 0 | 1 | 240-300 | 92 | IOP reduction of 3 mmHg at least; 1 medication reduction |
| Al-Haddad et al., 2007 | pediatric | 13,0 | 12 | 8 | 1,17 | 270 | 17 | IOP<=21; no complications; no further surgery |
| Carter et al., 2007 | aphakic and pseudophakic children | 12 | 34 | N/A | 1,8 | 180-270 | 53 | IOP<24; no complications; no further surgery |
| Murty et al., 2009 | all | 12,3 | 50 | 22 | N/A | 270-360 | 82,9 | IOP<22 |

Table 3. 810 nm diode laser ECP

retinal detachment. Kahook et al (Kahook et al., 2007) compared 2-incision ECP to 1-incision ECP, finding a success rate of 92% for 2-incision vs. 47% for 1-incision. No major complications have been reported.

## 5. Personal considerations and role of anti-VEGF and panfotocoagulation

We personally have experience with cyclocryotherapy, contact diode TSCP and ciliary ablation with ultrasound. We long ago abandoned the US ciliary ablation due to the difficulties of the treatment and some serious adverse events related to the difficulty of centering the ultrasound beam exactly on the ciliary body. We are not using anymore cyclocryotherapy mainly because of the inflammatory processes related to this method. Inflammatory processes might be present with diode laser TSCP as well if the treatment is not titrated. We are very concerned of possible adverse events related to cycloddestruction and with the diode laser we prefer to stay on the safe side at the eventual price of retreatment rather than risk serious complications. Our current protocol with the diode laser is to treat 180 degrees using the G-probe. The time is pre-set at 2 seconds and we generally start with a 1800 mW power. We increase the power until a bob can be appreciated and then we decrease the power by 100 mW and we continue the treatment. We pay a lot of attention to keep the probe strongly pressed on the globe in order to achieve a better conduction through the sclera. The number of applications is titrated on the basis of the IOP level and on the type of glaucoma. We generally give more applications if the IOP is elevated with the exception of uveitic and neovascular glaucoma where we never apply as first treatment more than 14 applications, because we fear that in this forms of secondary glaucoma there might coexist a lower acqueous production. Concerning the use of anti-VEGF, Although there are several reports that claim a resolution of IOP elevation, we cannot confirm these findings. Probably the patients that come to our Department present long standing forms of iris neovascularisation. Although some of our patients did not present a complete angle occlusion at gonioscopy, we never had a complete normalization of IOP by using intravitreal injections. In a few cases intravitreal ant-VEGF injection, nevertheless, allowed for a partial recovery of the glaucoma with some clearing of the cornea, which allowed us for starting a pan-retinal photocoagulation. Retinal cryotherapy is always added whenever the panretinal photocoagulation is impossible due to corneal decompensation, cataract or vitreous hemorrage.

## 6. Summary

Both 810 nm diode laser TSCPC and ECP are effective procedures for the treatment of refractory glaucoma. TSCPC is an extra-ocular procedure that has mainly been used in eyes that had received prior filtration surgeries or that had very limited visual potential. However, more recently, there has been a trend toward using 810 nm diode laser TSCPC as the primary surgery in eyes with relatively good vision. ECP is an intra-ocular surgery that has also been used as a primary procedure, often combined with phacoemulsification cataract extraction, but should probably be considered almost exclusively in eyes that have good potential vision. These relative indications for each type of CPC are guided by the possible complications of each procedure. TSCPC is a "blind" procedure that has significant rates of success, but also hypotony and/or phthisis, which may relate to its external approach. Greater energy is generally required to penetrate the sclera as compared with the

| STUDY | PROCEDURE | GLAUCOMA | F-UP (mo) | N (eyes) | VA LOSS (%) | N. TREAT | POWER (J) | DEGREES | N. SPOTS | SUCCESS (%) | SUCCESS CRITERIA |
|---|---|---|---|---|---|---|---|---|---|---|---|
| Yildirim et al., 2009 | TCP diode vs | neovascular | 24 | 33 | 18 | 1 | >1,5 | 270 | 17 | 61,2 | 5<IOP<21, no further surgery |
| Yildirim et al., 2009 | ahmed valve | neovascular | 24 | 33 | 27 | N/A | N/A | N/A | N/A | 59,2 | 5<IOP<21, no further surgery |
| Malik et al., 2006 | TCP diode vs | all | 35 | 28 | 46 | 2 | 1,75 - 2,5 | 360 | 24 | 64 | 6<IOP<21 |
| Malik et al., 2006 | molteno tube | all | 35 | 26 | 54 | N/A | N/A | N/A | N/A | 81 | 6<IOP<21 |
| Sood et al., 2009 | TCP diode vs | pediatric | 19,8 | 9 | 20 | 1 | 1 - 1,5 | 180-270 | 17 | 66,7 | IOP<22;no complications; no further surgery |
| Sood et al., 2009 | ahmed valve | pediatric | 26,3 | 8 | 75 | N/A | N/A | N/A | N/A | 75 (12mo); 62,5 (24mo) | IOP<22;no complications; no further surgery |
| Agarwal et al., 2004 | C TCP diode 830 nm vs. | all | 15,8 | 30 | 6 | 1,2 | 1,5 | 360 | 40 | 94 | IOP < 22 |
| Agarwal et al., 2004 | NC TCPdiode 830 nm | all | 15,8 | 30 | 6 | 1,6 | 1,5 | 360 | 40 | 90 | IOP < 23 |
| Youn et al., 1998 | TCP YAG vs. | all | 10,4 | 46 | 0 | 1,13 | 5,21 - 7,5 | 360 | 32 | 83 | 5<IOP<21 |
| Youn et al., 1998 | TCP diode | all | 10,4 | 49 | 8 | 1,2 | 1,75 - 3 | 360 | 25 | 71 | 5<IOP<22 |

Table 4. Comparing procedures

endoscopic approach. EPC allows the photocoagulation of the ciliary processes under direct visualization, but can also lead to the overtreatment of the ciliary tissues and surrounded structures, including the vascular structure of ciliary process, the pars plana, and the iris root, all of which may potentially predispose to phthisis or hypotony. The major disadvantage of ECP is that it is an intra-ocular procedure. Endophthalmitis, choroidal haemorrhage, and retinal detachment are rare, but remain potential serious complications. New transscleral 810 nm laser applications over the pars plana with a new micropulse laser emission mode, have been reported to result in effective IOP lowering, while avoiding most collateral problems of 810 nm continuous wave diode laser TSCPC and EPC (Tan et al., 2010).

## 7. References


Agarwal, H.C.; Gupta, V. & Sihota, R. (2004). Evaluation of contact versus non-contact diode laser cyclophotocoagulation for refractory glaucomas using similar energy settings. *Clin Experiment Ophthalmol.* Feb; 32(1):33-8.

Ansari, E. & Gandhewar, J. (2007). Long-term efficacy and visual acuity following transscleral diode laser photocoagulation in cases of refractory and non-refractory glaucoma. *Eye (Lond).* Jul; 21(7):936-40.

Ayyala, RS.; Pieroth, L.; Vinals, AF.; et al. (1998). Comparison of mitomycin C trabeculectomy, glaucoma drainage device implantation, and laser neodymium: YAG cyclophotocoagulation in the management of intractable glaucoma after penetrating keratoplasty. *Ophthalmology.* 105:1550–6.

Azuara-Blanco, A. & Dua, H.S. (1999). Malignant glaucoma after diode laser cyclophotocoagulation. *Am J Ophthalmol.* Apr; 127(4):467-9.

Bartamian, M. & Higginbotham, E.J. (2001). What is on the horizon for cycloablation? *Curr Opin Ophthalmol.* Apr; 12(2):119-23. Review.

Bechrakis, N.E.; Müller-Stolzenburg, N.W. ; Helbig, H. & Foerster, M.H. (1994). Sympathetic ophthalmia following laser cyclocoagulation. *Arch Ophthalmol.* Jan; 112(1):80-4. PubMed PMID: 8285899.

Bietti, G. (1950). Surgical intervention on the ciliary body: new trends for the relief of glaucoma. *JAMA.* 142:889–897.

Brancato, R.; Carassa, R.G.; Bettin, P.; Fiori, M. & Trabucchi, G. (1995). Contact transscleral cyclophotocoagulation with diode laser in refractory glaucoma. *Eur J Ophthalmol.* Jan-Mar; 5(1):32-9.

Carter, B.C.; Plager, D.A. Neely, D.E.; Sprunger, D.T.; Sondhi, N. & Roberts, G.J. (2007). Endoscopic diode laser cyclophotocoagulation in the management of aphakic and pseudophakic glaucoma in children. *J AAPOS.* Feb; 11(1):34-40.

Coleman, D.J.; Lizzi, F.L.; Driller, J. et al. (1985). Therapeutic ultrasound in the treatment of glaucoma. I. Experimental model. *Ophthalmology* 92:339–46.

Delgado, M.F.; Dickens, C.J.; Iwach, A.G.; Novack, G.D.; Nychka, D.S.; Wong, P.C. & Nguyen, N. (2003). Long-term results of noncontact neodymium:yttrium-aluminum-garnet cyclophotocoagulation in neovascular glaucoma. *Ophthalmology.* May; 110(5):895-9.

Egbert, P.R.; Fiadoyor, S.; Budenz, D.L. et al. (2001). Diode laser transscleral cyclophotocoagulation as a primary surgical treatment for primary open-angle glaucoma. *Arch Ophthalmol.* 119:345–50.

Frezzotti, P.; Mittica, V.; Martone, G.; Motolese, I.; Lomurno, L.; Peruzzi, S. & Motolese, E. (2010). Longterm follow-up of diode laser transscleral cyclophotocoagulation in the treatment of refractory glaucoma. *Acta Ophthalmol.* Feb; 88(1):150-5.

Ganesh, S.K. & Rishi, K. (2006). Necrotizing scleritis following diode laser trans-scleral cyclophotocoagulation. *Indian J Ophthalmol.* Sep; 54(3):199-200.

Gangwani, R.; Liu, D.T.; Congdon, N.; Lam, P.T.; Lee, V.Y.; Yuen, N.S. & Lam, D.S. (2011). Effectiveness of diode laser trans-scleral cyclophotocoagulation in patients following silicone oil-induced ocular hypertension in Chinese eyes. *Indian J Ophthalmol.* Jan-Feb; 59(1):64-6.

Ghosh, S.; Singh, D.; Ruddle, J.B.; Shiu, M.; Coote, M.A. & Crowston, J.G. (2010). Combined diode laser cyclophotocoagulation and intravitreal bevacizumab (Avastin) in neovascular glaucoma. *Clin Experiment Ophthalmol.* May; 38(4):353-7.

Grueb, M.; Rohrbach, J.M.; Bartz-Schmidt, K.U. & Schlote, T. (2006). Transscleral diode laser cyclophotocoagulation as primary and secondary surgical treatment in primary open-angle and pseudoexfoliatve glaucoma. Long-term clinical outcomes. *Graefes Arch Clin Exp Ophthalmol.* Oct; 244(10):1293-9.

Han, S.K.; Park, K.H.; Kim, D.M. & Chang, B.L. (1999). Effect of diode laser trans-scleral cyclophotocoagulation in the management of glaucoma after intravitreal silicone oil injection for complicated retinal detachments. *Br J Ophthalmol.* Jun; 83(6):713-7.

Heinz, C.; Koch, J.M. & Heiligenhaus, A. (2006). Transscleral diode laser cyclophotocoagulation as primary surgical treatment for secondary glaucoma in juvenile idiopathic arthritis: high failure rate after short term follow up. *Br J Ophthalmol.* Jun; 90(6):737-40.

Iliev, M.E. & Gerber, S. (2007). Long-term outcome of trans-scleral diode laser cyclophotocoagulation in refractory glaucoma. *Br J Ophthalmol.* Dec; 91(12):1631-5.

Kahook, M.Y.; Lathrop, K.L. & Noecker, R.J. (2007). One-site versus two-site endoscopic cyclophotocoagulation. *J Glaucoma.* Sep; 16(6):527-30.

Kaushik, S.; Pandav, S.S.; Jain, R.; Bansal, S. & Gupta, A. (2008). Lower energy levels adequate for effective transcleral diode laser cyclophotocoagulation in Asian eyes with refractory glaucoma. *Eye (Lond).* Mar; 22(3):398-405.

Kirwan, J.F.; Shah, P. & Khaw, P.T. (2002). Diode laser cyclophotocoagulation: role in the management of refractory pediatric glaucomas. *Ophthalmology.* Feb; 109(2):316-23.

Kramp, K.; Vick, H.P. & Guthoff, R. (2002). Transscleral diode laser contact cyclophotocoagulation in the treatment of different glaucomas, also as primary surgery. *Graefes Arch Clin Exp Ophthalmol.* Sep; 240(9):698-703.

Kwong, Y.Y.; Tham, C.C.; Leung, D.Y. & Lam, D.S. (2006). Scleral perforation following diode laser trans-scleral cyclophotocoagulation. *Eye (Lond).* Nov; 20(11):1316-7.

Lai, J.S.; Tham, C.C. ; Chan, J.C. & Lam, D.S. (2003). Diode laser transscleral cyclophotocoagulation in the treatment of chronic angle-closure glaucoma: a preliminary study. *J Glaucoma.* Aug; 12(4):360-4.

Lai, J.S.; Tham, C.C.; Chan, J.C. & Lam, D.S. (2005). Diode laser transscleral cyclophotocoagulation as primary surgical treatment for medically uncontrolled chronic angle closure glaucoma: long-term clinical outcomes. *J Glaucoma.* Apr; 14(2):114-9.

Lee, R.M.; Al Raqqad, N.; Gomaa, A.; Steel, D.H.; Bloom, P.A. & Liu, C.S. (2011). Endoscopic cyclophotocoagulation in osteo-odonto-keratoprosthesis (OOKP) eyes. *J Glaucoma.* Jan; 20(1):68-9; author reply 69.

Leszczyński, R.; Domański, R.; Formińska-Kapuścik, M.; Mrukwa-Kominek, E. & Rokita-Wala, I. (2009). Contact transscleral cyclophotocoagulation in the treatment of neovascular glaucoma: a five-year follow-up. *Med Sci Monit.* Mar; 15(3):BR84-7.

Lima, F.E.; Magacho, L.; Carvalho, D.M.; Susanna, R. Jr., & Avila, M.P. (2004). A prospective, comparative study between endoscopic cyclophotocoagulation and the Ahmed drainage implant in refractory glaucoma. *J Glaucoma*. Jun; 13(3):233-7.

Lin, P.; Wollstein, G.; Glavas, I.P. et al. (2004). Contact transscleral neodymium:yttrium-aluminum-garnet laser cyclophotocoagulation long-term outcome. *Ophthalmology*. 111:2137–2143. [Erratum in: *Ophthalmology*. 2005; 112:446.]

Lin, P.; Wollstein, G.; Glavas, I.P. & Schuman, J.S. (2005). Contact transscleral neodymium:yttrium-aluminum-garnet laser cyclophotocoagulation Long-term outcome. *Ophthalmology*. Nov; 111(11):2137-43. [Erratum in: Ophthalmology. 2005 Mar; 112(3):446.]

Lin, S.C. (2008). Endoscopic and transscleral cyclophotocoagulation for the treatment of refractory glaucoma. *J Glaucoma*. Apr-May; 17(3):238-47. Review.

Malik, R.; Ellingham, R.B.; Suleman, H. & Morgan, W.H. (2006). Refractory glaucoma--tube or diode? *Clin Experiment Ophthalmol*. Nov; 34(8):771-7.

Murphy, C.C.; Burnett, C.A.; Spry, P.G.; Broadway, D.C. & Diamond, J.P. (2003). A two centre study of the dose-response relation for transscleral diode laser cyclophotocoagulation in refractory glaucoma. *Br J Ophthalmol*. Oct; 87(10):1252-7.

Murthy, G.J.; Murthy, P.R.; Murthy, K.R.; Kulkarni, V.V. & Murthy, K.R. (2009). A study of the efficacy of endoscopic cyclophotocoagulation for the treatment of refractory glaucomas. *Indian J Ophthalmol*. Mar-Apr; 57(2):127-32.

Nabili, S. & Kirkness, C.M. (2004). Trans-scleral diode laser cyclophoto-coagulation in the treatment of diabetic neovascular glaucoma. *Eye (Lond)*. Apr; 18(4):352-6.

Noureddin, B.N.; Zein, W.; Haddad, C.; Ma'luf, R. & Bashshur, Z. (2006). Diode laser transcleral cyclophotocoagulation for refractory glaucoma: a 1 year follow-up of patients treated using an aggressive protocol. *Eye (Lond)*. Mar; 20(3):329-35.

Ocakoglu, O.; Arslan, O.S. & Kayiran, A. (2005). Diode laser transscleral cyclophotocoagulation for the treatment of refractory glaucoma after penetrating keratoplasty. *Curr Eye Res*. Jul; 30(7):569-74.

Pastor, S.A.; Singh, K.; Lee, D.A.; Juzych, M.S.; Lin, S.C.; Netland, P.A. & Nguyen, N.T. (2001). Cyclophotocoagulation: a report by the American Academy of Ophthalmology. Ophthalmology. 2001 Nov; 108(11):2130-8.

Preussner, P.R.; Ngounou, F. & Kouogan, G. (2010). Controlled cyclophotocoagulation with the 940 nm laser for primary open angle glaucoma in African eyes. *Graefes Arch Clin Exp Ophthalmol*. Oct; 248(10):1473-9. Epub 2010 May 2.

Raivio, V.E.; Immonen, I.J. & Puska, P.M. (2001). Transscleral contact krypton laser cyclophotocoagulation for treatment of glaucoma in children and young adults. *Ophthalmology*. Oct; 108(10):1801-7.

Raivio, V.E.; Puska, P.M. & Immonen, I.J. (2008). Cyclophotocoagulation with the transscleral contact red 670-nm diode laser in the treatment of glaucoma. *Acta Ophthalmol*. Aug; 86(5):558-64.

Rivier, D.; Paula, J.S.; Kim, E.; Dohlman, C.H. & Grosskreutz, C.L. (2009). Glaucoma and keratoprosthesis surgery: role of adjunctive cyclophotocoagulation. *J Glaucoma*. Apr-May; 18(4):321-4.

Rotchford, A.P.; Jayasawal, R.; Madhusudhan, S.; Ho, S.; King, A.J. & Vernon, S.A. (2010). Transscleral diode laser cycloablation in patients with good vision. *Br J Ophthalmol*. Sep; 94(9):1180-3.

Schlote, T.; Derse, M. & Zierhut, M. (2000). Transscleral diode laser cyclophotocoagulation for the treatment of refractory glaucoma secondary to inflammatory eye diseases. *Br J Ophthalmol*. Sep; 84(9):999-1003.

Schlote, T.; Grüb, M. & Kynigopoulos, M. (2008). Long-term results after transscleral diode laser cyclophotocoagulation in refractory posttraumatic glaucoma and glaucoma in aphakia. *Graefes Arch Clin Exp Ophthalmol.* Mar; 246(3):405-10.

Schuman, J.S.; Bellows, A.R.; Shingleton, B.J. & al. (1992). Contact transscleral Nd:YAG laser cyclophotocoagulation. Midterm results. *Ophthalmology.* 99:1089–94; discussion 1095.

Semchyshyn, T.M.; Tsai, J.C. & Joos, K.M. (2002). Supplemental transscleral diode laser cyclophotocoagulation after aqueous shunt placement in refractory glaucoma. *Ophthalmology.* Jun; 109(6):1078-84.

Sharkey, J.A. & Murray, T.G. (1994). Identification of the ora serrata and ciliary body by transillumination in eyes undergoing transscleral fixation of posterior chamber intraocular lenses [letter]. *Ophthalmic Surg.* 25:479–80.

Shields, M.B.; Wilkerson, M.H. & Echelman, D.A. (1993). A comparison of two energy levels for noncontact transscleral neodymium-YAG cyclophotocoagulation. *Arch Ophthalmol.* Apr; 111(4):484-7.

Sivagnanavel, V.; Ortiz-Hurtado, A. & Williamson, T.H. (2005). Diode laser trans-scleral cyclophotocoagulation in the management of glaucoma in patients with long-term intravitreal silicone oil. *Eye (Lond).* Mar; 19(3):253-7.

Sony, P.; Sudan, R.; Pangtey, M.S.; Khokhar, S. & Kumar, H. (2003). Iris retraction and retroflexion after transscleral contact diode laser photocoagulation. *Ophthalmic Surg Lasers Imaging.* Nov-Dec; 34(6):470-1.

Sood, S. & Beck, A.D. (2009). Cyclophotocoagulation versus sequential tube shunt as a secondary intervention following primary tube shunt failure in pediatric glaucoma. *J AAPOS.* Aug; 13(4):379-83.

Spencer, A.F. & Vernon SA. (1999). "Cyclodiode": results of a standard protocol. *Br J Ophthalmol.* Mar; 83(3):311-6.

Tan, A.M.; Chockalingam, M.; Aquino, M.C.; Lim, Z.I.; See, J.L. & Chew, P.T. (2010). Micropulse transscleral diode laser cyclophotocoagulation in the treatment of refractory glaucoma. *Clin Experiment Ophthalmol.* Apr; 38(3):266-72.

Vogt, A. (1936). Versuche zur intraokularen druckherabsetzung mittelst diathermieschädigung des corpus ciliare (Zyklodiathermiestichelung). *Klin Monatsbl Augenheilkd.* 97:672–3.

Walland, M.J. (1998). Diode laser cyclophotocoagulation: dose-standardized therapy in end-stage glaucoma. *Aust N Z J Ophthalmol.* May; 26(2):135-9.

Wilensky, J.T. & Kammer, J. (2004). Long-term visual outcome of transscleral laser cyclotherapy in eyes with ambulatory vision. *Ophthalmology.* Jul; 111(7):1389-92.

Yildirim, N.; Yalvac, I.S.; Sahin, A.; Ozer, A. & Bozca, T. (2009). A comparative study between diode laser cyclophotocoagulation and the Ahmed glaucoma valve implant in neovascular glaucoma: a long-term follow-up. *J Glaucoma.* Mar; 18(3):192-6.

Yip, L.W.; Yong, S.O.; Earnest, A.; Ji, J. & Lim, B.A. (2009). Endoscopic cyclophotocoagulation for the treatment of glaucoma: an Asian experience. *Clin Experiment Ophthalmol.* Sep; 37(7):692-7.

Youn, J.; Cox, T.A.; Allingham, R.R. & Shields, M.B. (1996). Factors associated with visual acuity loss after noncontact transscleral Nd:YAG cyclophotocoagulation. *J Glaucoma.* 5:390–4.

Youn, J.; Cox, T.A.; Herndon, L.W.; et al. (1998). A clinical comparison of transscleral cyclophotocoagulation with neodymium: YAG and semiconductor diode lasers. *Am J Ophthalmol.* 126: 640–7.

# 23

# Controlled Cyclophotocoagulation

Paul-Rolf Preußner
*University Eye Hospital, Langenbeckstr*
*Germany*

## 1. Introduction

Glaucoma treatments which partially destroyed the ciliary body started already in the thirthies of the 20th century. Heat and cold were used for this purpose, delivered from different devices such as hot needles, cryo applicators, ultrasound generators or radiation devices. All these methods were successful in lowering introcular pressure, but many eyes were lost and ended in a phthisis. The reasons of such disastrous outcomes is not fully investigated in all details, but it is mostly assumed that the production of aqueous humor has been reduced too much. In summary, the methods were called "cyclodestructive", a wording primarily related to the destruction of tissue in the ciliary body, but also making graphical the high destructive potential to the eye.

With the invention of lasers, many CW-lasers were utilized for tissue coagulation of the ciliary body, and the new word "cyclophotocoagulation" was created, also to distinguish photo- from cryocoagulation (1–13).

For a long time, current opinion was to restrict cyclophotocoagulation to intractable cases due to severe complications which had been observed by several authors (e.g. (14–21)). Meanwhile, however, transscleral cyclophotocoagulation is proposed also as primary therapy (22; 23).

An improvement of the coagulation was achieved by the introduction of contact methods (24), however, efforts undertaken in the past to optimize therapy parameters (25–29) including aspects of radiation transport (30; 31) could not solve the principal problem that the laser burns cannot be observed directly.

Without information about coagulation success, dosage cannot be adjusted to the individual situation which shows a strong inter- and intraindividual variation of optical properties of the corresponding tissue (32). For the reasons mentioned, we had developed a real-time control system (33; 34) to solve this problem.

## 2. Controlling device

During coagulation of the tissue, chemical and physical effects are induced which change the optical properties, i.e. the transmission, absorption and reflection in this material (35). For the ciliary body, this effect cannot be observed directly. However, the transmitted laser radiation produces diffuse stray light which is partly reflected from the fundus and can be observed from outside the eye by a sensor. The principle of the corresponding device is illustrated in fig. 1. The light intensity monitored by the sensor during the laser exposure depends on many

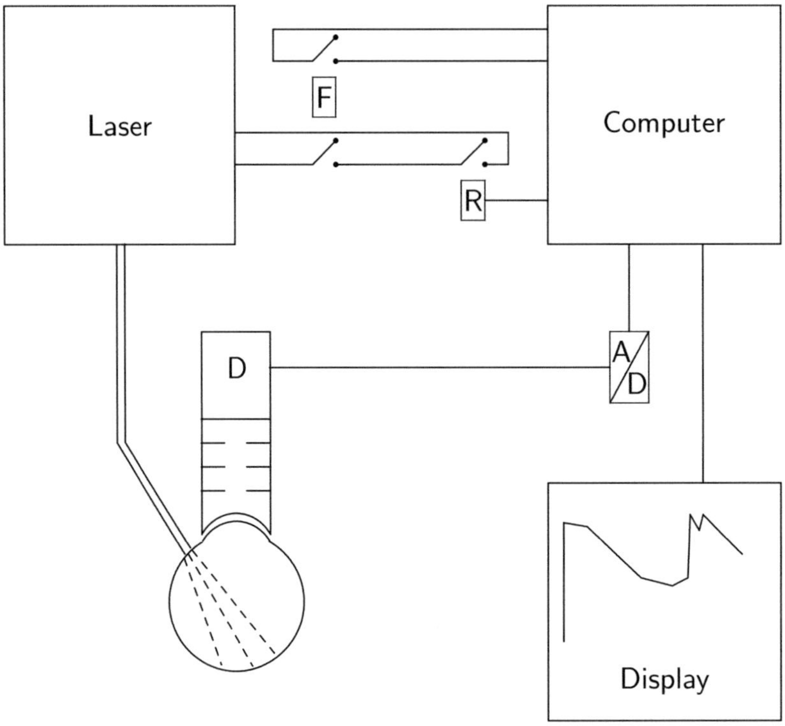


Fig. 1. Functional Diagram. *The laser radiation passing through sclera and ciliary body is partly reflected from the fundus and recorded by a detector* D. *The amplified electronical signal is digitized by an A/D-converter, recorded by a computer and displayed on a screen in real time. The whole process is initiated by pressing the foot-switch* F, *which starts the computer and closes* one *of the switches for the laser device. The* second one *is closed by a semiconductor-relay* R, *which is controlled by the computer. Exposure is stopped either if the operator (viewing the screen) releases his foot-switch* F *or if the computer opens the relay* R, *when the recorded signal has fulfilled certain programmable criteria.*

parameters such as fundus reflectivity, pupil width etc. and can therefore not be used directly as an *absolute* measure of the coagulation stage of the tissue. However, the coagulation process changes the light observed *as function of time* in any case. Therefore, this time dependence can be used to monitor the progress of coagulation. The electronic signal has to be normalized to its starting value, i.e., only *relative values* are used for further evaluation.
There are 2 ways the process can be controlled. First, the surgeon can interrupt the exposure if the displayed curve of changing transmission has a certain shape. This is possible, but difficult, because typical time scales are in the range of 0.1-0.5s, which is approximately the surgeon's own reaction time. As a second "operator", the computer can interrupt the exposure.

## 3. Physical parameters

### 3.1 Laser power

Laser power has to be adjusted in such a way that the target tissue is coagulated as selectively as possible, thereby saving all surrounding tissues. The physical parameters describing this

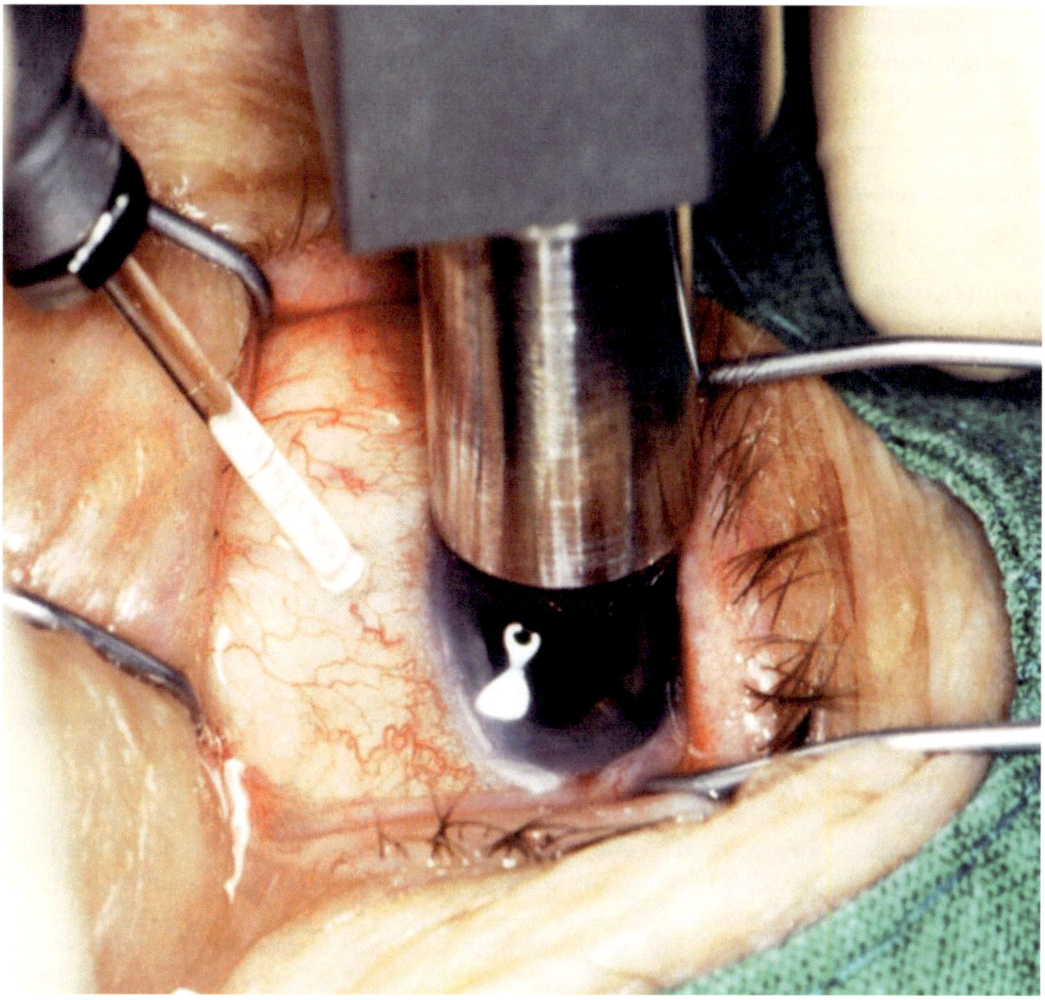

Fig. 2. Application to a Patient's Eye

in context are the *temperature gradient* and the *heat conduction*, which determine the *thermal relaxation time*. If laser power is too low, a long time is needed until coagulation starts. During this time, a high portion of heat is already dissipated into the surrounding tissue. This results in an unwanted large area of coagulated tissue, which can also be observed from the high value of the total energy, the product of power and time. A very high laser power, on the other hand, induces a steep temperature gradient with a higher risk of overheating parts of the target tissue before the rest is sufficiently coagulated. Such overheated tissue has a high probability of so-called "pop spots". A pop spot is a local overheating of the tissue in which the tissue membranes are disrupted by the steam pressure with an audible "pop" as in a pop corn.

As a compromise, we preferably use a laser power of 5W for the 810nm diode laser in Caucasian eyes and found the same value suitable for the 940nm laser in African eyes. Only in very rare cases of buphthalmos with very thin sclera this value has to be reduced to 3W.

### 3.2 Laser wavelength

The laser wavelength for transscleral cyclophotocoagulation must be selected in such a way that the laser light is *transmitted* through the conjunctiva, the sclera and the ciliary muscle, and that it is *absorbed* by the pigment epithelium of the ciliary body. These requirements, however, can only be fulfilled approximatively, depending on the spectral characteristics of the eye.
Caucasian and African eyes strongly differ in the absorption and transmission of visible and infrared radiation. If the absorption is too high, the fraction of energy already absorbed in conjunctiva, sclera or ciliary muscle causes an unwanted overheating of these tissues. Absorption and transmission of ocular tissues show a strong wavelength dependence (36). The spectra shown is this paper are consistent with the fact that the flux density needed for the 1064nm Nd:YAG laser is approximately 2-fold higher than with the 810nm diode laser. They also show that the same behavior as with the 810nm laser in Caucasian eyes could be expected with a 940nm laser in African eyes. In a few African eyes treated with the 810nm laser in Mainz University Eye Hospital, the abovementioned real-time control did not work, i.e. many pop spots occured. Therefore, after tests with African cadaver eyes in Ghana (43), the 940nm laser was clinically established in Cameroun.
Applications of shorter wavelengths for transscleral cyclophotocoagulation in the visible red range have been reported only by Scandinavian authors for a population with very lightly pigmented eyes (8; 37; 38), again consistent with the spectra in (36).

### 3.3 Location

As location, we chose the transition region between pars plicata and pars plana of the ciliary body, i.e., 3-3.5mm posterior to the limbus. We intend to coagulate at least a part of the secreting tissue, but care should be taken of the ciliary muscle including fixation of zonula fibers (which could be disintegrated), because the procedure should also be applicable to phakic, accommodating eyes. The effectiveness of even higher limbus distances has been proven by other authors (39). Fortunately, our real-time control shows optimal performance just in the chosen limbus distance.
Normally, 360° are treated. The only exceptions are scleral lesions / thinned sclera, particularly the areas of previous trabeculectomies.

### 3.4 Optic of the laser applicator

The laser applicator (the tip directly pressed on the eye) should be designed in such a way that the optical power density at the conjunctiva is minimal and the power density in the target tissue (ciliary body) is maximal. Focussing therefore seems to be a reasonable procedure. Unfortunately, the outcome of focussing is rather poor. If a (spherical) lens is used, even for a material with a high refractive index a relatively long focal width results, because the refractive index of the sclera is similar to that of water, i.e., much larger than one. This problem could be solved in principle by a so-called "gradient index lens" (40), for which the focal width can be set to any position. But, our own measurements and calculations (31) also with such optical devices have shown that diffuse multiple scattering in scleral tissue largely neutralises the focussing effect. Fortunately, radiation transport can be optimised by an appropriate choice of the diameter of the optical tip. As shown in (31), this diameter should be larger than or at least equal to the thickness of the sclera. On the other hand, a smaller tip diameter theoretically causes a higher pressure on the sclera leading to an improved optical transmission (41; 42). Thus, both effects have to be balanced against each other by an optimal tip diameter. Tests in Caucasian and African cadaver eyes showed that a tip diameter of 1.5mm was optimal for Caucasian and of 1.95mm for African eyes.

### 3.5 Shape of transmission curves

Typical curves resulting from coagulation in porcine eyes, Caucasian cadaver eyes and in the eyes of Caucasian patients are in detail reported in (33), see fig.3 for an example. The curves of African eyes principally show the same shape, but with slightly different amplitudes from minimum to maximum which therefore needed different software settings.

The shape of these curves (see fig.3) corresponds to the temperature change in the target tissue: In the first, horizontal part (1), no irreversible chemical or physical effects occur, therefore the transmission in the tissue remains constant. The temperature may increase to about 45-50°C. In the second, decreasing part (2), the transmission is reduced mainly by shrinkage of the tissue. The temperature further increases to about 60-70°C. After that, only minor changes in the transmission occur (3), but the temperature increases to a value above 100°C. Trapped, overheated steam then disrupts tissue membranes in the "pop spot". Since for the "wanted" effect of irreversible coagulation, a temperature of about 55-60°C is sufficient, the process should be interrupted at the end of phase two. This is normally less than 1/3 of the time to pop spot, because at the beginning of the coagulation, the temperature raise is steeper than at the end due to heat dissipation to the neighbourhood. Fortunately, further heating above 60°C but well below 100°C is not critical, thus giving a relative safe "therapeutic window" before a pop spot occurs.

## 4. Clinical applications

### 4.1 Indication

Controlled cyclophotocoagulation is indicated in all open angle glaucomas in which eye drops do not effectively reduce the intraocular pressure. This includes cases of insufficient compliance in industrial countries as well as developing countries in which eye drops are not available or not effordable. In severe cases of hemorrhagical secondary glaucoma in blind eyes even repeated controlled cyclophotocoagulation may be insufficient and should be replaced by cryocoagulation.

### 4.2 Preoperative preparation and anesthesia

It is recommended to dilate the pupil preoperatively because it increases the signal-to-noise-ratio of the detector of the real time control, but when the pupil cannot be dilated, the procedure can be applied anyway.

Anesthesia can be a para- or retrobulbar injection, or a general anesthesia, or a combination of topical anesthesia by eye drops and general analgesia (e.g. Propofol combined with a short acting opioid). Topical anesthesia alone with eye drops is insufficient. In case of para- or retrobulbary injections, it should be kept in mind that the risk of these injections is higher than that of the controlled cyclophotocoagulation. Analgesia alone needs very high drug doses when the simulataneous topical anesthesia is omitted.

### 4.3 Treatment

Generally, 16 spots are applied over 360°. A larger number (24 spots) did not result in a significantly higher IOP reduction, but in a significantly higher and longer lasting

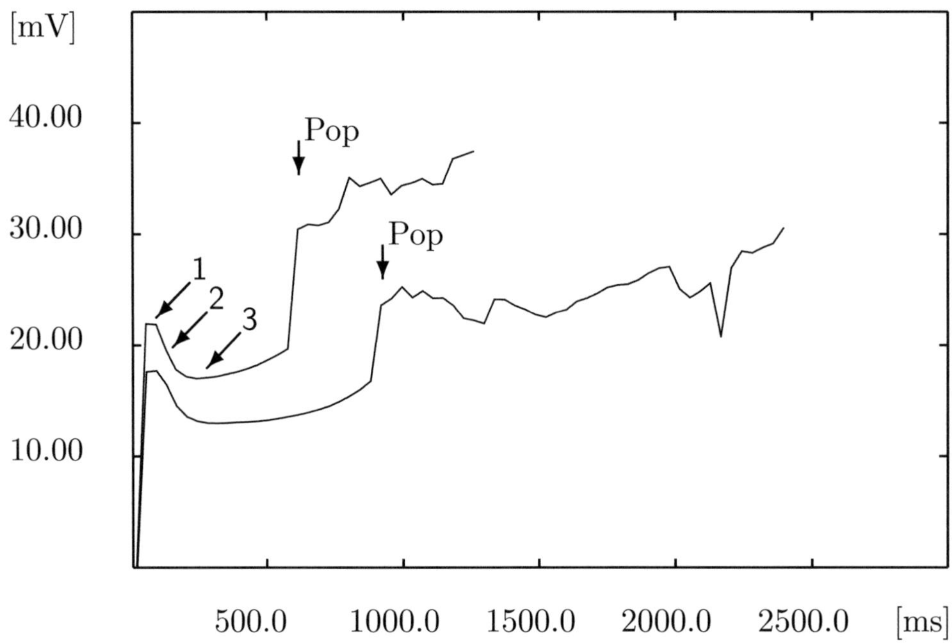


Fig. 3. Typical Transmission Curves. *The recordings are from porcine eyes. The numbers (1,2,3) and their meaning are explained in the text.*

inflammation reaction (cells). An integrated instrument comprising laser source and computer and its application in Cameroun is shown in fig.4.

#### 4.4 Postoperative medication

After surgery, local antibiotics are applied once in order to prevent infections based on minor (and prehaps overlooked) corneal or conjinctival lesions. Local steroids and Scopolamin or Homatropine are applied until there are no more signs of inflammation (cells) visible at the slitlamp.

#### 4.5 Complications

Major complications such as intraocular bleedings, shallow anterior chamber, chorioideal detachment, ocular hypotension <7mmHg or phthisis have not been observed during more than 2000 treatments of Caucasian patients with the 810nm laser in the university eye hospital of Mainz, Germany, nor in more than 1000 treatments of African patients with the 940nm laser in the eye clinic at Acha Bafoussam, Cameroun. Such complications also did not come to our knowledge from other hospitals using this method.
Some minor complications can happen from time to time:
Conjunctival hemorrhages can occur at the locations where the tip is placed on the conjunctiva, particularly in patients with systemic anticoagulation. Depending on the surgeons' experience and care also corneal erosions can be produced. Intraocular iritis (cells)

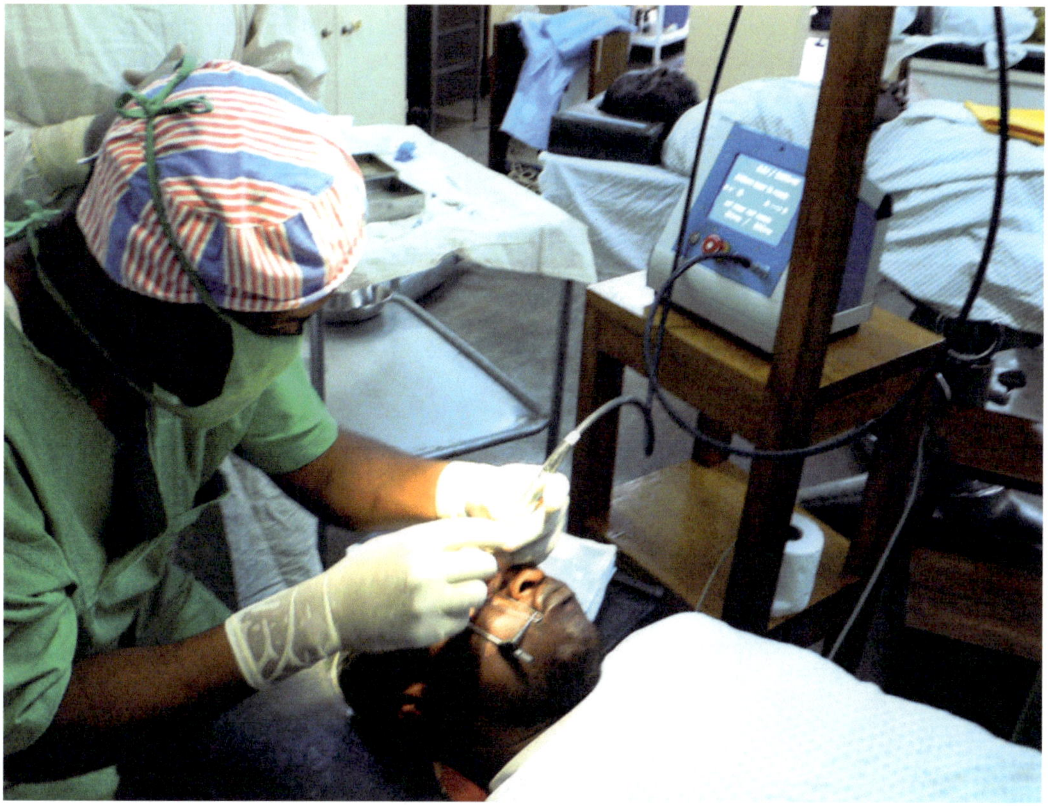

Fig. 4. Application in Camerounian Patients

mostly disappear after one or two days, and higher degrees of inflammation (fibrin exudation) is extremely rare (<1% of the treatments).

In our opinion, also pop spots should be looked at as complications. Even if the probability of pop spots is highly reduced by the real-time control of the coagulation, this probability is not zero. In Caucasian eyes one or more pop spots occur in ≈20% of the eyes, in African eyes in ≈30%.

Even if *visual acuity* as a measure of unwanted side effects has been recorded pre- and postoperatively, the data have not been evaluated systematically. They are often incomplete and biased by the often unknown refraction and by additional reasons (e.g. cataract) that worsens visual acuity. Nevertheless, a significant decrease following the treatment did not occur. It did, however, in Mainz University eye hospital in one case that was treated with 24 spots in the starting phase. The reason was a macula edema. With the generally recommended protocol of 16 spots no further macula edema was observed.

### 4.6 Influence on Intraocular Pressure (IOP)

#### 4.6.1 Caucasian eyes

Despite the high treatment numbers in the University Eye Hospital Mainz, these patients could not be followed up systematically because of the deduction rules of the health insurance. Patients are referred from other doctors to the University Hospital, but seen again only in case of complications or isufficient treatment. Fig.5 shows the IOP of another German hospital which could do a systematic follow-up without selection bias.

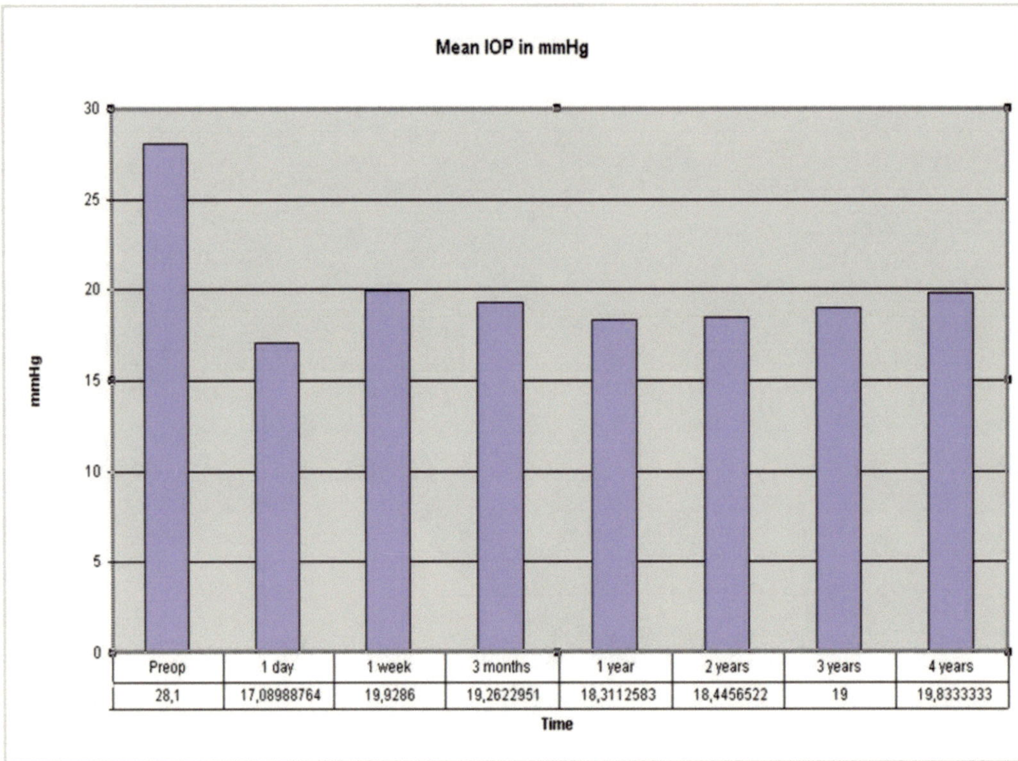


Fig. 5. Intraocular Pressure in European Eyes. *The IOP of 40 eyes in which controlled cyclophotocoagulation was the 1st and only glaucoma surgery is shown as function of the follow-up time of 4 years. The numbers on the bottom of each column show the averages. (Picture by courtesy of Dr. Gerl, Dr. Schmickler, Augenklinik Ahaus, Germany)*

### 4.6.2 African eyes

272 eyes of 188 patients with primary open angle glaucoma were treated in the eye hospital of Bafoussam, Cameroun. Follow-ups were scheduled for 1 day, 1 week, 1 month, 3 months, 6 months and 1 year after surgery. But mostly, patients were unable to meet such fixed dates. Instead, if at all, they appeared more or less at random times after surgery. All individual IOP changes at all recording times are shown in figs. 6 and 7.

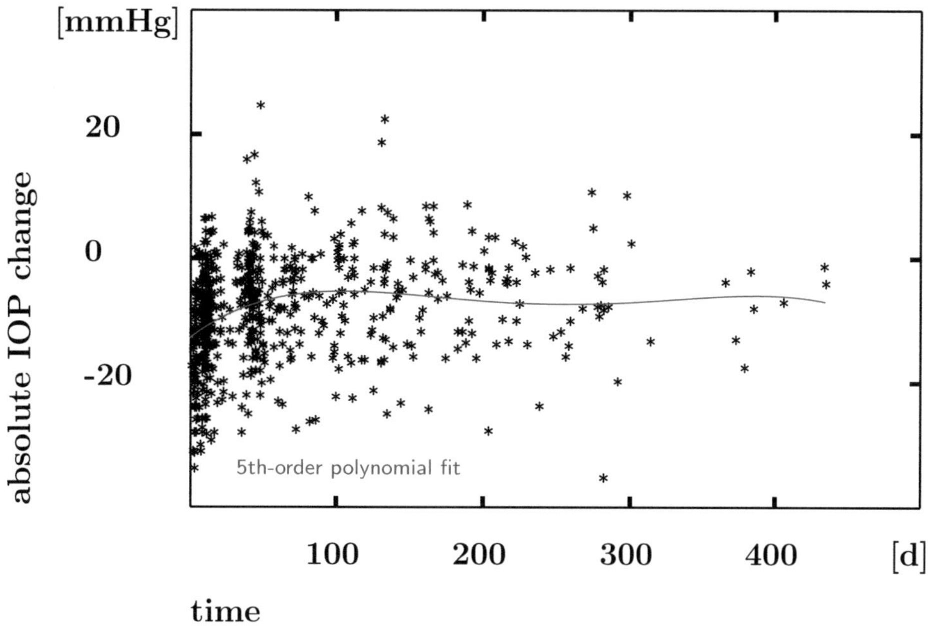


Fig. 6. Absolute Change in IOP *The average of the starting IOP was 28.5mmHg.*

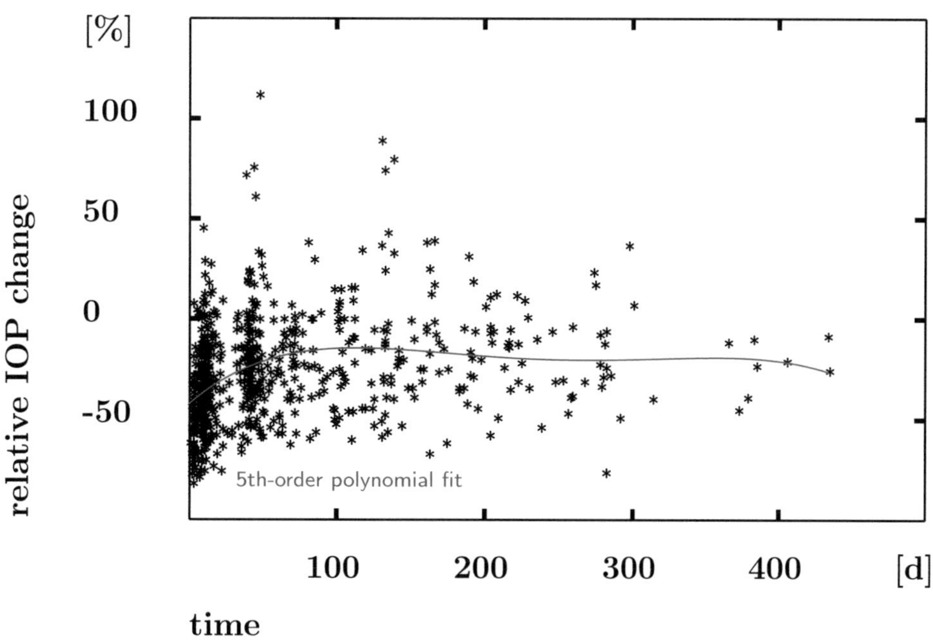


Fig. 7. Relative Change in IOP

## 5. Discussion

Controlled cyclophotocoagulation with the 810nm laser for Caucasian and with the 940nm laser for African glaucoma eyes is a method with nearly negligible complications. However, the individual IOP reduction is not predictable.
Re-treatments are possible, but an interval of at least 4 weeks is recommended, because a significant prostaglandine release for at least 2 weeks is an unavoidable concomittant of the coagulation (45). The maximum number of re-treatments performed so far was 13 in an eye in which no other glaucoma surgery was possible (only functioning eye of this patient, and this eye had already multiple surgeries). The function of the eye could be preserved at an IOP that finally reached 8mmHg. Even if not explicitely shown for humans, at least a partial recovery must be assumed for the coagulated tissue.
The low complication risk can be understood as a result of the low energy load compared with the uncontrolled coagulation. In Caucasian eyes, the energy per spot is $\approx$1.5J and in Africans $\approx$1.0J, which is to be compared with the much higher values reported from other authors: 3.6J (13) or 2.2J to 3.3J (30) in Caucasians and 2.25 to 3.125J in Africans (22). Nd:YAG-laser values are even higher (44).
In Africans, IOP reduction is obviously higher and complication rate lower compared to the uncontrolled coagulation with the 810nm laser (22).
As a consequence of the high power (5W) and low exposure time ($\approx$0.2s in Africans and $\approx$0.3s in Caucasians), the major fraction of energy is thermalized in the highest absorbing tissue, i.e. in the (black) pigmented ciliary epithelium, thus causing a selective coagulation of this target tissue.
As a major drawback, cyclophotocoagulation in general may result in conjunctival scarring which interferes with other procedures such as trabelectomy or shunt tube placement. However, the probability of such conjunctival scarring is reduced by a more selective approach.
To apply such a high power without the risk of very many pop spots, the real time control is an indispensable necessity of the device.

## 6. References


[1] Weekers R, Lavergne G, Watillon M, Gilson M, Legros AM (1961) Effects of photocoagulation of the ciliary body upon ocular tension. Am J Ophthalmol 52:156-163

[2] Beckman H, Kinoshita A, Rota AN, Sugar HS (1972) Transscleral ruby laser irradiation of the ciliary body in the treatment of intractable glaucoma. Trans Am Acad Ophthal Otol 76:423-436

[3] Beckman H, Sugar HS (1973) Neodymium laser cyclophotocoagulation. Arch Ophthalmol 90:27-28

[4] Hampton C, Shields MB, Miller KN, Blasini M (1990) Evaluation of a protocol for transscleral neodymium:YAG cyclophotocoagulation in one hundred patients. Ophthalmology 97:910-917

[5] Brooks AMV, Gillies WE (1991) The use of YAG cyclophotocoagulation to lower pressure in advanced glaucoma. Aust NZ J Ophthal 19:207-210

[6] Heidenkummer HP, Mangouritsas G, Kampik A (1991) Klinische Anwendungen und Ergebnisse der transskleralen Nd:YAG-Zyklophotokoagulation bei therapierefraktärem Glaucom. Klin Mbl Augenheilk 198:174-180

[7] Wright MM, Grajewski AL, Feuer WJ (1991) Nd:YAG cyclophotocoagulation: outcome of treatment for uncontrolled glaucoma. Ophthalmic Surg 22:279-283

[8] Immonen IJ, Puska P, Raitta C (1994) Transscleral contact krypton laser cyclophotocoagulation for treatment of glaucoma. Ophthalmology 101:876-882
[9] Brancato R, Carassa RG, Bettin P, Fiori M, Trabucchi G (1995) Contact transscleral cyclophotocoagulation with diode laser in refractory glaucoma. Eur J Ophthalmol 5:32-39
[10] Hamard P, Kopel J, Valtot F, Quesnot S, Hamard H, Haut J (1995) Traitement des glaucomes réfractaires par cyclophotocoagulation au laser à diode. J Fr Ophthalmol 18:447-454
[11] Hawkins TA, Stewart WC (1993) One-year results of semiconductor transscleral cyclophotocoagulation in patients with glaucoma. Arch Ophthalmol 111:488-491
[12] Hennis HL, Stewart WC (1992) Semiconductor diode laser transscleral cyclophotocoagulation in patients with glaucoma. Am J Ophthalmol 113:81-85
[13] Omofolasade K, Gaasterland DE, Pollack IP, Enger CL (1996) Long-term outcome of initial ciliary ablation with contact diode laser transscleral cyclophotocoagulation for severe glaucoma. Ophthalmology 103:1294-1302
[14] Maus M, Katz LJ (1990) Choroidal detachment, flat anterior chamber, and hypotony as complications of neodymium:YAG laser cyclophotocoagulation. Ophthalmology 97:69-72
[15] Smith RS, Stein MN (1969) Ocular hazards of transscleral laser radiation: II. Intraocular injury produced by ruby and neodymium lasers. Am J Ophthalmol 67:100-110
[16] Hamada M, Suzuki R, Kurimoto S (1991) Transient complete visual loss during transscleral cyclophotocoagulation. Jap J Clin Ophthalmol 45:949-951
[17] Edwards DP, Brown SV, Higginbotham E (1989) Sympathetic ophthalmia following Nd:YAG cycloptherapy. Ophthalmic Surg 20:544-546
[18] Bechrakis NE, Müller-Stolzenburg NW, Helbig H (1994) Sympathetic ophthalmia following laser cyclocoagulation. Arch Ophthalmol 112:80-84
[19] Geyer O, Neudorfer M, Lazar M (1993) Retinal detachment as a complication of neodymium:yttrium:aluminium garnet laser cyclocoagulation. Ann Ophthalmol 25:170-172
[20] Johnson SM (1998) Neurotrophic corneal defects after diode laser cycloablation. Am J Ophthalmol 126:725-727
[21] Sabry K, Vernon SA (1999) Scleral perforation following trans-scleral cyclodiode. Br J Ophthalmol 83:502-503
[22] Egbert PR, Fiadoyor S, Budenz DL, Dadzie P, Byrd S (2001) Diode laser transscleral cyclophotocoagulation as a primary surgical treatment for primary open-angle glaucoma. Arch Ophthalmol 119:345-350
[23] Kramp K, Vick HP, Guthoff R (2002) Transscleral diode laser contact cyclophotocoagulation in the treatment of different glaucomas, also as primary surgery. Graefes Arch Clin Exp Ophthalmol 240:698-703
[24] Federman JL, Ando F, Schubert HD, Eagle RC (1987) Contact laser for transscleral photocoagulation. Ophthalmic Surg 18:183-184
[25] Allingham RR, Kater AW de, Bellows AR, Hsu J (1990) Probe placement and power levels in contact transscleral neodymium:YAG cyclophotocoagulation. Arch Ophthalmol 108:738-742
[26] England C, Van der Zypen E, Fankhauser F, Kwasniewska S (1988) A comparison of optical methods used for transscleral cyclophotocoagulation in rabbit eyes produced with the Nd:YAG laser: a morphological physical and clinical analysis. Lasers Light Ophthalmol 2:87-102

[27] Kwasniewska S, Fankhauser F, Van der Zypen E, Rol P, Henchoz PD, England C (1988) Acute effects following transscleral contact irradiation of the ciliary body and the retina/choroid with the cw Nd:YAG laser. Lasers Light Ophthalmol 2:25-34
[28] Schuman JS, Noecker RJ, Puliafito CA, Jacobsson JJ, Shepps GJ, Wang N (1991) Energy levels and probe placement in contact transscleral semiconductor diode laser cyclophotocoagulation in human cadaver eyes. Arch Ophthalmol 109:1534-1538
[29] Takahashi H, Okisaka S (1991) Safety and effectiveness of contact transscleral cyclophotocoagulation with continuous-wave Nd:YAG laser. Jap J Clin Ophthalmol 45:1233-1237
[30] Roider J, Schmidt-Erfurth U, El-Hifnawi E, Herboth T, Hoerauf H, Birngruber R, Laqua H (1996) Zyklophotokoagulation mit dem Diodenlaser im Kontaktverfahren mit einer neuen fokussierenden Sonde. Ophthalmologe 93:576-580
[31] Preußner PR, Schwenn O (1995) Steps to optimize transscleral photocoagulation. Graefes Arch Clin Exp Ophthalmol 233:302-306
[32] Echelman DA, Stern RA, Shields SR, Simmons RB, Shields MB (1995) Variability of contact transscleral neodymium:YAG cyclophotocoagulation. Invest Ophthalmol Vis Sci 36:497-502
[33] Preußner PR, Boos N, Faßbender K, Schwenn O, Pfeiffer N (1997) Real-time control for transscleral cyclophotocoagulation. Graefes Arch Clin Exp Ophthalmol 235:794-801
[34] Preußner PR (1998) Kontrollierte Zyklophotokoagulation. Ophthalmologe 95:645-650
[35] Francis A. L'Esperance, Ophthalmic lasers, 3rd ed., Mosby, 1989.
[36] Geeraets WJ, Williams RC, Chan G, Ham WT, Guerry D, Schmidt FH (1960) The loss of light energy in retina and choroid. Arch Ophthalmol 64: 606-615
[37] Raivio VE, Immonen IJ, Puska PM (2001) Transscleral contact krypton laser cyclophotocoagulation for treatment of posttraumatic glaucoma. J Glaucoma 10:77-84
[38] Raivio VE, Vesaluoma MH, Tervo TM, Immonen IJ, Puska PM (2002) Corneal innervation, corneal mechanical sensitivity, and tear fluid secretion after transscleral contact 670nm diode laser cyclophotocoagulation. J Glaucoma 11:446-453
[39] Liu GJ,Mizukawa A, Okisaka S (1994) Mechanism of intraocular pressure decrease after contact transscleral continuous-wave Nd:YAG laser cyclophotocoagulation. Ophthalmic Res 26:65-79
[40] Schröder G (1990) Technische Optik. Kamprath-Reihe, Vogel, Würzburg, ISBN 3-8023-0067-X
[41] Rol P, Niederer P, Dürr U, Henchoz PD, Fankhauser F (1990) Experimental investigations on the light scattering properties of the human sclera. Laser and Light in Ophthalmol 3:201-212
[42] Vogel A, Dlugos C, Nuffer R, Birngruber R (1991) Die optischen Eigenschaften der menschlichen Sklera und deren Bedeutung für transsklerale Laseranwendungen. Fortschr Ophthalmol 88:754-761
[43] Holbach M, Fiadoyor S, Preußner PR. Controlled cyclophotocoagulation for the therapy of primary open angle glaucoma in African eyes. Presentation on the 101. congress of the Deutsche Ophthalmologische Gesellschaft (DOG), Berlin, 25.-28.09.2003
[44] Krott R, Diestelhorst M, Zollweg M, Krieglstein GK (1997) Zur Dosis-Wirkungs-Beziehung der transskleralen Kontaktzyklophotokoagulation. Ophthalmologe 94:273-276
[45] Nasisse MP, McGahan MC, Shields MB, Echelman D, Fleisher LN (1992) Inflammatory effects of continuous-wave neodymium:yttrium aluminum garnet laser cyclophotocoagulation. Invest Ophthalmol Vis Sci 33:2216-2223

# Part 3

# Clinical Concepts – Specific Glaucoma Entities

# 24

# Congenital Glaucoma

Jair Giampani Junior and Adriana Silva Borges Giampani
*Federal University of Mato Grosso,*
*Brazil*

## 1. Introduction

### 1.1 Terminology, epidemiology and heredity

Congenital glaucoma is a major cause of blindness in children, despite its low incidence (1:10,000 births)[1]. This category includes isolated congenital glaucoma (also called primary congenital glaucoma) and glaucomas associated with other developmental anomalies, either systemic or ocular.

Juvenile glaucoma is the term used to designate cases in which the pressure rise develops after the third birthday but before the age of 16 years.[2] The enlargement of the eye (buphthalmos) is least common, despite the elevated intraocular pressure. Gonioscopy is normal or reveals trabeculodysgenesis. This condition may simulate the primary open-angle glaucoma.

The eyes with primary congenital glaucoma have an isolated maldevelopment of the trabecular meshwork not associated with others developmental ocular anomalies or ocular diseases that can raise intraocular pressure. It's the most common glaucoma of infancy, occurring in about 1: 30,000 live births[1].

Primary congenital glaucoma is a bilateral disease in about 75% of cases, with males accounting for approximately 65% of cases. [2] Most cases are sporadic in occurrence, with no evident hereditary pattern. In approximately 10% in which a hereditary pattern is evident, it generally is believed to be autosomal recessive. Many authors believe the inheritance pattern is polygenic.[1]

### 1.2 Pathogenesis

Clinical evidence supports the theory that the obstruction to aqueous flow, with a resultant increase in intraocular pressure, is located at the trabecular sheets. This obstruction is caused by maldevelopment of the anterior chamber angle, unassociated with any other major ocular anomalies (isolated trabeculodysgenesis).[2]

Clinically, trabeculodysgenesis is characterized by absence of the angle recess, with the iris inserted into the surface of the trabeculum in one of two configurations:[2]

a. Flat iris insertion: the iris inserts flatly into the thickened trabeculum at or anterior to the scleral spur.
b. Concave iris insertion: is less common. The plane of the iris is well posterior to the normal position of the scleral spur. However, the anterior iris stroma continues upward and over the trabecular meshwork, obscuring the scleral spur and the others angular structures.

### 1.3 Clinical presentation

Frequently, the first symptoms of primary congenital glaucoma are epiphora, photophobia and blepharospasm. These symptoms occur secondary to the corneal epithelial edema caused by elevated intraocular pressure.

The elevated intraocular pressure also causes an enlargement of the eye (buphthalmos) (Figure 1), mainly at the corneoscleral junction. Stretching of the zonules can cause lens subluxation.[3]

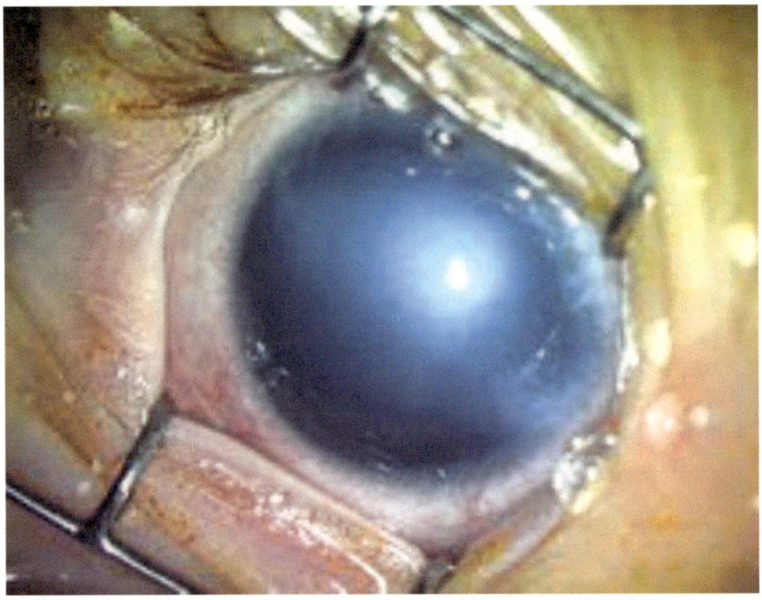

Fig. 1. Buphthalmos and corneal edema (Courtesy Prof. Augusto Paranhos Jr.)

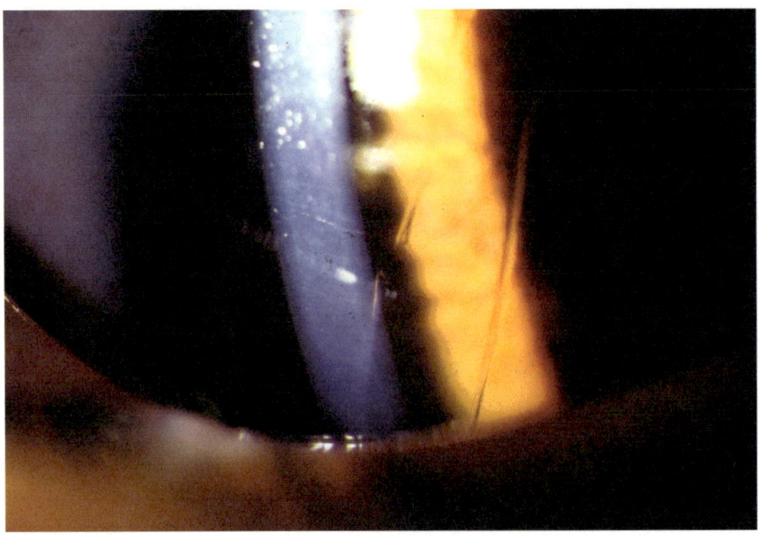

Fig. 2. Haab's striae (Courtesy Prof. Ernst Oltrogge)

As the cornea stretches, ruptures of the Descemet´s membrane allow influx of aqueous into the corneal stroma and epithelium, causing an increase in edema and haze. The breaks in Descemet´s membrane (Haab´s striae - Figure 2) are single or multiples, and appear as elliptical parallel ridges on the posterior cornea.[3] The Haab's striae are usually horizontal or oblique in contrast to traumatic Descemet's tears that are vertically oriented. Progressive myopia may occur if the elevated intraocular pressure persists.

Pain is unusual in the older child with glaucoma, unless corneal erosion or ulceration appear.

In contrast to the adult eye, the scleral canal in the infant eye enlarges as part of the generalized enlargement of the globe, and the lamina cribrosa may bow posteriorly, in response to elevated intraocular pressure. Therefore, cup size may be increased from neuronal loss, enlargement of the scleral canal, or both.[2]

### 1.4 Initial evaluation and follow-up (Flowchart 1)

Depending on the patient's age and ability to cooperate, either an office examination or an examination using general anesthesia with intravenous ketamine is required to evaluate the child with glaucoma.[3]

Examination of the corneal diameter should be undertaken first, followed by applanation tonometry, slit lamp examination, gonioscopy and evaluation of the optic discs.

a. corneal diameter should be measured in both vertical and horizontal meridians with calipers. The horizontal diameter is usually easier to measure and more accurate than the vertical, due an excessive corneal limbus stretching in this meridian. A diameter > 12 mm prior to the age of one year should be viewed with suspicion.[4]

b. Intraocular pressure could be measure with a Goldmann tonometer, Perkins tonometer or Tono-Pen. Elevated intraocular pressure by itself, unless extreme, is not sufficient to confirm a diagnosis of glaucoma. It is necessary to depend on signs such as increased corneal diameter and corneal thickness, increased cup-disc ratio or evidence of trabeculodysgenesis to confirms the diagnosis.

   The normal intraocular pressure in children under general anesthesia is unknown. Some authors consider glaucoma suspects children with IOP above 14 mm Hg.[4] Nevertheless, its important to remember the major of anesthetics reduces the intraocular pressure, while ketamine may increase intraocular pressure.[4]

c. The slit lamp examination may reveal corneal edema, haze and ruptures of the Descemet´s membrane (Haab´s striae). The anterior chamber is deep, with iris hypoplasia sometimes showing the iris pigment epithelium.[4] Stretching of the zonules can cause lens subluxation.

d. Gonioscopy should be performed with a Koeppe lens or one of the others goniolenses. Gonioscopy of the eye with congenital glaucoma reveals an anterior insertion of the iris directly into the trabecular meshwork. This insertion most commonly is flat (Figure 3), although a concave insertion may also be seen. The level of the iris insertion may vary at different areas of the angle. No pigment band is present, but a thin section of ciliary body can be seen through the thickened trabeculum. The peripheral iris may show a thinning of the anterior stroma.

e. Opthalmoscopy of the eye with congenital glaucoma may be impossible in some cases, due corneal edema and/or haze. The infant glaucomatous cup usually has a configuration different from that of an adult glaucomatous cup. It's more commonly round, steep walled and central.[1] The cup tends to enlarge circumferentially with progression of the glaucoma. In the very young, cupping can decrease after intraocular pressure is brought under control. To provide records for future comparison, it is best to take photographs of the optic nerve head, whenever possible.

f. Auxiliary exams: the measurement of axial length by A-scan ultrasonography has been recommended by some authors for routine use in the diagnosis and follow-up of congenital glaucoma.[4] The eyes with congenital glaucoma commonly present an elevated axial length due the elevated intraocular pressure.

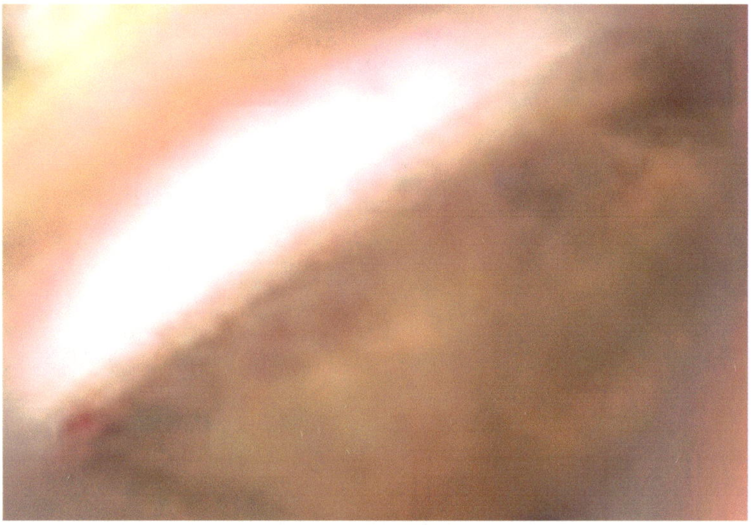

Fig. 3. Gonioscopy showing the flat iris configuration (Courtesy Prof. Augusto Paranhos Jr.)

The standard automated perimetry may be useful in the diagnosis and follow-up of congenital glaucoma patients above 7 years old.[4] Unfortunately, there is not adequate software to analyze children in any automated perimeters.

Patients with congenital glaucoma require follow-up examinations for life. The IOP measure, ophthalmoscopy and visual field analysis, when it is possible, must be realized at least every 3 to 6 months, depending the glaucoma severity. The long-term prognosis for intraocular pressure control in successfully treated cases of congenital glaucoma appears excellent. However, the visual outcome and IOP control in unsuccessfully treated cases after one or two surgical procedures, may be poor.

### 1.5 Differential diagnosis

Many conditions may confuse the primary congenital glaucoma diagnosis and present corneal edema, epiphora, corneal enlargement or elevated intraocular pressure. [2]

a. Cloudy cornea at birth: trauma with breaks in the Descemet´s membrane, intrauterine rubella, metabolic disorders (mucopolysaccharidoses) and congenital hereditary endothelial dystrophy.
b. Corneal enlargement: megalocornea and high myopia.
c. Epiphora: congenital obstruction of the nasolacrimal duct.
d. Secondary infantile glaucoma: trauma, ectopia lentis, uveitis, tumors, retinopathy of prematurity and persistent hyperplastic primary vitreous, corticosteroid-related glaucoma.

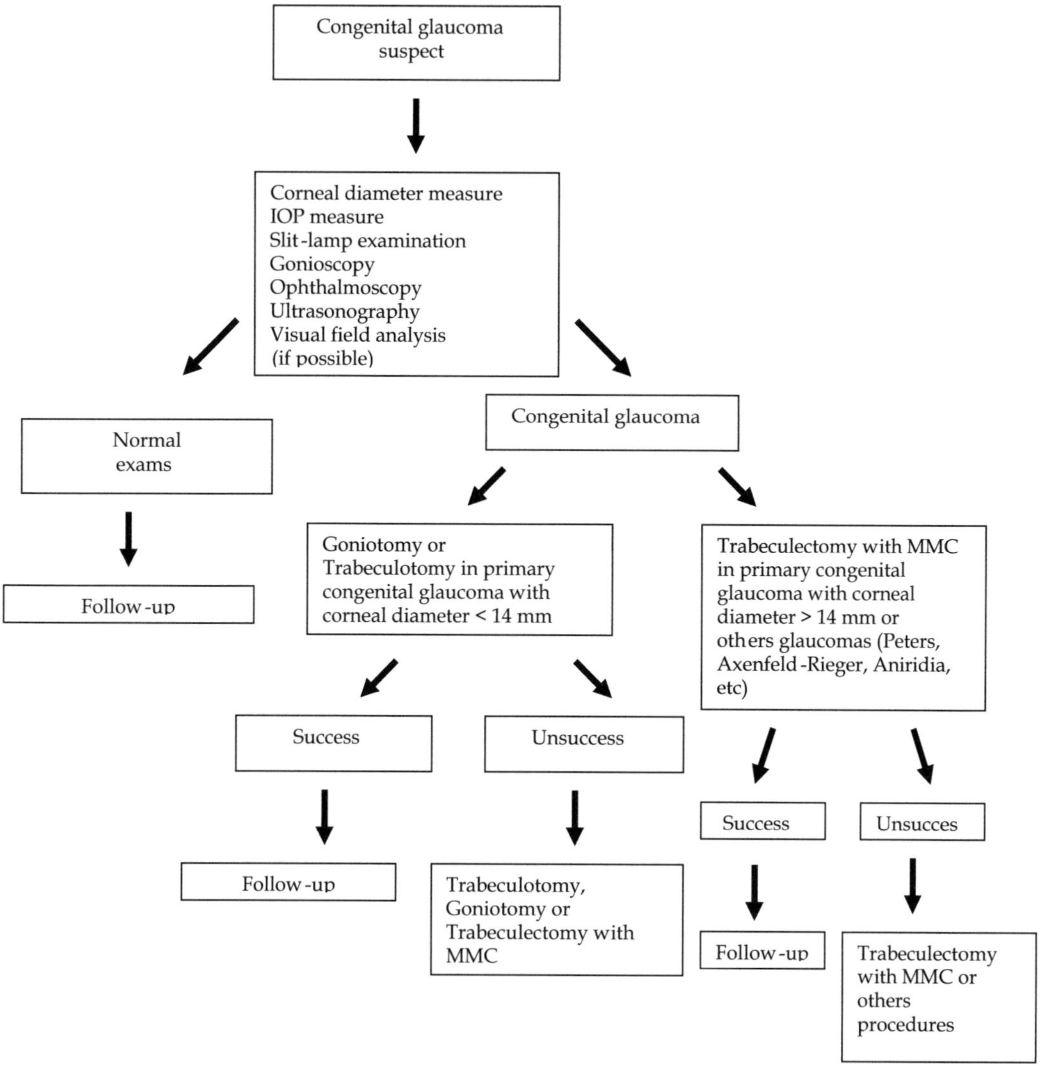


Flowchart 1. congenital glaucoma management and follow-up

### 1.6 Management

Congenital glaucoma is essentially a surgical disease, in which surgery must be performed as early as possible. Goniotomy and trabeculotomy are usually the first procedures of choice (Flowchart 1).[1] Both are safe and have a low incidence of complications. Factors that can decrease the success rate of initial trabeculotomy are the association of CG with others ocular anomalies (Peters, Sturge-Weber, Aniridia, etc.) and a corneal diameter of > 14 mm.[2] Usually, trabeculectomy is the option when previous goniotomies or trabeculotomies failed. Glaucoma drainage implants, non-penetrating surgery and cyclodestructive procedures are options also.

Surgery is preferred for several reasons, including problems with compliance to medications, lack of knowledge about the systemic effects of medications in the infant and poor response

to clinical treatment in infants. Moreover, surgery has a high success rate and low incidence of complications.
Neither goniotomy nor trabeculotomy should be performed by surgeons inexperienced with the procedure. The first operation, whether goniotomy or trabeculotomy, has the greatest chance of success.

*a) Goniotomy*

Goniotomy is a very safe procedure when performed skillfully. Goniotomy is commonly the procedure of choice when corneal transparency permits adequate visualization of the angle (Figures 4 and 5). Corneal clouding only rarely prevents performance of goniotomy, particularly if cloudy epithelium is removed.[4]

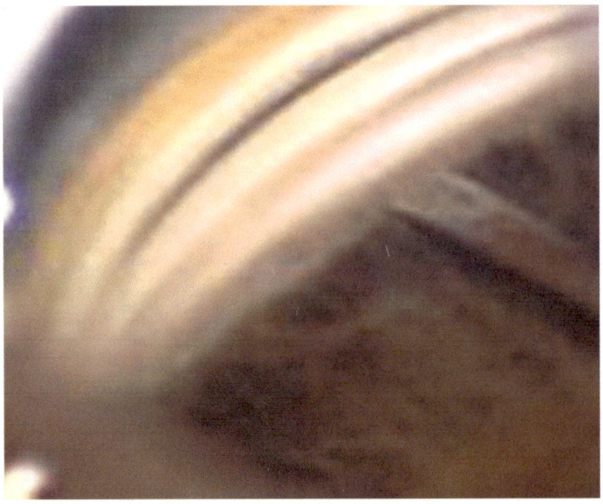

Fig. 4. Goniotomy (Courtesy Prof. Augusto Paranhos Jr.)

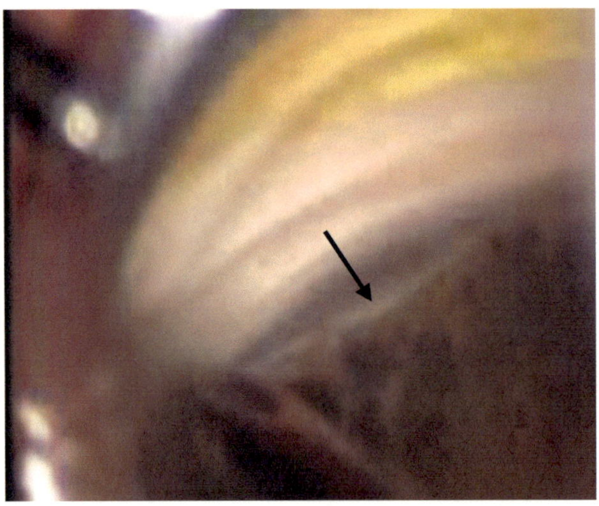

Fig. 5. Goniotomy: see the iris configuration after incision (arrow) (Courtesy Prof. Augusto Paranhos Jr.)

It is necessary a goniolenses, like the Worst lens, to performed the goniotomy through direct visualization of the angle.
Shaffer[5] reported in a study on a series of 287 eyes, one or two goniotomies cured 94% of patients diagnosed between 1 month and 24 months of age. Goniotomy is unlikely to be effective if corneal diameter exceeds 14 mm, since in such eyes the Schlemm´s canal is obliterated.[2]

*b) Trabeculotomy*

Trabeculotomy may be necessary if corneal clouding prevents visualization of the angle (Figures 6 and 7). It was described initially by Burian in 1964, and posteriorly improved by Harms and Machensen.[4]

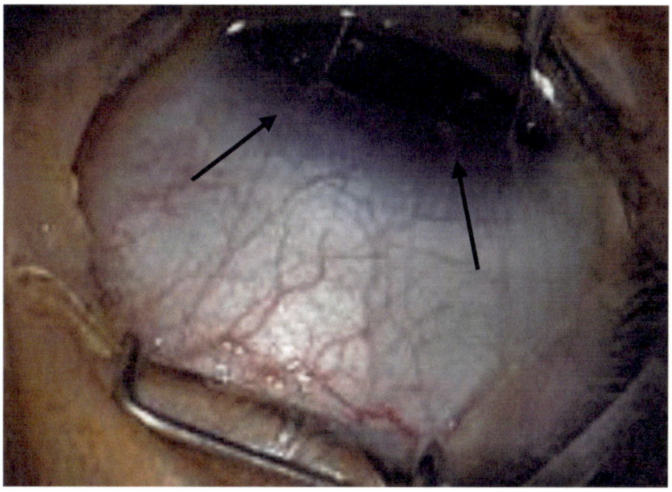

Fig. 6. Trabeculotomy: see the enlargement of the corneoscleral junction (arrows) (Courtesy Prof. Augusto Paranhos Jr.)

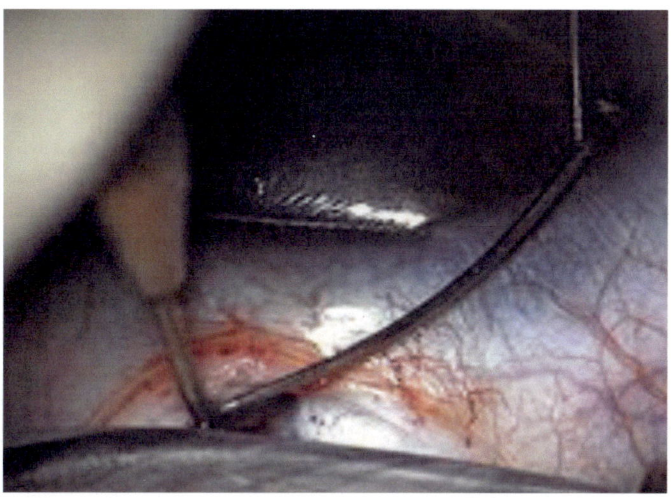

Fig. 7. Trabeculotomy: see the trabeculotome position (Courtesy Prof. Augusto Paranhos Jr.)

Trabeculotomy also has a high success rate, with most studies citing an 80% to 90% success rate.[6] The incidence of complications is low, and includes hyphema, tears in Descemet´s membrane, ciclodialysis, iridodialysis and synechiae.[3]

*c) Update in trabeculectomy in congenital glaucoma*

Usually, trabeculectomy is the option when previous goniotomies or trabeculotomies failed. It has been reported that trabeculectomy without adjunctive antimetabolites in pediatric patients (less than 18 years of age) has a successful outcome in 30 % to 50% of cases.[7-9] The 50% rate is from a study with relatively short follow-up (mean 15.5 months).[7] Studies with longer follow-up report a success rate of 30% to 35%. [8-9]

Mitomycin C (MMC) is a more potent inhibitor of fibroblast proliferation comparing to 5-fluorouracil, and can be used intraoperatively, making it an attractive alternative for children in which previous surgery have failed. Clinical studies comparing the two antifibrotic agents have demonstrated a greater success rate and a greater degree of IOP with MMC.[10-13]

Susanna et al. [14] had an overall success rate of 67% with a mean follow-up of 17 months in a series of 56 patients (79 eyes) with primary congenital glaucoma or developmental glaucomas underwent to trabeculectomy and adjunctive MMC. This success rate is better than it described for Giampani Jr et al.[15] (55.26 %), probably because their longer follow-up (61.16 months).

Beck et al.[16] described a success rate of 58% after 24 months follow-up, although they had a large number of aphakic patients and a mean age of 91.2 months (7.6 years old). Sidoti et al. [17] showed a success rate of 59% in a case series with 29 eyes, with a mean follow-up time of 25.1 +/- 16 months. Giampani Jr et al.[15] described a success rate of 90.2 % at 24-month, 78.7% at 36-month, 60.7 % at 48-month and 50.8 % at 60-month.

A very high success rate (95%) was described by Mandal et al. in a series of 19 mitomycin C trabeculectomies (Table 1).[18] However, this study had only one patient under 1 year of age, which may be an important factor in that study's superb success rate. Miller and Rice also showed a better prognosis for surgeries performed in older children.[19]

Susanna et al. noted no changes in success rate when comparing eyes that had previous glaucoma surgery with those eyes that had no prior surgery.[14] They suggested that the results of the group that had no prior glaucoma surgery were skewed by the presence of more eyes with poor prognoses, namely Axenfeld-Rieger syndrome, Sturge-Weber syndrome, and Aniridia. Beck et al.[16] demonstrated a lower success rate for the group that had prior glaucoma surgery (55% compared with 70%), but without statistically significant difference. Giampani Jr et al. observed that the success rate was also higher in the group with no previous glaucoma surgery (64.28% compared with 51.21 %), but without statistically significant difference also (p= 0.32).[15]

Endophthalmitis is a major complication associated with trabeculectomy, and it has been reported in children who have had trabeculectomy with mitomycin C.[20] Giampani Jr et al. observed eight eyes with endophthalmitis in a total of 164 operated eyes (4.88 %).[15] Beck and associates[16] reported a higher endophthalmitis rate (8%), while Susanna et al[14] reported one case in 79 eyes, and Wallace and associates[21] noted one case in a series of 16 eyes. Mandal et al. had no cases of endophthalmitis in 19 eyes.[18] Sidoti et al. described the highest infection complication rate of any reported series (10% of blebitis and 7% of endophthalmitis).[17] Probably, the higher MMC concentration utilized for them (0.5 mg/mL) explained, in part, that rate. In adults, the endophthalmitis rate after use of antimetabolites range from 2% to 9%.[22-24]

Others complications, like overfiltration and hypotony maculopathy, are rarely observed after trabeculectomy with adjunctive mitomycin C in primary congenital glaucomas.[15]

| Authors | Success rate (%) | Follow-up (months) |
|---|---|---|
| *Giampani Jr. et al.*[15] | 55.26% | 61.16 |
| *Beck et al* [16] | 58% | 24 |
| *Sidoti et al.*[17] | 59% | 25.1 |
| *Susanna et al.*[14] | 67% | 17 |
| *Mandal et al.*[18] | 95% | 19.52 |

Table 1. Trabeculectomy success rate in congenital glaucoma

*a) Aqueous drainage device surgery in congenital glaucoma*

Aqueous drainage devices were recommended in congenital glaucoma treatment when others procedures, like goniotomy, trabeculotomy and trabeculectomy failed (Figures 8 and 9). Unfortunately, the long-term successful rate is generally poor.[4]

O´Malley et al. described, in a chart review including 38 eyes with congenital glaucoma, a success rate about only 42% after 10 years follow-up.[25] Khan et al. observed, in a small sample of 11 eyes with congenital glaucoma, a success rate of 90.9% after 2 years follow-up, using the silicone Ahmed valve.[26] A long -term study using this device is needed to determine whether or not silicone as a good option in congenital glaucoma patients.

The most common complications in congenital glaucoma patients are tube malpositioning with corneal touch, tube exposure, endophthalmitis, retinal detachment and ocular motility abnormalities.[27]

*b) Cyclodestructive procedures*

Cyclocryotherapy may be used when repeated surgery to improve outflow has failed. Transscleral cyclophotocoagulation has been used to produce thermal damage to the ciliary body and processes to decrease aqueous production. This method can have the advantage of less pain and inflammation than with cyclocryotherapy, but it still usually is reserved for cases in which surgery to improve aqueous outflow has failed.[3]

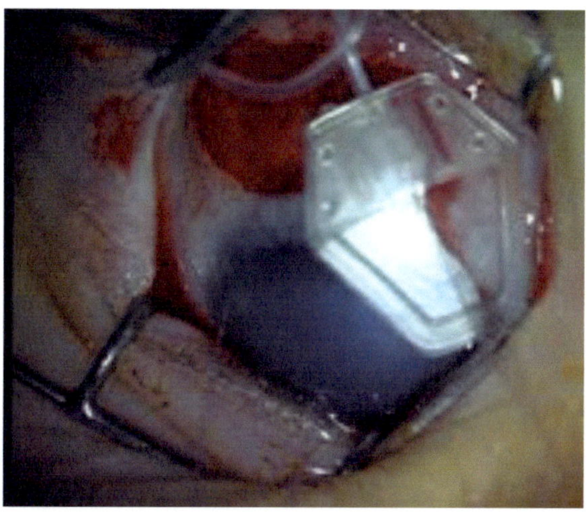

Fig. 8. Ahmed valve in primary congenital glaucoma (Courtesy Augusto Paranhos Jr.)

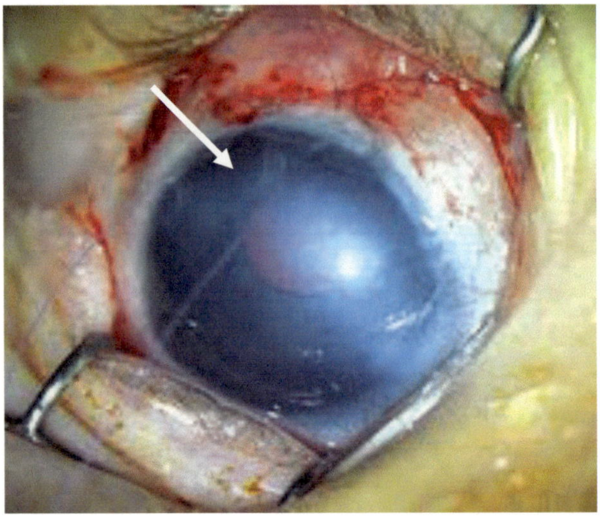

Fig. 9. Ahmed valve: see the tube in the anterior chamber (arrow) (Courtesy Augusto Paranhos Jr.)

*c) Novel surgical procedures*

Viscocanalostomy was recently described as a novel surgical procedure to improve the aqueous outflow in congenital glaucoma patients. Kay et al. reviewed 39 eyes that underwent dilation and probing of Schlemm´s canal and viscocanalostomy. Surgical success was achieved in 27 of 39 eyes (69%) with an average follow-up of 22 months. In patients without history of previous surgery and the diagnosis of primary congenital or juvenile glaucoma, surgical success was achieved in 17 of 19 eyes (89%) with an average follow-up of 20 months. There were no serious surgical complications associated with this procedure in this study.[28]

Nouredin et al. studied the effectiveness of viscocanalostomy in patients with primary congenital glaucoma and compared it with trabeculotomy ab externo. Eight patients with bilateral primary congenital glaucoma were enrolled in the study. After establishing the diagnosis, the more severely affected eye was randomly selected to undergo either trabeculotomy ab externo or viscocanalostomy, whereas the second eye underwent the other surgery 2 weeks after the first. The mean standard deviation (SD) follow-up period was 12.5 (1.86) months. A drop in IOP was noted in both groups at week 1, month 6 and at the last follow-up visit ($p<0.001$).[29] Viscocanalostomy proved to be as effective as trabeculotomy ab externo in lowering IOP in this small sample study. Nevertheless, long-term follow-up studies using viscocanalostomy are required to determine it as a good option in congenital glaucoma patients.

## 2. Glaucomas associated with congenital anomalies

### 2.1 Iridocorneal dysgenesis

Iridocorneal dysgenesis consists of overlapping rare congenital disorders involving the cornea and the iris, some of which may be associated with glaucoma. These conditions occur as a result of abnormal neural crest cell development and are: Axenfeld-Rieger syndrome, Peters anomaly and aniridia.[30]

*a) Axenfeld-Rieger syndrome*

This syndrome is characterized by a mesodermal dysgenesis with different degrees of presentation. The Axenfeld anomaly shows a prominent and anteriorly displaced Schwalbe´s line (called posterior embryotoxon) onto which are attached strands of peripheral iris tissue (Figure 10). The secondary glaucoma is rare in this condition. On the other hand, the Rieger anomaly is an autosomal dominant condition with a high degree of penetrance, where mutations in PITX2 and FOXC1 genes were described.[31] Involvement is usually bilateral but not always symmetrical. The slit-lamp biomicroscopy may show posterior embryotoxon, iris stromal hypoplasia, corectopia, pseudopolycoria and ectropion uveae (Figure 11). The gonioscopy in mild cases shows Axenfeld anomaly. In severe cases, broad leaves of the iris stroma adhere to the corneal anterior to Schwalbe´s line. Glaucoma develops in about 50% of cases, usually during the early childhood.[4]

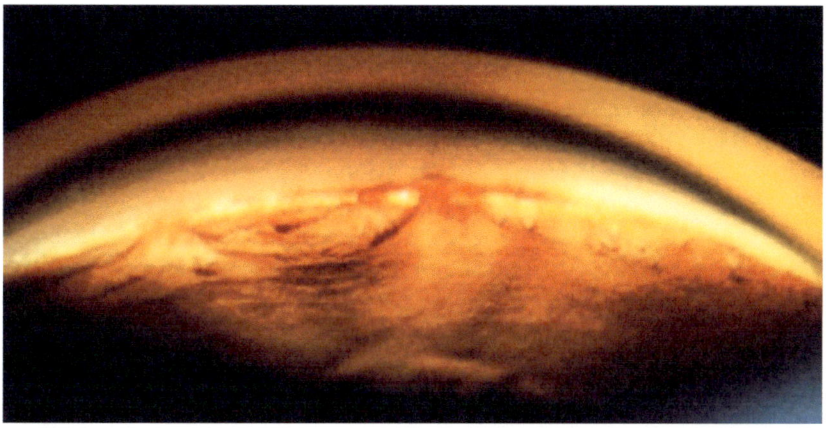

Fig. 10. posterior embryotoxon onto which are attached strands of peripheral iris (Courtesy Prof. Ernst Oltrogge)

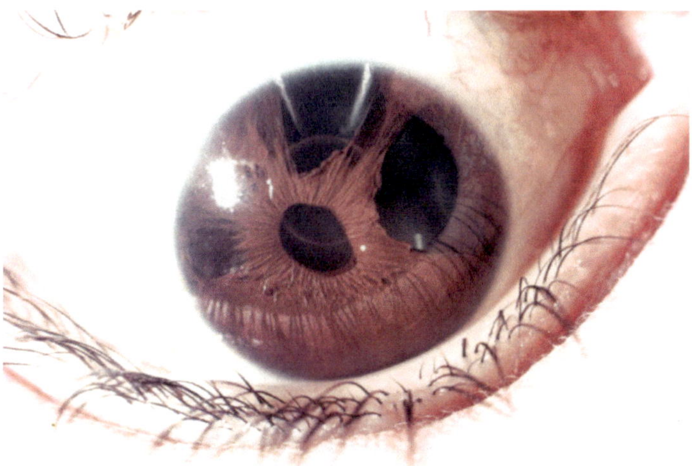

Fig. 11. Rieger´s anomaly showing corectopia and pseudopolycoria (Courtesy Prof. Celso Antonio de Carvalho)

The Rieger´s syndrome consists of Rieger´s anomaly in association with systemic malformations, like hypodontia (a decrease in the number of teeth), microdontia (a decrease in the teeth size) and facial malformations, including hypoplasia of the maxilla, a broad flat nasal bridge, telecanthus (a lateral displacement of the medial canthus) and hypertelorism (an increased distance between the bony orbits).[30] Others anomalies include redundant paraumbilical skin.

Some authors proposed the term Axenfeld-Rieger syndrome for all clinical variations within this spectrum of developmental disorders.[4]

The glaucoma treatment is surgical in the most cases of these disorders. Options of incisional surgery include goniotomy, trabeculotomy and trabeculectomy. The first two procedures have been used in infants with limited success. Trabeculectomy with adjunctive mitomycin C is the surgical procedure of choice for most patients with glaucoma associated with Axenfeld-Rieger syndrome. The long-term successful rates, however, are poor.[14,15]

*b) Peters anomaly*

This anomaly is characterized by a congenital central cornea leukoma associated with a defect in the corresponding posterior stroma and Descemet´s membrane, with synechiae extending from the central iris to the periphery of the corneal opacity (Figure 12).[32] Some patients may have a central keratolenticular adherence with shallowing of the anterior chamber, whereas others may have an anterior polar cataract. A variety of less commonly associated ocular findings include microcornea, microphthalmia, cornea plana, aniridia, sclerocornea and corectopia. An association between Peters anomaly and the systemic alterations seen in Axenfeld-Rieger syndrome is not uncommon.[4]

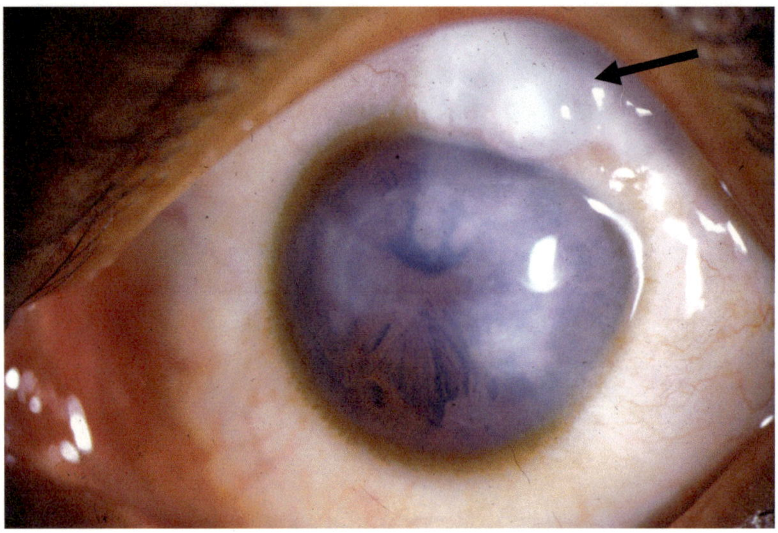

Fig. 12. Peters anomaly after trabeculectomy with MMC (see the bleb – arrow) (Courtesy Prof. Ernst Oltrogge)

Most cases are sporadic, although autosomal recessive inheritance and chromosomal defects have been described. About 80% percent of cases are bilateral. The pathogenesis involve a defect neural crest cell migration in the sixth to eight weeks of fetal development, during which time the anterior segment of the eye is formed.[30]

Glaucoma occurs in 50% to 70% of cases. Elevated intraocular pressure unresponsive to topical medications should be treated surgically, before penetrating keratoplasty is performed. Trabeculectomy with use of antimetabolites is the procedure of choice in these cases.[32] Unfortunately, the long-term visual outcome and glaucoma control are usually poor.[4]

*c) Aniridia*

It is a bilateral condition with life-threatening associations. It occurs as a result of abnormal neuroectodermal development secondary to a mutation in the PAX6 gene linked to 11p13.[30] This gene controls the development of a number of structures, hence the broad nature of ocular and systemic manifestations. The inheritance is autosomal dominant in most cases.

The aniridia is variable in severity, ranging from minimal to total (Figure 13). However, even eyes with total involvement usually show a residual iris tissue in the angle on gonioscopy. Others ocular findings include corneal lesions (leukomas, microcornea and sclerocornea), cataract, aphakia and lens subluxation, foveal hypoplasia, choroidal coloboma and optic nerve hypoplasia. The systemic manifestations include Wilm´s tumor, genitourinary anomalies, mental retardation and cerebellar ataxia.

Glaucoma occurs in approximately 2/3 of cases and usually presents in late childhood and adolescence.[4] The intraocular pressure control is usually difficult, and the medical therapy is inadequate in most cases. The surgical procedures, like goniotomy and trabeculotomy, show poor long-term results. The trabeculectomy with adjunctive antimetabolites is the procedure of choice is most cases. However, the long-term results are also disappointing.[14-16]

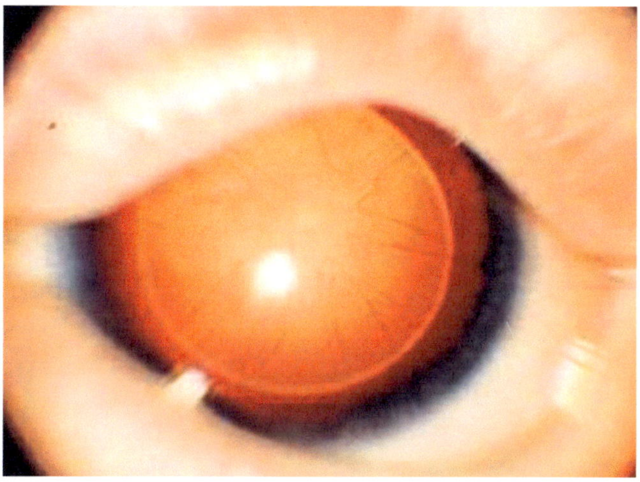

Fig. 13. Total aniridia (Courtesy Prof. Ernst Oltrogge)

## 2.2 Phacomatoses

The Phacomatoses are characterized by the formation of hamartias and hamartomas in the eye, central nervous system, skin and viscera. They are hereditary disorders with variable penetrance and expressivity.

*a) Sturge-Weber syndrome*

Also called encephalotrigeminal angiomatosis is characterized by facial haemangioma (naevus flammeus -Figure 14), choroidal haemangioma and intracranial meningeal angiomata. The haemangioma usually involves the first and second divisions of the trigeminal nerve. The disease has little familial tendency, and no sexual or racial predisposition. Chromosomal abnormalities have been reported in some patients, and the disorder may be a dominant trait with incomplete penetrance.[33]

Glaucoma develops in about 30% of patients, ipsilateral to the facial haemangioma, especially if the lesion affects the upper eyelid.

The glaucoma pathogenesis involves a trabeculodysgenesis and an elevated episcleral venous pressure. The medical treatment with prostaglandin analogues (enhancing uveo-scleral outflow) may be useful in some cases. Nevertheless, surgical approach is necessary in most cases. The goniotomy may be successful in eyes with angle anomalies (trabeculodysgenesis). The combined trabeculotomy-trabeculectomy gives good results in early-onset cases, before the buphthalmos appearing. Surgery always carries a high risk of choroidal effusion and suprachoroidal haemorrhage. Adverse consequences of this may be minimized by performing a posterior sclerotomy before opening the eye.[34]

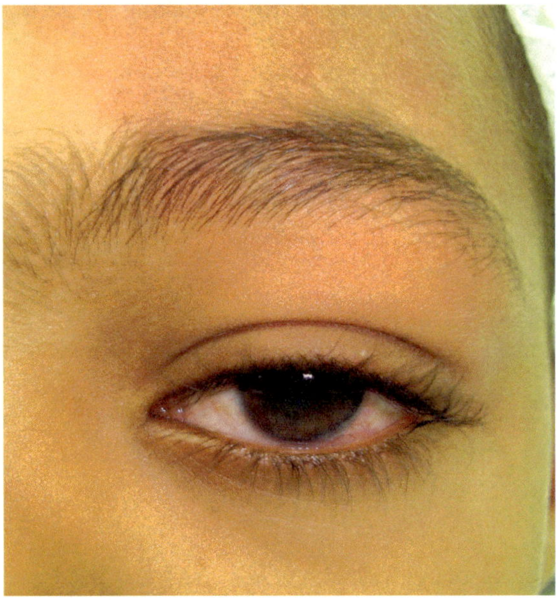

Fig. 14. Naevus flammeus in Sturge-Weber syndrome

*b) Neurofibromatosis*

It is a neuroectodermal dysplasia characterized by tumor-like formations (neurofibromas) derived from the proliferation of peripheral nerve elements. The neurofibromas can occur in the central nervous system, central and peripheral nerves, as well in skin and mucus membranes. Inheritance is autosomal dominant with irregular penetrance and variable expressivity. Glaucoma is uncommon, usually unilateral and congenital. Classically, neurofibromatous involvement of the upper lid is present. Glaucoma is present in 50% of all eyes with plexiform neuroma.[4]

Many mechanisms have been postulated as causes of glaucoma in neurofibromatosis. The elevated intraocular pressure may occur secondary to obstruction of aqueous outflow by neurofibromatous tissue, developmental angle anomaly or angle closure caused by neurofibromatous thickening of the ciliary body or synechiae.

Many surgical procedures, like goniotomy, trabeculotomy, trabeculectomy and cyclodestructive procedures have been reported for the glaucoma treatment. [35] However, the overall rate of success of surgery in literature is much lower than that for primary congenital glaucoma.[33]

## 3. Secondary infantile glaucoma

The secondary infantile glaucomas may be associated with non-hereditary congenital diseases, trauma or intraocular tumors. The secondary glaucoma after congenital cataract surgery is usually a disease with poor visual outcome. Fortunately, the modern cataract surgery and the novels topical anti-inflammatory drugs reduced the complications after congenital cataract surgery, like vitreous loss, retinal detachment and glaucoma. Nevertheless, the treatment of elevated intraocular pressure after congenital cataract surgery is usually difficult and a trabeculectomy with adjunctive antimetabolite may be necessary. [4] Others secondary infantile glaucoma causes include persistent hyperplastic primary vitreous, retrolental fibroplasia, corticosteroid-related glaucoma and retinoblastoma.

## 4. References

[1] Dickens CJ., Hoskins JR HD. Epidemiology and Pathophysiology of Congenital Glaucoma. In The Glaucomas. Ritch R, Shields MB, Krupin T. Mosby, second edition, 729-738; 1996.
[2] Kanski J. J. Primary Congenital Glaucoma. In Clinical Ophthalmology. Butterworth-Heinemann, fifth edition, 245-248; 2003.
[3] Dickens CJ, Hoskins JR HD. Diagnosis and Treatment of Congenital Glaucoma. In The Glaucomas. Ritch R, Shields MB, Krupin T. Mosby, second edition, 739-749; 1996.
[4] Betinjane, AJ. Glaucoma Infantil. In Glaucoma. Susanna Jr R. Cultura Médica. 145-179; 1999.
[5] Shaffer RN. Prognosis of goniotomy in primary infantile glaucoma. Trans Am Ophthalmol Soc 80:321; 1982.
[6] Anderson DR. Trabeculotomy compared to goniotomy for glaucoma in children. Ophthalmology 90: 805; 1983.
[7] Beauchamp GR, Parks MM. Filtering surgery in children: barriers to success. Ophthalmology 1979, 86: 170-80.
[8] Inaba Z. Long-term results of trabeculectomy in the japanese: an analysis by life-table method. Jpn J Ophthalmol 1982, 26: 361-73.
[9] Gressel MG, Heuer DK, Parrish II RK. Trabeculectomy in young patients. Ophthalmology 1984, 91: 1242-6.
[10] Katz GJ, Higginbotham EJ, Lichter PR et al. Mitomycin C versus 5-fluorouracil in high-risk glaucoma filtering surgery. Ophthalmology 1995; 102: 1263-9.
[11] Kitazawa Y, Kawase K, Matsushita H, Minobe M. Trabeculectomy with mitomycin. A comparative study with Fluorouracil. Arch Ophthalmol 1991; 109: 1693-8.
[12] Lamping KA, Belkin JK. 5-Fluorouracil and Mitomycin C in pseudophakic patients. Ophthalmology 1995; 102: 70-5.
[13] Prata JA Jr, Minckler DS, Baerveldt G et al. Trabeculectomy in pseudophakic patients: postoperative 5-fluorouracil versus intraoperative mitomycin C antiproliferative therapy. Ophthalmic Surg 1995; 26: 73-7.
[14] Susanna R, Oltrogge EW, Carani JCE, Nicolela MT. Mitomycin as adjunct chemotherapy in congenital and developmental glaucoma. J Glaucoma 1995; 4: 151-7.

[15] Giampani J; Borges-Giampani AS; Carani JC; Oltrogge EW; Susanna R. Efficacy and safety of trabeculectomy with mitomycin C for childhood glaucoma: a study of results with long-term follow-up. Clinics 63(4): 421-6; 2008.
[16] Beck AD, Wilson WR, Lynch MG, Lynn MJ, Noe R. Trabeculectomy with adjunctive mitomycin C in pediatric glaucoma. Am J Ophthalmol 1998; 126: 648-57.
[17] Sidoti PA, Belmonte SJ, Liebmann JM, Ritch R. Trabeculectomy with Mitomycin-C in The Treatment of Pediatric Glaucomas. Ophthalmology 2000; 107: 422-9.
[18] Mandal AK, Walton DS, John T, Jayagandan A. Mitomycin C-augmented trabeculectomy in refractory congenital glaucoma. Ophthalmology 1997; 104: 996-1001.
[19] Miller MH, Rice NS. Trabeculectomy combined with β-irradiation for congenital glaucoma. Br J Ophthalmol 1991; 75: 584-90.
[20] Wahee US, Ritterband DC, Greenfield DS, Liebmamm JM, Sidoti AO, Ritch R. Bleb-related ocular infection in children after trabeculectomy with mitomycin C. Ophthalmology 1997; 104: 2117-20.
[21] Wallace DK, Plager DA, Synder SK, Raiesdana A, Helveston EM, Ellis FD. Surgical results of secondary glaucomas in childhood. Ophthalmology 1998; 105: 101-111.
[22] Wolner B, Liebmann JM, Sassani JW, Ritch R, Speaker M, Marmor M. Late bleb-related endophthalmitis after trabeculectomy with adjunctive 5-fluorouracil. Ophthalmology 1991; 98: 1053-60.
[23] Higginbotham EJ, Stevens RK, Musch DC, et al. Bleb-related endophthalmitis after trabeculectomy with mitomycin C. Ophthalmology 1996; 103: 650-6.
[24] Greenfield DS, Suver IJ, Miller MP, Kangas TA, Palmberg PF, Flynn HW. Endophthalmitis after filtering surgery with mitomycin. Arch Ophthalmol 1996; 114: 943-9.
[25] O'Malley Schotthoefer E; Yanovitch TL; Freedman SF. Aqueous drainage device surgery in refractory pediatric glaucomas: I. Long-term outcomes. AAPOS; 12(1): 33-9; 2008.
[26] Khan AO; Al-Mobarak F. Comparison of polypropylene and silicone Ahmed valve survival 2 years following implantation in the first 2 years of life. Br J Ophthalmol; 93(6):791-4; 2009.
[27] Khan AO; Al-Mobarak F. Comparison of polypropylene and silicone Ahmed valve survival 2 years following implantation in the first 2 years of life. Br J Ophthalmol 93(6): 791-4; 2009.
[28] Kay JS; Mitchell R; Miller J. Dilation and Probing of Schlemm´s Canal and Viscocanalostomy in Pediatric Glaucoma. J Pediatr Ophthalmol Strabismus 48(1): 30-7; 2011.
[29] Noureddin BN; El-Haibi CP; Cheikha A; Bashshur ZF. Viscocanalostomy versus trabeculotomy ab externo in primary congenital glaucoma: 1-year follow-up of a prospective controlled pilot study. Br J Ophthalmol; 90(10): 1281-5; 2006.
[30] Kanski JJ. Iridocorneal dysgenesis. In Clinical Ophthalmology. Butterworth-Heinemann, fifth edition, 248-252; 2003.
[31] Borges AS, Susanna Jr. R, Carani JCE, Betinjane AJ, Alward WL, Stone EM, Sheffield VC, Nishimura DY. Genetic analysis of PITX2 and FOXC1 in Rieger Syndrome patients from Brazil. J Glaucoma 11(1): 51-56; 2002.
[32] Shottenstein EM. Peters anomaly. In The Glaucomas. Ritch R, Shields MB, Krupin T. Mosby, second edition, 887-897; 1996.
[33] Weiss JS, Ritch R. Glaucoma in the Phacomatoses. In The Glaucomas. Ritch R, Shields MB, Krupin T. Mosby, second edition, 899-924; 1996.
[34] Bellows AR. Choroidal effusion during glaucoma surgery in patients with prominent episcleral vessels. Arch Ophthalmol 97: 793; 1979.
[35] Bost M. Congenital glaucoma and von Recklinghausen disease. Pediatrie 40:207; 1985.

25

# Primary Angle Closure Glaucoma

Michael B. Rumelt
*Washington University Deparment of Ophthalmology and Visual Sciences*
*St. Louis, Missouri*
*USA*

## 1. Introduction

Glaucoma, a leading cause of blindness world wide, may be classified into two main types based on the anatomy of the anterior chamber angle: open angle, which is generally a chronic disease and narrow angle glaucoma, which can be an acute medical emergency. An acute primary angle closure glaucoma attack presents with a painful, inflamed eye, cloudy cornea, fixed mid dilated pupil, reduced vision, high intraocular pressure, and possibly nausea and vomiting. If not diagnosed or untreated promptly and appropriately, the attack can result in severe damage and possibly blindness.

## 2. Epidemiology

It is estimated that by 2020 in the United States 3 million persons will have glaucoma, approximately 10% to 16% will have narrow angle glaucoma. World wide by 2020 it is estimated almost 80 million persons will have glaucoma. Angle closure glaucoma accounts for as much as half of blindness from glaucoma cases in other nations (particularly Asian countries). Four million are bilaterally blind. (1)
Risk is higher older individuals, individuals with high hyperopic refractive error (2), and diabetes.
The ethnic risks for acute angle closure glaucoma is approximately 1 in 1000 for Caucasians (3-11), 1 in 100 for Hispanics and Asians (12-20); 2-4 in 100 for Inuits (21-23). Primary narrow angle closure glaucoma is three times more frequent in Caucasian females over age fifty, less frequent in African Americans or native Americans, and is very common in India with intumescent lenses a frequent component.

## 3. Genetics

Genetics may play a role in the genesis of primary angle closure glaucoma in some situations. Autosomal dominant nanophthalmos (NNO1) with high hyperopia and angle closure glaucoma (51) maps to chromosome 11. An autosomal recessive form of nanophthalmos has been found in an Amish-Mennonite family (NNO2) and analysis found the mutation to be a frameshift insertion, 1143C in the membrane frizzled-related protein (MFRP) gene is located at cytogene location (11q23.3) and encodes a member of the frizzeled related proteins family, some of which may play a role in eye development.

Axenfeld-Rieger ocular dysgenesis is associated with mutations of the Human Pituitary Homeobox 2 (PITX2) and forkhead box C1 (FOXC1) genes (52).

### 3.1 Classification of angle closure glaucoma

A new definition and classification of angle closure glaucoma based on population and epidemiologic studies has been developed to allow comparison between the studies. It has the following types: Primary Angle closure suspect; Primary angle closure; Primary Angle closure glaucoma; Primary Acute Angle Closure Glaucoma Crisis attack. The term glaucoma is not applied unless there is glaucomatous optic nerve damage, characteristic visual field changes, and specific gonioscopic criteria. The terms chronic, intermittent, and subacute are eliminated.

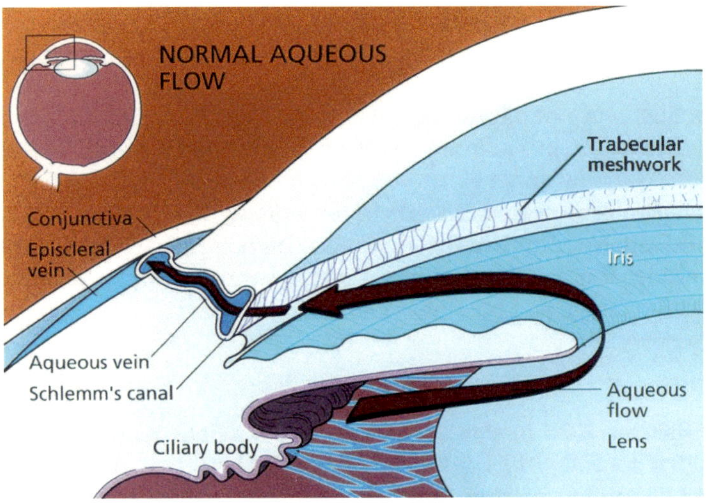


Fig. 1. Normal angle anatomy

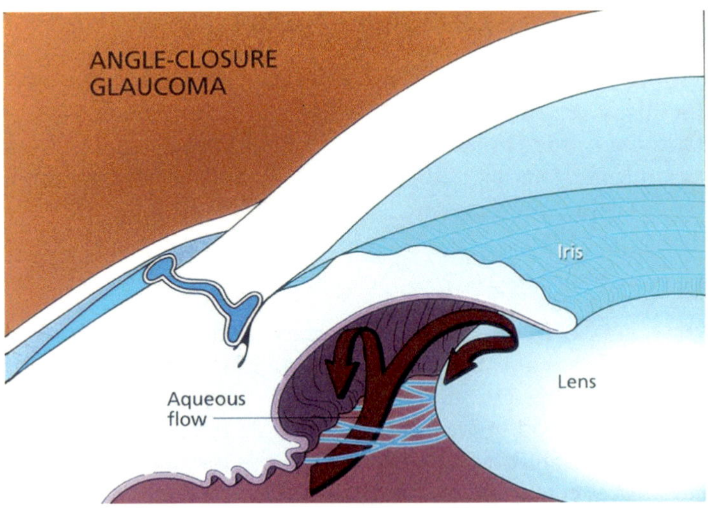


Fig. 2. Anatomy of primary angle closure glaucoma

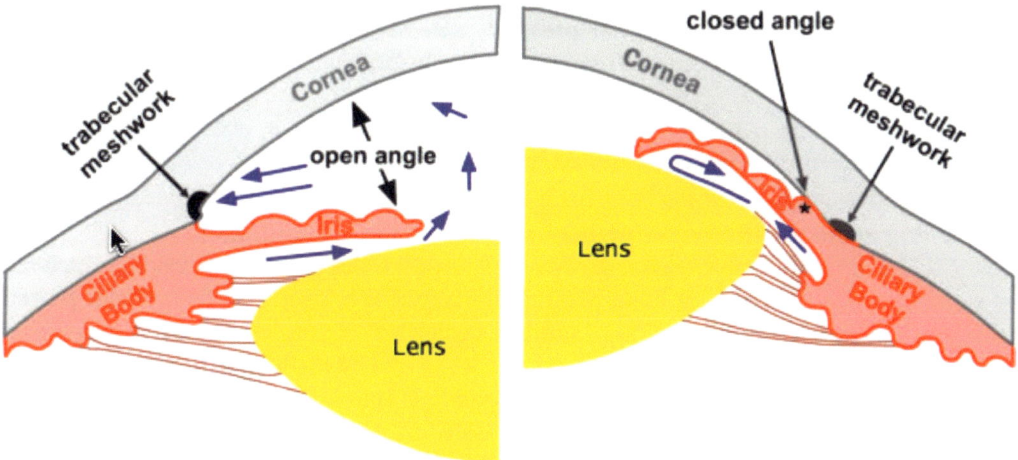


Fig. 3. The perheral iris in apposition to the trabecular meshwork blocking flow with an resultant increase intraocular pressure

### 3.2 Primary angle closure suspect

Anatomically narrow angles, normal IOP, absence of peripheral anterior synechiae, absence of glaucomatous optic neuropathy, and normal visual fields. (25) Patients should be warned of the symptoms of angle closure, drugs that may precipitate an attack, and the importance of a prompt evaluation by an ophthalmologist. They should be followed at appropriate intervals determined by the clinical expertise of the ophthalmologist, with gonioscopy and intraocular pressure monitoring performed at each visit, at least once a year. (56) If the patient is to be traveling to or living in a remote area where medical and/or ophthalmological may be unavailable for lengthy periods of time or transportaion may be delayed if an emergency arises, consideration of prophylactic laser peripheral iridotomies may be discussed with the patient (along with risks of the procedure).

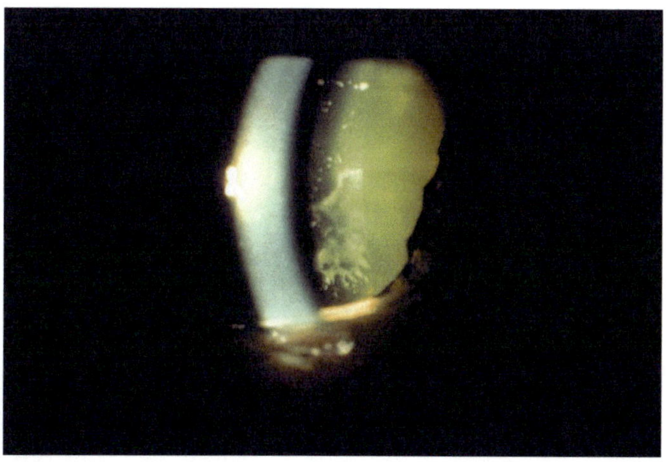

Fig. 4. Glauckomaflecken

**Primary angle closure glaucoma**: narrow angles, peripheral anterior synechiae, iris changes, glaucomaflecken, elevated intraocular pressure, excessive pigmentation in the trabeculum, no optic nerve damage, and normal visual fields. (26-28) They should be followed at least annually.

Primary angle closure glaucoma narrow angles, peripheral anterior synechiae, glaucomatous optic neuropathy, and characteristic visual findings. (29)

### 3.3 Primary acute angle closure glaucoma crisis attack presentation

About 10% of patients with closed angles present with acute angle closure crises characterized by sudden ocular pain, seeing halos around lights, red eye, very high intraocular pressure (>30 mmHg), nausea and vomiting, sudden decreased vision, and a fixed, mid-dilated pupil. Acute angle closure is an ocular emergency. Primary angle closure glaucoma occurs when the peripheral iris blocks the access of aqueous humor to the trabecular meshwork. Continued production of aqueous humor results in elevated intraocular pressure and damage to the nerve. In plateau iris, mild dilation of the pupil results in similar blockage of the angle. If not diagnosed promptly and treated appropriately, severe damage or blindness may result with either anatomical condition. (30)

An attack may present with headache and vomiting, and can be misdiagnosed as neurological or gastrointestinal in origin. If the attack occurs in a setting where either the patient can't communicate or an ophthalmologic consultation is unavailable or delayed, damage to the eye may be severe. Examples are demented patients in a nursing home, in post operative recovery, or the intensive care unit where the patient is sedated or receiving pain medication. Patients may choose self-diagnosis or treatment with over the counter medications to reduce healthcare costs and thus delay diagnosis and treatment.

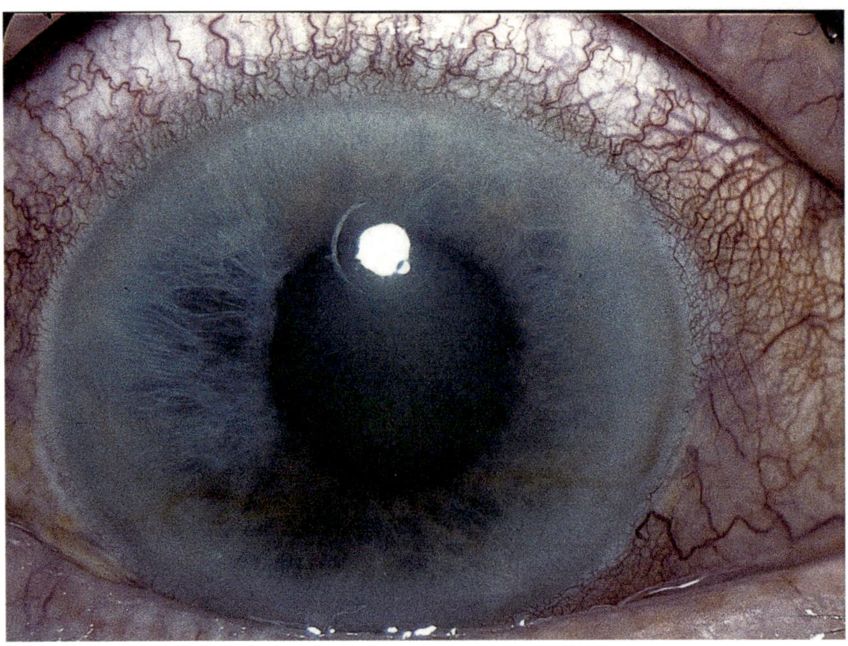

Fig. 5.

### 3.4 Example of a medical treatment regimen for acute primary angle closure glaucoma crisis attack

1. Topical brimonidine tartrate (Aphagan P®) x1 and timolol maleate-dorzolaminde HCL (Cosopt®) x1 (and an instruction for bid, unless there are contraindications).
2. IV acetazolamide (Diamox®) 500 mg (and an instruction for acetazolamide 250 mg tid).
3. PO glycerol 50% 100cc (1.5gr/kg) or isosorbide 25% for patients without diabetes mellitus.
4. In IOP below 60 mm Hg adding topical pilocarpine 2% x1.
5. IOP measurement after 30 min. If the IOP decreased, adding an instruction for pilocarpine 2% qid.
6. Massage with glass rod over the center of the cornea to force aqueous into the angle.
7. Analgesics and an antiemetic if necessary for pain and vomiting respectively up to every 4-6 hours.
8. Nd:YAG laser iridotomy in both eyes a day after. Adding topical apraclonidine (Iopidine®) 0.25% x1 and prednisolone acetate (Pred Forte®) qid for a week.
9. Indentation: it may be possible to break an attack by pressing with a four-mirror gonioscope lens, which may deepen the chamber angle and break peripheral anterior synechiae by hydraulic forces. Alternatively one may press firmly with a muscle hook or glass rod to accomplish the same goal: to flatten the cornea and compress aqueous humor into the anterior chamber angle to release fresh peripheral anterior synechiae. This may decrease the likelihood of developing chronic angle closure glaucoma.
10. Corneal edema may preclude gonioscopy and thus oral glycerin or topical glycerin may be useful in clearing the cornea.
11. The use of miotics like pilocarpine should be delayed until there is a drop in iop, generally less than 40 mm Hg so ischemia of the pupillary sphincter can resolve and the pupillary sphincter can function. Miotics may cause thickening of ciliary body and forward displacement of the ciliary body, thus worsening pupillary block but its use is still recommended.

If intervention is rapid enough, the attack may be broken and vision saved.
An attack that doesn't resolve may require filtering surgery, but operating on an inflamed eye with high intraocular pressure can be fraught with severe complications, including malignant glaucoma.

### 3.5 Etiology of angle closure

#### 3.5.1 Primary angle closure

**Pupillary block**

Anatomically narrow angle: iris bombe, chronic progressive angle closure in which peripheral anterior synechiae gradually occlude the angle generally in an asymptomatic fashion and thus may be mis-diagnosed as open angle glaucoma if gonioscopy is omitted.

**Ciliary block**

Pan retinal photocoagulation can cause swelling of the ciliary body, scleral buckles, some drugs.
**Plateau iris** has a relatively deep mid anterior chamber with narrowing at the angle the severity of potential apposition or closure depending upon where the iris root inserts on the angle structures.

### 3.5.2 Secondary angle closure

Due to forces that pull the iris-lens diagphragm foreward such as uveitis with iris bombe, diabetic neovascular glaucoma, forces pushing iris lens forward such as swollen lens, tumor, and malignant glaucoma following intraocular surgery. Malignant glaucoma first described by von Graefe (31) in 1869 in the classical form has elevated intraocular pressure, shallow or flat anterior chamber in the presence of a patent iridectomy. It occurs rarely after filtering surgery for angle closure glaucoma, with an incidence of 0.6 to 4%. The mechanism proposed is blockage of aqueous flow at the iris lens anterior vitreous face. Aqueous is misdirected into the vitreous cavity and displaces the iris-lens diaphragm forward resulting in shallow or flat anterior chamber. A newer theory (32) postulates that choroid expansion is involved. Many entities have been associated with malignant glaucoma: intraocular surgery, glaucoma drainage devices, various laser surgeries, (Neodynium-doped Yttrium Garnet) Nd:YAG cyclophotocoagulation, and other causes. Diagnosis is facilitated by Ultrasound BioMicroscopy). Treatment consists of phenylephrine to tighten zonules, topical beta-blockers, alpha agonists, and carbonic anhydrase inhibitors (topical and systemic) to reduce aqueous production. Prostaglandin analogues may be helpful by increasing uveoscleral outflow with reduction of intraocular pressure. If medical therapy fails, Nd:YAG laser might disrupt the vitreious face and allow normal flow of aqueous. If that fails, pars plana vitrectomy with or without lensectomy may disrupt the anterior vitreous face restoring normal flow. In pseudophakic patients, lens remnants should be removed and the vitreous face disrupted.

### 3.5.3 Secondary angle closure due to lens factors such as intumescent cataracts.

**Drug induced angle closure glaucoma.**

Anticholinergic are the most common for inducing "pupillary block" angle-closure glaucoma adrenergic agents, certain beta(2)-adrenergic agonists and anticholinergic agents may induce pupillary dilation and precipitate angle-closure glaucoma in susceptible patients: locally administered phenylephrine drops, nasal ephedrine, nebulized salbutamol or systemically administered (epinephrine for anaphylactic shock). Other drugs that can induce pupillary dilation and precipitate angle-closure glaucoma due to anticholinergic effects include tropicamide and atropine drops, tri and tetracyclic antidepressants, antihistamines, mydriatics, and phenothiazines. A novel anticholinergic form follows the use of periocular botulinum toxin diffusing back to the ciliary ganglion inhibiting the pupillary sphincter.

Sulfa based drugs (33) (acetazolamide, hydrochlorothiazide, cotrimoxazole, and topiramate (34)) induce "non-pupillary block" angle-closure glaucoma as an idiosyncratic reaction to the drug, cause swelling of the ciliary body with anterior rotation of the iris-lens diaphragm, and lead to the development of angle-closure glaucoma.

## 4. History of gonioscopy and concepts of angle closure glaucoma

In the modern eye clinic, the ease of use of the slit lamp microscope and various diagnostic contact lenses can lead one to take for granted the technological advance that each represents. Examination of the anterior chamber by gonioscopy, described in 1907, only became commonly used in the 1950's. It is instructive to learn about the history of gonioscopy and evolving understanding of the pathophysiology of angle closure. The work of Dellaporta(36) provides an excellent review and source of much of the following information.

Until the middle of the twentieth century, glaucoma was classified into congestive and non-congestive. Treatment included bleeding, purging, leeches, counter-irritation and injecting mercury into an eye with chronic glaucoma to cause systemic inflammation, which would hopefully counteract the inflammation caused by glaucoma.

Herman von Helmholtz revolutionized the field of ophthalmology in 1851 with the invention of the ophthalmoscope.

Albrect von Graefe noted in 1856 that scleral ectasias in glaucoma often became smaller after iridectomy. He deduced that IOP could be lowered by this procedure.

Examination of the anterior chamber angle dates back to 1875 when Alexios Trantas, a Greek ophthalmologist living in Istanbul until 1922 when he was forced to resettle in Athens due to political repression, was the first to examine the angle in a living person. In a 1907 presentation to the French Ophthalmological Society, he described his observations of the angle and his method, direct gonioscopy, that used digital pressure on the limbal area to indent the eye and allow visualization of the angle with a direct ophthalmoscope and a plus lens, power ranging from plus four to plus fourteen diopters. The term gonioscopy (which derives from the Greek and means observe the angle (36)) was first used by him, in the body of a paper (not the title) published in 1915 (35), but lost until after the end of the First World War.

Maximilian Salzmann's papers on gonioscopy and the angle, were published independently of Trantas in 1915. He tried direct ophthalmoscopy first but then found indirect ophthalmoscopy with a contact lens to be more satisfactory. He initially used Adolf Eugen Fick's scleral contact lens, first described in a paper published in 1888 (37). Salzmann later used a customized Zeiss scleral contact lens with a smaller diameter, that made gonioscopy easier.

In 1893 Theodor Leber (38-39) showed that the aqueous flows from the posterior chamber to the anterior chamber through the pupil. He and his collaborators injected various substances, including fine India ink, into the vitreous or anterior chamber of freshly enucleated eyes or those scheduled to undergo medically necessary enucleation and demonstrated the materials in the anterior chamber, iris, and Schlemm's canal.

The development of the slit lamp microscope by Zeiss in 1920 further advanced gonioscopy.

Leonhard Koeppe examined patients sitting at the slit lamp with the contact lens he developed, held in position by a bandage, allowing viewing of the nasal and temporal aspects of the angle.

Later Karl Wolfgang Ascher examined patients in the supine position, and used the Keoppe lens, thus adding views of the superior and inferior angle. Ascher also identified episcleral veins near the limbus which carried clear fluid and when compressed with a small glass rod demonstrated the flow of aqueous from the anterior chamber into the blood vessels. He subsequently named them "aqueous veins".

In 1920, Edward James Curran described relative pupillary block and its treatment by peripheral iridectomy for the first time. Edward James Curran's observations were not accepted for many years.

Manuel Uribe Tronosco in 1925 invented a self illuminating monocular gonioscope (40), developed a version of the Koeppe lens made of polymethylmethacrylate rather than glass, and then a binocular microscope. In 1947 Edward James Curran published a book on gonioscopy.

Little progress was made until the 1936 publication of Otto Barkan's landmark paper, "On the Genesis of Glaucoma" (41), based on his observations made possible by modifications to the technique of gonioscopy, that allowed him to differentiate glaucoma into open angle and narrow angle glaucoma. His appreciation of the importance of pupillary block to angle closure glaucoma was a vital advance in gonioscopy and the understanding of the mechanism of glaucoma. Otto Barkan's ingenious innovation was to combine a handheld Zeiss binocular microscope suspended from the ceiling, an intensely bright source of illumination, the Koeppe lens, and finally the patient in a supine position. This process allowed great mobility, direct visualization of the entire angle, and manipulation of the eye. As important as Barkan's method of gonioscopy was, the widespread adoption by non glaucoma eye care specialists, was limited by the cumbersome details of the setup. Barkan also invented goniotomy for congenital glaucoma, facilitated by direct ophthalmoscopy using a special lens flattened on one edge to allow passage of a goniotomy knife

Because it was not efficient to apply direct gonioscopy to every patient, it became necessary to triage which patient would be examined. Wiliam van Herick (42) devised a method to identify patients with possibly narrow angles. He described positioning the slit beam at the temporal limbus angled sixty degrees to the side of the observer. If the space between the anterior iris stroma and the corneal endothelium was less than one fourth of the thickness of the cornea, those individuals would receive direct gonioscopy.

The development of the Goldmann indirect gonioscope lens (43), a contact lens incorporating one or more mirrors allowed examination of the entire angle with a patient seated before the slit lamp microscope. Two artifacts impact the utility of the lens: the requirement to use methylcellulose gel to eliminate air bubbles and if the lens was tiled, it could possibly indent the globe and falsely indicate a narrowing of the angle. The Koeppe lens won't indent the globe unless tilted and pressure applied, but with the patient in the supine position the chamber could deepen under the influence of gravity.

The development of the Zeiss 4-mirror and other similar lenses (44) which incorporated mirrors facilitated examination of the entire anterior chamber angle because these lenses were smaller in diameter than the cornea, used the tear film rather than methylcellulose to allow placement of the lens on the cornea, and had a handle which allowed indentation of the cornea to determine if apposition of the peripheral iris to the trabecular meshwork was permanent with synechiae or temporary and whether pressing with the contact lens could open the angle.

The technique of indenting the cornea was taught by Bernard Becker and Robert Moses at Washington University School of Medicine (45). Bernard Becker demonstrated the reduction of intraocular pressure by acetazolamide in 1954, a major advance in the treatment of glaucoma.

Glaucoma was officially divided into wide and narrow-angle types at the American Academy of Ophthalmology in 1948.

In the 1950s many advances in understanding angle closure glaucoma were made: Paul Chandler rediscovered Edward James Curran's work, and advanced the concept of pupillary block; Joseph Haas and Harold Scheie described angle opening after peripheral iridectomy and postulated resistance to the forward flow of aqueous lead to bowing of the peripheral iris; Otto Barkan supported Edward James Curran and Paul Chandler's concept; Chandler, Shaffer and Barkan described malignant glaucoma; and Tornquist described plateau iris.

Gerd Myer-Schwikerath in 1956 introduced Xenon photocoagulation of the iris but corneal and lens damage limited its use. It was replaced by laser iridotomies, first with the ruby, then with development of Argon and Neodynium-doped Yttrium aluminium garnet (ND:YAG) lasers. Iridectomy became noninvasive and moved from the operating room to the office.

The 1980's and 1990's saw the development of the concept of pupillary block, the concept of complete and incomplete plateau iris syndrome and the advent of laser iridoplasty, to shrink the peripheral iris to open the angle.

In the 2000's produced advances in instrumentation capable of non-contact anterior segment biometry: ultrasonic Biomicroscopy (UBM) (which does not require a clear cornea), ocular coherence tomography (OCT), and Pentascan using the Scheimpflug principle.

## 5. Examination of the angle to assess risk of closure

### Gonioscopy

Because of total internal reflection of light, it is impossible to see angle structure and anatomy without other means. To overcome this problem, special contact lenses called goniocopy lenses are utilized. The examiner must be careful not to incorrectly estimate angle depth when illumination passes through the pupil because miosis might deepen the angle.

### Direct gonioscopy

One looks through a contact lens to the meridian of interest in the eye with a Koeppe lens, requires methylcellulose, supine position, an assistant to hold lens in place with a q-tip, after the examination, vision may be blurred due to methylcellulose.

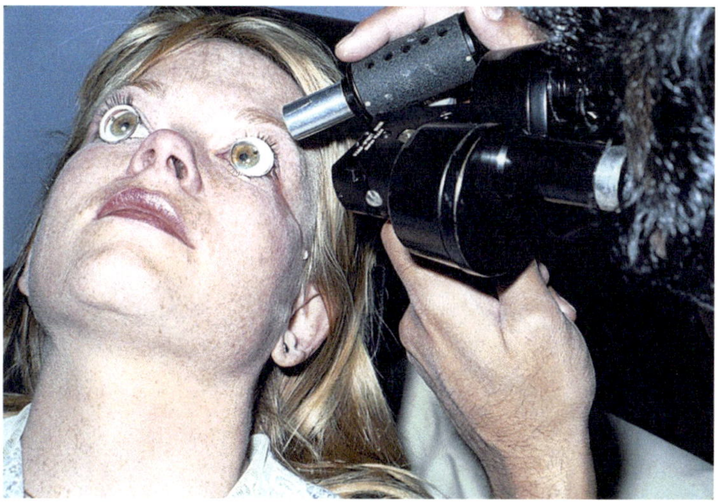

Fig. 6. Koeppe lens, hand held illuminator, microscope, supine patient

### Indirect gonioscopy

To see a particular meridian of the angle, a contact lens with a mirror or series of mirrors is used. Examination of the angle anatomy is done at the slit lamp with either a Zeiss four mirror gonioscopy lens or a Goldmann lens, which requires methylcellulose gel to eliminate air bubbles and can blur vision after the exam for a period of time. Goldmann lenses are larger than the diameter of cornea and may be uncomfortable for the patient. Zeiss or Posner four mirror lenses do not require methylcellulose and rely on the tear film to allow placement of the lens without air bubbles. They have a smaller diameter compared to other type of contact lens and can be used to do indentation gonioscopy to determine if a narrowed angle can be opened or synechiae can be broken.

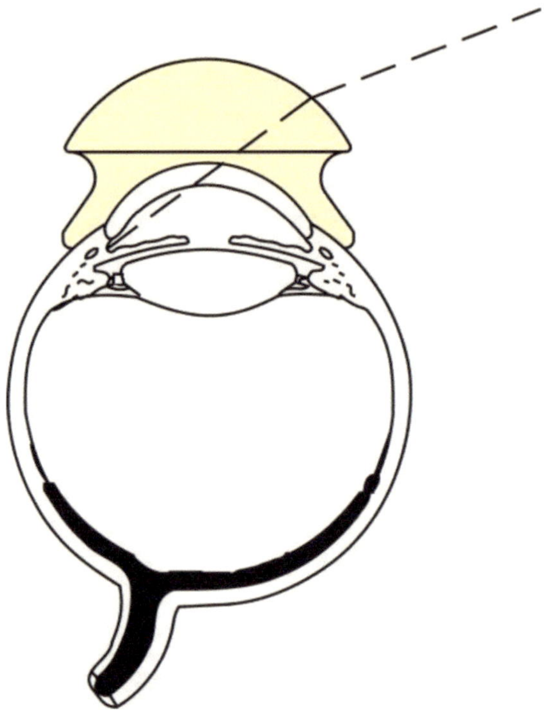

Fig. 7. Illustration of koeppe lens

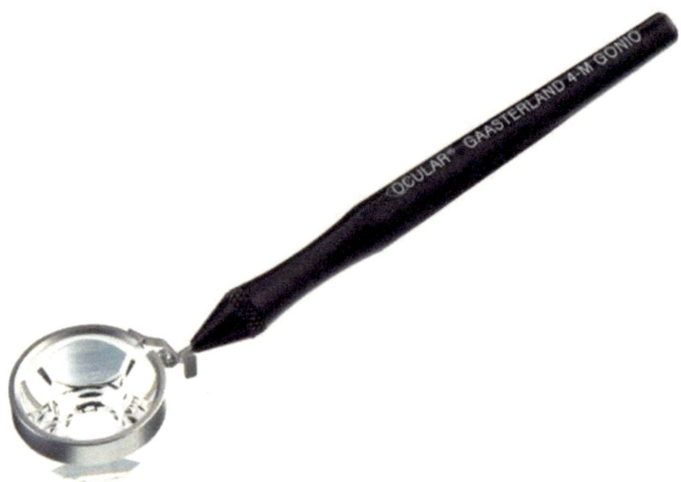


Fig. 8. Mirror gonioscope lens

### 5.1 Grading the anterior chamber depth with gonioscopy

At the bedside with the flashlight test, a flashlight beam is directed parallel to the iris from the temporal side. If the crescentic iris shadow thus formed is less than half to one-third or no shadow the eye is considered to have a narrow angle and merit further examination.
At the slit lamp William van Herick's (42) method of grading peripheral anterior chamber depth at the slit lamp consists of placing the slit beam at an angle of 60 degrees, just inside limbus, magnification 15, low to medium illumination, observe the space between corneal endothelium and front surface of iris. If the space (PAC) was less than one fourth of the thickness of the cornea (CT) the angle was considered possibly narrow and should be evaluated with gonioscopy.

**Van Herick grading (42)**

| | | |
|---|---|---|
| Grade 4 | angle is wide open | PAC >CT |
| Grade 3 | angle is narrow | PAC= 1/4 to 1/2 CT |
| Grade 2 | angle dangerously narrow | PAC=1/4 CT |
| Grade 1 | angle narrow or closed | PAC<CT |

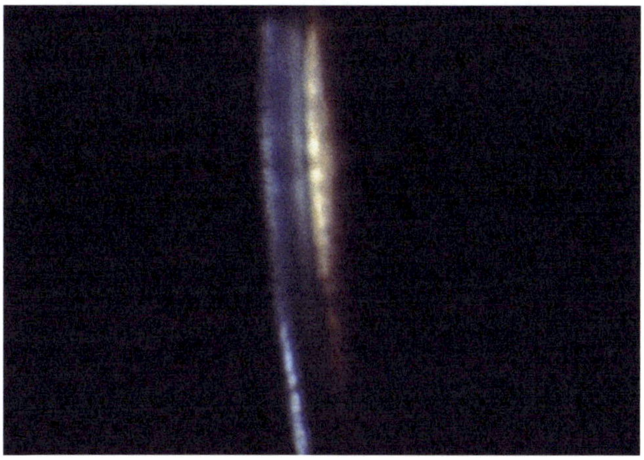

Fig. 9. Van Herick grade 1

**Scheie grading (46)**

Scheie proposed a grading system in which Roman numerals describe the degree of angle closure based upon the examiner's visualization of the anterior chamber angle's structures;

| | |
|---|---|
| Grade I | all structures visible |
| Grade II | iris root visible |
| Grade III | posterior trabeculum obscured |
| Grade IV | only Schwalbe's line visible |

**Shaffer grading (47)**

Shaffer graded the angle of iris insertion with plane of trabecular meshwork:

| | | |
|---|---|---|
| Grade 4 | 45 to 35 degree angle | wide open |
| Grade 3 | 35 to 20 degree angle | wide open |
| Grade 2 | 20 degree angle | narrow |
| Grade 1 | <10 degree angle | extremely narrow |
| Slit | 0 degree angle | narrowed to slit |

Shaffer grading system of depth of anterior chamber showing angle between iris and trabeculum

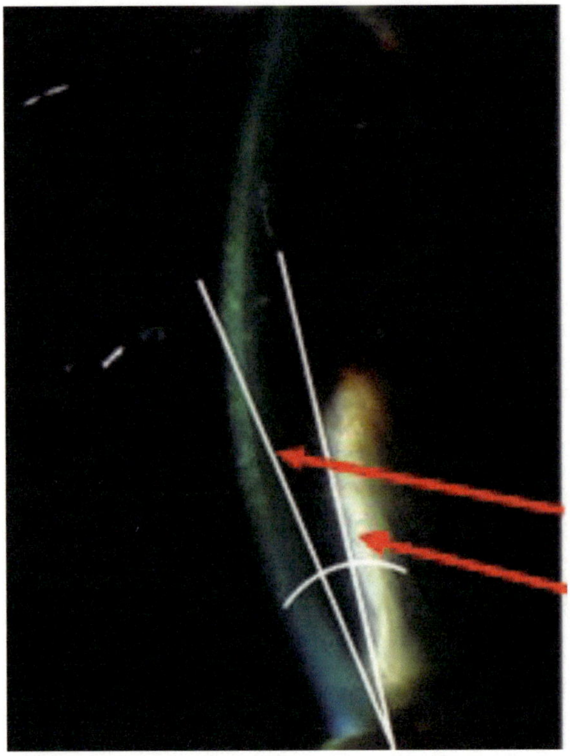


Fig. 10.

**Spaeth's grading (48)**

Spaeth's grading scheme is as follows
Iris insertion
A anterior to Schwalbe's line
B between Schwalbe's line and slceral spur
C scleral spur visibile
D deep with ciliary body visible
E very deep with >1 mm of ciliary body visible
Peripheral iris
F flat
B bowed anteriorly
P pleateau iris
C concave
Pigmentation of trabecular meshwork
0 no pigment
1+ minimal
2+ mild
3+ moderate
4+ intense

**Provocative testing** such as dark room prone provocative testing is rarely utilized. A positive test is helpful, but a negative test does not guarantee that a particular individual with narrow angles will not suffer a future attack.

**Optical coherence tomography** of the anterior segment (OCT) is a non contact imaging system that can show detailed images of the anatomy including the anterior chamber angle. It can't acquire images behind the heavily pigmented posterior iris epithelium because the coherent light is absorbed by the iris pigment epithelium and thus may not be adequate for study of the ciliary body, zonules, posterior chamber, or anterior vitreous. The size of the pupil may be affected by ambient light and constrict falsely indicating a deeper chamber. The following illustration demonstrates crowding of the angle by peripheral iris with a dilated pupil.

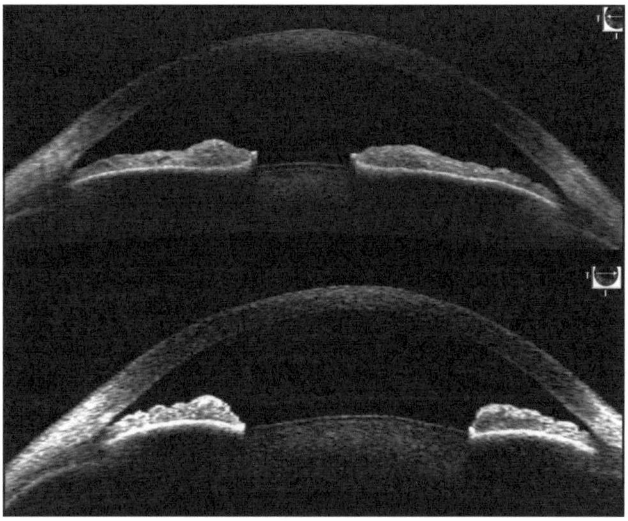

Fig. 11.

**High resolution ultrasonography** of the anterior segment, known as Ultrasound BioMicroscopy (UBM), is a contact imaging technique that can assess and display anterior chamber depth, configuration of the angle, lens position, iris thickness, and the ciliary body which may be thickened, rotated forward, have masses or cysts, or other anomalies presenting with angle closure in the presence of a cloudy cornea. UBM uses a higher frequency transducer (20-80 Mhz) than A-scan or B-scan (10 Mhz). Modifications in the system to apply the probe to the cornea eliminate the acoustic dead zone in front of the probe and allow the study to be performed sitting or supine.

Recent studies have suggested that increased iris thickness and cross-sectional area are associated with increased risk of angle closure glaucoma, there may be increased accumulation of proteins in iris in other cases. Another study comparing gonioscopy and UBM assessment of anterior chamber depth in Asian and Indian eyes found a very close correlation.

**Central corneal thickness** will affect Goldmann tonometry, since a thicker than "normal" cornea may be associated with a falsely higher pressure measurement and conversely measuring the intraocular pressure in a patient with a thinner cornea may underestimate the true intraocular pressure (49). A study comparing Pentacam Scheimpflug camera with ultrasonic pachymetry and noncontact specular microsopy in measuring central corneal thickness showed the values obtained are similar but the methods are not interchangeable (50).

**A-scan biometry** of the axial length of the eye will reveal those eyes that are very short such as in nanophthalmos and at risk of angle closure glaucoma.

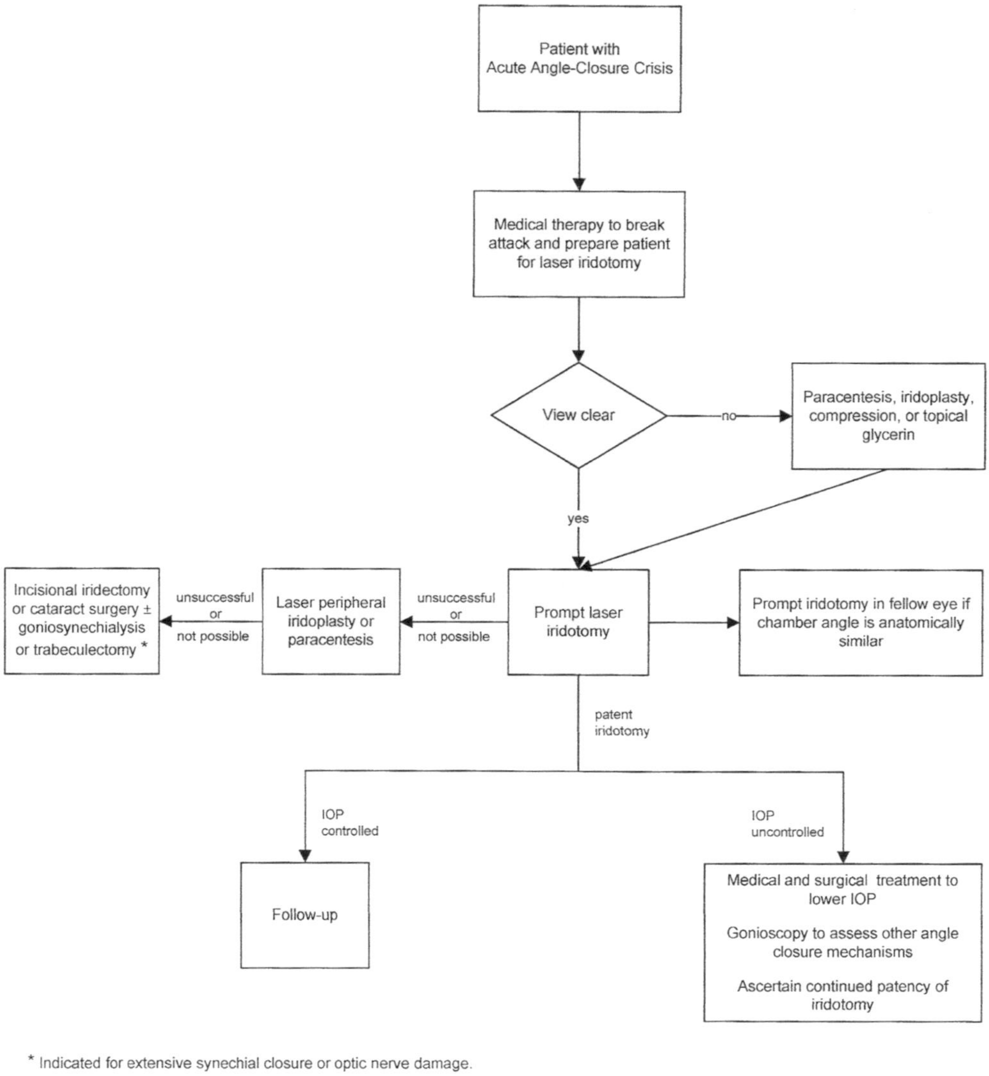


Fig. 12. Algorithm for the management of patients with acute angle-closure crisis American Academy of Ophthalmogy preferred practice pattern 2010

## 6. Management of chronic angle-closure glaucoma (CACG)

The first step in the chronic angle-closure glaucoma (CACG) is often a surgical procedure to open up, as far as possible, those segments of the drainage angle that are appositionally closed or narrow. Options may include laser peripheral iridotomy, argon laser peripheral iridoplasty, and lens extraction. Intraocular pressure (IOP) may, however, remain increased after these procedures, which may be the result of extensive residual synechial angle closure. IOP-lowering medications are indicated if a safe IOP level cannot be reached after angle-opening procedures. In the past, timolol and pilocarpine were extensively used in CACG. Once-daily prostaglandin analogue regimes are generally well tolerated by patients with CACG, and have become an important member in the medical arsenal against CACG. If the intraocular pressure remains elevated, or there is evidence of optic nerve damage, and/or significant visual field defects, then follow up intervals are similar to those when following an open angle glaucoma patient.

## 7. Medications available to treat elevated intraocular pressure

It is important to have a thorough knowledge of the patient's allergies, medical and surgical history, and a list of current medications to anticipate drug interactions or harmful side effects.

**Alpha2-adrenergic receptor agonists:** brimonidine tartrate 0.2%, 0.5%, 0.1% (Alphagan®, (Alphagan®P®), apraclonidine 0.5%, 1% (Iopidine®).

These medications may decrease IOP by reducing aqueous humor production and increase uveoscleral outflow.

The recommended dose is one drop of Alphagan®P® in the affected eye(s) twice daily, approximately 12 hours apart.

Use with precautions in coronary insufficiency, chronic renal failure, recent myocardial infarction, cerebrovascular disease, Raynaud disease, thromboangiitis obliterans, and patients with depression. A moderate risk of allergic response to this drug exists. Caution should be used in individuals who have developed an allergy to Iopidine. The brand Alphagan-P contains the preservative Purite and has been shown to be much better tolerated than its counterpart Alphagan. Coadministration with topical beta blockers may further decrease intraocular pressure; tricyclic antidepressants may decrease effects of brimonidine; CNS depressants such as barbiturates, opiates, and sedatives may potentiate effects of brimonidine. Contraindications if documented hypersensitivity and patients receiving Monoamine Oxidase Inhibitors inhibitors therapy.

**Beta-adrenergic blocking agents:** timolol maleate 0.25%,0.5% (Timoptic® Timoptic-XE®, Betimol®, Istalol®), levobunolol 0.25%, 0.5% (Betagan®), carteolol 1% (Ocupress®).

Beta-adrenergic receptor antagonists decrease aqueous humor production by the ciliary body and possibly increased outflow.

Treatment can be initiated at one drop of 0,25% Timoptic® solution in each affected eye twice a day.

These medications may cause bradycardia, bronchospasm, obstructive pulmonary disease, cardiac failure, may contain sulfites and cause allergic reactions. Use with caution in patients with cerebrovascular insufficiency; in myasthenic syndromes, may potentiate muscle weakness; patients with an anaphylactic reaction may be unresponsive to usual dose of epinephrine. The product may cause depression, confusion, hallucinations, and psychosis, especially in the elderly. These effects may occur suddenly and are typically reversible upon discontinuation; some have sulfites, which may cause allergic-type reactions in susceptible patients. Punctal occlusion after dosing may reduce systemic absorption.

**Topical carbonic anhydase inhibitors**: brinzolamide 1%(Azopt®) dorzolamide 2%(Trusopt®). Dosage is 1 drop in affected eye tid.
The mechanism of action is to reduce secretion of aqueous humor by inhibiting carbonic anhydrase in ciliary body, causing a decrease in intraocular pressure. May use concomitantly with other topical ophthalmic drug products to lower intraocular pressure.
Local ocular adverse effects, primarily conjunctivitis and lid reactions may occur with chronic administration.
**Systemic carbonic anhydase inhibitors:** acetzolamide 125mg, 250 mg tablet (Diamox®), 500mg extended release capsule (Diamox Sequels®); 25 mg, 50mg methazolamide) Neptazane®).
Dosage Acetazolamide tablet (Diamox®) dosage 250 mg tablet qDay/bid/tid/qid; (Diamox Sequels®) 500 mg po bid; 25, 50 mg Methazolamide (Neptazane®) dosage 50-100 mg po bit/tid.
Systemic absorption can affect carbonic anhydrase in the kidney, reducing hydrogen ion secretion at renal tubule, and increasing renal excretion of sodium, potassium bicarbonate, and water.
Systemic administration of carbonic anhydrase inhibitors may have potential serious side effects. They may decrease levels of lithium, alter excretion of amphetamines, quinidine, phenobarbital, and salicylates by alkalinizing urine. Derived chemically from sulfa drugs. Boxed warning: rare fatalities have occurred because of severe reactions to sulfonamides resulting in Stevens-Johnson syndrome, toxic epidermal necrolysis, fulminant hepatic necrosis, agranulocytosis, aplastic anemia, and other blood dyscrasias; reports of anorexia, tachypnea, lethargy, coma, and death with concomitant high-dose aspirin may cause substantial increase in blood glucose in some diabetic patients; may result in loss of potassium.
**Miotic agents (parasympathomimetics):** pilocarpine ophthalmic 0.5%, 1%,2%,4%, Gel; 4% (Isopto Carpine®, Pilopine HS Gel®).
Dosage is 1 gtt tid/qid, gel apply 0.5 inch ribbon in lower cul de sac q hs.
A naturally occurring alkaloid, pilocarpine mimics muscarinic effects of acetylcholine at postganglionic parasympathetic nerves, directly stimulate cholinergic receptors in the eye, decreasing resistance to aqueous humor outflow. Miotics cause the pupilary sphincter to contract, mechanically pulling the aris away from the trabecular meskwork and open the angle, and cause the ciliary muscle to contract increasing trabecular outflow. They may be ineffective when used concomitantly with nonsteroidal anti-inflammatory agents, are contraindicated with documented hypersensitivity and acute inflammatory disease of anterior chamber. In pregnancy, the risk to fetus not established or studied in humans but may be used if benefits outweigh risk to fetus. Use with caution in acute cardiac failure, peptic ulcer, hyperthyroidism, GI spasm, bronchial asthma, Parkinson disease, recent MI, urinary tract obstruction, and hypertension or hypotension.
**Prostaglandin analogs:** travoprost 0.004% (Travatan®, Travatan Z®), latanoprost 0.005% (Xalatan®), bimatoprost 0.01%,0.03% (Lumigan®).
Dosage 1 gtt in affected eye a Day.
Exact mechanism of action unknown but believed to reduce IOP by increasing uveoscleral outflow. Another mechanism of action may be through induction of metalloproteinases in ciliary body, which breaks down extracellular matrix, thereby reducing resistance to outflow through ciliary body.

Commonly causes ocular hyperemia; may cause permanent increases in brown pigment in iris and eyelid; eyelash growth may increase; bacterial keratitis may occur; use with caution in uveitis or macular edema (Prostaglandins may aggravate or induce cystoid macular edema); do not instill if wearing contact lenses. Co-administration with eye drops, containing the preservative thimerosal, may reduce effects (administer at intervals of 5 min between applications. Contraindicated if there is documented hypersensitivity; signs of inflammation. Use with caution in pregnant patients.

**Topical hyperosmotic agents:** glycerin (Ophthalgan®) One or two drops of applied to the cornea prior to gonioscopy may facilitate gonioscopy by clearing corneal edema.

**Systemic hyperosmotic agents**: mannitol (Osmitrol®), Ismotic® (isosorbide) Solution 45% w/v, glycerin (Osmoglyn®)

Prior to intravenous administration, assess for adequate renal function in adults by administering a test dose of 200 mg/kg IV over 3-5 min. Should produce a urine flow of at least 30-50 mL/h of urine over 2-3 h. If safe to administer, then administer 1.5-2 g/kg body weight IV over 30-60 minutes;

Isosorbide 45% soution, (Ismotic®) oral dosage 1-2 gm/kg body weight (55);

Glycerin (Osmoglyn®) oral dosage 1 ml/kg body weight (55).

Osmotic agents lower IOP by creating an osmotic gradient between ocular fluids and plasma.

Assess for adequate renal function in adults or children. Carefully evaluate cardiovascular status before rapid administration of mannitol since a sudden increase in extracellular fluid may lead to fulminating congestive heart failure; If blood is given simultaneously with mannitol, add at least 20 mEq of sodium chloride to each liter of mannitol solution to avoid pseudoagglutination. Consultation with specialists in internal medicine is strongly advised.

## 8. Neuroprotective agents

The use of neuroprotective agents may facilitate recovery of function or at least attenuation of damage. The results of studies of brimonidine and memantidine as potential neuroprotective agents are encouraging (54).

## 9. Surgical treatment

Surgical treatment may consist of laser iridotomies, laser iridoplasties to shrink the peripheral plateau iris, surgical iridectomies, and filtering procedures.

Argon laser peripheral iridotomy in eyes with light blue or green irides includes the following steps. After informed consent is obtained, Topical anesthetic (proparacaine 0.5%), topical alpha-agonist (apraclonidine or brimonidine), and pilocarpine 1% are placed on the eye. To perform laser peripheral iridotomy (LPI). Either the Abraham lens or equivalent lens, is placed on the cornea with the magnifying bubble rotated to an upper nasal position and the patient instructed to fixate with the opposite on an appropriate target. The lenses stabilize the eye, act as a speculum, reduce power due to the magnifying portion of the lens, and absorb heat to reduce the chances of burning of the cornea. The location of the treatment should be upper and nasal near the arcus sinelis in a spot where the iris appears thinner, such as an iris crypt. By placing the spot thusly, one may avoid annoying optical effects due to light entering the iridotomy, a rare occurrence requiring a large iridotomy opening or extremely observant patient. Suggested starting settings for the Argon laser are as follows:

Spot size - 50 mm Duration - 0.03-0.04 seconds Power - 900 mW. These may be adjusted depending on iris color and thickness of the iris stroma. Each surgeon should determine appropriate parameters for each clinical situation and adjust them accordingly. Prednisolone acetate 1% is started (4 times a day for 5-7 d). Follow up examination is in one hour to avoid missing any spike in intraocular pressure, which must be treated appropriately. The patient is seen in one week, one month, then at three to six months, then at least annually.

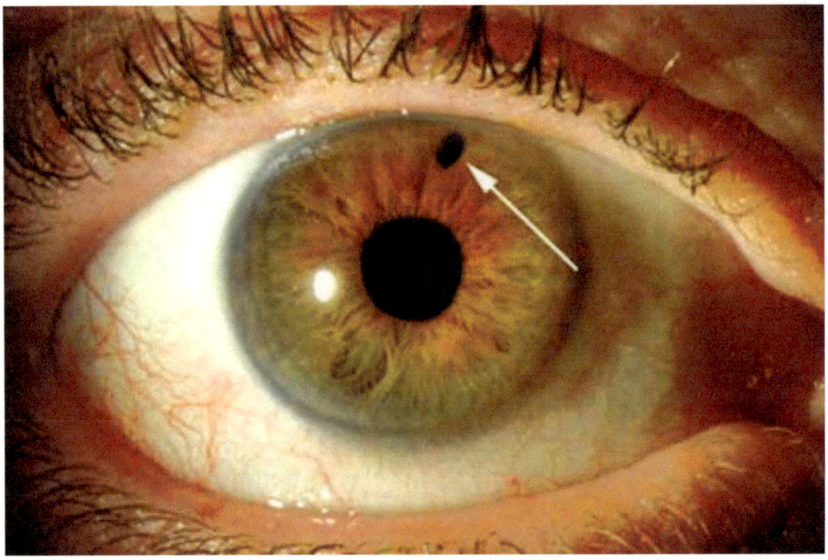

Fig. 13. Argon laser peripheral iridotomy is illustrated

ND: Yag laser peripheral iridotomy is indicated in eyes that have thick dark brown irides. After similar preparatory steps as above, the proposed treatment site is thinned with the Argon laser, and then the iris perforated with the ND:Yag with starting settings: power 1.7-3 mJ, pulses per burst 2. Follow up examination in one hour to avoid missing any spike in intraocular pressure, which must be treated appropriately. The patient is seen in one week, one month, then at three to six months.

The number of surgical iridectomies has declined dramatically with the introduction of laser procedures which are noninvasive and thus avoid the potential and real complications of intraocular surgery. Lensectomy with posterior chamber intraocular lenses for intumescent or dislocated cataracts has been reported to have good clinical results with deepening of the anterior chamber. However, results of clinical trials to determine the true value of this procedure are pending.

One type of patient with narrow angles deserves special attention: the rare individual with nanophthalmos. These highly hyperopic eyes with very short axial lengths and proportionally large lenses, are prone to very serious complications during and after intraocular surgery such as vitreous loss during surgery and post operative hypotony with effusions in the suprachoroidal space culminating in huge choroidal detachments that in extreme cases seem to fill the eye. Corrective surgery is difficult and may involve vitrectomy, removing sclera surrounding vortex veins, and drainage of the choroidals. Posterior sclerotomy prior to trabeculectomy has some but does have not widespread support. (58)

## 10. Financial cost of glaucoma

In the United States of America in 2006, approximately eighty five thousand laser iridotomies and three thousand laser iridoplasties were reimbursed by Medicare for payment (53).
The total financial burden of adult major visual disorders is estimated to be 25.4 billion, with more than $2.9 billion due to glaucoma. Outpatient medical and pharmaceutical costs accounted for the bulk of glaucoma expenditure. In 1996 the cost of Social Security benefits, lost income tax revenues, and healthcare expenditures was considered to be 1.5 billion dollars (USD). In 2003 it was estimated that blindness and vision loss were responsible $2.14 billion in non eye related costs.
There is also a cost to society in terms of quality of life and supportive care for the blind. Individuals with impared vision are at risk of falls, auto accidents, require more care, and may have reduced life expectancy.
Should the fellow eye be treated if it has not suffered an attack? It is usually warranted since both angles usually have similar structures. In the United States of America, medical liability may be a risk for not treating the fellow eye for blinding condition. The management of patients who are anatomically at risk who have not suffered an attack presents a dilemma: should they be treated or should treatment be delayed until the attack occurs. The cost of treatment must be factored into the decision with the knowledge that failure to diagnose primary angle closure glaucoma carries a risk of harm to the patient and malpractice litigation.

## 11. Prognosis

### 11.1 Acute angle closure

After the the acute attack is over, eyes should be examined for degree of angle closure, presence of peripheral anterior synechiae (PAS), and optic disc and visual field damage. Intraocular pressure (IOP) should be checked often to detect asymptomatic rise in IOP. The second eye should be assessed and treated to prevent attack. (59)
The prognosis is favorable if the IOP can be controlled. IOP is reported to be controlled with laser peripheral iridotomy alone in 42% to 72%, in whites more often then in Asians. (60) (61)

### 11.2 Angle closure glaucoma

Progressive visual deterioration may be prevented if control of the IOP can be achieved. Whether or not peripheral iridotomy alone can control the IOP depends the underlying mechanism and the stage of the disease when diagnosed. (62)
If more PAS, a higher IOP, and a larger cup-to-disc ratio are found, there is a likelyhood of poor pressure control following iridotomy. (63) Once glaucomatous optic neuropathy has developed most patients will require further treatment to control IOP. (64)
*Clinical clues for non-ophthalmologists* that an individual may be having an attack of angle closure glaucoma. If a patient, who may or may not be able to communicate, has an inflamed eye with oval pupil and hazy cornea with loss of clarity, the diagnosis of angle closure glaucoma should be entertained. If the patient wears thick glasses that magnify objects, the patient may be far sighted or hyperopic with a small eye at risk of angle closure glaucoma. The flashlight test may point to narrow angles if a bright light is positioned to shine on the eye from the ear side and only a temporal crescent is lit up and the rest of the

iris is in shadow, instead of the entire iris being illuminated. A detailed medical is important to learn of prior eye problems, a family history of glaucoma, prior eye surgery, and a complete list of all medications both prescription and over the counter.

## 12. Summary

A significant number of individuals world wide are at risk of blindness from angle closure glaucoma. Acute angle closure glaucoma crises attacks are relatively easy to diagnose. The challenge is identification and examination of patients at risk of angle closure glaucoma, those with anatomically narrow angles who have not suffered an acute attack, those with evidence of subclinical attacks, symptoms of headache, blurry vision, halos around lights, narrowed angles, peripheral anterior synechiae, and the fellow eye of one that has suffered an attack of acute angle closure. Signs of a prior attack to look for include glaukomaflecken, Iris atrophy, ovoid pupil, and peripheral anterior synechiae.

The methods of grading the depth of the anterior chamber at the slit lamp (van Herick), indirect gonioscopy (Shaffer, Spaeth), and new non contact methods (UBM, anterior segment OCT, Scheimpflug, Pentascan) can be helpful in identifying patients who may be at risk of angle closure glaucoma and treated before they progress to optic nerve damage, visual field defects, and blindness.

## 13. Future directions in diagnosis and management of patients at risk of or suffering from angle closure glaucoma

The large numbers of individuals at risk of developing or those with eyes already damaged demonstrate the need for early detection and treatment, particularly in underdeveloped countries. A hand held self contained UBM or OCT would greatly facilitate the identification of those at risk. Such a portable device could scan the eye and wirelessly transmit data to a smart phone to store and display the results. The information could then be uploaded to a central health agency's website for further action.

To facilitate iridotomies in the field a hand held self contained portable ND:Yag laser would useful.

Current imaging methods analyze the optic nerve, nerve fiber layer, and other structures. Perhaps a future method could image nerve impulses traveling along the ganglion cell axons to provide information about their functional status, identify unhealthy ones, allow mapping, and help suggest when appropriate treatment should be started.

Study of the genetic machinery involved in the embryologic development of the eye might identify the genes and other process involved and enable restarting the genetic machinery in damaged or blind eyes to regenerate or rebuild damaged retina and optic nerves. This assumes that the genes involved are turned on for a period of time, then silenced, are not removed from the genome, but persist in all cells and could be restarted.

## 14. References

[1] Quigley H. A. Number of people with glaucoma worldwide. Br J Ophthalmolol. 1996, 80: 389-393.

[2] Noecker, Robert J., and Lauri Graham. "Acute Angle-Closure Glaucoma." *eMedicine Consumer Health*. Eds. Richard W. Alliinson, et al. 18 Nov. 2005. Medscape. 30 Oct. 2009.
[3] Bonomi L., Marchini G., Marraffa M., et al. Prevalence of glaucoma and intraocular pressure distribution in a defined population. The Egna-Neumarkt Study. Ophthalmology 1998; 105:209-15.
[4] Mitchell P., Smith W., Attebo K., Healey P. R. Prevalence of open-angle glaucoma in Australia. The Blue Mountains Eye Study. Ophthalmology 1996; 103:1661-9.
[5] Bankes JL, Perkins ES, Tsolakis S, Wright JE. Bedford glaucoma survey. Br Med J 1968; 1:791-6.
[6] Coffey M., Reidy A., Wormald R., et al. Prevalence of glaucoma in the west of Ireland. Br J Ophthalmol 1993; 77:17-21.
[7] Hollows F. C., Graham P. A. Intra-ocular pressure, glaucoma, and glaucoma suspects in a defined population. Br J Ophthalmol 1966; 50:570-86.
[8] Wensor M. D., McCarty C. A., Stanislavsky Y. L., et al. The prevalence of glaucoma in the Melbourne Visual Impairment Project. Ophthalmology 1998; 105:733-9.
[9] Klein B. E., Klein R., Sponsel W. E., et al. Prevalence of glaucoma. The Beaver Dam Eye Study. Ophthalmology 1992; 99:1499-504.
[10] Dielemans I., Vingerling J. R., Wolfs R. C., et al. The prevalence of primary open-angle glaucoma in a population-based study in The Netherlands. The Rotterdam Study. Ophthalmology 1994; 101:1851
[11] Bengtsson B. The prevalence of glaucoma. Br J Ophthalmol 1981; 65:46-9.
[12] Casson R. J., Newland H. S., Muecke J., et al. Prevalence of glaucoma in rural Myanmar: the Meiktila Eye Study. Br J Ophthalmol 2007; 91:710-4.
[13] Salmon J. F., Mermoud A., Ivey A., et al. The prevalence of primary angle closure glaucoma and open angle glaucoma in Mamre, western Cape, South Africa. Arch Ophthalmol 1993; 111:1263-9.
[14] Dandona L., Dandona R., Mandal P., et al. Angle-closure glaucoma in an urban population in southern India. The Andhra Pradesh eye disease study. Ophthalmology 2000; 107:1710-6.
[15] Bourne R. R., Sukudom P., Foster P. J., et al. Prevalence of glaucoma in Thailand: a population based survey in Rom Klao District, Bangkok. Br J Ophthalmol 2003; 87:1069-74.
[16] Vijaya L., George R., Arvind H., et al. Prevalence of angle-closure disease in a rural southern Indian population. Arch Ophthalmol 2006; 124:403-9.
[17] Ramakrishnan R., Nirmalan P. K., Krishnadas R., et al. Glaucoma in a rural population of southern India: the Aravind comprehensive eye survey. Ophthalmology 2003; 110:1484-90.
[18] Rahman M. M., Rahman N., Foster P. J., et al. The prevalence of glaucoma in Bangladesh: a population based survey in Dhaka division. Br J Ophthalmol 2004; 88:1493-7.
[19] Shiose Y., Kitazawa Y., Tsukahara S., et al. Epidemiology of glaucoma in Japan--a nationwide glaucoma survey. Jpn J Ophthalmol 1991; 35:133-55.
[20] Yamamoto T., Iwase A., Araie M., et al. The Tajimi Study report 2: prevalence of primary angle closure and secondary glaucoma in a Japanese population. Ophthalmology 2005; 112:1661-9.

[21] Van Rens G. H., Arkell S. M., Charlton W., Doesburg W. Primary angle-closure glaucoma among Alaskan Eskimos. Doc Ophthalmol 1988; 70:265-76.

[22] Arkell S. M., Lightman D. A., Sommer A., et al. The prevalence of glaucoma among Eskimos of northwest Alaska. Arch Ophthalmol 1987; 105:482-5.

[23] Bourne R. R., Sorensen K. E., Klauber A., et al. Glaucoma in East Greenlandic Inuit--a population survey in Ittoqqortoormiit (Scoresbysund). Acta Ophthalmol Scand 2001; 79:462-7.

[24] Seah S. K., Foster P. J., Chew P. T., et al. Incidence of acute primary angle-closure glaucoma in Singapore. An island-wide survey. Arch Ophthalmol 1997; 115:1436-40.

[25] Weinreb R. N., Friedman D. S., eds. Angle Closure and Angle Closure Glaucoma. World Glaucoma Association Consensus Series-3. The Netherlands: Kugler Publications, 2006.

[26] Anderson D. R., Jin J. C., Wright M. M. The physiologic characteristics of relative pupillary block. Am J Ophthalmol 1991;111:344-50.Tiedeman JS. A physical analysis of the factors that determine the contour of the iris. Am J Ophthalmol 1991; 111:338-43.

[27] Jin J. C., Anderson D. R. The effect of iridotomy on iris contour. Am J Ophthalmol 1990; 110:260-3.

[28] Seah S. K., Foster P. J., Chew P. T., et al. Incidence of acute primary angle-closure glaucoma in Singapore. An island-wide survey. Arch Ophthalmol 1997; 115:1436-40.

[29] American Academy of Ophthalmology Glaucoma Panel. Preferred Practice Pattern® Guidelines. Primary Open-Angle Glaucoma. San Francisco, CA: American Academy of Ophthalmology; 2010. Available at: www.aao.org/ppp.

[30] Aung T., Husain R., Gazzard G., et al. Changes in retinal nerve fiber layer thickness after acute primary angle closure. Ophthalmology 2004; 111:1475-9.

[31] von Graefe, A.,Beitragezur Pathol und Therapiedes Glaucoma, Arch. f. Ophth., 15:i 8,i869.

[32] Quigley H. A., Angle-Closure Glaucoma-Simpler Answers to Complex Mechanisms: LXVI Edward Jackson Memorial Lecture. Am J Ophthalmol 2009; 118:657-669. Panday V. A, Rhee D. J.

[33] Review of sulfonamide-induced acute myopia and acute bilateral angle-closure glaucoma. Compr Ophthalmol Update 2007; 8:271-6.

[34] Fraunfelder F. W., Fraunfelder F. T., Keates E. U. Topiramate-associated acute, bilateral, secondary angle-closure glaucoma. Ophthalmology 2004; 111:109-11.

[35] A. Trantas: Sur la gonioscopie (Ophtal- moscopie de l'angle iridocorneen). Arch Ophtalmol (Paris) 45:616, 1928.

[36] Dellaporta A. Historical notes on gonioscopy. Surv Ophthalmol 1975; 20:137–49.

[37] Salzmann M. Nachtrag zu ophthalmoskopie der kammerbucht. Z Augenheilk 1915; 34: 160–2.

[38] Blum, M., et al, Theodor Leber: a founder of ophthalmic research, Surv Ophthalmol, 1992: p. 83-8.

[39] Jaeger, W. The foundation of experimental ophthalmology by Theodor Leber. Doc Ophthal. 1988 Jan-Feb; 68:71-7.

[40] Troncoso M. U. Gonioscopy with the Electric Ophthalmoscope. New York, NY: New York Academy of Medicine; 1921.

[41] Barkan O., Boyle S. F., Maisler S. On the genesis of glaucoma. An improved method based on slit lamp microscopy of the angle of the anterior chamber. Am J Ophthalmol 1936; 19:209–15.
[42] Van Herick W., Shaffer R. N., Schwartz A. Estimation of width of angle of anterior chamber. Incidence and significance of the narrow angle. Am J Ophthalmol 1969; 68:626–9.
[43] Goldmann H. Zur Technik der Spaltlampenmikroskopie. Ophthalmologica 1938; 96:90–7.
[44] Allen L, Braley A. E, Thorpe H. E. An improved gonioscopic contact prism. AMA Arch Ophthalmol 1954; 51:451–5.
[45] Forbes M. Gonioscopy with corneal indentation. A method for distinguishing between appositional closure and synechial closure. Arch Ophthalmol 1966; 76:488–92.
[46] Scheie H. G. Width and pigmentation of the angle of the anterior chamber; a system of grading by gonioscopy. AMA Arch Ophthalmol 1957; 58:510–2.
[47] Shaffer R. N. Stereoscopic Manual of Gonioscopy. St. Louis, MO: Mosby; 1962.
[48] Spaeth G. L. The normal development of the human anterior chamber angle: a new system of grading. Trans Ophthalmol Soc UK 1971; 91:709–39.
[49] James D. Brandt, M. D., 1 Julia A. Beiser, M. S., 2 Michael A. Kass, M. D., 2 Mae O. Gordon, PhD,2and the Ocular Hypertension Treatment Study (OHTS). Group Central Corneal Thickness in the Ocular Hypertension Treatment Study (OHTS). *Ophthalmology 2001*; 108: 1779–1788
[50] Fujioka M., Nakamura M., Tatsumi Y., Kusuhara A., Maeda H., Negi A. Comparison of Pentacam. Scheimpflug camera with ultrasound pachymetry and noncontact specular m.icroscopy in measuring central corneal thickness. Curr Eye Res. 2007 Feb; 32:89-94.
[51] M. I. Othman, S. A. Sullivan, G. L. Skuta, D. A. Cockrell, H. M. Stringham, C. A. Downs, A. Forne, A. Mick M. Boehnke, 2 D. Vollrath, and J. E. Richards, Autosomal Dominant Nanophthalmos (*NNO1*) with High Hyperopia and Angle-Closure Glaucoma Maps to Chromosome 11. Am. J. Hum. Genet. 63:1411–1418, 1998.
[52] Fred B. Berry, Matthew A. L., J. Martin, Tim Footz D. Alan Underhill, Philip J. Gage and Michael A. Walter, Functional interactions between FOXC1 and PITX2 underlie the sensitivity to FOXC1 gene dose in Axenfeld-Rieger syndrome and anterior segment dysgenesis. Human Molecular Genetics, 2006, Vol. 15, No. 6 doi: 10.1 093/hmg/ddl008
[53] Jordana K. Schmier, M. A; David W. Covert, M. B. A; Edmund C. Lau, M. S; Alan L. Robin, M. D. Trends in Annual Medicare Expenditures for Glaucoma Surgical Procedures From 1997 to 2006. *Arch Ophthalmol.* 2009; 127:900-905.
[54] R H W Funk E-M Kniep and C Röhlecke. Detecting the effects of neuroprotection in living cells. *Eye* (2007) 21, S38–S41; doi:10.1038/sj.eye.6702887
[55] Kolker, A. E. Symposium on glaucoma The Association for Research in Ophthalmology and the National Society for the Prevention of Blindness.
[56] Hyperosmotic agents in glaucoma. Investigative Ophthalmology Volume 9 Number 6 June 1970 418-423.
[57] Primary Angle Closure Preferred Practice Pattern October 2010.
[58] Eibschitz-Tsimhoni M, Lichter P, Del Monte M, et al. Assessing the need for posterior sclerotomy at the time of filtering surgery in patients with Sturge-Weber syndrome. *Ophthalmology* 2003; 110:1361-1363.

[59] Hollows F. C, Graham P. A. Intra-ocular pressure, glaucoma, and glaucoma suspects in a defined population. Br J Ophthalmol. 1966; 50:570-586.
[60] Wishart P. K., Atkinson P. L. Extracapsular cataract extraction and posterior chamber lens implantation in patients with primary chronic angle-closure glaucoma: effect on intraocular pressure control. Eye. 1989; 3:706-712.
[61] Gunning F. P., Greve E. L. Lens extraction for uncontrolled glaucoma. J Cataract Refract Surg. 1998; 24:1347-1356.
[62] Ang L. P., Aung T., Chua W. H., et al. Visual field loss from primary angle-closure glaucoma: a comparative study of symptomatic and asymptomatic disease. Ophthalmology. 2004; 111:1636-1640.
[63] Salmon J. F. Long-term intraocular pressure control after Nd:YAG laser iridotomy in chronic angle-closure glaucoma. J Glaucoma. 1993; 2:291-296.
[64] Rosman M., Aung T., Ang L. P., et al. Chronic angle-closure with glaucomatous damage: longterm clinical course in a North American population and comparison with an Asian population. Ophthalmology. 2002; 109:2227-2231.

# 26

# Plateau Iris

Yoshiaki Kiuchi, Hideki Mochizuki and Kiyoshi Kusanagi
*Hiroshima University*
*Japan*

## 1. Introduction

Primary angle-closure glaucoma (PACG) is a common form of glaucoma in Asia (Foster & Johnson, 2001). It is associated with a high risk of visual loss (Congdon et al., 1992; Foster et al., 1996). PACG was estimated to blind 5 times more people than primary open-angle glaucoma (Quigley et al. 2001). The original concept of primary angle closure glaucoma was a pupil- block angle-closure mechanism occurring in predisposed eyes with shallow anterior chamber angles. Peripheral iridectomy prevents the progression of primary angle closure glaucoma (Lowe, 1964). However, many patients experienced recurrent angle-closure glaucoma attacks after iridectomy (Wand et al., 1977). The occurrence of narrow angle in eyes with relatively normal depth in the anterior chamber and a relatively flat iris plane had been noted as early as 1940 (Gradle & Sugar, 1940). Chandler presented the case of a patient with repeated intermittent angle-closure glaucoma attacks despite a patent iridectomy, who was successfully treated with pilocarpine (Wand et al., 1977). Those cases were considered to be different from ordinary cases of narrow angle glaucoma. They were particularly found

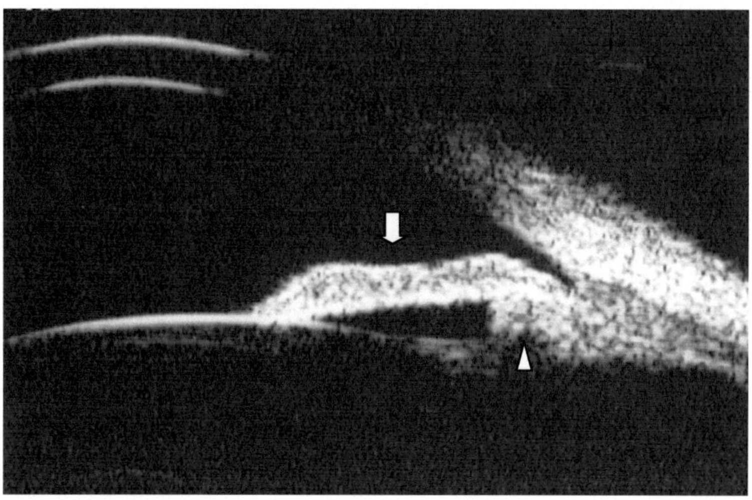

Fig. 1. Plateau iris configuration. Ultrasound biomicroscopy image shows a flat iris plane (⇩) accompanied by a narrow or closed anterior chamber angle. Plateau iris configuration is caused by anteriorly located ciliary processes (△), which close the ciliary sulcus and provide support to the peripheral iris

in younger patients in whom a peripheral iridectomy is often ineffective. These patients had a flat iris and a narrow angle secondary to an abrupt angulation at the root of the iris. This iris shape was called a plateau iris configuration.
The concept of the plateau iris was introduced in a publication by Shaffer (Shaffer, 1960). Primary angle closure includes those that are caused by a pupillary block and plateau iris configuration (Tarongoy et al., 2009).

## 2. Plateau iris configuration and plateau iris syndrome

Wand et al. reported that the plateau iris syndrome should be differentiated from the plateau iris configuration, to avoid confusion. Native plateau iris configuration refers to a preoperative (iridectomy or iridotomy) condition, in which angle-closure glaucoma is confirmed by gonioscopy, but the iris is flat and the anterior chamber is not shallow (Wand et al., 1977). One third of all patients demonstrating primary angle closure were estimated to have plateau iris configuration (Kumar et al., 2009, Mochizuki et al., 2010).
Plateau iris syndrome refers to the development of angle closure in an eye with plateau iris configuration. The intraocular pressure (IOP) increases because of angle closure after pupillary dilation. Plateau iris configuration can be diagnosed before iridotomy. However, plateau iris syndrome is normally diagnosed after laser iridotomy. Plateau iris syndrome is rare. Less than 10 % of all patients with primary angle closure are considered to have plateau iris syndrome.
The prevalence of angle closure attack in plateau iris syndrome is not known.

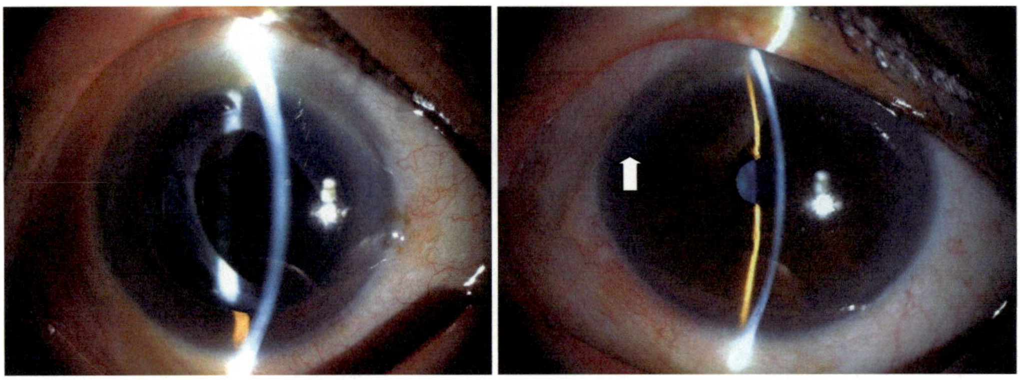

Fig. 2. Slit lamp photograph of an eye with a re-attack of acute closer attack and the patient's opposite eye. Right eye; Pupil is dilated after the second attack. Left eye; The laser iridotomy hole (⇧ ) is observed at 10 o'clock

The right eye developed acute closed-angle attack on December 2005. After successful treatment by laser iridotomy patients had a re-attack on October 2006. This patient underwent cataract surgery for the relief of the angle closure attack. Cataract surgery stabilized the IOP in the right eye.
Plateau iris syndrome is classified into two groups. Complete syndrome has a high plateau and covers the chamber angle after dilation and causes elevation of the IOP. Incomplete Syndrome partially covers the chamber angle after dilation of the pupil. The IOP will not elevate after dilating the pupil. However, the peripheral anterior synechia (PAS) increases

over time (Wand et al., 1977). Many people tend to confuse incomplete plateau syndrome with plateau iris configuration.

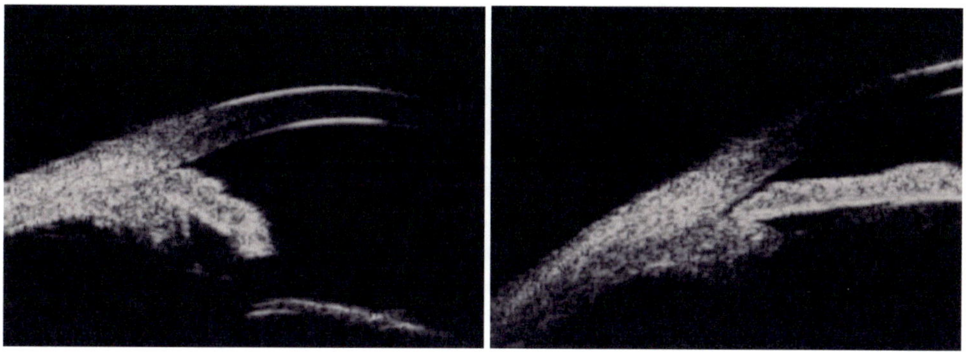

Right eye Left eye

Fig. 3. Ultrasound biomicroscopy image of Figure 2

## 3. Diagnosis

### 3.1 Gonioscopic findings

Generally, the diagnosis of a plateau iris configuration is based on typical gonioscopic findings. A plateau iris configuration is defined as a flat iris plane accompanied by a narrow or closed anterior chamber angle. Some patients with a plateau iris configuration show an increased intraocular pressure after the pupils are dilated by angle closure even after laser iridotomy.

Indentation gonioscopy of eyes with a plateau iris configuration following patent iridotomy reveals a sine-shaped curve of the iris surface. Indentation presses the iris surface backward. The deepest point of indentation is not at the iris periphery, but at approximately two-thirds of the distance between the center of the pupil and the iris root. The iris rises again from this point to the site of appositional closure. This shape is called a double hump sign.

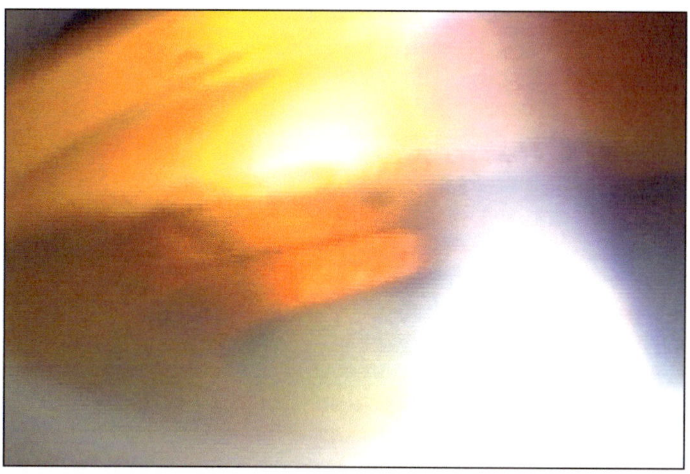

Fig. 4. Double hump sign after indentation

A double hump sign observed on indentation gonioscopy was strongly correlated with the presence of a plateau iris, and is, therefore a useful indicator of a plateau iris configuration. Therefore, a plateau iris configuration can be detected in many cases, without using a UBM (Kiuchi et al., 2009; Ritch, 1992).

### 3.2 Ultrasound biomicroscopy (UBM) findings

UBM provides detailed sub surface images of the angle region. This method showed that plateau iris configuration is caused by anteriorly located ciliary processes, which close the ciliary sulcus and provide support to the peripheral iris (Roberts et al., 2008). The ciliary processes were situated anteriorly in all the plateau iris configuration patients in comparison to the position in normal subjects and in patients with angle closure caused by pupillary block. The ciliary processes provide structural support beneath the peripheral iris, preventing the iris root from falling away from the trabecular meshwork after iridotomy (Pavlin et al., 1992).

Observation with a slit lamp causes miosis and thus the iris becomes thinner. An unintentional indentation and/or miosis induced by the slit-lamp light might prevent the identification of appositional angle closure during regular gonioscopic examination (Sakata et al., 2006). The importance of the diagnosis of plateau iris configuration by UBM resides in the fact that the plateau iris configuration can be detected without any interference from the effect of the lighting. Provocative tests were not usually helpful for detecting plateau iris syndrome (Ritch et al., 2009).

## 4. Gender and age

Women from Japan, Israel, Finland, and Thailand showed a consistently more frequent occurrence of PACG (Yamamoto et al., 2005). One study found no sexual predisposition for plateau iris configuration (Ritch, 1992). Others report that most patients with plateau iris were female and younger than those with pupillary block. The average age of the patients studied by Diniz et al. was 60.1 years old (Diniz et al., 2010). This is consistent with the results of the study by Mandell et al (Mandell et al., 2003), in which the plateau iris configuration patients averaged 57.5 years old.

Ritch, et al. evaluated the findings in patients 40 years of age or younger with angle closure. Sixty-seven patients (49 females, 18 males) met the entry criteria. Plateau iris configuration was found in 35 patients (52.2%) (Ritch et al., 2003).

On the other hand, the prevalence of PACG significantly increases with age in population based epidemiological studies (Yamamoto et al., 2005). Pupillary block angle closure is a disease of older persons, peaking in incidence between 55 and 70 years of age (Suzuki et al., 2008).

### 4.1 Prevalence of plateau iris configuration

Kumar et al. used standardized UBM criteria and found plateau iris in about one third of PACS eyes after laser iridotomy (Kumar et al., 2008, 2009). Mochizuki et al. conducted a study under the same criteria used by Kumar et al. to determine the prevalence of plateau iris configurations in acute angle-closure, chronic angle-closure glaucoma, and open-angle glaucoma eyes using ultrasound biomicroscopy The study included fellow eyes from 27 acute angle-closure patients, 26 open-angle glaucoma patients, and 26 chronic angle-closure glaucoma patients with no history of acute angle-closure. Plateau iris configurations were found in the opposite eyes of 10 (37.0%) of 27 patients with acute angle-closure, 9 (34.6%)of 26 patients with chronic angle-closure glaucoma, and 5 (19.2%) of 26 patients with open-angle glaucoma (Mochizuki et al., 2010). Filho also reported that plateau iris configuration in 10.2% of patients with open-angle glaucoma (Diniz Fiho et al., 2010). The clinical significance of plateau iris configurations in open-angle glaucoma eyes is unclear. Open-angle glaucoma eyes do not have plateau iris configurations high enough to occlude the trabecular meshwork, which is associated with the elevation of IOP or other clinical events. However, lower plateau iris configuration may become higher over time due to increased thickness and anterior movement of the lens, which would consequently result in angle closure.

### 4.2 Prevalence of plateau iris syndrome

Cases of recurrent angle-closure glaucoma after iridectomy, as a result of plateau iris syndrome are relatively rare. Plateau iris syndrome is believed to constitute a small percentage of eyes with plateau iris configuration. A study of eyes that had experienced angle-closure episodes was conducted to determine the relative frequency of plateau iris syndrome. All of the patients had undergone peripheral iridectomy. The IOP increased more than 8 mmHg after topical application of homatropine in 4 (6.2%)of the 65 eyes. Those 4 eyes were classified as the iris plateau type of angle –closure glaucoma (Godel et al., 1968). Saitoh reported that five of 50 iridectomized PACG eyes developed complete closure of the angle with an increase in the IOP exceeding 10 mmHg following the administration of homatropine which acts on the sphincter muscle located at the pupillary margin. However, those 5 subjects did not show IOP elevation after topical application of phenilephrine hydrochloride (alpha adrenergic stimulator) Phenilephrine acts on the iris dilator muscle which is located just above the iris pigment epithelium. Homatropine and phenilephrine act on different muscles in the iris, and the difference in the distribution of the dilator muscle and the sphincter muscle causes the different morphological changes in the iris after application of the midriatic agents. This may explain the difference in IOP response after dilation of pupil by midriatic agents (Saitoh, 1974).

### 4.3 Biometrics of plateau iris configuration

Historically, plateau iris configuration is regarded as angle closure with normal anterior chamber depth and flat iris plane. Mandel et al. reported that all plateau iris configuration eyes showed biometric parameters that were completely different for those of normal eyes, except for the peripheral iris thickness at 500 µm from the scleral spur. The eyes with plateau iris configuration showed a shallower anterior chamber depth than normal eyes (Mandell et al., 2003). The mean anterior chamber depth in patients with plateau iris syndrome (2.04 +/- 0.30 mm) was significantly smaller than the hypothesized normal anterior chamber depth (3 mm). The mean anterior chamber depth in patients with pupillary block (2.17 +/- 0.30 mm) was also significantly smaller than the hypothesized normal anterior chamber depth. Although a review of the literature suggested that patients with plateau iris had a normal or deeper axial anterior chamber depth in comparison to those with pupillary block, the mean anterior chamber depth in patients with plateau iris syndrome was significantly smaller than the anterior chamber depth in patients with pupillary block in the report by Mandell et al (Mandell et al., 2003).

There is one more report related to the biometrics of plateau iris configuration. Kiuchi et al. reported that patients with plateau iris configuration had deeper anterior chamber and longer axial length than chronic angle closure patients without plateau iris configuration (Kiuchi et al., 2009). Further study is necessary to clarify this issue.

### 4.4 Changes in the biometrics of plateau iris configuration after intervention

Palvin et al. used ultrasound biomicroscopy to image angles in the dark, in the light, and following pilocarpine administration to clarify factors that produce angle opening changes in this syndrome. Changes in angle opening in dark and light were solely related to changes in iris thickness. Their results were consistent with the concept that the space between the ciliary processes and trabecular meshwork constitutes a passageway of fixed dimension. An increase in iris thickness resulted in a decrease in angle opening, and a decrease in iris thickness resulted in an increase in angle opening. Angle closure occured if the iris thickness fills the space between the ciliary processes and the trabecular meshwork (Pavlin & Foster, 1999).

## 5. The cause of plateau iris configuration

The cause of the plateau iris configuration is not known. The anomaly of the pars plicata position could be developmental or acquired. Ciliary processes develop during the 24$^{th}$ week of embryogenesis and initially overlap the trabecular meshwork but later recede to a position behind the scleral spur. This repositioning is thought to be due to a differential growth rate of the various tissue elements. The specific features of the ciliary processes in the eyes with plateau iris might be due to the failure of the ciliary processes to separate from the posterior iris surface. The displacement of the pars plicata from the peripheral iris to the iris root during embryogenesis may be incomplete in eyes with a shorter axial length. However, incomplete cleavage between the iris and ciliary body is unlikely (Razeghinejad & Kamali-Sarvestani, 2007; Tran et al., 2003).

Tran and associates (Tran et al., 2003) examined the anterior segments of 6 patients with plateau iris syndrome before and after cataract surgery. They found that irido-ciliary apposition persisted after extracapsular cataract extraction, thus indicating that the age related growth of the lens (i.e., acquired changes in the zonular fibers stretched by cataract formation) does not induce a reversible anterior pulling and or rotation of the ciliary body processes.

Etter investigated the prevalence of plateau iris syndrome in the first-degree relatives of patients affected with plateau iris syndrome. They found a high prevalence of plateau iris configuration in family members of patients with plateau iris syndrome. Five of the 10 participating patients (50%) were found to have at least 1 first-degree family member with plateau iris configuration. The presence of plateau iris configuration in successive generations, where there was not consanguineous marriage, therefore suggested that it might be inherited in an autosomal dominant manner with incomplete penetrance (Etter et al., 2006).

## 6. Differential diagnosis

### 6.1 Iris cyst

Tanihara et al. reported a case of high, broad, peripheral anterior synechiae caused by multiple, bilateral iridociliary cysts. The peripheral anterior synechia extended to the corneal endothelium beyond Schwalbe's line. Ultrasound biomicroscopic imaging showed that multiple, bilateral iridociliary cysts causes elevation of the iris structure (Tanihara et al., 1997). This report showed that an iris cyst could cause the pseudo-plateau configuration. The incidence and sector distribution of ciliary body cysts in normal subjects is not low. A UBM study conducted by Kunimatsu et al. showed that cysts were detected in 63 (54.3%) of the 116 subjects. The number and diameter of the cysts decreased with age. Gender and refractive error did not affect the incidence and distribution. A significant bilateral correlation was found in the number, incidence, and distribution of ciliary body cysts (Kunimatsu et al., 1999). There was a high prevalence of iris cysts in young subjects. Younger subjects with a bumpy peripheral iris have a higher likelihood of a diagnosis of pseudo-plateau iris (Shukla et al., 2008).

### 6.2 Others

Any disorder that causes swelling of the ciliary body or forward rotation of the ciliary body can create a pseudo-plateau iris configuration. Sulfa based compounds like hydrochlorothiazide, oral acetazolamide, supra ciliary effusions and ciliary body thickening after scleral buckling procedures can cause ciliary swelling and precipitate angle closure glaucoma.(Geason & Perkins, 1995; Palvin et al., 1997; Tripathi et al., 2003)

## 7. Management

### 7.1 Miotics

Miotic therapy is one option for plateau iris configuration. One drop of pilocarpine causes significant changes in the anterior eye segment morphology. This decreases the pupillary diameter and the iris thickness (Németh et al., 1996-1997). A single drop of 2% pilocarpine is an effective agent for thinning the iris and opening the angle in plateau iris syndrome. The ability to visualize the degree of angle opening produced by pilocarpine can be helpful in predicting the efficacy of this therapy (Pavlin and Foster, 1999). There are two problems associated with pilocarpine treatment for glaucoma associated with plateau iris configuration. Most patients are relatively young in age in comparison to the usual angle-closure glaucoma patients, and therefore, are unhappy with pilocarpine- induced myopia and miosis. These side effects may decrease the compliance (adherence) to the medical therapy.

Yasuda et al. examined the long-term effects of topical pilocarpine on IOP control in primary angle-closure glaucoma without iridectomy. Six (43%) out of 14 eyes with acute PACG under topical pilocarpine therapy had re-attacks while one eye (7%) developed increased IOP. Twelve of 47 fellow eyes of patients with acute PACG (26%) developed acute attacks while 3 eyes (6%) showed increased IOP. They concluded that long-term medical therapy for PACG is unsatisfactory. A single drop of pilocarpine works only for 6 hours. Short acting duration of pilocarpine and poor compliance (adherence) may play some role in this result. They included all types of angle closure glaucoma in their study. Patients with plateau iris configuration might yield the same results (Yasuda & Kageyama, 1988).

### 7.2 Laser treatment

#### 7.2.1 Laser iridotomy

Laser iridotomy (LI) is the appropriate treatment for angle closure glaucoma due to primary pupillary block. UBM studies in patients with pupillary block glaucoma post-LI demonstrated substantial increases in the anterior chamber angle aperture following laser iridotomy. Previous studies have also shown that in eyes with an acute attack, the angle widened in the first 2 weeks after LI, but did not change thereafter over 1 year, and the amount of peripheral anterior synechia (PAS) remained stable throughout. The results indicate the effectiveness of LI in preventing progressive closure of the angle in the first year after the angle closure attack (Porikoff et al., 2005). However, laser iridotomy is insufficient to treat glaucoma associated with plateau iris. Many patients with a patent iridotomy hole experienced acute angle-closed attacks. Polikoff et al. also examined the effect of laser iridotomy on anterior segment anatomy of patients with plateau iris configuration. Iridotomy will remove any contribution from pupillary block in these patients, but the angle will remain narrow because the anteriorly positioned ciliary processes prevent the peripheral iris from moving posteriorly. This report also showed that pupil block and plateau iris configuration coexists in many cases (Polikoff et al., 2005). Approximately one of three of the eyes showed PAS progression during a 3-year follow-up period after LI. The probability of progression was found to be high in the eyes that exhibited plateau iris (Choi & Kim, 2005). These data show that laser iridotomy alone is not an effective treatment for glaucoma with plateau iris configuration.

### 7.2.2 Argon laser peripheral iridoplasty

Argon laser peripheral iridoplasty can effectively eliminate residual appositional closure after laser iridotomy caused by plateau iris syndrome, and the effect is maintained for years. Argon laser iridoplasty may also prove valuable in the treatment of plateau-like iris configuration resulting from iridociliary cysts (Crowston et al., 2005). Rich et al. documented the long-term effect of argon laser iridoplasty in patients with plateau iris syndrome. A total of 26 argon laser iridoplasty procedures were performed in 23 eyes of 14 patients. The angle remained open in 20 of 23 (87.0%) eyes after only 1 treatment with Argon laser iridoplasty over a follow-up period of 78.9 ± 8.0 months (range, 72–188 months). They concluded that Argon laser iridoplasty could effectively eliminate residual appositional closure after laser iridotomy caused by plateau iris syndrome (Ritch et al., 2004). However, there are no other reports that indicate the effectiveness of laser peripheral iridoplasty.

### 7.2.3 Cataract surgery

Hayashi showed that the anterior chamber depth and angle width in angle closure glaucoma eyes approximates that of POAG eyes and control eyes without glaucoma after phaco-emulsification and posterior chamber intraocular lens implantation (Hayashi et al., 2000). They thought that these changes contribute to the significant IOP reduction seen in the postoperative follow-up period of 12 months. Tran et al. evaluated the ultrasound biomicroscopic appearance of the anterior segment before and after cataract extraction in eyes with plateau iris syndrome. None of the six eyes with plateau iris syndrome in their study showed a change in the configuration of the ciliary body after IOL implantation. However, the anterior chamber depth increased and the angle opened further after cataract surgery. The persistent iridociliary apposition after cataract surgery suggests that the iris and pars plicata appear to move together (Tran et al., 2003). Nonaka et al. reported cataract surgery for angle closure including plateau configuration opened the angle concomitant with attenuation of the anterior positioning of the ciliary processes. Cataract surgery would contribute to postoperative widening of the angle not only by completely removing the lens

volume and pupillary block, but also by attenuating the anterior positioning of the ciliary processes in eyes with primary angle closed eyes (Nonaka et al., 2006). There are currently no randomized controlled trials supporting the use of clear lens extraction as the treatment of choice for PACG. However, the potential of obtaining some benefit from this procedure is considered to be biologically plausible (Thomas et al., 2011).
Phacoemulsification and goniosynechialysis (PEGS) is also effective in managing acute and subacute primary angle closure including patients plateau iris (Harasymowycz et al., 2005). Topical application of miotic agents, laser peripheral iridoplasty and cataract surgery seem to be effective for glaucoma with plateau iris configuration. There is a lack of well-designed, randomized, controlled trials to assess the effect as a therapeutic modality for glaucoma with plateau iris configuration, because the occurrence of plateau iris is relatively rare.

## 8. Conclusions

A plateau iris configuration is defined as a flat iris plane accompanied by a narrow or closed anterior chamber angle. Pathological and physiological data of plateau iris configuration and plateau iris syndrome are increasing. However, we do not have enough information related to plateau iris configuration and syndrome to manage them. The prognosis of this disorder compared to pupillary block angle closure glaucoma also remains to be elucidated. There are no quantitative diagnosis criteria, yet. This condition confuse the interpretation of the data appeared at the journals. The best therapeutic protocol should be established in future. New imaging technology will help us to obtain the new information.

## 9. References

Choi, JS. & Kim, YY. (2005). Progression of peripheral anterior synechiae after laser iridotomy., *American Journal of Ophthalmology*, Vol.140, No.6, (2005), pp.1125-1127

Congdon, N., Wang, F., & Tielsch, JM. (1992). Issues in the epidemiology and population-based screening of primary angle-closure glaucoma, *Survey of Ophthalmology*, Vol.36, No.11, (1992), pp.411-423

Crowston, JG., Medeiros, FA. Mosaed, S., & Weinreb, RN. (2005). Argon laser iridoplasty in the treatment of plateau-like iris configuration as result of numerous ciliary body cysts, *American Journal of Ophthalmology*, Vol.139, No.2, (2005), pp.381-383

Diniz Filho, A., Cronemberger, S., Ferreira, DM., Mérula, RV., & Calixto, N. (2010). Plateau iris configuration in eyes with narrow-angle: an ultrasound biomicroscopic study, *Arquivos brasileiros de oftalmologia*, Vol.73, No.2, (2010), pp.155-160

Etter, JR., Affel, EL., & Rhee, DJ. (2006). High prevalence of plateau iris configuration in family members of patients with plateau iris syndrome, *Journal of Glaucoma*, Vol.15, No.5 (2006), pp.394-398

Foster, PJ., Baasanhu, J., Alsbirk, PH., Munkhbayar, D., Uranchimeg, D., & Johnson, J. (1996). Glaucoma in Mongolia: a population-based survey in Hovsgol province, northern Mongolia, *Archives of Ophthalmology*, Vol.114, No.10, (1996), pp.1235-1241

Foster, PJ. & Johnson, GJ. (2001). Glaucoma in China: how big is the problem?, *British Journal of Ophthalmology*, Vol.85, No.11, (2001), pp.1277-1282

Geanon, JD. & Perkins, TW.(1995). Bilateral acute angle-closure glaucoma associated with drug sensitivity to hydrochlorothiazide, *Archives of Ophthalmology*, Vol.113, No.10, (1995), pp.1231-1232

Godel, V., Stein, R., & Feiler-Ofry, V. (1968). Angle-closure glaucoma: following peripheral iridectomy and mydriasis, *American Journal of Ophthalmology*, Vol.65, No.4, (1968), pp.555-560

Gradle, HS. & Sugar, HS. (1940). Concerning the chamber angle. III. A clinical method of goniometry, *American Journal of Ophthalmology*, Vol.23, (1940), pp.1135-1139

Harasymowycz, PJ., Papamatheakis, DG., Ahmed, I., Assalian, A., Lesk, M., Al-Zafiri, Y., Kranemann, C., & Hutnik, C. (2005). Phacoemulsification and goniosynechialysis in the management of unresponsive primary angle closure, *Journal of Glaucoma*, (2005), pp.186–189

Hayashi, K., Hayashi, H., Nakao, F., & Hayashi, F. (2000). Changes in anterior chamber angle width and depth after intraocular lens implantation in eyes with glaucoma, *Ophthalmology*, Vol.107, No.4, (2000), pp.698-703

Kiuchi, Y., Kanamoto, T., & Nakamura, T. (2009). Double hump sign in indentation gonioscopy is correlated with presence of plateau iris configuration regardless of patent iridotomy, *Journal of Glaucoma*, Vol.18, No.2, (2009), pp.161–164

Kumar, RS., Baskaran, M., Chew, PT., Friedman, DS., Handa, S., Lavanya, R., Sakata, LM., Wong, HT., & Aung ,T.(2008) . Prevalence of plateau iris in primary angle closure suspects an ultrasound biomicroscopy study, *Ophthalmology*, Vol.115, No.3, (2008), pp.430–434

Kumar, RS., Tantisevi, V., Wong, MH., Laohapojanart, K., Chansanti, O., Quek, DT., Koh, VT., MohanRam, LS., Lee, KY., Rojanapongpun, P., & Aung, T. (2009). Plateau iris in Asian subjects with primary angle closure glaucoma, *Archives of Ophthalmology*, Vol.127, No.10, (2009), pp.1269-1272

Kunimatsu, S., Araie, M., Ohara, K., & Hamada, C. (1999). Ultrasound biomicroscopy of ciliary body cysts, *American Journal of Ophthalmology*, Vol.127, No.1, (1999), pp.48–55

Lim, LS., Aung, T., Husain, R., Wu, YJ., Gazzard, G., & Seah, SK. (2004). Acute primary angle closure: configuration of the drainage angle in the first year after laser peripheral iridotomy, *Ophthalmology*, Vol.111, No.8, (2004), pp.1470–1474

Lowe, RF. (1964). Primary angle-closure glaucoma. Investigation after surgery for pupil block, *American Journal of Ophthalmology*, Vol.57, (1964), pp.931-938

Mandell, MA., Pavlin, CJ., Weisbrod, DJ., & Simpson, ER. (2003). Anterior Chamber Depth in Plateau Iris Syndrome and Pupillary Block as Measured by Ultrasound Biomicroscopy, *American Journal of Ophthalmology*, Vol.136, No.5, (2003), pp.900–903

Mochizuki, H., Takenaka, J., Sugimoto, Y., Takamatsu, M., & Kiuchi, Y. (2010). Comparison of the Prevalence of Plateau Iris Configurations Between Angle-closure Glaucoma and Open-angle Glaucoma Using Ultrasound Biomicroscopy, *Journal of Glaucoma*, (2010)

Németh, J., Csákány, B., & Pregun, T. (1996-1997). Ultrasound biomicroscopic morphometry of the anterior eye segment before and after one drop of pilocarpine, *International Ophthalmoogyl*, Vol.20, No.1-3,(1996-1997), pp.39-42

Nonaka, A., Kondo, T., Kikuchi, M., Yamashiro, K., Fujihara, M., Iwawaki ,T., Yamamoto, K., & Kurimoto, Y. (2006). Angle widening and alteration of ciliary process configuration after cataract surgery for primary angle closure. *Ophthalmology*, Vol.113, No.3, (2006), pp.437–441

Pavlin,CJ & Foster, FS.(1999). Plateau iris syndrome: changes in angle opening associated with dark, light, and pilocarpine administration, *American Journal of Ophthalmology*, Vol.128, No.3, (1999), pp.288-291

Pavlin, CJ., Ritch R., & Foster, FS. (1992). Ultrasound biomicroscopy in plateau iris syndrome, *American Journal of Ophthalmology*, Vol.113, No. 4, (1992), pp.390-395

Pavlin, CJ., Rutnin, SS., Deveny R., Wand, M. & Foster, FS.(1997). Supraciliary effusions and ciliary body thickening after scleral buckling procedures, *Ophthalmology*, Vol.104, No. 3, ( 1997), pp.433-438

Polikoff, LA., Chanis, RA., Toor, A., Ramos-Esteban, JC., Fahim, MM., Gagliuso, DJ., & Serle, JB. (2005). The effect of laser iridotomy on the anterior segment anatomy of patients with plateau iris configuration, *Journal of Glaucoma*, Vol.14, No.2, (2005), pp.109-113

Quigley, HA., Congdon, NG., & Friedman, DG. (2001). Glaucoma in China (and worldwide): changes in established thinkingwill decrease preventable blindness, *British Journal of Ophthalmology*; Vol.85, No.11, (2001), pp.1271-1272

Razeghinejad, MR. & Kamali-Sarvestani,E. (2007). The plateau iris component of primary angle closure glaucoma: developmental or acquired, *Medical Hypotheses*, Vol. 69, No.31, (2007), pp.95-98

Ritch, R. (1992). Plateau iris is caused by abnormally positioned ciliary processes, *Journal of Glaucoma*, Vol.1, (1992), pp.23-26

Ritch, R., Aung, T., & Lam, DS. (2009). Angle-closure Glaucoma, *Journal of Glaucoma*, Vol.18, No.7, (2009), pp.567-570

Ritch, R., Chang, BM., & Liebmann, JM. (2003). Angle closure in younger patients, *Ophthalmology*, Vol.110, No.10, (2003), pp.1880-1889

Ritch, R., Tham, CC., & Lam DS (2004). Long-term success of argon laser peripheral iridoplasty in the management of plateau iris syndrome, *Ophthalmology*, Vol.111, No.1, (2004), pp.104-108

Roberts, DK., Ayyagari, R., & Moroi, SE. (2008). Possible association between long anterior lens zonules and plateau iris configuration, *Journal of Glaucoma*, Vol.17, No.5, (2008), pp.393-396

Saitoh, S. (1974). Midriasis test in primary angle-closure glaucoma, *Nippon Ganka Gakkai Zasshi*, Vol.78, No.11, (1974), pp.1179-1185

Sakata, LM., Sakata, K.,& Susanna, R Jr. (2006). Long ciliary processes with no ciliary sulcus and appositional angle closure assessed by ultrasound biomicroscopy, *Journal of Glaucoma*, Vol. 15, No.5, (2006), pp.371-379

Shaffer, RN. (1960). Primary Glaucomas. Gonioscopy, ophthalmoscopy and perimetry, *Transactions - American Academy of Ophthalmology and Otolaryngology*, Vol.64, (1960), pp.112-127

Shukla, S., Damji, KF., Harasymowycz, P., Chialant, D., Kent, JS., Chevrier, R., Buhrmann, R., Marshall, D., Pan, Y., & Hodge, W. (2008). Clinical features distinguishing angle closure from pseudoplateau versus plateau iris, *British Journal of Ophthalmology*, Vol. 92, No.3, (2008), pp.340-344

Suzuki, Y., Yamamoto, T., Araie, M., Iwase, A., Tomidokoro, A., Abe, H., Shirato, S., Kuwayama, Y., Mishima, HK., Shimizu, H., Tomita, G., Inoue, Y., & Kitazawa, Y. (2008). Tajimi Study review, *Nippon Ganka Gakkai Zasshi*, Vol.112, No.12, (2008), pp.1039-1058

Tanihara, H., Akita, J., Honjo, M., & Honda, Y. (1997). Angle closure caused by multiple bilateral iridociliary cysts, *Acta ophthalmologica Scandinavica*, Vol. 75, No.2, (1997), pp.216–217

Tarongoy, P., Ho, CL., & Walton, DS. (2009). Angle-closure glaucoma: the role of the lens in the pathogenesis, prevention, and treatment, *Survey of Ophthalmology*, Vol.54, No. 2, (2009), pp.211--225

Tran, HV., Liebmann, JM., & Ritch, R. (2003). Iridociliary apposition in plateau iris syndrome persists after cataract extraction, *American Journal of Ophthalmology*, Vol.135, No.1, (2003), pp.40–43

Tripathi, RC., Tripathi, BJ., Haggerty C. (2003). Drug-induced glaucomas: mechanism and management, *Drug safety*, Vol. 26, No.11, (2003), pp.749–767

Wand, M., Grant, WM., Simmons, RJ., & Hutchinson, BT. (1977). Plateau iris syndrome, *Transactions. Section on Ophthalmology. American Academy of Ophthalmology and Otolaryngology*, Vol. 83, No. 1, (1977), pp.122-130

Yamamoto, T., Iwase, A., Araie, M., Suzuki, Y., Abe, H., & Shirato, S. (2005). The Tajimi Study report 2: prevalence of primary angle closure and secondary glaucoma in a Japanese population, *Ophthalmology*, Vol. 112, No.10,(2005), pp.1661–1669

Yasuda, N. & Kageyama, M. (1988). The long-term effects of local medication on intraocular pressure control in primary angle-closure glaucoma, *Nippon Ganka Gakkai Zasshi*, Vol.92, No.10, (1988), pp.1644-1649

# 27

# Normal-Tension (Low-Tension) Glaucoma

Tsvi Sheleg
*Department of Ophthalmology, Western Galilee – Nahariya Medical Center, Nahariya, Israel*

## 1. Introduction

Normal-tension glaucoma, also known as low-tension glaucoma, is defined as glaucomatous damage to the optic nerve and visual fields with normal diurnal values of intraocular pressure (IOP). The term 'low-tension glaucoma' is not often used because in most patients with normal-tension glaucoma, the IOP is within the higher range of normal values and rarely low. The diagnosis is insidious in many cases and requires a complete and thorough work-up to exclude other causes for optic disc and visual field abnormalities. The definition is problematic because the normal limits of IOP have a wide Gaussian curve range and their effect on the development of glaucoma varies. Some patients may retain a high IOP for many years without any glaucomatous damage, while others with low values of IOP may suffer from ongoing progressive glaucomatous disease. IOP is considered as a risk factor for the advancement of glaucoma even in patients with normal values of IOP, and lowering the IOP often protects the optic nerves (Collaborative Normal Tension Glaucoma Study Group [CNTGSG], 1998). Some optic nerves are more vulnerable even to low levels of IOP than others (Drance et al, 1973). Though many factors have been suspected and investigated, it appears that in addition to variability of the structure of the lamina cribrosa, vascular and genetic factors are most likely involved. Most authors consider normal-tension glaucoma to be a variant of primary open angle glaucoma (POAG) (Caprioli & Spaeth, 1984; Chumbley & Brubaker, 1976); others rely on characteristic clinical features of many normal-tension glaucoma patients to consider it a distinct entity (Caprioli & Spaeth, 1984; Shields, 2008). The debate is ongoing and will probably continue to be the subject of research for many years.

## 2. Pathogenic theories

The optic nerve damage in normal-tension glaucoma, as in POAG, follows a cascade of pathophysiological events that includes impaired axonal transport, ischemia and free radical formation that leads to apoptosis (Harris et al., 2005). The mechanical theory is based on the assumption that high IOP reduces the axoplasmic axonal flow by causing direct pressure on the axons, resulting in damage to the nerves. Structural differences in the appearance of the optic nerve discs and elastin fibers in glaucoma patients also support the mechanical theory (Dandona et al., 1990; Quigley et al., 1994). The pressure gradient over the optic disc should also be considered, as chronic low intra-cranial pressure may result in a pressure difference that can affect the axoplasmic outflow and lead to glaucomatous progression in normal-tension glaucoma patients.

On the other hand, the vascular ischemic theory suggests that low perfusion to the optic nerve is a major factor in the process of glaucomatous damage. This is supported by many articles that emphasize the importance of low ocular perfusion pressure and blood pressure in the development of POAG (Caprioli & Coleman, 2010). Blood supply to the optic nerve is derived through the ophthalmic artery mainly through the pial system and posterior ciliary arteries, but also from the central retinal artery. Several methods have been used to evaluate the blood flow and resistance of the ophthalmic artery and choroidal vessels, and their relationship with glaucomatous disease progression in POAG and in normal-tension glaucoma patients. Ultrasound Doppler has been used to show correlation between low blood flow and high resistance of the ophthalmic artery, to visual field progression in POAG patients (Galassi et al., 2003). Scanning laser ophthalmoscope demonstrated larger fluorescein filling defects, correlated with low blood flow in the central retinal artery and choroidal vessels of normal-tension glaucoma patients compared with controls (Plange et al., 2003). Heidelberg retinal flowmetry has detected a reduction in neuroretinal rim blood flow in conjunction with visual field defects in normal-tension glaucoma patients (Sato et al., 2006). The future of understanding the ischemic aspect in the development of glaucoma may be by optical measurement of retinal vessel oxygenation. Oxygenation of retinal arteries was found to be lower in normal-tension glaucoma patients than in healthy subjects (Michelson et al., 2006). Other factors influence the perfusion of the optic nerve and participate in the development and progression of the disease. Hypertension leads to a greater resistance in small blood vessels and causes atherosclerotic changes. Hypotension, especially in the presence of insufficient vascular autoregulation, may participate in the development of the ischemia (Goldberg et al., 1981). Circadian fluctuation of mean ocular perfusion pressure was found to be an important clinical risk factor for severity of glaucoma in eyes with normal-tension glaucoma (Choi et al., 2007). Nocturnal dips have also been evaluated and are thought to play a role in the development of normal-tension glaucoma (Bechetoille et al., 1995; Graham et al., 1995). Another observation that indirectly supports the vascular theory is that many normal-tension glaucoma patients suffer from vasospastic diseases such as migraine (Corbett et al., 1985; Phelps & Corbett, 1985) and Raynaud disease (Broadway & Drance, 1998). However, other studies found no difference in the prevalence of atherosclerotic vascular disease in NTG and POAG patients (Klein et al., 1993; Leighton & Phillips, 1972). The role of vascular disease in the pathogenesis of NTG is probably related to the reduction of optic nerve resistance to the IOP and this may precedes changes in vasculature that occur also in POAG. Many believe that both theories have a part in the pathogenesis and their importance in the advancement of the disease varies from patient to patient.

## 3. Epidemiology

Normal tension glaucoma has been found to be common in many population-based studies, though the numbers vary in different studies and populations. The main reasons for the variation are the difference in normal IOP range in different populations and the difficulty in making the diagnosis. Ruling out high-tension glaucoma by diurnal measurements was not performed in most of these studies. Other causes of "burned out" secondary glaucoma such as steroid-induced or uveitis-related glaucoma were not diagnosed and excluded in some studies. Large epidemiological studies in North America, Europe and Australia estimated the prevalence of normal-tension glaucoma to be up to half that of POAG (Leibowitz et al., 1980; Sommer et al., 1991). The Beaver Dam Eye Study estimated the prevalence of normal-tension glaucoma to be up to 1.6% in patients over 75 years of age

(Klein et al., 1992). In Japan the prevalence is considerably higher. The Tajimi eye study assessed the prevalence of POAG in patients over 40 years and found it to be 3.9%, in 92% the IOP was 21 mmHg or lower (Iwase et al., 2004). A nationwide survey estimated the normal-tension glaucoma with (IOP under 21mmHg) prevalence to be 3.5 times that of POAG, but these numbers are thought to be biased since normal IOP in Japan is lower than in the western population, averaging 10-18 mmHg. The prevalence of normal tension glaucoma is higher in women than in men, this and other risk factors will be discussed later in this chapter. Whatever the prevalence of normal tension glaucoma is in various populations, it is obvious that the numbers are higher than once assumed, and patients are actually diagnosed only when optic disc and visual field abnormalities are already present.

## 4. Genetic considerations

Family history is a major risk factor in glaucoma ,and genetic mutations related to specific phenotypes of glaucoma are under investigation. Such information can help diagnose and classify subtypes of glaucoma, and perhaps even to clarify the pathogenesis. Research may find ways to repair mutation in utero or early in life, before glaucomatous damage has occurred. Genetic research has found transmission of a NTG phenotype in only a few families, all of them are autosomal dominant (Bennett et al., 1989). Of the seven gene loci that have been linked to POAG, two genes have been identified and named TIGR/ Myocilin and Optineurin (Optic Neuropathy-Inducing Protein - ONTP). A specific mutation GLC1E locus of the ONTP was found in location 10p14-15, with autosomal dominant inheritance as in all POAG locui that were identified (Sarfarazi et al., 1998). ONTP is expressed in the retina and was found to be involved in apoptosis. The Blue Mountains Eye Study in Australia found that the prevalence of mutation in the ONTP gene was higher in POAG than in healthy subjects but the difference was not statistically significant (Baird et al., 2004). Reports found the ONTP mutation associated with high prevalence of POAG and NTG in adult Japanese patients, suggesting it may be involved in the pathogenesis of both entities (Fuse et al., 2004; Umeda et al., 2004). Other reports could not find OPTN mutations in NTG (Toda et al., 2004). Genetic screening for the gene is not an option because of the low incidence of the mutation. Recently another locus GLCA3 was investigated for association with NTG, but no statistically significant relationship was found (Kamio et al., 2009).

## 5. Diagnosis and differential diagnosis

The diagnosis of normal-tension glaucoma is illusive and requires a high degree of suspicion. Since IOP measurements are usually in the high teens in normal-tension glaucoma, routine IOP screening measurement may be deceiving. Often, the first sign is an abnormal optic disc or disk asymmetry suspicious of glaucomatous damage. In up to half of the patients repeated measurements or daily IOP curve discovers high IOP, and the diagnosis of POAG is made (Ito et al., 1991; Perkins, 1973). The significance of a daily IOP curve in the diagnosis of NTG is crucial. Few other factors must be considered. Pachymetry should be performed to adjust the difference between measured IOP by Goldman tonometry and true IOP. Ocular hypertension study (OHTS) highlighted the importance of thin corneas in the diagnosis of glaucoma. Thinner corneas can lead to underestimation of IOP, and misdiagnosis has occurred in many NTG patients compared with POAG patients (Morad et al., 1998). The effect of corneal hysteresis and scleral rigidity should be considered and Ocular Response Analyzer (ORA) can help in estimating the true IOP (Morita et al.,

2010). Thin corneas following corneal refractive surgery and in patients after penetrating or lamellar keratoplasty can make the task of IOP estimation more challenging (Papastergiou et al., 2010; Sanchez-Naves et al., 2008). Other factors such as refraction and astigmatism should also be considered and ORA may achieve a better estimation of the true IOP in these patients (Hagishima et al., 2010).

The controversy of whether NTG is different from POAG is demonstrated in many articles regarding optic disc appearance. While some studies show no difference in the optic disc appearance between NTG and POAG (Tomita, 2000), others found distinct characteristics such as thin rim that can help distinguish NTG (Caprioli & Spaeth, 1985). OCT plays a major role in the diagnosis and monitoring of glaucoma especially when the diagnosis is not certain. Measuring the RNFL thickness, optic disk cupping and their correlation with visual field abnormalities is a powerful tool. Recently a study comparing the optic discs using optical coherence tomography (OCT) and Heidelberg retina topography (HRT) supports some of the differences (Shin et al., 2008). Disc appearance in NTG is traditionally divided into two sub-groups. The more common is the senile sclerotic group, which is characterized by a pale shallow sloping neuroretinal rim. These patients are often older in age and suffer from vascular diseases. The other group, focal ischemic, is characterized by deep focal notching of the rim. Splinter hemorrhages are a typical finding in NTG and imply in most cases a progressive disease (Drance et al., 2001; Jonas & Xu, 1994). Beta zone peripapillary atrophy has also been suggested related to optic nerve damage in NTG (Xia et al., 2005). The site of the hemorrhage may predict an area of notch development with a correlated visual field loss (Chumbley & Brubaker, 1976; Siegner & Netland, 1996; Tomita, 2000). Visual field patterns in NTG are similar to the ones seen in POAG, still some articles found differences in the distribution and shape of the scotomas. Scotomas observed in NTG visual fields often tend to be deeper, steeper and closer to fixation than in POAG patients (Caprioli & Spaeth, 1984; Harrington, 1960). Some articles mainly from japan found that scotomas in NTG may be more predominant in the lower hemifield (Araie, 1995).

The ophthalmologist should rule out "burned out" secondary glaucoma and other misleading diagnosis. Careful history and meticulous ophthalmic examination should look for previous trauma, uveitis, glaucomatocyclitic crisis, pigmentary glaucoma, previous topical or systemic steroid treatment, previous acute angle closure attack and the use of systemic medication that lowers IOP (e.g., beta-blockers). Compliance should be appreciated to rule out the possibility that the patient takes his anti-glaucoma medications only before the ophthalmologist examination in order to "please" their doctor. Non-glaucomatous optic disc abnormalities such as congenital colobomas, optic nerve pit, anterior ischemic optic neuropathy, traumatic optic neuropathy, optic nerve or chiasm compressing lesion, and various retinal abnormalities should be considered and revoked. The diagnosis and follow-up of NTG is more challenging with hypoplastic and myopic tilted discs. Systemic evaluation is advised to identify diseases that are more frequent in NTG patients, and when the diagnosis is difficult. Blood pressure, ischemic vascular disease, perfusion pressure, vasospastic disorders (migraine, Raynaud phenomenon) and obstructive sleep apnea should be assessed in selected cases. Some cases may require neurological evaluation and hematological work-up to search for various neurological conditions or coagulopathies. Generally, systemic evaluation is reserved for atypical cases when the optic disc appearance and visual field do not correlate with glaucomatous damage, when glaucomatous damage is found with IOP lower than the high teens before treatment or when other neurological symptoms are present. Neurological examination is vital in all cases of NTG with atypical clinical manifestation. Lesions such as meningiomas, craniopharingiomas, pituitary adenomas, and compressive vascular lesions such as aneurisms can mimic NTG. Some ophthalmic signs are more suggestive of a neurological disease and should prompt a neurological evaluation. Perhaps the most important of them is a rapid progression of the disease despite low IOP with or without treatment. Other signs that should raise suspicion are pale optic disks and poor best corrected visual acuity. Needless to say any neurologic symptoms prompt neurologic workup. Some authors believe that it is important in all cases of NTG to perform a CT scan (Gutman et al., 1993), though others found no value for a routine neurological examination in NTG patients (Kesler et al., 2010).

Risk factors for the development of NTG in untreated patients that were found in the Collaborative Normal Tension Glaucoma Study (CNTGS) are migraine, female gender and splinter disc hemorrhage at the diagnosis (Drance et al., 2001). Age over 60 years is common (Klein et al., 1992), and a high prevalence was found in Japanese as mentioned earlier (Iwase et al., 2004; Shiose et al., 1991). Other risk factors found to be more prevalent in NTG than in POAG patients were ischemic vascular disease, obstructive sleep apnea, autoimmune diseases, and coagulopathies, but their effect on development of NTG was not consistent.

The progression of glaucomatous damage in NTG is usually very slow. Collaborative Normal Tension Glaucoma Study (CNTGS) showed that half of the untreated patients did not progress in 5 years, and in most cases the progression was slow (Anderson, 2003). In some of these patients a previous hypotensive crisis from a massive bleeding or arrhythmia resulted in optic disk cupping. (Drance, 1977). In patients without a subsequent hypotensive crisis the glaucoma is not expected to progress. Other cases such as steroid responders or "burned out" pigmentary or uveitic glaucoma may not progress at all. Despite their effect as risk factors for the development of NTG, neither age nor untreated level of IOP affected the risk for progression in untreated eyes (Anderson, 2003). Disc hemorrhages, as mentioned earlier, where also found to be related to the progression of glaucomatous damage (Ishida et al., 2000).

## 6. Practical steps for diagnosis

It is difficult to diagnose NTG if the cup to disc ratio is over 0.5 even if the differences in cupping are 0.2 or higher in the presence of normal IOP. At this stage, the visual fields are usually normal. If the cornea is thin, POAG may be suspected after correction of the IOP according to the corneal thickness. But if the corneal thickness is normal, the diagnosis of NTG cannot be established. Those patients may stay with the diagnosis of glaucoma suspects until new signs of disk abnormalities appear that correlate with the glaucomatous visual field defects. Although these patients may deteriorate slowly, other glaucoma patients may deteriorate rather quickly. Therefore, it is recommended to follow individuals over the age of 40, glaucoma suspects and individuals with family history, at least every 6 months. There have been cases were glaucoma appeared and progressed within less than a year, and this is the reason for a 6 months routine follow-up. Preperimetric normal tension glaucoma should be evaluated using FDT or Swap when available.

The diagnosis is made when optic disc cupping and glaucomatous visual field defects are found in conjunction with normal IOP. POAG should be ruled out by corneal pachymetry and adjustment of the IOP to the corneal thickness. Other causes for optic disc cupping and visual field defects should be ruled out by detailed anamnesis (e.g., episodes of major blood loss) and further analysis (e.g., brain computed tomography to rule out tumors as mentioned earlier).

## 7. Treatment

The decision to treat a patient suspected with NTG must include the patient's age and all aspects of the disease, its extent, pathogenic factors and especially the rate of progression. If the patient's disease seems not to be progressive, monitoring of the disease is advised. When the disease is bilateral and not severe, treatment in one eye may be suitable. Careful follow-up and comparison of both eyes for progression is essential. Some patients suffer from visual field loss and disc damage and require prompt therapy. As in POAG, it is customary to begin with medical therapy, but laser and even surgical treatment should be considered for advanced cases. The target IOP was recommended to be 30% reduction by CNTGS and this reduces the progression from 35% in untreated patients to 12% in the treated group. Approximately two-thirds of the patients that did not receive any therapy did not progress (Drance et al., 2001). Target IOP was reached with medication and laser trabeculoplasty in half of CNTGS patients. This was achieved without beta-blockers or prostaglandin analogs. Currently the available drugs are thought to produce better effects on lowering the IOP, better compliance and better results in preventing disease progression. Still some patients continue to deteriorate after proper IOP reduction.

Some drops especially brimonidine were found to have neuroprotective effects in animal models (Vidal et al., 2010; Wolde Mussie et al., 2001). The research to achieve better control of glaucoma using a mechanism other than lowering IOP is promising. Unfortunately, neuroprotection by preventing the death of retinal ganglion cells, and vision preservation have not yet been proven in humans (Saylor et al., 2009). Long-term follow-up should determine whether or not neuroprotective agents may be beneficial for glaucoma patients (Sena et al., 2010). A low-tension glaucoma study LoGTS is currently underway comparing timolol and brimonidine treatment in NTG patients. The authors believe the neuroprotective effect of brimonidine will provide better results in preventing the disease progression. Dorzolamide, betaxolol, and latanaprost were considered to increase blood flow around the optic nerve (Harris et al., 1996, 2000), but newer published studies suggest that the effect, if exists at all, is minor (Bergstrand et al., 2002; Harris et al., 2003). Calcium channel blockers treatment was proved to be beneficial (Koseki et al., 2008; Netland et al., 1993). The treatment is recommended especially if a vasospastic disorder is diagnosed. Systemic side effects of calcium channel blockers such as flushing, edema, hypotension, headaches and reflex tachycardia requires careful selection of patients for this therapy.

In patients with low compliance or troubling side effects, laser treatment should be considered. Selective laser trabeculoplasty has promising results on lowering IOP and is considered a safe and reproducible treatment for NTG (El Mallah et al., 2010; Realini, 2008). Argon laser trabeculoplasty was studied as treatment for normal-tension glaucoma patients. The results varied from little to no effect (Schulzer, 1992; Sharpe & Simmons, 1985). SLT is considered a safe and effective treatment for lowering IOP, especially in noncompliant patient and in patients with severe side effects from topical or systemic drug treatment.

Trabeculectomy was found to lower IOP and slow the progression after long term follow-up (Bhandari et al., 1997; Shigeeda et al., 2002). Both medical and surgical treatments increase the risk for cataract formation. Cataract development was more frequent in patients undergoing trabeculectomy than in patients receiving only medical treatment (Drance et al., 2001). Follow-up and cataract extraction is advisable to improve visual acuity and follow-up reliability. Finally any systemic disease that can affect optic nerve perfusion such as systemic hypertension, congestive heart failure, arrhythmia and anemia, should be treated (Chumbley & Brubaker, 1976).

## 8. References

Anderson, D.R. Normal Tension Glaucoma Study. (2003). Collaborative Normal Tension Glaucoma Study. *Current Opinion in Ophthalmology*, Vol.14, No.2, pp. 86-90

Araie, M. (1995). Pattern of Visual Field Defects in Normal-Tension and High-Tension Glaucoma. *Current Opinion in Ophthalmology*, Vol.6, No.2, pp. 36-45

Baird, P.N., Richardson, A.J., Craig, J.E., Mackey, D.A., Rochtchina, E., & Mitchell, P. (2004). Analysis of Optineurin (OPTN) Gene Mutations in Subjects With and Without Glaucoma: The Blue Mountains Eye Study. *Clinical and Experimental Ophthalmology*, Vol.32, No.5, pp. 518-522

Bechetoille, A. & Bresson-Dumont, H. (1994). Diurnal and Nocturnal Blood Pressure Drops in Patients with Focal Ischemic Glaucoma. *Graefes' Archive for Clinical and Experimental Ophthalmology*, Vol. 232, No. 11, pp. 675-679

Bennett, S.R., Alward, W.L., & Folberg, R. (1989). An Autosomal Dominant Form of Low Tension Glaucoma. *American Journal of Ophthalmology*, Vol.108, pp. 238–244

Bergstrand, I.C., Heijl, A., & Harris, A. (2002). Dorzolamide and Ocular Blood Flow in Previously Untreated Glaucoma Patients: A Controlled Double-Masked Study. *Acta Ophthalmologica Scandinavica*, Vol.80, No.2, pp. 176-182

Bhandari, A., Crabb, D.P., Poinoosawmy, D., Fitzke, F.W., Hitchings, R.A., & Noureddin, B.N. (1997). Effect of Surgery on Visual Field Progression in Normal-Tension Glaucoma. *Ophthalmology*, Vol.104, No.7, pp. 1131-1137

Broadway, D.C. & Drance, S.M. (1998). Glaucoma and Vasospasm. *British Journal of Ophthalmology*, Vol.82, No.8, pp. 862-870

Caprioli, J. & Spaeth, G.L. (1984). Comparison of Visual Field Defects in the Low-Tension Glaucomas with Those in the High-Tension Glaucomas. *American Journal of Ophthalmology*, Vol.97, No.6, pp. 730-737

Caprioli, J. & Spaeth, G.L. (1985). Comparison of the Optic Nerve Head in High- and Low-Tension Glaucoma. *Archives of Ophthalmology*, Vol.103, No.8, pp. 1145-1149

Caprioli, J. & Coleman, A.L. (2010). Blood Pressure, Perfusion Pressure, and Glaucoma. *American Journal of Ophthalmology*, Vol.149, No.5, pp.704-712

Choi J, Kim, K.H., Jeong, J., Cho, H.S., Lee, C.H., & Kook, M.S. (2007). Circadian Fluctuation of Mean Ocular Perfusion Pressure is a Consistent Risk Factor for Normal-Tension Glaucoma. *Investigative Ophthalmology & Visual Science*, Vol.48, pp. 104-111

Chumbley, L.C. & Brubaker, R.F. (1976). Low-Tension Glaucoma. *American Journal of Ophthalmology*, Vol.81, No.6, pp. 761-767

Collaborative Normal Tension Glaucoma Study Group. (1998). The Effectiveness of Intraocular Pressure Reduction in the Treatment of Normal Tension Glaucoma. *American Journal of Ophthalmology*, Vol.126, pp. 498-505

Corbett, J.J., Phelps, C.D., Eslinger, P., & Montague, P.R. (1985). The Neurologic Evaluation of Patients with Low-Tension Glaucoma. *Investigative Ophthalmology & Visual Sciences*, Vol. 26, No.8, pp. 1101-1104

Dandona, L., Quigley, H.A., Brown, A.E., & Enger, C. (1990). Quantitative Regional Structure of the Normal Human Lamina Cribrosa. A Racial Comparison. *Archives of Ophthalmology*, Vol.108, pp. 393-398

Drance, S.M., Sweeney, V.P., Morgan, R.W., & Feldman, F. (1973). Studies of Factors Involved in the Production of Low Tension Glaucoma. *Archives of Ophthalmology*, Vol. 89, No.6, pp. 457-465

Drance, S.M. (1977). The Visual Field of Low Tension Glaucoma and Shock-Induced Optic Neuropathy. *Archives of Ophthalmology*, Vol. 95, No. 8, pp. 1359-1361

Drance, S., Anderson, D.R., & Schulzer, M. Collaborative Normal-Tension Glaucoma Study Group. (2001). Risk Factors for Progression of Visual Field Abnormalities in Normal-Tension Glaucoma. *American Journal of Ophthalmology*, Vol.131, No.6, pp. 699-708

El Mallah, M.K., Walsh, M.M., Stinnett, S.S., & Asrani, S.G. (2010). Selective Laser Trabeculoplasty Reduces Mean IOP and IOP Variation in Normal Tension Glaucoma Patients. *Clinical Ophthalmology*, Vol. 4, pp. 889-893

Fuse, N., Takahashi, K., Akiyama, H., Nakazawa, T., Seimiya, M., Kuwahara, S., & Tamai, M. (2004). Molecular Genetic Analysis of Optineurin Gene for Primary Open-Angle and Normal Tension Glaucoma in the Japanese Population. *Journal of Glaucoma*, Vol. 13, No. 4, pp. 299-303

Galassi, F., Sodi, A., Ucci, F., Renieri, G., Pieri, B., & Baccini, M. (2003). Ocular Hemodynamic and Glaucoma Prognosis. A Color Doppler Imaging Study. *Archives in Ophthalmology*, Vol. 121, No. 12, pp. 1711-1715

Goldberg, I., Hollows, F.C., Kass, M.A., & Becker, B. (1981). Systemic Factors in Patients with Low Tension Glaucoma. *British Journal of Ophthalmology*, Vol. 65, No. 1, pp. 56-62

Graham, S.L., Drance, S.M., Wijsman, K., Douglas, G.R., & Mikelberg, F.S. (1995). Ambulatory Blood Pressure Monitoring in Glaucoma. The Nocturnal Dip. *Ophthalmology*, Vol.102, No.1, pp.61-69

Gutman I, Melamed S, Ashkenazi I, Blumenthal M. Optic nerve compression by carotid arteries in low-tension glaucoma. *Graefes Arch Clin Exp Ophthalmol*. 1993 Dec; 231(12):711-7.

Hagishima, M., Kamiya, K., Fujimura, F., Morita, T., Shoji, N., & Shimizu, K. (2010). Effect of Corneal Astigmatism on Intraocular Pressure Measurement Using Ocular Response Analyzer and Goldmann Applanation Tonometer. *Graefes Archive in Clinical and Experimental Ophthalmology*, Vol. 248, No. 2, pp. 257-262

Harrington, D.O. (1960). Pathogenesis of the Glaucomatous Visual Field Defects: Individual Variations in Pressure Sensitivity, In: Newell FW, editor: *Conference on Glaucoma. Transactions of the Fifth Josiah Macy Conference*, F.W. Newell, (ed.), Josiah Macy Foundation, New York

Harris, A., Arend, O., Arend, S., & Martin, B. (1996). Effects of Topical Dorzolamide on Retinal and Retrobulbar Hemodynamics. *Acta Ophthalmologica Scandinavica*, Vol. 74, No. 6, pp. 569-572

Harris, A., Arend, O., Chung, H.S., Kagemann, L., Cantor, L., & Martin, B. (2000). A Comparative Study of Betaxolol and Dorzolamide Effect on Ocular Circulation in Normal-Tension Glaucoma Patients. , *Ophthalmology*, 2000, Vol. 107, No. 3, pp. 430-434

Harris, A., Migliardi, R., Rechtman, E., Cole, C.N., Yee, A.B., & Garzozi, H.J. (2003). Comparative Analysis of the Effects of Dorzolamide and Latanoprost on Ocular Hemodynamics in Normal Tension Glaucoma Patients. *European Journal of Ophthalmology*, Vol. 13, No. 1, pp. 24-31

Harris, A., Rechtman, E., Siesky, B., Jonescu-Cuypers, C., McCranor, L., & Garzozi, H.J. (2005). The Role of Optic Nerve Blood Flow in Pathogenesis of Glaucoma. *Ophthalmology Clinics of North America*, Vol. 18, No. 3, pp. 345-353

Ishida, K., Yamamoto, T., Sugiyama, K., & Kitazawa, Y. (2000). Disk Hemorrhage is a Significantly Negative Prognostic Factor in Normal-Tension Glaucoma. *American Journal of Ophthalmology*, Vol. 129, No. 6, pp. 707-714

Ito, M., Sugiura, T., & Mizokami, K. (1991). A Comparative Study on Visual Field Defect in Low-Tension Glaucoma. *Nippon Ganka Gakkai Zasshi*, Vol. 95, pp. 790-794

Iwase, A., Suzuki, Y., Araie, M., Yamamoto, T., Abe, H., Shirato, S., Kuwayama, Y., Mishima, H.K., Shimizu, H., Tomita, G., Inoue, Y., & Kitazawa, Y. Tajimi Study Group, Japan Glaucoma Society. (2004). The Prevalence of Primary Open Angle Glaucoma in Japanese: The Tajimi Study. *Ophthalmology*, Vol. 111, No. 9, pp. 1641-1648

Jonas, J.B. & Xu, L. (1994). Optic Disk Hemorrhages in Glaucoma. *American Journal of Ophthalmology*, Vol. 118, pp. 1-8

Kamio, M., Meguro, A., Ota, M., Nomura, N., Kashiwagi, K., Mabuchi, F., Iijima, H., Kawase, K., Yamamoto, T., Nakamura, M., Negi, A., Sagara, T., Nishida, T., Inatani, M., Tanihara, H., Aihara, M., Araie, M., Fukuchi, T., Abe, H., Higashide, T., Sugiyama, K., Kanamoto, T., Kiuchi, Y., Iwase, A., Ohno, S., Inoko, H., & Mizuki, N. (2009). Investigation of the Association Between the GLC3A Locus and Normal Tension Glaucoma in Japanese Patients by Microsatellite Analysis. *Clinical Ophthalmology*, Vol.3, pp. 183-188

Kesler, A., Haber, I., & Kurtz, S. (2010). Neurologic Evaluations in Normal-Tension Glaucoma Workups: Are They Worth the Effort? *Israel Medical Association Journal*, Vol. 12, No. 5, pp. 287-289

Klein, B., Klein, R., Sponsel, W.E., Franke, T., Cantor, L.B., Martone, J., & Menage, M.J. (1992). Prevalence of Glaucoma: The Beaver Dam Eye Study. *Ophthalmology*, Vol. 99, No. 10, pp. 1499–1504

Klein, B.E., Klein, R., Meuer, S.M., & Goetz, L.A. (1993). Migraine Headache and Its Association with Open-Angle Glaucoma. The Beaver Dam Eye Study. *Investigative Ophthalmology and Visual Sciences*, Vol. 34, No. 10, pp. 3024-3027

Koseki, N., Araie, M., Tomidokoro, A., Nagahara, M., Hasegawa, T., Tamaki, Y., & Yamamoto, S. (2008). A Placebo-Controlled 3-year Study of a Calcium Blocker on Visual Field and ocular Circulation in Glaucoma with Low-Normal Pressure. *Ophthalmology*, Vol. 115, No. 11, pp. 2049-2057

Leighton, D.A. & Phillips, C.I. (1972). Systemic Blood Pressure in Open-Angle Glaucoma, Low Tension Glaucoma and the Normal Eye, *British Journal of Ophthalmology*, Vol. 56, pp. 447-53

Leibowitz, H.M., Krueger, D.E., Maunder, L.R., Milton, R.C., Kini, M.M., Kahn, H.A., Nickerson, R.J., Pool, J., Colton, T.L., Ganley, J.P., Loewenstein, J.I., & Dawber, T.R. (1980). The Framingham Eye Study Monograph: An Ophthalmological and

Epidemiological Study of Cataract, Glaucoma, Diabetic Retinopathy, Macular Degeneration, and Visual Acuity in a General Population of 2631 Adults, 1973-1975. *Survey of Ophthalmology*, Vol. 24 (Suppl), pp. 335-610

Michelson, G. & Scibor, M. (2006). Intravascular Oxygen Saturation in Retinal Vessels in Normal Subjects and Open-Angle Glaucoma Subjects. *Acta Ophthalmologica Scandinavica*, Vol. 84, No. 3, pp. 289-295

Morad, Y., Sharon, E., Hefetz, L., & Nemet, P. (1998). Corneal Thickness and Curvature in normal-Tension Glaucoma. *American Journal of Ophthalmology*, Vol. 125, No. 2, pp. 164-168

Morita, T., Shoji, N., Kamiya, K., Hagishima, M., Fujimura, F., & Shimizu, K. (2010). Intraocular Pressure Measured by Dynamic Contour Tonometer and Ocular Response Analyzer in Normal Tension Glaucoma. *Graefes Archive of Clinical and Experimental Ophthalmology*, Vol. 248, No. 1, pp. 73-77.

Netland, P.A., Chaturvedi, N., & Dreyer, E.B. (1993). Calcium Channel Blockers in the Management of Low-Tension and Open-Angle Glaucoma. *American Journal of Ophthalmology*, Vol. 115, No. 5, pp. 608-613

Papastergiou, G.I., Kozobolis, V., & Siganos, D.S. (2010). Effect of Recipient Corneal Pathology on Pascal Tonometer and Goldmann Tonometer Readings in Eyes after Penetrating Keratoplasty. *European Journal of Ophthalmology*, Vol. 20, No. 1, pp. 29-34

Perkins, E.S. (1973). The Bedford Glaucoma Survey. I. Longterm Followup of Borderline Cases. *British Journal of Ophthalmology*, Vol. 57, No. 3, pp. 179-185

Phelps, C.D. & Corbett, J.J. (1985). Migraine and Low-Tension Glaucoma. A Case-Control Study. *Investigative Ophthalmology and Visual Sciences*, Vol. 26, No. 8, pp. 1105-1108

Plange, N., Remky, A., & Arend, O. (2003). Colour Doppler Imaging and Fluorescein Filling Defects of the Optic Disc in Normal Tension Glaucoma. *British Journal of Ophthalmology*, Vol. 87, No. 6, pp. 731-736.

Quigley, H., Pease, M.E., & Thibault, D. (1994). Change in the Appearance of Elastin in the Lamina Cribrosa of Glaucomatous Optic Nerve Heads. *Graefes Archive of Clinical and Experimental Ophthalmology*, Vol. 232, pp. 257-261

Realini, T. (2008). Selective Laser Trabeculoplasty: A Review. *Journal of Glaucoma*, Vol. 17, No. 6, pp. 497-502.

Sánchez-Navés, J., Furfaro, L., Piro, O., & Balle, S. (2008). Impact and Permanence of LASIK-Induced Structural Changes in the Cornea on Pneumotonometric Measurements: Contributions of Flap Cutting and Stromal Ablation. *Journal of Glaucoma*, Vol. 17, No. 8, pp. 611-618

Sarfarazi, M., Child, A., Stoilova, D., Brice, G., Desai, T., Trifan, O.C., Poinoosawmy, D., & Crick, R.P. (1998). Localization of the Fourth Locus (GLC1E) for Adult-Onset Primary Open-Angle Glaucoma to the 10p15-p14 Region. *American Journal of Human Genetics*, Vol. 62, No. 3, pp. 641-652

Sato, E.A., Ohtake, Y., Shinoda, K., Mashima, Y., & Kimura, I. (2006). Decreased Blood Flow at Neuroretinal Rim of Optic Nerve Head Corresponds with Visual Field Deficit in Eyes with Normal Tension Glaucoma. *Graefes Archive of Clinical and Experimental Ophthalmology*, Vol. 244, No. 7, pp. 795-801

Saylor, M., McLoon, L.K., Harrison, A.R., & Lee, M.S. (2009). Experimental and Clinical Evidence for Brimonidine as an Optic Nerve and Retinal Neuroprotective Agent: An Evidence-Based Review. *Archives of Ophthalmology,* Vol. 127, No. 4, pp. 402-406

Schulzer, M. (1992). The Normal-Tension Glaucoma Study Group: Intraocular Pressure Reduction in Normal-Tension Glaucoma Patients. *Ophthalmology,* Vol. 99, pp. 1468-1470

Sena, D.F., Ramchand, K., & Lindsley, K. (2010). Neuroprotection for Treatment of Glaucoma in Adults. *Cochrane Database of Systematic Reviews,* Vol. 17, CD006539

Shields, M.B. (2008). Normal-Tension Glaucoma: Is It Different From Primary Open-Angle Glaucoma? *Current Opinion in Ophthalmology,* Vol. 19, No. 2, p. 85-88

Sharpe, E.D. & Simmons, R.J. (1985). Argon Laser Trabeculoplasty as a Means of Decreasing Intraocular Pressure from "Normal" Levels in Glaucomatous Eyes. *American Journal of Ophthalmology,* Vol. 99, No. 6, pp. 704-707

Shigeeda, T., Tomidokoro, A., Araie, M., Koseki, N., & Yamamoto, S. (2002). Long-Term Follow-Up of Visual Field Progression After Trabeculectomy in Progressive Normal-Tension Glaucoma. *Ophthalmology,* Vol. 109, No. 4, pp. 766-770

Shin, I.H., Kang, S.Y., Hong, S., Kim, S.K., Seong, G.J., Tak, M.K., & Kim, C.Y. (2008). Comparison of OCT and HRT Findings Among Normal, Normal Tension Glaucoma, and High Tension Glaucoma. *Korean Journal of Ophthalmology,* Vol. 22, No. 4, pp. 236-241

Shiose, Y., Kitazawa, Y., Tsukahara, S., Akamatsu, T., Mizokami, K., Futa, R., Katsushima, H., & Kosaki, H. (1991). Epidemiology of Glaucoma in Japan: A Nationwide Glaucoma Survey, *Japan Journal of Ophthalmology,* Vol. 35, No. 2, pp. 133-155

Siegner, S.W. & Netland, P.A. (1996). Optic Disc Hemorrhages and Progression of Glaucoma. *Ophthalmology,* Vol. 103, No. 7, pp. 1014-1024

Sommer, A., Tielsch, J.M., Katz, J., Quigley, H.A., Gottsch, J.D., Javitt, J., & Singh, K. (1991). Relationship Between Intraocular Pressure and Primary Open Angle Glaucoma among White and Black Americans. The Baltimore Eye Survey. *Archives of Ophthalmology,* Vol. 109, No. 8, pp. 1090-1095

Toda, Y., Tang, S., Kashiwagi, K., Mabuchi, F., Iijima, H., Tsukahara, S., & Yamagata, Z. (2004). Mutations in the Optineurin Gene in Japanese Patients with Primary Open-Angle Glaucoma and Normal Tension Glaucoma. *American Journal of Medical Genetics A,* Vol. 125, No. 1, pp. 1-4

Tomita, G. (2000). The Optic Nerve Head in Normal-Tension Glaucoma. *Current Opinion in Ophthalmology,* Vol. 11, No. 2, pp. 116-120

Umeda, T., Matsuo, T., Nagayama, M., Tamura, N., Tanabe, Y., & Ohtsuki, H. (2004). Clinical Relevance of Optineurin Sequence Alterations in Japanese Glaucoma Patients. *Ophthalmic Genetics,* Vol. 25, pp.:91

Vidal, L., Díaz, F., Villena, A., Moreno, M., Campos, J.G., & Pérez de Vargas, I. (2010). Reaction of Müller Cells in an Experimental Rat Model of Increased Intraocular Pressure Following Timolol, Latanoprost and Brimonidine. *Brain Research Bulletin,* Vol. 82, No. 1-2, pp. 18-24

WoldeMussie, E., Ruiz, G., Wijono, M., & Wheeler, L.A. (2001). Neuroprotection of Retinal Ganglion Cells by Brimonidine in Rats with Laser-Induced Chronic Ocular

Hypertension. *Investigative Ophthalmology and Visual Sciences*, Vol. 42, No. 12, pp. 2849-2855

Xia, C.R., Xu, L., & Yang, Y. (2005). A Comparative Study of Optic Nerve Damage Between Primary Open Angle Glaucoma and Normal Tension Glaucoma. *Zhonghua Yan Ke Za Zhi*, Vol. 41, No. 2, pp. 136-140

# 28

# Drug-Induced Glaucoma (Glaucoma Secondary to Systemic Medications)

Eitan Z. Rath
*Department of Ophthalmology, Western Galilee – Nahariya Medical Center, Israel*

## 1. Introduction

Glaucoma comprises a group of diseases that have in common a characteristic optic nerve and visual field damage and elevated intraocular pressure (IOP) is the main risk factor. The IOP depends on the balance between the formation and drainage of aqueous humor. The glaucoma can be classified into four main groups: open-angle (OAG), acute angle-closure (ACG), secondary and developmental glaucoma. The first two refer to the pathophysiology of the disease.

Drug-induced glaucoma is a form of secondary glaucoma induced by topical and systemic medications. The most common one is glucorticoid OAG. Several drugs like antidepressants, anticoagulants, adrenergic antagonists, sulpha -based drugs and antiepileptic dugs have been reported to produce an acute ACG and especially in those with predisposed angle closure.

Bilateral simultaneous ACG is extremely a rare entity. Drug-induced uveal effusion causing secondary ACG have been reported[1-9] involving medications such as topiramate,[2,4,6,9] trimethoprin[1] and venlafaxine.[3] The mechanism of secondary OAG is usually the microscopic obstruction of the trabecular meshwork whereas ACG is induced by uveal effusion. The treatment of these two entities is similar to OAG and, it could be medically as well as surgical.

The differential diagnosis, prognosis and several future directions for research will be discussed.

Ophthalmologists should be aware of these types of glaucoma, which to my opinion are becoming more common in a busy glaucoma clinic.

## 2. Epidemiology

Armaly as shown that within the general population 5 to 6 % of the healthy subjects will develop marked elevation of IOP, 4 to 6 weeks after administration of topical dexamethasone or betamethasone eye drops.[12] These studies have also shown that these numbers are directly related to the frequency of the administration and duration of usage of this medication. Increasing usage is related to the increased risk for elevated IOP. At higher risk are patients with primary open-angle glaucoma, their first-degree relatives, diabetic patients, highly myopic individuals, and patients with connective tissue disease, specifically rheumatoid arthritis. In addition, patients with angle recession glaucoma are more susceptible to corticosteroid-induced glaucoma.

## 3. Mechanisms of IOP elevation in drug-induced glaucoma

### 3.1 Open-angle

Corticosteroid is a group of drugs that may produce IOP elevation by open-angle mechanism. Not all the patients taking steroid will develop this glaucoma. The risk factors include preexisting primary open-angle glaucoma, a family history of glaucoma, high myopia, diabetes mellitus and young age.[13] It has been shown that 18-36% of the general population and 46–92% of patients with primary open-angle glaucoma respond to topical ocular administration of corticosteroids with an elevation of IOP, usually within 2–4 weeks after therapy has been instituted.

Topically applied eye drops and creams to the periorbital area and intravitreal injections are more likely to cause IOP elevation than intravenous, parenteral and inhaled forms. Since IOP elevation can be gradual and asymptomatic, patients on chronic corticosteroid therapy may remain undiagnosed, which can result in glaucomatous optic nerve damage. Steroid-induced IOP elevation typically occurs within a few weeks after commencing steroid therapy. In most cases, IOP returns spontaneously to the baseline within a few weeks to months upon discontinuing the steroid (steroid responders). In rare situations, the IOP remains high (steroid-induced glaucoma) that may require prolonged glaucoma medication or even surgery. This subject is discussed in details in the chapter on steroid-induced glaucoma.

### 3.2 Closed-angle

Some drugs have contraindications or adverse effects that are related to acute angle-closure glaucoma. These drugs will incite an attack in individuals with very narrow anterior chamber angles that are prone to occlusion, especially when the pupils are dilated. The classes of medications that have the potential to induce angle-closure are topical anticholinergic or sympathomimetic pupil dilating drops, tricyclic antidepressants, monoamine oxidase inhibitors, antihistamines, anti-Parkinson drugs, antipsychotic medications and antispasmolytic agents.

Sulfonamide-containing medications may induce an ACG by a different mechanism, involving the anterior rotation of the cilliary-body. Typically, the angle-closure is bilateral and occurs within the first few doses. Patients with narrow or wide open angles are potentially susceptible to this rare and idiosyncratic reaction.

## 4. Pathophysiology of drug-induced glaucoma

### 4.1 Open-angle

The exact pathophysiology of steroid-induced glaucoma is unknown. It is known that steroid-induced IOP elevation is secondary to increased resistance to aqueous outflow. Some evidence shows that there could be an increased accumulation of glycosaminoglycans or increased production of trabecular meshwork-inducible glucocorticoid response (TIGR) protein, which could mechanically at microscopic level obstruct the aqueous outflow. Other evidence suggests that the corticosteroid-induced cytoskeletal changes could inhibit pinocytosis of aqueous humour or inhibit the clearing of glycosaminoglycans, resulting in the accumulation of this substance and blockage of the aqueous outflow.

### 4.2 Closed-angle

Aqueous humor is secreted by the ciliary body and circulates through the pupil to reach the anterior chamber angle. (Fig. 1) The pathophysiology of angle-closure glaucoma is usually due to pupillary block, i.e. iris-lens contact at the pupillary border resulting from pupillary dilation.

People at risk for Angle Closure Glaucoma (ACG) are those with hypermetropia, microphthalmus and nanophthalmos. Medications have a direct or indirect effect, either in stimulating sympathetic or inhibiting parasympathetic activation causing pupillary dilation, which can precipitate an acute angle-closure in patients with occludable anterior chamber angles. These agents include adrenergic agonists (e.g. β2-specific adrenergic agonists (e.g. salbutamol), non-catecholamine adrenergic agonists (e.g. amphetamine, dextroamphetamine, methamphetamine and phendimetrazine) and anticholinergics (e.g. tropicamide). Histamine H1receptor antagonists (antihistamines) and histamine H2 receptor antagonists (e.g. cimetidine and ranitidine) have weak anticholinergic adverse effects. Antidepressants such as fluoxetine, paroxetine, fluvoxamine and venlafaxine also have been associated with acute angle-closures, which is believed to be induced by either the anticholinergic adverse effects or the increased level of serotonin that cause mydriasis.

Sulfa-containing medications may result in acute angle-closures by a different mechanism. This involves the anterior rotation of the ciliary body with or without choroidal effusions, resulting in a shallow anterior chamber and blockage of the trabecular meshwork by the iris. Pupillary dilation and a preexisting shallow anterior chamber angle are not necessary. The exact reason for ciliary body swelling is unknown but it occurs in susceptible individuals. Topiramate is a sulfa-containing anticonvulsant. There were reports about patients on topiramate developing acute angle-closure. However, a pilot study was conducted in the Hong Kong Eye Hospital and the Prince of Wales Hospital recently, which showed that short-term use of topiramate, did not induce an asymptomatic angle narrowing. Therefore, it was suggested that topiramate induced secondary angle-closure glaucoma may be an all-or-none phenomenon.

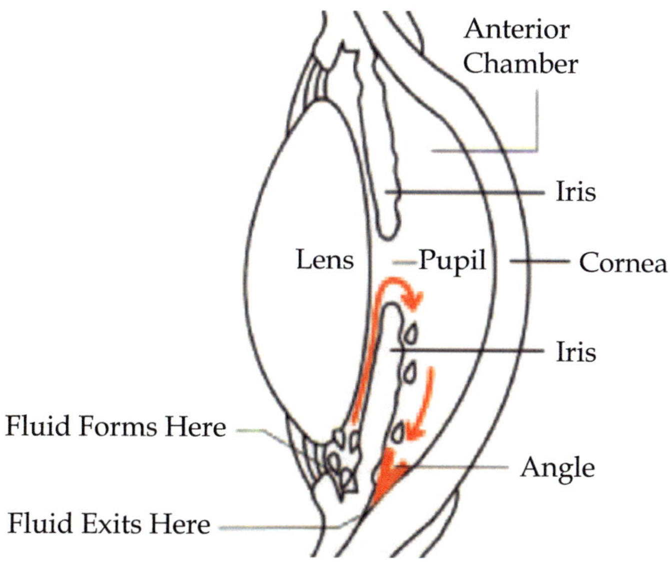


Fig. 1. Aqueous humor flow

Carbamazepine is also an anticonvulsive medication and a mood stabilizer and is primarily used in treating of epilepsy, bipolar disorders and trigeminal neuralgia.[10] It stabilizes and

inactivates the sodium Chan resulting in fewer active channels and fewer excited brain cells. It was only reported once as causing this disorder.[8]
We had two cases that developed simultaneously acute angle-closure glaucoma 4-6 weeks after intake of PO carbamazepine.

**Case no. 1**

A 58-year-old woman presented with a bilateral acute ACG. Her medical history included epilepsy treated with carbamazepine (Novartis Pharma BU (Novolog), Basel, Switzerland) 200 mg once a day for 4 weeks to stabilize her medical status. Eleven years earlier she underwent thyroidectomy due to hyperthyroidism.
The best-corrected visual acuity (BCVA) was 20/80 (with +3.75D) OD and 20/100 (with +4.25D) OS. The intraocular pressure (IOP) was 54 OD and 46mmHg OS. Both corneas were edematous and the anterior chambers were shallow. Gonioscopy revealed angle closure in both eyes and fixed, mid-dilated pupils. Ultrasound biomicroscopy (UBM) showed an anterior displaced crystalline lens with extensive irido-lenticular contact and peripheral anterior synechiae OU. The axial length was 21.35 mm OD and 21.30 mm OS. B-Scan ultrasound showed normal posterior segment OU.
The patient was treated systemically with PO acetazolamide 250mg, topical timolol maleate - dorzolamide HCl and brimonidine tartrate twice a day and the IOP decreased to 18mmHg OD and 16mmHg OS .Neodymium: Yttrium-Aluminum-Garnet (Nd: YAG) laser iridotomy was successfully performed OU. A week later, the BCVA improved to 20/80 OD and 20/60 OS, on ocular examination, potent iridotomies, mid dilated pupils with sphincter atrophy, mild nuclear sclerosis and normal optic discs were noted. The anterior chamber depth measured by Scheimpflug imaging (Pentacam®, Oculus Optikgerate GmbH, Wetzlar, Germany) was 1.54mm OD and 1.67mm OS and the volume was 90mm$^3$ and 76mm$^3$ respectively. The pachymetry was 572µm OD and 568µm. The visual fields 30-2 (Humphrey II® automatic perimeter, Allergan-Humphrey, San Leandro, CA) performed two months later showed inferior nasal step OU.

**Case no. 2**

A 53-year-old female was admitted due to high IOP simultaneously in both eyes. She was hypermetropic since childhood and had amblyopic OS. She suffered from epilepsy and had two attacks four and six weeks before being hospitalized for which she received PO carbamazepine 200mg/d for five weeks. A day before admission, she experienced severe bilateral ocular pain, vomiting and decrease in visual acuity OU.
Her BCVA was 20/40 with +5.50D OD and 20/100 with + 7.50D OS. The IOP was 54 mmHg OD and 49 mmHg OS. Both eyes had edematous cornea, very shallow anterior chamber, iris bombe and mid-dilated pupil that were not reacting to light. The anterior chamber had a narrow angle 360 degrees OU on UBM (Fig. 2). The posterior poles were normal. The patient was treated with topical pilocarpine 2% qid and PO acetazolamide 250mg bid.
The patient underwent Nd: YAG laser iridotomy OU. Three days later, the BCVA improved to 20/25 OD and 20/60 OS. The IOP decreased to 8mmHg OD and 6mmHg OS. The anterior chambers' depth was deepened and patent iridotomies, mild-dilated pupil, clear lens and posterior pole with normal optic discs were observed.
The mechanism of these agents causing bilateral AACG has been attributed to ciliochoroidal effusion, which causes forward rotation of the lens-iris diaphragm resulting in a secondary angle-closure and increased IOP. This medication and others can produce an excessive

amount of aqueous production as well as causing culinary body edema. The common denominator to our patients was hypermetropia. Indeed, patients with short axial length, such as nanophthalmos and hyperopia have a tendency to develop thickened uvea, which can be aggravated by intraocular procedures such as cataract surgery resulting in acute ACG.[11]

## 5. Non-steroidal agents associated with glaucoma

Unlike corticosteroid agents, the list of non-steroidal agents associated with glaucoma is wide and diverse (Table 1). [14] The causes of glaucoma associated with these agents are also varied. The largest single cause of glaucoma in these patients appears to be an atropine-like effect, eliciting pupillary dilatation. This class of agents includes antipsychotropics, antidepressants, monoamine oxidase (MAO) inhibitors, antihistamines, antiparkinsonian agents, antispasmolytic agents, mydriatic agents, sympathetic agents, and botulinum toxin. The pupillary dilatation seen in these cases may be enough to precipitate an attack of angle-closure glaucoma in patients with narrow angles.

Concerning open-angle glaucoma, the causes of elevated IOP are much more varied, including the release of pigment during the pupillary dilation with subsequent obstruction of the trabecular meshwork, and a possible increase of inflow during papillary dilation. As an alternative, some agents have been documented to produce an idiopathic swelling of the lens, associated with angle closure glaucoma. These agents include the antibiotics sulfa, quinine, and aspirin. Some agents directly obstruct the trabecular meshwork, such as the viscoelastic agents and silicone oil.

### 5.1 The role of psychotropic agents

Of the antipsychotropic agents on the market today, only perphenazine (Trilafon®) and fluphenazine decanoate (Prolixin®) have been documented to cause glaucoma. In both instances these were attacks of angle-closure glaucoma. These episodes were felt to reflect the anticholinergic effect of these agents on the eyes.

### 5.2 The role of antidepressant agents

Amitryptiline (Elavil® and Amitril®) and imipramine (Tofranil®), which are antidepressant tricyclic agents, have been shown to produce attacks of an angle-closure glaucoma. Of the non-tricyclic drugs, fluoxetine (Prozac®) and mianserin hydrochloride (Bolvidon®) [15] have been documented to be associated with attacks of angle-closure glaucoma.

### 5.3 The role of mood-altering agents, such as minor tranquilizers, sedatives, and stimulants

This is a rather diverse class of agents including sedatives such as diazepam (Valium®), morphine, barbiturates, and stimulants such as amphetamine and methylxanthines such as caffeine and theophylline. Diazepam has been reported to be taken by some patient having an attack of angle-closure glaucoma, in the literature there it is believed that this drug accentuate the anti cholinergic action on the eye in some rare cases with predisposed ACG . Barbiturates, morphine, para-aldehyde, meperidine, reserpine, and phenytoin have not been reported to produce an elevated IOP. The amphetamines have not been documented to produce an elevated IOP in any patient.

### 5.4 The role of antibiotics

#### Sulfa drugs

Agents that contain sulfa have been well documented to produce an idiosyncratic swelling of the lens associated with shallowing of the anterior chamber, retinal edema, and elevated IOP. These episodes do not involve the pupil and are not responding to cycloplegic agents. This observation has been confirmed by A-scan measurements of the eye during such an attack[16].

**Antipsychotropic agents**
Phenothiazines
Perphenazine (Trilafon), fluphenazine decanoate (Prolixin)

**Antidepressants**
Tricyclic agents
Amitryptiline (Elavil), imipramine (Tofranil)
Nontricyclic agents
Fluoxetine (Prozac), mianserin HC1 (Bolvidin)

**Monoamine oxidase (MAO) inhibitors**
Phenylzine sulfate (Nardil)
Tranylcypromine sulfate (Parnate)

**Antihistamines**
Ethanolamines
Orphenadrine citrate (Norgesic)

**Antiparkinsonian agents**
Trihexyphenidyl HC1 (Artane)

**Antispasmolytic agents**
Propantheline bromide (Pro-Banthine)
Dicydomine HC1 (Bentyl)

**Antibiotics**
Sulfa, quinine

**Sympathomimetic agents**
Epinephrine, ephedrine
Phenylephrine
Amphetamine
Hydroxyamphetamine

**Mydriatic agents**
All agents
Surgical agents
Viscoelastic agents, silicone oil

**Botulin toxin**
**Cardiac agents**
Disopyramide phosphate (Norpace)

Table 1. Non-steroidal agents

### 5.5 The role of antiparkinsonian agents

The anti-Parkinson agents act through two mechanisms: (1) Replenishing diminished stores of dopamine in the corpus striatum, and (2) Acting as a strong anticholinergic. Indeed, trihexyphenidyl
HCl (Artane)[17] has been documented to precipitate angle-closure glaucoma. This finding is felt to reflect the anticholinergic effect of this agent.

### 5.6 The role of antispasmolytic agents

These agents act to reduce both the gastrsecretion and the motility of the stomach. Their effect directly reflects their anticholinergic power. Although no attacks of angle-closure glaucoma are documented with these agents, propantheline bromide (Pro-Banthine®) and dicyclomine HCl (Bentyl®) [18] have been documented to raise the IOP in patients with open-angle glaucoma probably because of their anticholinergic effect.

### 5.7 The role of anesthetic agents

General anesthesia has always entailed an increased risks to the patient, including the risk of elevated IOP and glaucoma. It has always been difficult to separate the various risk factors to the patient undergoing general anesthesia. The induction of general anesthesia itself may be associated with an elevated IOP from laryngeal spasm, coughing, and wheezing associated with endotracheal intubation. Specifically, succinylcholine, ketamine and chloral hydrate have been well documented to raise IOP. This effect is felt to be due to an increased extra-ocular muscle tone from these agents. [19] The preoperative use of atropine, scopalmine, and ephedrine associated with attacks of angle-closure glaucoma following general anesthesia.

### 5.8 The role of antihistamines in inducing glaucoma

The antihistamines are a diverse group of agents that can be divided into two classes the H1 and the H2 antihistamines. The H1 antihistamines block the action of histamine on capillary permeability and vascular, bronchial, and other smooth muscles.[20] The H2 antihistamines block the effect of histamine on the smooth muscle in peripheral blood vessels and secretion of gastric acid. This group is important because of their anticholinergic effect of these agents. Although the anticholinergic action is mild, orphenadrine citrate (Norgesic®), an H1 antihistamine, has been documented to precipitate an attack of angle-closure glaucoma. It should also be noted that the H1 antihistamine promethazine HCl (Phenergan®) has been shown to produce an idiopathic swelling of the lens as documented with the sulfa agents. These agents exert only a weak response but should be approached with caution in the patient at risk for glaucoma.

### 5.9 The role of inhalation agents in inducing glaucoma

As mentioned above ,a wide variety of agents are found as inhalation products, including sympathomimetic and parasympathomimeric agents. Salbutamol and ipratropium (used in combination for chronic obstructive airway) have also been documented to precipitate attacks of angle-closure glaucoma due to the anticholinergic effect of ipratropium in combination with the effect of salbutamol (a β2 adreno receptor agonist) on increrasing aqueous humor production.[21] Therefore, these agents should be used with caution in patients at risk for such an attack of glaucoma.

### 5.10 The role of cardiac agents in inducing glaucoma

The traditional cardiac agents including digitalis and quinidine do not appear to have any effect on the IOP. However, disopyramide phosphate (Norpace®) does appear to have some anticholinergic activity and has indeed been documented to produce an attack of angle-closure glaucoma.[22]

### 5.11 The role of botulinum toxin (Oculinum)

Botulinum toxin has become popular for the treatment of essential blepharo-spasm and extraocular muscle palsy; this injectable agent has been documented to produce an acute attack of angle closure glaucoma. The effect of this drug is on the ciliary ganglion, producing pupillarymydriasis.[23]

### 5.12 The role of avastin and lucentis

A series of patients that developed sustained elevation of intraocular pressure (IOP) after intravitreal anti-VEGF injection for the treatment of neovascular age-related macular degeneration (AMD) is presented un numerous of recent publications[24] IOP reflects a balance between the rate that fluid flows into the eye and the rate that it exits the eye. If inflow increases or outflow decreases, then IOP will go up. Intravitreal injection of drugs, such as Lucentis (ranibizumab) or Avastin (bevacizumab), increases the amount of fluid within the eye, and hence will increase IOP. Normally, as the excess fluid gradually exits the eye over a period of time, the IOP returns to normal. However, there are a growing number of cases of patients undergoing Lucentis and Avastin therapy that develop elevation of IOP that does not return to normal.

In a recent study four out of 116 patients with AMD (3.45%) developed sustained elevated intraocular pressure (IOP) after multiple intravitreal injections of Avastin (1.5 mg/0.06 mL) and/or Lucentis (0.5 mg/0.05 mL). An analysis of 4 cases revealed: None of the patients had a previous diagnosis or family history of glaucoma/OHT. Two patients had both bevacizumab and ranibizumab injections. Two patients developed OHT after recent intravitreal ranibizumab and 2 patients after recent intravitreal Avastin injection. It appears that anti-VEGF drugs may, in some persons, lead to sustained elevation of IOP and possible glaucoma. It is not clear why this occurs, nor have any risk factors for this adverse effect, such as family history of glaucoma, been identified. Nor is it clear whether the IOP elevation is permanent, or whether IOP may return to normal after cessation of anti-VEGF injections. Glaucoma medications can lower IOP after it has been elevated by anti-VEGF drug use.

There are some publictions[25] which describe the decrease of rubeosis iridis in patients with neo-vascular after intra- vitreal Avastin injection and can lead to decrease in IOP within 48 hours.

## 6. Treatment of drug-induced glaucoma

### 6.1 Medical: Open-angle

If the patient's underlying medical condition can tolerate discontinuation of corticosteroids, then its discontinuation will usually result in normalization of IOP. In case of topical corticosteroid drops, using a lower potency steroid medication, such as the phosphate forms of prednisolone and dexamethasone, loteprednol etabonate or fluorometholone should be considered. These drugs have a lesser chance to increase the IOP, but they are usually not as effective as others. Topical non-steroidal anti-inflammatory medications (e.g., diclofenac, ketorolac) are other alternatives do not cause IOP elevation, but they have only a limited anti-inflammatory activity to treat the patient's underlying condition. In the occasional cases in which the patient's IOP does not normalize upon the cessation of the steroid or in those patients who must continue with treatment, topical anti-glaucoma medications are considered.

### 6.2 Medical: Closed-angle

If the etiology of closed angle glaucoma is sulfa containing medications, the increase in IOP generally will resolve upon discontinuing the agent. However, severe cases of sulfonamide-induced angle-closure (i.e. IOP >45 mm Hg) may not respond to discontinuing the offending agent. They may respond to intravenous mannitol. Other etiologies of drug-induced angle-closure are treated similar to primary acute angle-closure glaucoma with topical beta-blockers, prostaglandin analogues, cholinergic agonists and often oral acetazolamide.

### 6.3 Laser treatment

For open-angle steroid-induced glaucoma, selective laser trabeculoplasty or Argon laser trabeculoplasty (Fig. 3) can be applied in the absence of intraocular inflammation if the IOP is suboptimal with medication.

In closed-angle glaucoma, an Argon laser peripheral iridoplasty or YAG laser iridotomy may be performed to widen the angle and deepen the anterior chamber. Laser iridotomy can be performed to reverse pupillary block or to prevent further pupillary block. Laser Irididotomies can be performed as a preventive procedure in hepermetropic naophthalmic and microphthalmic eyes. Fig. 4 shows the effect of Argon laser laser iridotomy. When medical and laser therapy are ineffective in lowering the IOP to target pressure or the patient is intolerant to medical therapy, surgical therapy is indicated. Usually, trabeculectomy, a guarded filtration procedure, with or without intraoperative anti-metabolites, is the primary procedure. In cases of eyes with active neovascularization or inflammation, a glaucoma drainage implant may be used as the primary procedure.

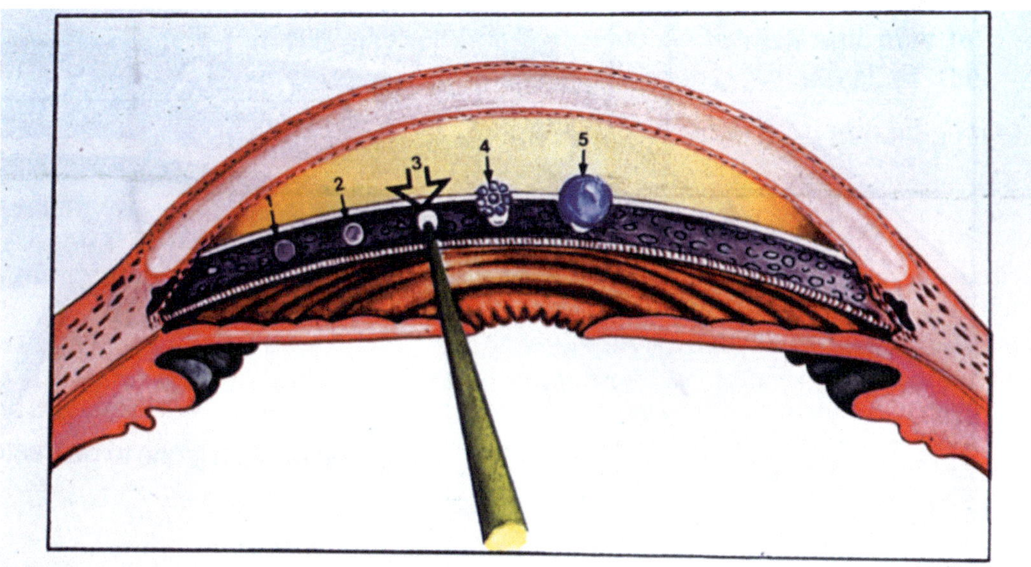


Fig. 2. ALT Argon Laser Trabeculoplasy

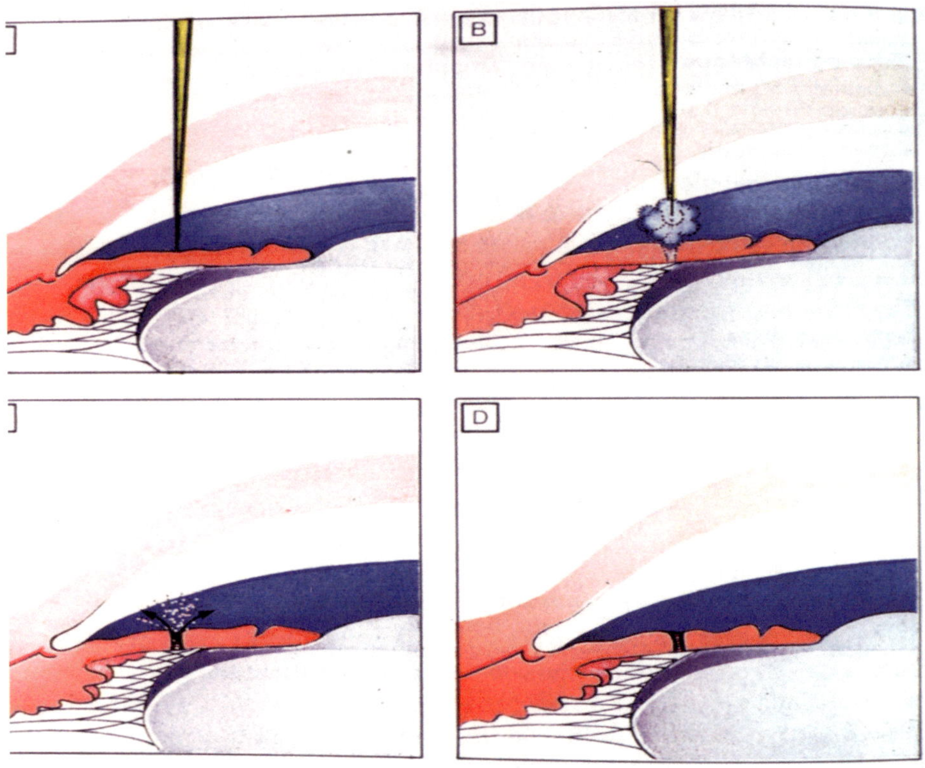


Fig. 3. LI Laser Iridotomy

### 6.4 Surgical: Closed-angle

Trabeculectomy can also be performed with similar indications as open-angle glaucoma. However, the surgery is more difficult since the anterior chamber is shallower and the cornea is usually hazier due to the acute IOP rise.

## 7. Prevention of drug induced glaucoma

### 7.1 Open-angle

Unnecessary prolonged use of cortcosteroid should be avoided. Ophthalmic evaluation is recommended for patients treated with long-term steroids especially with risk factors such as family history of primary open-angle glaucoma.

### 7.2 Closed-angle

Prophylactic laser iridotomy may be performed in patients requiring frequent mydriasis such as frequent fundus examinations for diabetic retinopathy. Agents causing secondary angle-closure should be avoided in susceptible individuals as far as possible.

## 8. Conclusion

Drugs that cause or exacerbate open-angle glaucoma are mostly glucocorticoids. Several classes of drugs, including adrenergic agonists, cholinergics, anticholinergics, sulpha-based drugs, selective serotonin reuptake inhibitors, tricyclic and tetracyclic antidepressants, anticoagulants and histamine H(1) and H(2) receptor antagonists, have been reported to induce or precipitate acute angle-closure glaucoma, especially in individuals predisposed with narrow angles of the anterior chamber. In some instances, bilateral simultaneous development of acute ACG occurs after carbamazepine and topiramate intake may occur especially in eyes with short axial length such as hypermetropia, microphthalmia and nanophthalmos. Clinicians should be mindful of the possibility of drug-induced glaucoma, whether or not the drug is listed as a contraindication and if in doubt, consult an ophthalmologist. Patients should visit an ophthalmologist routinely twice a year after the age of 40 and inform him about their different medications.

## 9. Acknowledgment

I acknowledge the support of Tradis Gat Ltd. in publication of this chapter.

## 10. References

[1] Matz T, Abbott L. Bilateral acute angle-closure glaucoma. *Resident and Staff Physician* 2008; 54:3.

[2] Kakaria V, Chalam, Tillis T, Farhana S, Brar SA. Acute bilateral simultaneous angle closure glaucoma Topiramate administration: a case report. *J Med Case Reports* 2008; 2:1.

[3] GuMHP, Thiagalingam S, Ong P, Goldberg I. Bilateral acute angle closure caused by supraciliary effusion associated with Velafaxine intake. *MJA* 2005; 182:121-123.

[4] Nemet A, Nesher R, Almog Y, Assia E. Bilateral acute angle closure glaucoma following Topiramate treatment. *Harefuah* 2002; 141:597-9.

[5] Ates H.; Kay O., Lu K., Andac K. Bilateral angel closure glaucoma following general anesthesia: *International Ophthalmology* 1999; 23:129-30.

[6] Singh SK, Thapa SS, Badhu BP. Topiramate induced bilateral angle-closure glaucoma. *Kathmandu University Medical Journal* 2007; 5:234-.

[7] Lachkar Y, Bouassida W. Drug-induced acute angle closure glaucoma. *Curr Opin Ophthalmol* 2007; 18:129-33.

[8] Chan KCY, Sachdev N, Wells AP. Bilateral acute angle closure secondary to uveal effusions associated with Flucloxacillin and Carbamazepine. *Br J Ophthalmol* 2008; 92:428-430.

[9] Levy J, Yagev R, Petrova A, Lifshitz T. Topiramate - induced bilateral angle-closure glaucoma. *Can J Ophthalmol* 2006; 41:221-5.

[10] Sean Sweetman (Ed.). Martindale-the complete drug reference, 36th edition, 471-477.

[11] Brockhurst RJ. Nanophthalmos with uveal effusion: A new clinical entity. *Trans Am Ophthalmol Soc* 1974; 72:371-403.

[12] Arnnaly MF. Statistical attributes of the steroid hypertensive response in the clinically normal eye. I. the demonstration of three levels of response. *Invest Ophthalmol* 1965; 4:187.

[13] Stewart RH, Kimbrough RL .Intraocular pressure response to topically administered fluorometholone. *Arch. Ophthalmol* 1979; 97:2139.

[14] Mandelkom R. Drug induced Glaucoma, clinical pathway in glaucoma, in :Zimmerman and Kooner, New York: Thieme Medical Publishers inc. 2001 350-333

[15] Kinek M .Glaucoma following the antidepressant mianserin. Harefuah 1990:118-699.
[16] Hook SR, Holladay JI, Perager TC, Goosey JD. Transient myopia induced by sulphonamides. *Am J Ophthalmol* 1986; 101:495.
[17] Friedman Z, Neuman E. Benzhexalol induced blindness in Parkinson's disease. *Br Med J* 1972; 1:605.
[18] Mody MV, Keeney AH. Propantheline (probanthine) bromide in relation to normal and glaucomatous eyes: effects on intraocular tension and pupillary size. *JAMA* 1955; 159:1113.
[19] Katz RI, Eakins KB. Mode of action of succinylcholine on intraocular pressure. *J Pharmacol Exp Ther* 1968; 162:1.
[20] Bard L.A. Transient myopia associated with promethazine (phenergan) therapy: report of a case. *Am J Ophthalmol* 1964; 58:682?
[21] Malawi JT, Rhobinson GM, Seneviratne H. Ipratropium bromide induced angle closure glaucoma (letter). *NZ Med J* 1982; 95:759.
[22] Monica ML, Hesse RJ, Messerli FH .The effect of a calcium channel blocking agent on intraocular pressure. *AM J Ophthalmol* 1983; 96:814.
[23] Kupfer C. Selective block of synaptic transmission in ciliary ganglion by type A botulinum toxin in Rabbits. *Proc Soc Exp Biol Med* 1958; 99:474.
[24] Adelman RA, Zheng Q. Mayer HR. Persistent ocular hypertension following intravitreal bevacizumab and ranibizumab injections. *J Ocul Pharmacol Ther*. 2010 Feb; 26(1):105-10.
[25] Milko E. Iliev, Diego Doming, Ute , Sebastin Wolf, Intravitreal Bevacizumab (Avastin®) in the Treatment of Neovascular Glaucoma. *AJO* Volume 142, Pages 1054-56, Dec. 2006.

# 29

# Steroid Induced Glaucoma

Avraham Cohen
*Western Galilee Hospital,*
*Department Of Ophthalmology*
*Israel*

## 1. Introduction

Increased intraocular pressure and glaucoma following corticosteroid therapy are well known issues for the ophthalmologist for more than 50 years. Corticosteroids use has gained popularity in ophthalmology as anti-inflammatory and anti-allergic agents but can have important consequences and should be used only with judicious monitoring. The therapeutic use of corticosteroids can lead to the development of ocular hypertension and iatrogenic open-angle glaucoma in susceptible individuals. It can occur in any age group, either gender and from steroid therapy for any ocular or systemic disease and by any route of administration: topical, systemic or inhaled.

## 2. Epidemiology

About one in every three people is considered a potential "steroid responder", but only a small percentage will have a clinically significant elevation in intraocular pressure. 5-6% of the normal population develops a marked increase in intraocular pressure of more than 31 mmHg after 4-6 weeks of topical corticosteroids therapy. 33% are moderate responders (elevation of 6-15 mmHg) and the remaining are considered non responreds (less than 6mmHg of elevation in intraocular pressure). Although approximately 30%-40% of the normal population are "steroid responders" (i.e., develop reversible steroid-induced ocular hypertension), most of primary open angle glaucoma patients or with a family history are steroid responders. Normal individuals who are steroid responders are at higher risk for subsequently developing primary open angle glaucoma. In one study, high corticosteroid responders (intraocular pressure greater than 31 mm Hg during dexamethasone administration qid for 6 weeks), 13.0% developed glaucomatous visual field loss during the follow-up period of 5 years. In steroid induced glaucoma patients, glaucoma is triggered by steroid treatment, and intraocular pressure will not decrease after cessation of steroid application. Thus, steroid induced glaucoma patients necessitate anti-glaucoma medications to control intraocular pressure. Steroid responsiveness appears to be heritable, however low concordance of pressure response in monozygotic twins to topical testing may indicate a limited role for a genetic basis. In addition highly myopic patients and diabetic patients have a higher rate of elevated intraocular pressure response to topical steroids.

Age is also an important factor. In pediatric patients taking oral prednisone for inflammatory bowel disease 32% were steroid responders. When children younger than 10 years of age where treated with topical instillation of dexamethasone, marked elevation in intraocular pressure was noted. A dose-dependent hypertensive pressure response occurs more frequently, more severely and more rapidly in children than in adults.

## 3. Pathophysiology

There have been reports suggesting that endogenous cortisol may play a role in the pathogenesis of primary open angle glaucoma. Excess endogenous production of glucocorticosteroids (Cushing's syndrome) can also cause increase in intraocular pressure.
Glucocorticosteroids alter several trabecular meshwork cellular functions including inhibition of cellular proliferation, migration, phagocytosis, and increased cell and nucleus size. Glucocorticosteroids also increase extracellular matrix synthesis and decrease its turnover.
Many mechanisms have been proposed to explain the elevated intraocular pressure in response to glucocorticosteroids. One hypothesis is that glucocorticosteroids protect the lysosomal membrane and thus inhibit release of hydrolases responsible of depolimerization of glycosaminoglycans. Accumulated glycosaminoglycans in the ground substance of the outflow pathways retain water and narrow the trabecular spaces, causing increase in outflow resistance. In steroid-induced glaucoma there is also an increase in fine fibrillar material in the subendothelial region of Schlemm's cannal. These fibrils are deposited underneath the inner wall endothelium. The main finding in steroid-induced glaucoma is an accumulation of basement membrane-like material staining for type IV collagen. These accumulations are found throughout all layers of the trabecular meshwork.
There are multiple isoforms of the glucocorticoid receptor (GR) a ligand-dependent transcriptional factor that activates or represses gene transcription. GRα is the ligand binding form of the receptor that is responsible for the physiologic and pharmacological effects of glucocorticosteroids. Most of the physiological and pharmacological effects of glucocorticosteroids are directly mediated by GRα. GRα resides predominantly in the cytoplasm in the absence of ligand as a multiprotein heterocomplex that contains Hsp 90, Hsp 70 and other proteins. Steroid binding to GRα causes a conformation change and activation of the receptor. Activated GRα can alter gene expression via GRE-dependent (classical) and GRE-independent (nonclassical) mechanisms. In the GRE-dependent pathway activated GRα translocates to the nucleus along microtubules. GRα bind to specific palindromic DNA sequence (GRE) as a homodimer on the promoter region of target genes to induce transcription. In addition, GRα functions as a negative regulator of transcription in a specific subset of genes that contains a negative GRE. The GRE-independent pathway is an additional way to inhibit gene expression. GRα physically interacts with other transcription factors to prevent them from binding to their response elements of genes that encode for proinflammatory cytokines. The anti-inflammatory and immune suppression are mediated via this GRE-independent pathway. GRβ is an alternatively spliced form of the receptor, that resides in the nucleus, which lacks the conventional ligand binding domain, does not bind glucocorticosteroids, and acts as a dominant negative regulator of glucocorticosteroids activity. Increased expression of GRβ appears to be responsible for unresponsiveness to anti-inflammatory therapy for asthma, inflammatory bowel disease rheumatoid arthritis and ulcerative colitis. Recent work has shown that glaucomatous trabecular meshwork cells have lower levels of GRβ compared with normal trabecular meshwork cells, and this appears to be responsible for increased glucocorticosteroids sensitivity in the glaucomatous trabecular meshwork cells. In primary open angle glaucoma

an abnormal accumulation of dihydrocortisol may potentiate exogenous glucocorticosteroids activity and increased intraocular pressure.

Changes in protein synthesis have also been implicated in steroid induced glaucoma. *MYOC* gene, located on chromosome 1, encodes a secretory glycoprotein of 504 amino acids named Myocilin, and is the first gene to be linked to juvenile open-angle glaucoma and some forms of adult-onset primary open-angle glaucoma. The gene was identified as an up regulated molecule in cultured trabecular meshwork cells after treatment with dexamethasone and was originally referred to as trabecular meshwork-inducible glucocorticoid response (*TIGR*). Interestingly, the profile of *MYOC* up regulation by dexamethasone is in a dose- and time-dependent manner very similar to the course of development of steroid induced glaucoma. This led many investigators to believe that an increased *MYOC* level is a cause of glaucoma. However, a putative association between *MYOC* induction and primary open angle glaucoma has not been firmly established.

Glucocorticosteroids inhibit prostaglandin synthesis by trabecular cells. Prostaglandins $E_2$ and $F_{2a}$ normal function is to lower the intraocular pressure by increasing the outflow facility. Endothelial cells of the trabecular meshwork can act as phagocytes of debris. Glucocorticosteroids can suppress phagocytic activity causing accumulation of debris in the trabecular meshwork and decrease in outflow facility.

In a study on rabbit eyes, after topical treatment with dexamethasone, Transmission electron microscopy showed increased abnormality of nucleus of the trabecular meshwork cells, microfilament and microtubules among interstitial cells also increased, cytoplasmic vacuolation, rough endoplasmic reticulum expansion, as well as an increase in intercellular amorphous material. The mechanism of elevated intraocular pressure is thought to be increased aqueous outflow resistance owing to an accumulation of extracellular matrix material in the trabecular meshwork (fig 1).

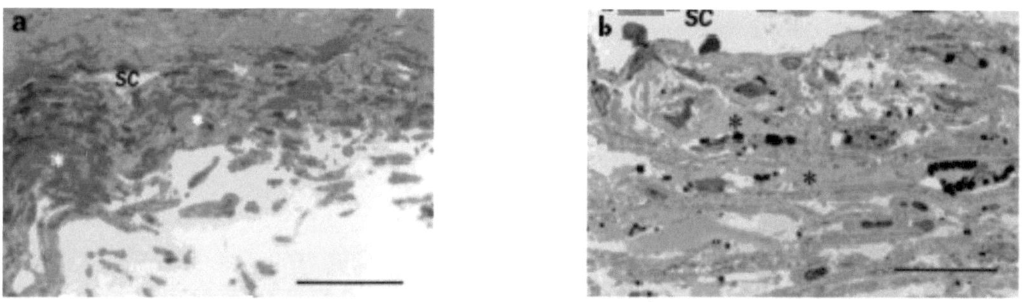


Fig. 1. Light microscopic pictures of the trabecular meshwork from steroid-induced glaucoma (SG). a) (Right eye in case 1), b) (Case 2): Schlemm's canal (SC) is open. The intertrabescular spaces in the outer part of the TM are filled with the homogeneous extracellular matrix (ECM) (asterisks). Azure II staining. Scale bars indicate 50 µm for a) and 20 µm for b)

Effects of Glucocorticosteroids are mediated by the Glucocorticosteroids receptor, which is a ligand-dependent transcription factor altering the expression of trabecular meshwork genes. Glucocorticosteroids increase the expression of extracellular matrix (collagen, fibronectin, laminin), proteinase inhibitor genes (Serpina3) and decreased expression of proteinase genes (MMP1, TPA). Altered expression of cytoskeletal genes (ACTA2, FLNB, and NEBL) may be associated with Glucocorticosteroids mediated reorganization of trabecular meshwork cell microfibrils and microtubules. Glucocorticosteroids reorganizes the actin cytoskeleton to form cross-linked actin networks (CLANs) in cultured trabecular meshwork cells, and is reversible after Glucocorticosteroids withdrawel. In addition Glucocorticosteroids alters microtubules to form microtubule tangles.

## 4. Routes of corticosteroid administration

### 4.1 Topical route

Topical route includes ocular drops and ointments. Of various routes of administration, topical therapy most commonly induces elevated intraocular pressure and correlates with the duration and frequency of administration. Dexamethasone and prednisolone increase intraocular pressure more frequently than loteprendol (Lotemax), fluorometholone (FML), rimexolone (Vexol) or hydrocortisone. Fluorometholone (FML) in particular is less likely to increase intraocular pressure but is also a less potent steroid (table 1). Rimexolone has a low intraocular pressure elevating potential comparable to that of fluorometholone in adults. The chemical structure is responsible to the lower propensity to increase intraocular pressure of some steroids. Loteprendol is a site-active steroid that contains an ester rather than a ketone group at the C-20 position, rendering de-esterification to an inactive metabolite. It is highly lipid-soluble, with enhanced penetration into cells. Loteprendol appears to have an improved safety profile compared with ketone corticosteroids. Fluorometholone is deoxygenized at the C-21 position. Rimexolone lacks a hydroxyl substituent at the C-21 position. It has lower aqueous solubility and increased lipophilicity. It appears that the potency of topical steroids is directly correlated with the propensity to elevate intraocular pressure. Intraocular pressure elevation almost never occurs in less than 5 days and rarely in less than 2 weeks of steroid treatment. However, late rise in ocular pressure is not uncommon, even if intraocular pressure has been within normal limits during a treatment course of 6 weeks.

### 4.2 Intraocular route

Before the advent of anti VEGF, intravitreal steroid injections have been used largely in the treatment of exudative age related macular degeneration, chronic cystoid macular edema, proliferative diabetic vitreoretinopathy, retinal vascular occlusion and chronic uveitis. Rise in intraocular pressure is dependent on dose, presence of aphakia or pseudophkaia and a history of vitrectomy, facilitating penetration of the drug into the anterior segment. Intraocular pressure may rise in 30-50 % of patients as soon as 1-4 weeks after intravitreal injection of triamcinolone acetonide (Kenalog) and often returns to baseline several months after injection. It is advisable to perform a trial of topical prednisolone acetate before intravitreal triamcinolone acetonide injection is performed.

Fluocinolone acetonide intravitreal implants are an effective therapy for non-infectious posterior uveitis. However, patients receiving this treatment are at high risk for development of vision-threatening increased intraocular pressure. Therefore, patients treated with these implants should have frequent intraocular pressure monitoring. Intractable glaucoma may necessitate removal of the depot by pars plana vitrectomy to lower intraoculare pressure. In the SCORE study grid photocoagulation and repeated injections of triamcinolone acetonide 1 or 4 mg seemed to be equally effective in producing improvements in best corrected visual acuity in patients with macular edema due to branch retinal vein occlusion. 41% of patients treated with triamcinolone acetonide 4 mg initiated intraocular pressure lowering medications during the 12 months study. In patient with central retinal vein occlusion 35% of the patients receiving 4 mg triamcinolone acetonide initiated glaucoma medications. Ozurdex is a slow release intravitreal implant of dexamethasone currently under clinical trials for the treatment of macular edema in retinal vein occlusion disease. It appears that the dexamethasone implant is well tolerated, producing transient, moderate and readily managed increase in intraocular pressure in less than 16% of eyes.

### 4.3 Periocular route

Subconjunctival, sub-Tenon and retrobulbar injections of triamcinolone acetonide may cause dangerous and prolonged elevation of intraocular pressure because of their long duration of action. Surgical excision of sub-Tenon triamcinolone acetonide deposit should be considered if the primary treatment for steroid-induced glaucoma is refractory to medical treatment.
The application of topical corticosteroids to the eyelids and periorbital region, in the treatment of atopic dermatitis, even over long periods of time, was not related to the development of glaucoma or cataracts.

### 4.4 Systemic route

Systemic administration includes ingestion, inhalation and nasal spray. It is less likely to cause intraocular elevation. However, intraocular pressure may rise weeks to years after treatment. When administrated concurrently with topical steroids it may have an additive effect and higher intraocular pressure than a single route.
Intranasal corticosteroids have become a gold standard in therapy for allergic rhinoconjunctivitis and recent evidence indicates that may be effective at alleviating ocular symptoms as well. Intranasal corticosteroids are absorbed systemically in small measurable amounts. Some studies suggest a relationship between intranasal steroids and increased intraocular pressure.
Aerosolized drugs delivered with a facemask may inadvertently deposit in the eyes, raising concerns about ocular side effects. Inhaled corticosteroids have been associated with an increased risk of skin thinning, bruising, cataracts and possibly glaucoma in adults. The risks increase with advanced age, higher doses, and longer duration of use. In children, the risks of cataracts and glaucoma were negligible with inhaled corticosteroids, whether a mouthpiece or a mask interface was used. It is not known whether exposed children will have increased risks from inhaled corticosteroids later in life. Therefore, it is wise to avoid face and eye deposition when possible, to use the minimally effective dose and a regular follow up of intraocular pressure.

### 4.5 Endogenous route

Elevated blood levels of corticosteroids of endogenous production, as seen in adrenal hyperplasia or neoplasia (Cushing syndrome) can also cause increase in the intraocular pressure. After adrenalectomy, increased intraocular pressure may retune to normal values

## 5. Clinical course

An increase in intraocular pressure may occur days to weeks and even months after the administration of steroids. The increase in intraocular pressure depends on potency, penetration, frequency and route of administration. Individual susceptibility, older age and ocular disease are also important factors. An acute presentation may occur after intense systemic steroid therapy. Patient may complain on pain, decreased vision and conjunctival hyperemia. In infants the clinical picture may resemble that of congenital glaucoma. Signs are tearing, Descement's membrane breaks, corneal edema, enlarged corneal diameter, elevated intraocular pressure and optic disc cupping. Unlike congenital glaucoma, the anterior chamber angle is normal.

| Potency | Steroid | Glaucoma risk |
|---|---|---|
| High | Betamethasone<br>Clobetasol propionate<br>Dexamethasone<br>Flucinonide | ↑ |
| Medium | Triamcinolone acetonide<br>Loteprendole etabonate<br>Dexamethasone sodium phosphate<br>Fluormethalone | |
| Low | Hydrocortisone<br>Rimexolone<br>Medrisone | |

Table 1. Comparison of anti-inflamatory and intraocular pressure elevating potencies

Additional ocular findings from topical steroids include corneal ulcers, exacerbation of bacterial and viral infections, posterior subcapsular cataracts, mydriasis, delayed wound healing, scleral melting ptosis and skin atrophy and depigmentation of the eyelids. Systemic steroids side effects are suppression of the pituitary-adrenal axis, Cushinoid facies, buffalo hump, truncal obesity, hirsutism, cutaneous striae, easy bruisability, delayed wound healing, osteoporosis, aseptic necrosis of the hip, peptic ulcers, diabetes, hypertension, insomnia and psychiatric disorders.

## 6. Management

This secondary glaucoma clinically mimics many features of primary open angle glaucoma. Currently, the propensity to develop steroid-induced ocular hypertension must be determined empirically. Therefore, all patients on protracted steroid therapy should have their intraocular pressure monitored periodically.

Steroid induced glaucoma usually responds to cessation of steroid therapy and to topical anti-glaucoma medication. In steroid responders the intraocular pressure generally returns to normal within few days to weeks after discontinuation of steroids. Rarely, intraocular pressure remains elevated despite steroid cessation and may result from damage to outflow channels. In these cases management is similar to that of open angle glaucoma patients.

If anti-inflammatory therapy is needed in known steroid responders or glaucoma patients, treatment with FML 0.1% or medrisone (MHS) are possible options. Loteprendol (Lotemax) and Rimexolone (Velox) are potent anti-inflammatory corticosteroids with reduced propensity to raise intraocular pressure.

Alternative topical anti-inflammatory agents are the nonsteroidal anti-inflammatory agents (NSAIDs), such as diclofenac (Voltaren), ketorolac tromethamine (Acular LS) and bromfenac (Xibrom). NSAIDs do not induce increase in intraocular pressure but their anti-inflammatory potential is lower than that of corticosteroids.
When indicated, topical anti-glaucoma medications should be used. Prostaglandins should be used with caution as they may have pro-inflammatory effect. If intraocular pressure remains intractable despite maximal tolerated medical therapy, Argon laser trabeculoplasty and Nd:YAG laser selective trabeculoplasty (SLT) have variable success and patients required additional surgical procedures. Repeat SLT treatments may be necessary. SLT is a temporizing procedure to consider in patients with steroid-induced elevated IOP.
A possible new treatment under investigation is anecortave acetate injection into the anterior sub-Tenon space in eye with uncontrolled steroid-related ocular hypertension following intravitreal or sub-Tenon injections of triamcinolone acetonide. Anecortave acetate is a synthetic molecule derived from cortisol. The resulting molecule is referred to as a cortisene. The modification renders the molecule free of all glucocorticoid and mineralocorticoid activity. Anecortave acetate possesses antiangiogenic activity via inhibition of the proteases necessary for vascular endothelial cell migration and has been evaluated as a potential therapy for neovascular age-related macular degeneration. In one preliminary, uncontrolled study a rapid and sustained reduction of intraocular pressure was noted as soon as 1 week after treatment. The mechanism by which anecortave acetate lowers intraocular pressure in eyes with steroid-related ocular hypertension is unknown. With glucocorticoid treatment, trabecular meshwork cells increases the expression of plasminogen activator inhibitor-1, a protein that inhibits activation of extracellular proteinases and leads to enhanced extracellular matrix deposition. Recent studies have shown that anecortave acetate blocks glucocorticoid induction of plasminogen activator inhibitor-1, which may be partially responsible for anecortave acetate's intraocular pressure lowering activity.
Surgical treatments include filtration surgery, tube shunt, excision of the sub-Tenon steroid depot, explantation of steroid implant and pars plana vitrectomyfor the removal of the intravitreal depot.

## 7. References


Armaly MF. The heritable nature of dexamethasone-induced ocular hypertension. Arch Ophthalmol. 1966; 75:32–5.

Bamberger CM, Bamberger AM, de Castro M, Chrousos GP. Glucocorticoid receptor beta, a potential endogenous inhibitor of glucocorticoid action in humans. J Clin Invest. 1995; 95:2435–41.

Bartlett JD, Woolley TW, Adams CM. Identification of high intraocular pressure responders to topical ophthalmic corticosteroids. J Ocul Pharmacol. 1993; 9:35–45.

Becker B, Chevrette L. Topical corticosteroid testing in glaucoma siblings. Arch Ophthalmol. 1966; 76:484–7.

Becker B. Diabetes mellitus and and primary open angle glaucoma. Am J Opphthalmol. 1971; 71:1.

Bregmann J, Witmer MT, Slonim CB. The relationship of intranasal steroids to intraocular pressure. Curr Allergy Asthma Rep. 2009 Jul; 9(4):311-5.

Duma D, Jewell CM, Cidlowski JA. Multiple glucocorticoid receptor isoforms and mechanisms of post-translational modification. J Steroid Biochem Mol Biol. 2006; 102:11–21.

Fautsch MP, Bahler CK, Jewison DJ, et al. Recombinant TIGR/MYOC increases outflow resistance in the human anterior segment. Invest Ophthalmol Vis Sci 2000; 41:4163–8.

Gould DB, Miceli-Libby L, Savinova OV, et al. Genetically increasing MYOC expression supports a necessary pathologic role of abnormal proteins in glaucoma. Mol Cell Biol 2004; 24:9019–25.

Haeck IM, Rouwen TJ, Timmer-de Mik L, de Bruin-Weller MS, Bruijnzeel-Koomen CA. Topical corticosteroids in atopic dermatitis and the risk of glaucoma and cataracts. J Am Acad Dermatol. 2011 Feb; 64(2):275-81.

Hass JS, NootensRH: Glaucoma secondary to benigne adrenal adenoma. Am J Ophthalmol 1974; 78:497.

Jilani FA, Khan AM, Kesharwani RK: Study of topical corticosteroid response in glaucoma suspects and family members of established glaucoma patients. Indian J Ophthalmol 1987; 35:141.

Jonas JB, Degenring RF, Kreissig I, Akkoyun I, Kamppeter BA. Intraocular pressure elevation after intravitreal triamcinolone acetonide injection. Ophthalmology. 2005;112(4):593-598.

Jonas JB. Intravitreal triamcinolone acetonide: a change in a paradigm. Ophthalmic Res. 2006;38(4):218-245.

Jones R 3rd, Rhee DJ. Corticosteroid-induced ocular hypertension and glaucoma: a brief review and update of the literature. . Curr Opin Ophthalmol. 2006 Apr; 17(2):163-7.

Julia A. Haller et al for the OZURDEX GENEVA Study Group. Randomized, sham controlled trial of dexamethasone intravitreal implant in patients with macular edema due to retinal vein occlusion. Ophthalmology 2010;117:1134-46.

Kitazawa Y, Horie T. The prognosis of corticosteroid-responsive individuals. Arch Ophthalmol. 1981; 99:819–23.

Kwok AK, Lam DS, Fan DS, et al. Ocular hypertensive response totopical steroids in children. Ophthalmol1997; 104:2112.

Lewis JM, Priddy T, Judd J, Gordon MO, Kass MA, Kolker AE, Becker B. Intraocular pressure response to topical dexamethasone as a predictor for the development of primary open-angle glaucoma. Am J Ophthalmol. 1988; 106:607–12.

Lutjen-Drecoll E, May CA, Polansky JR, et al. Localization of the stress proteins alpha B-crystallin and trabecular meshwork inducible glucocorticoid response protein in normal and glaucomatous trabecular meshwork. Invest Ophthalmol Vis Sci 1998; 39:517–25.

McCarty GR, Schwartz B. Increased plasma noncortisol glucocorticoid activity in open-angle glaucoma. Invest Ophthalmol Vis Sci. 1991; 32:1600–8.

Mindel JS, Tavitian HO, Smith H, Jr, et al. Comparative ocular pressure elevation by medrysone, fluorometholone, and dexamethasone phosphate. Arch Ophthalmol 1980; 98:1577–8.

NG JS, Fan DS, young AL et al,Ocular hypertensive response to topical dexamethasone in children: a dose-dependent phenomenon. Ophthalmol 2000; 107:2097.

Nguyen TD, Chen P, Huang WD, et al. Gene structure and properties of TIGR, an olfactomedin-related glycoprotein cloned from glucocorticoid-induced trabecular meshwork cells. J Biol Chem 1998; 273:6341–50.
Oakley RH, Sar M, Cidlowski JA. The human glucocorticoid receptor beta isoform. Expression, biochemical properties, and putative function. J Biol Chem. 1996; 271:9550–9.
Ohji M, Kinoshita S, Ohmi E, Kuwayama Y. marked intraocular response to instillation of corticosteroids in children. Am J Ophthalmol 1191; 112:450.
Okka M, Bozkurt B, Kerimoglu H, Ozturk BT, Gunduz K, Yılmaz M, Okudan S. Control of steroid-induced glaucoma with surgical excision of sub-Tenon triamcinolone acetonide deposits: a clinical and biochemical approach. Can J Ophthalmol. 2010 Dec; 45(6):621-6.
Robin AL, Suan EP, Sjaarda RN, Callanan DG, Defaller J; Alcon Anecortave Acetate for IOP Research Team. Reduction of intraocular pressure with anecortave acetate in eyes with ocular steroid injection-related glaucoma. Arch Ophthalmol. 2009 Feb; 127(2):173-8.
Rozsival P, Hampl R, Obenberger J, Starka L, Rehak S. Aqueous humour and plasma cortisol levels in glaucoma and cataract patients. Curr Eye Res. 1981; 1:391–6.
Rubin B, Taglienti A, Rothman RF, Marcus CH, Serle JB. The effect of selective laser trabeculoplasty on intraocular pressure in patients with intravitreal steroid-induced elevated intraocular pressure. J Glaucoma. 2008 Jun-Jul;17(4):287-92.
Schwartz JT, Reuling FH, Feinleib M et al. Twin study on ocular pressure after topical dexamethasone. I. frequency distribution of pressure response. Am J Ophthalmol 1973; 76:126.
Schwartz JT, Reuling FH, Feinleib M et al. Twin study on ocular pressure folloing topically applied dexamethasone. II. Inheritance of variation in pressure response. Arch Ophthalmol 1973; 90:281.
SCORE Study Research Group. A randomiezed trial compering the efficacy and safety of intravitreal triamcinolone with standard care to treat vision loss associated with macular edema secondary to central retinal vein occlution: the Standard Care vs Corticosteroid for Retinal Vein Occlusion (SCORE) Study report 5. Arch Ophthalmol 2009;127:1101-14.
SCORE Study Research Group. A randomiezed trial compering the efficacy and safety of intravitreal triamcinolone with standard care to treat vision loss associated with macular edema secondary to branch retinal vein occlution: the Standard Care vs Corticosteroid for Retinal Vein Occlusion (SCORE) Study report 6. Arch Ophthalmol 2009;127:1115-28.
Smithen LM, Ober MD, Maranan L, Spaide RF. Intravitreal triamcinolone acetonide and intraocular pressure. Am J Ophthalmol. 2004;138(5):740-743.
Southren AL, Gordon GG, Weinstein BI. Genetic defect in cortisol metabolism in primary open angle glaucoma. Trans Assoc Am Physicians. 1985; 98:361–9.
Stone EM, Fingert JH, Alward WL, et al. Identification of a gene that causes primary open angle glaucoma. Science 1997; 275:668–70.
Tawara A, Tou N, Kubota T, Harada Y, Yokota K. Immunohistochemical evaluation of the extracellular matrix in trabecular meshwork in steroid-induced glaucoma. Graefes Arch Clin Exp Ophthalmol. 2008 Jul;246(7):1021-8.

Tektas OY, Lütjen-Drecoll E. Structural changes of the trabecular meshwork in different kinds of glaucoma. Exp Eye Res. 2009 Apr;88(4):769-75.

Tripathi RC, Kirschner BS. Kipp M. et al. corticosteroid treatment for inflammatory bowel disease in pediatric patients increases intraocular pressure. Gastroenterology 1992; 102:1957.

Wang RF, Guo BK. Steroid-induced ocular hypertention in high myopia. Chin Med J 1984; 97:24.

Wang X, Johnson DH. mRNA in situ hybridization of TIGR/MYOC in human trabecular meshwork. Invest Ophthalmol Vis Sci 2000; 41:1724–9.

Zhang X, Clark AF, Yorio T. Regulation of glucocorticoid responsiveness in glaucomatous trabecular meshwork cells by glucocorticoid receptor-beta. Invest Ophthalmol Vis Sci. 2005; 46:4607–16.

Zhang X, Ognibene CM, Clark AF, Yorio T. Dexamethasone inhibition of trabecular meshwork cell phagocytosis and its modulation by glucocorticoid receptor beta. Exp Eye Res. 2007;84(2):275-284.

Zhao J, Zhang Q. Ultrastructural changes of the trabecular meshwork in glucocorticoid induced glaucoma. Yan Ke Xue Bao. 2010 Nov; 25(2):119-124.

Zillig M, Wurm A, Grehn FJ, et al. Overexpression and properties of wild-type and Tyr437His mutated myocilin in the eyes of transgenic mice. Invest Ophthalmol Vis Sci 2005; 46:223–34.

# 30

# Glaucoma in Cases of Penetrating Keratoplasty, Lamellar Procedures and Keratoprosthesis

Shimon Rumelt
*Department of Ophthalmology,*
*Western Galilee – Nahariya Medical Center, Nahariya,*
*Israel*

## 1. Introduction

The two main issues that concern glaucoma patients before and after penetrating keratoplasty and posterior lamellar procedures and patients that develop glaucoma after surgery are the risks of graft failure and the aggravation of the glaucoma. Failure of the corneal graft may require regrafting, which increases the risk of developing or aggravating glaucoma, while uncontrolled glaucoma may result in graft failure and further damage to the optic disc and visual field. These two problems may lead to each other creating a vicious circle. They should be treated by glaucoma and corneal specialists or by someone who is expert with both.

Glaucoma was found in 10-42% of the patients with a single corneal transplantation, 0-27% of them had preoperative glaucoma.[1-6] Preexisting glaucoma was usually a result of an initial insult such as chemical burn or secondary glaucoma. In repeated corneal transplantation, the incidence of postoperative glaucoma was higher (14-47%) than in primary transplantation.[7-12] It increases with increased number of regrafts and in aphakia. Corneal graft failure 3 years after keratoplasty occurred in 29-47% when glaucoma was present, compared with 9-30% when it was absent.[13,14]

Patients requiring penetrating keratoplasty and lamellar procedures (deep lamellar keratoplasty, Descemet's stripping (automated) endothelial keratoplasty, Descemet's membrane endothelial keratoplasty) may suffer from preexisting various types of open and closed angle glaucomas, which may be primary or secondary. Primary open angle and primary closed angle glaucomas may preexist and corneal surgery may be required for unrelated disorders such as Fuchs' corneal dystrophy. Secondary glaucomas may occur due to open and closed globe injuries. In those injuries, the glaucoma may be of open angle and caused by obstruction of the trabecular meshwork by red blood cells (from hyphema), ghost cells (ghost cell glaucoma) or tearing of the meshwork (angle recession). It may also be closed-angle caused by peripheral anterior synechiae. Corneal transplantation may also be required in chemical burns especially alkali. In these cases, the cornea may be opaque because of chronic edema and scarring. Secondary glaucoma may also be associated with corneal abnormalities such as anterior mesenchymal dysgenesis (e.g., Peter's and Axenfeld-Rieger's anomalies). In these disorders, in addition to corneal opacity due to scarring, the angle may be poorly formed. The common features for all these conditions are persistent corneal edema and scarring due to endothelial decompensation. The decompensation is a result of a combination of damaged or compromised endothelium (whether by trauma or other corneal disorders) and increased intraocular pressure (IOP) that contributes to egress of aqueous humor into the corneal layers. Corneal opacity due to persistent edema and scarring is more common in these conditions than in normal population.

Repeated or even primary corneal transplantation may also result in secondary glaucoma. The attributing factors for secondary glaucoma include 1. Donors button undersizing, which results in corneal graft over-stretching, causing corneal flattening and angle closure. 2. Trauma to the angle by the inadvertent touch by surgical instruments. The damage might be micro or macroscopic. 3. Corticosteroid-induced glaucoma, since topical and sometimes systemic corticosteroids are being frequently use after transplantation to decrease the risk for corneal graft rejection or to treat it. 4. Posterior synechiae that may develop due to postoperative intraocular inflammation especially if the angle is traumatized or becomes shallow. The most common forms of post-keratoplasty glaucoma in single and repeated corneal transplantation are chronic angle closure followed by steroid-induced glaucoma.

## 2. Assessment of patients requiring penetrating keratoplasty

The preoperative office evaluation of patients requiring penetrating keratoplasty or lamellar procedure whether or not having glaucoma includes defining the primary indication for surgery. Certain indications may require certain precautions or additional treatment to prevent loss of the graft clarity. For example, corneal transplantation for infectious diseases such as herpetic, fungal or acanthamebic keratitis require prolonged postoperative anti-herpetic, fungal or acanthamebic treatment to prevent reactivation. Defining the associated ocular disorders of the recipient and donor is paramount.[12] Corneal vascularization increases the risk of corneal graft rejection especially if involves three or more quadrants and requires prolonged use of corticosteroids as well as immuno-suppressants. Ocular surface disorders such as entropion and trichiasis also increase the likelihood of graft loss due to persistent rubbing of the ocular surface that results in corneal epithelial defects and ulcers that may lead to perforation.[15] Limbal cell deficiency in corneal cicatricial disorders such as ocular cicatricial pemphigoid and erythema multiforme (Steven Johnson disease) provides poor supporting environment to the graft, while dry eyes do both (poor supporting and increased friction upon blinking). Poor blinking and lagophthalmos may also cause dryness of the ocular surface resulting in persistent epithelial defects, ulcers and even perforation. These findings should be pretreated.

Cataract, glaucoma and retinal disorders may be associated with poor visual prognosis despite of clear corneal graft and should be evaluated before any corneal procedure. Defining the associated systemic disorders in recipient and donor are also essential. Diabetes mellitus is also manifested as fragile epithelium and slow epithelial healing, which could endanger the corneal graft.

Before any corneal surgery, best-corrected visual acuity of each eye should be obtained and recorded. This will assist in surgery decision making. Ultrasound is part of the evaluation if the cornea is severely opaque and fundus cannot be evaluated. It is used to rule out retinal detachment and intraocular masses (e.g., choroidal melanoma). When ocular disorders other than corneal disease exist, such as glaucoma and retinal disorders, they should be evaluated for their contribution to visual acuity. The evaluation includes potential acuity meter (PAM), Lambda and laser interferometry. With these instruments, if the visual acuity is improved, the eye has a potential for visual recovery and a corneal surgery should be attempted. In non-verbal patients as children or in patients with mental retardation, a less accurate method to evaluate the potential for visual recovery is electroretinography (ERG). When anamnesis cannot be obtained, poor prognostic factors for visual improvement are nystagmus, which develops in the first 3 postnatal months, and esotropia that develop in the first 6 postnatal months and indicate severe irreversible amblyopia. Exotropia on the other hand may be acquired at older age and therefore, with poor anamnesis is not a poor prognostic factor for visual recovery.

The preoperative evaluation should include a complete ocular examination including examining the anterior chamber angle, especially following ocular trauma, burns, preexisting glaucoma and candidates for large diameter grafts. If the cornea is opaque, ultrasound biomicroscopy (UBM) is a good alternative for gonioscopy. In presence of shallow anterior chamber, peripheral anterior synechiae or partially closed angle even with normal IOP, placement of anterior chamber IOL is contraindicated in triple procedures, because it may result in the development of secondary glaucoma.

## 3. Preoperative tips

Consider alternative treatment options for penetrating keratoplasty, especially if glaucoma exists. If the corneal opacity is central and localized (e.g., in Peter's anomaly), optical iridectomy may be a better surgical alternative. Rotational autokeratoplasty is an alternative for eccentric. If the corneal opacity is minimal, surgery may not be warranted. It is always imperative to consider whether the expected visual acuity will be better than the preoperative visual acuity. If not, it is better to avoid surgery.

It is important to perform complicated surgical procedures such as filtration surgery in uncontrolled and controlled glaucoma patients before corneal transplantation or posterior lamellar procedures. The IOP should be controlled at time of the penetrating keratoplasty or posterior lamellar procedures. Otherwise, the graft may become edematous and lost. In patients with glaucoma, any procedure should spare the limbus and conjunctiva as much as possible to allow glaucoma filtration surgery.

## 4. Surgical steps of penetrating keratoplasty to increase the success rate

Oversized donor corneal button is always required to decrease the risk for development of secondary glaucoma and aggravating a preexisting one. The details for oversizing are described below.

Specular microscopy of the donor button to ensure an endothelial cell count of more than 2,000 $mm^2$ without endothelial polymegatism or pleomorphism will at least guarantee that the corneal graft has safety margins and that the risk of endothelial decompensation will be decreased.

Pretreatment of preexisting glaucoma is a crucial step in successful penetrating and posterior lamellar procedures. Therefore, it is important recognizing the type and the etiology of preexisting glaucoma. Surgical pretreatment should be considered even in medically controlled glaucoma, because these patients may become uncontrolled after surgery and this may endanger the transparency of the corneal graft. Trabeculectomy is the treatment of choice for primary open angle glaucoma. Antimetabolites such as mitomycin-C (MMC) are indicated for all patients under the age of 55 even in primary surgery, for repeated surgery and for combined procedures. Trabeculectomy should be preferred over glaucoma drainage devices in triple procedures and in the presence of corneal graft. MMC should be applied in all cases of secondary glaucomas, triple procedure or in the presence of corneal graft although potential diffusion of the drug may endanger the endothelium. MMC 0.04% is soaked by a small piece of sponge and is placed under the scleral flap before penetrating into the anterior chamber or under the conjunctival flap for 2min avoiding its edges. It should not be placed over corneal button–recipient bed interface. Such a low concentration and short exposure minimize the risks for complications such as poor healing, scleral melting, anterior chamber reaction and increased IOP.

In angle closure glaucoma, laser iridotomy and laser iridoplasty or synechiolysis are warranted. Laser iridotomy may facilitate aqueous flow from the posterior into the anterior chamber and deepen the anterior chamber. Laser iridoplasty causes shrinkage of the peripheral iris and retracts the base of the iris to open the angle, while, synechiolysis has a similar effect by breaking peripheral anterior synechiae and opening the angle. The last two procedures are beneficial if peripheral anterior synechiae have been present for less than 6 months. Peripheral iridectomy may replace laser iridotomy only if iridotomy cannot be performed due to corneal opacity, thick iris or when laser in unavailable. The procedures are described below.

Penetrating keratoplasty should be delayed until the intraocular inflammation subsides and the IOP is stable within the target pressure range. This should be at least 3 months after any intraocular surgery.

## 5. Prevention of secondary glaucoma

Several precautions should be employed to prevent a secondary glaucoma. As mentioned, preoperative evaluation of the anterior chamber angle is essential especially in patients with preexisting glaucoma. If the angle is already compromised (close, narrow or has peripheral anterior synechiae), the risks of development of glaucoma or aggravation of preexisting one increase. It is important to oversize corneal donor button by 0.5-0.75 mm. In keratoconus or keratoglobus, an over-sizing of 0.25 mm is sufficient to decrease the risk of postoperative angle closure, while preventing too steep postoperative graft. For large graft diameter (8.0-9.5 mm) that is required sometimes for corneal perforations, large descematocele or widespread disease, an over-sizing of 0.75-1.0 mm is advocated. Avoiding manipulations near the angle with surgical instruments is important. The only exception is when synechiolysis is performed. The angle may also be filled with viscoelastic agent to protect it during the procedure, but the viscoelastic material should be aspirated at the conclusion of the surgery to prevent postoperative high IOP. To decrease damage to the trabecular meshwork, preoperative and postoperative intraocular inflammation should be controlled. This may be done by topical corticosteroids with high corneal penetrance such as prednisolone acetate (Pred Forte®). The frequency of drop instillation depends on the degree of inflammation and it is tapered gradually according to the response. Additional systemic corticosteroids may be employed for severe or recurrent sterile uveitis. Usually, 1 gr/kg/day of prednisone is sufficient.

## 6. Post-keratoplasty glaucoma

If glaucoma develops after corneal surgery, a distinction between immediate postoperative and late postoperative glaucoma should be made. Immediate postoperative glaucoma develops within a week after surgery in 42-55% of the primary keratoplasties. The causes for its development include viscoelastic agent left in the anterior chamber and blocking the drainage of the aqueous humor through the angle and corticosteroid-induced glaucoma. The later develops after the initiation of corticosteroid treatment and occurs at least in 20-30% of the patients. It can occur with any form of corticosteroid although it occurs more often after topical use. The increase in IOP in these cases is usually reversible if diagnosed early and if corticosteroids are discontinued. Therefore, topical and if necessary systemic corticosteroids should be replaced immediately with non-steroidal anti-inflammatory (NSAID) medications. Corticosteroid-induced glaucoma may be avoided by employment of topical NSAID such as ketorolac tromethamine 0.5% (Acular® or Tradol®), diclofenac sodium (Voltaren® (0.1%), Solaraze® (3%)) or indomethacin 1% (Indoptic®). Its incidence is also lowered with IOP sparing corticosteroids such as loteprednol etabonate 0.5% (Lotemax®) or rimexolone 1% (Vexol®) but because of their low potency, they may be more frequently required.

Late postoperative glaucoma may develop weeks or months after surgery. The incidence of this complication is 10-42% after primary keratoplasty. The risk factors for its development include preexisting glaucoma in 27-80% of the cases, aphakia in 20-39%, semi-flexible, closed-loop anterior chamber IOL in 23-50%, regrafting in 43% and wound dehiscence in 50%. Anterior mesenchymal disorders are risk factors for glaucoma in 50-90% of the patients, while open or closed globe injury in 31-77%. Glaucoma may be encountered in up to 47% of the patients with pseudophakic or aphakic bullous keratopathy, and the corneal edema may be a result of it. Certain old types of IOLs have also been associated with late postoperative glaucoma including iris-fixed anterior chamber IOL due to uveitis-glaucoma-hyphema (UGH) syndrome, caused by rubbing of the IOL against the iris. Large corneal grafts and posterior lamellar grafts may also increase the risk for glaucoma development because they may interfere with the angle. The same may occur from the sutures if they are long, tight and full thickness The causes for late postoperative glaucoma include synechial angle closure, changes in angle ultrastructure, direct mechanical damage to angle by surgical instruments, chronic postoperative inflammation causing toxic effects and presence of vitreous in the angle. Immune graft rejection was found to be more common in patients developing postoperative glaucoma than in those who did not develop it.[16,17] The glaucoma also increases with the number of corneal transplantation procedures.[17]

## 7. Post-keratoplasty evaluation of preexisting and secondary glaucoma

The evaluation of the anterior chamber is important not only before corneal transplantation and other posterior lamellar procedures but also after surgery, because if there is a progressive closure of the angle or formation of peripheral anterior synechiae, they may be treated before the development of glaucoma or to prevent its worsening. Periodic gonioscopy for development of anterior chamber angle closure is performed with gonioscopic lens when the peripheral cornea is clear. A 4 mirror hand-held lens has the advantages of avoiding viscoelastic material and of short diameter that allow indentation of the cornea. This allows distinguishing between apposition of the iris against the angle and true closure. It also allows breaking of fresh anterior synechiae if present. Indentation should be performed cautiously immediately after surgery, because it can result in wound dehiscence. Other gonioscopic lenses include the Goldman three and four mirror lenses, which have a broader base (diameter) and cannot indent only the cornea. They also require viscoelastic agent. Newer imaging modalities of the anterior chamber angle include the anterior segment optical coherence tomography (OCT) using 1310nm wavelength, which has a resolution of 10µm and Scheimpflug camera (Pentacam®) that has UV-free blue light source of 475nm with a similar resolution. Scheimpflug camera requires a clear cornea and direct visualization of the angle is still a better choice. When the peripheral cornea is opaque, ultrasound biomicroscopy (UBM) is the imaging of choice. It may also assists in evaluation of the ciliary body for congestion as part of uveal effusion syndrome and for aqueous misdirection. Thus, it may elucidate the mechanism of closed angle glaucomas.

Periodic IOP measurements are essential to disclose the development of glaucoma or aggravation of preexisting one. They should be performed in scheduled meetings during different hours of the day to reveal high IOP spikes in patients with high diurnal variations. In cases of doubt, a diurnal IOP curve is indicated and is usually performed every 4 hours between 8:00 and 20:00, but may be performed more frequently (i.e., every 2 hours) and during nighttime as well. IOP measurements should be especially performed when a patient is treated with topical and/or systemic corticosteroids or receives corticosteroid in other forms (e.g., inhalations). If newly IOP elevation is disclosed, recognizing the type of secondary glaucoma is important in treatment decision making (see above). IOP measurements of with Goldmann applanation tonometry may be challenging, because of corneal graft edema, which underestimate the real IOP and corneal graft astigmatism that distorts the image. When measured with Goldmann, the prism may be rotated to aim the red mark on it to the least curved corneal meridian (the negative axis). To overcome the astigmatism, the IOP may be measured twice, one in 90 degrees from the other, and the mean IOP may be calculated from these two measurements. IOP measurements may be performed by pneumatic tonometer, Tono-Pen or Mackay-Marg tonometer if they are impossible to be obtained with Goldmann. Alternatively, the IOP may be qualitatively estimated with a glass rod or by digital palpation. In eyes with corneal scarring, the IOP is overestimated.

When the diagnosis of postoperative or secondary glaucoma is established and the patient is being treated, it is important to avoid discontinuation of the anti-glaucoma medications, unless the patient is closely being followed-up. The course of postoperative glaucoma may be unpredictable and unstable. There might be high long-term fluctuations; i.e. cycles of normal IOP may alternate with increased IOP and the ophthalmologist may mislead to think that the glaucoma has resolved.

Actually, when a diagnosis of secondary glaucoma is made, the patient should always be on anti-glaucoma medications, unless he/ she develops excessive low IOP or intermittent ocular hypotony. In such cases, the anti-glaucoma medications should be discontinued while the patient is followed- up closely. These cases may represent a transition to phthisis bulbi. In cases of ocular hypotony, corticosteroids either topically or systemically may induce some IOP elevation, but if this does not result, pars plana vitrectomy with silicone oil injection into the vitreous might prevent phthisis. Pars plana vitrectomy with silicone oil injection is indicated for chronic ocular hypotony even if the visual acuity is no light perception, because it may prevent phthisis bulbi.

## 8. Treatment of progressive angle closure

The treatment of postoperative progressive angle closure even with normal IOP includes peripheral laser iridotomy and topical corticosteroids to control anterior chamber inflammation. If the IOP increases, a prompt surgical synechiolysis is warranted.

## 9. Treatment of secondary glaucoma

Open angle glaucoma is treated in the following order. The first line of treatment is medical with alpha-agonists (brimonidine tartrate) and beta-blockers (timolol maleate, betaxolol). In phakic eyes, prostaglandin analogs (latanoprost) and adrenergic agents (dipivefrin, epinephrine) may be added. In aphakic and pseudophakic eyes, prostaglandin analogs and adrenergic agents may induce cystoid macular edema (CME), which may result in a decrease in visual acuity, and therefore should be avoided. Topical carbonic anhydrase inhibitors (dorzolamide, brinzolamide) may cause graft failure due to toxicity to endothelial cells. Miotics may initiate intraocular inflammation by breaking the blood-aqueous barrier and may increase the likelihood of corneal graft rejection. In aphakic eyes, the risk of retinal detachment also increases. Therefore, these agents should be spared if possible.

The adverse effects of beta-blockers include superficial punctate keratopathy, corneal anesthesia and dry eyes. Alpha-adrenergic agents may also cause superficial punctate keratopathy and dry eyes.

If medical treatment fails, trabeculectomy with MMC (option for two such procedures) should be considered (Figure 1). However, some authors suggested that the prognosis might be poorer than for placement of a glaucoma drainage implant. If a trabeculectomy is performed, a soaked sponge (WekCel) of MMC 0.2-0.4 mg/ml under the scleral flap before penetrating the anterior chamber (or under the conjunctiva avoiding its edge) for 2-3 min should be added. The MMC should not be placed over corneal button–recipient bed interface. Then the area should be copiously irrigated with balanced salt solution or saline. This procedure may be repeated if it failed once. In some cases, the filtration procedure may be functioning well causing a decrease in IOP, but to insufficient level (above the target pressure). In such a case, an additional trabeculectomy rather than anti-glaucoma medications may be successful decreasing further the IOP to the desired level because they may diminish the filtration through the trabeculectomy resulting in its failure for long term. Also, with a successful second trabeculectomy, the patient may not need long-term topical medications, which are a burden. An alternative for MMC is 5-fluorouracil (5FU). Five-mg may be injected subconjunctivally before or at intervals after surgery, but is less potent. Another option is to place 50mg/ml of 5-FU over or under the scleral flap intraoperatively. It inhibits epithelial proliferation, while MMC is better against fibrous proliferation. Both drugs may be injected in conjunction.

The complications of trabeculectomy with MMC in the presence of corneal graft are similar to those without a graft, but in addition, damage to the endothelium may be caused by the MMC, if it penetrates into anterior chamber. The same precautions that apply for placing MMC during surgery for primary open angle glaucoma should be applied here.

If one or two trabeculectomies with MMC have been failed or as a first surgical option, glaucoma shunt tube may be performed. Anterior or posterior drainage devices are available. Anterior drainage devices connect the anterior chamber with the subconjunctival space. Schlemm's canal or suprachoroidal space are easier to implant and require only limited healthy conjunctiva to function. Among the anterior drainage devices are Ex-Press,

Solx Gold shunt and iStent. Posterior drainage devices also drain the anterior chamber through a silastic tube, but the tube is connected to a plate that is placed under the conjunctiva posteriorly. This is the reason that they are called posterior devices. Two types of posterior shunt tubes exist. The first type is with control of the flow (with a "valve" or flow resistance) includes Ahmed (New World Medical, Rancho Cucamonga, CA) and Krupin-Denver (Hood Laboratories, Pembroke, MA) drainage implants. The second type is without pressure control and includes Molteno single or double plate (IOP, Inc., Costa Mesa, CA, USA, and Molteno Ophthalmic Limited, Dunedin, New Zealand), Baerveldt (Advanced Medical Optics, Santa Ana, California, USA), Shocket (self-assembled) and Eagle Vision (Eagle Vision, Inc. Memphis, TN, USA) implants. The later require blocking the aqueous flow for a few days externally by temporary suture or internally by passing a suture through the lumen of the tube or injecting viscoelastic agent. The implantation may also be performed as a two-stage implantation, to decrease the risk for postoperative hypotony. Ahmed and Krupin implants should be preferred over the implants without a valve, because the risk for postoperative overflow and hypotony that may result in endothelial-iris and lens touch is decreased. Ahmed has a convenient plate to implant and suture in variable sizes including for pediatric population.

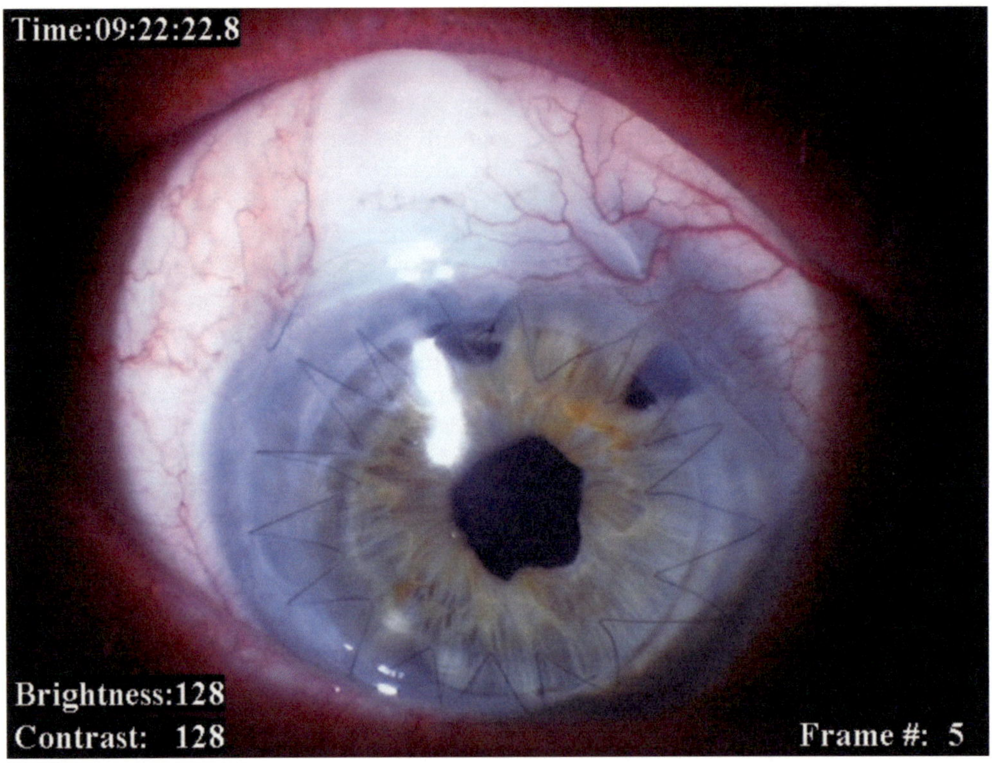


Fig. 1. Trabeculectomy in presence of clear corneal graft in a pseudophakic eye. Note the two patent peripheral iridectomies

The experience with anterior drainage devises is limited to a short follow-up, since they are relatively new. Results with Ex-press are promising.[18] The success rate defined as IOP below 21mmHG in 15 corneal transplanted eyes with closed angle glaucoma was 87% over a mean follow-up of 12 months, but a longer follow-up is required. The implantation is performed under 5x5mm partial thickness scleral flap similar to limbal-based trabeculectomy and MMC 0.05% is applied for 3min and rinsed after it. No data exist yet concerning the other anterior devices. In cases of corneal transplantation or posterior lamellar procedure, the position of the shunt tube may play a critical role in preservation of clear graft. In phakic eyes, the tube is usually placed through the anterior chamber angle. This results in control of the glaucoma in 68-96%.[19-25] However, placement of the tube into the anterior chamber may endanger the transparency of the graft due to tube-endothelial touch or turbulent flow of aqueous through the tip even in the absence of touch. Additional causes include eye rubbing and pressure on the cornea on sleeping. This complication is unique for corneal grafts and for compromised corneas (e.g., in Fuchs' endothelial dystrophy), since it has been demonstrated that progressive endothelial cell lost is observed after placement of glaucoma drainage tube into the anterior chamber angle, and this may occur even in the absence of endothelial-tube touch. Forty-two percent of the eyes with corneal transplants develop corneal decompensation.[23]

It is possible to redirect the tube placed into the anterior chamber angle through an existing iridectomy to the posterior chamber in aphakic or pseudophakic eyes as long as the iris would not block it. Another alternative in pseudophakic or aphakic eyes, is to place the tube into the posterior chamber through the ciliary sulcus, by an incision made 1mm posterior to the limbus.[26] This procedure is especially advantageous in eyes with corneal transplants or which are candidates for corneal transplantation or posterior lamellar grafts, Fuchs' corneal dystrophy, shallow anterior chamber and extensive synechial angle closure. A meticulous anterior vitrectomy is required if cases of vitreous loss.

For placement of glaucoma shunt tube into the ciliary sulcus, limbal peritomy is performed in the upper temporal (or if not feasible, inferonasal) quadrant and dissection is carried posteriorly over the sclera. The drainage plate is secured to the sclera with 6-0 polyester sutures 8 to 10mm posterior to the limbus between the superior and the horizontal recti muscles. A 2 to 5mm-long scleral tunnel is fashioned with angled crescent knife and the drainage tube is passed beneath it. Alternatively, the tube may be covered with scleral, corneal, pericardial or dural patch adjacent to the external sclerostomy. The tube is passed into the ciliary sulcus through a sclerostomy performed 1mm posterior to the limbus at 11 or 1 o'clock position under a half-thickness, limbal based scleral flap of 3x3mm. The sclerostomy is performed with a myringotomy blade that is inserted with its shaft perpendicular to the limbus and beveled parallel to the iris plane (as performed for scleral-fixated intraocular lens). The position of the tip of the blade is observed through the dilated pupil to confirm its position and avoid ciliary body separation. The edge of the tube is protruding 3mm into the posterior chamber. It should not exceed the dilated pupil margin to avoid glare and should not be too short to avoid blockage by ciliary processes. The fornix-based conjunctival flap is secured to the limbus with 7-0 polygalactin sutures (Figures 2,3). At the conclusion of the surgery betamethasone acetate 3mg and gentamicin sulfate 20mg are injected subconjunctivally 180° away from the implant plate. Topical corticosteroid, antibiotic and cycloplegic are prescribed and tapered gradually. The main potential complications include ciliary body separation and suprachoroidal hemorrhage. These were not observed in a series of patients that underwent this procedure.[26-28] The corneal grafts remained clear for years of follow-up and the glaucoma was controlled following this procedure. Placement of the shunt tube into the posterior chamber through the ciliary sulcus is contraindicated in phakic eyes because it may endanger the integrity of the crystalline lens.

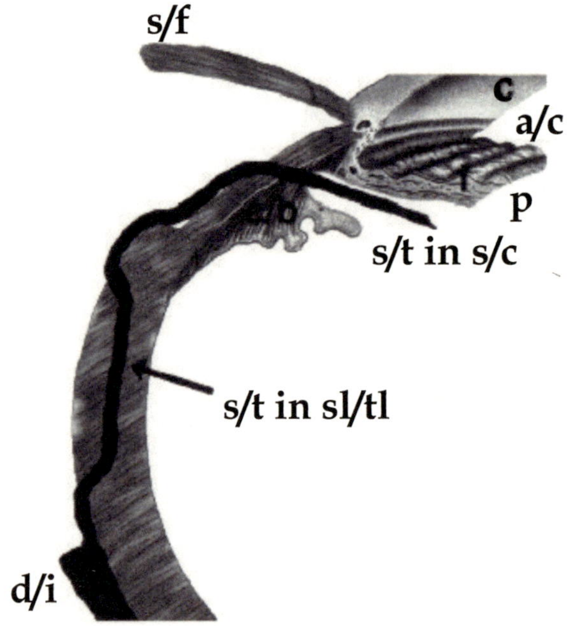


Fig. 2. A diagram showing a side view of placement of a glaucoma drainage device in the ciliary sulcus. c - cornea, a/c - anterior chamber, I - iris, p - pupil, s/f - scleral flap, c/b - ciliary body, s/t in c/s - shunt tube in the ciliary sulcus, s/t in sl/tl - shunt tube in scleral tunnel, d/i - implant disc

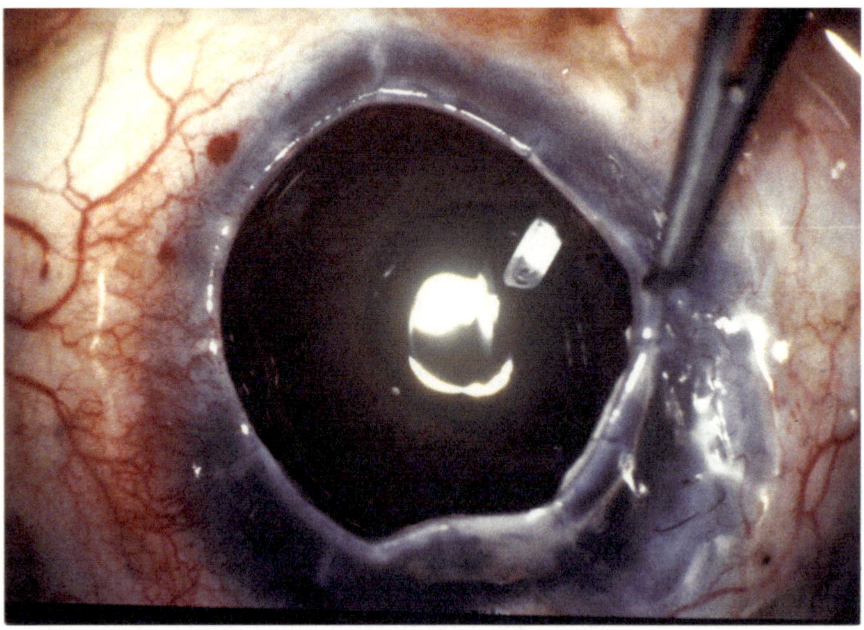

Fig. 3. The tip of ciliary sulcus glaucoma shunt tube behind the iris during surgery before placing a corneal graft

In cases of posterior segment disorders, when pars plana vitrectomy is required, the tube may be placed into the vitreous cavity through it.[30,31] A meticulous vitrectomy is a prerequisite so vitreous strands will not block the tube. The common feature for placement of the shunt tube into the posterior chamber through the ciliary sulcus or into the vitreous cavity through the pars plana is placing the tip of the tube away from the corneal graft, which decreases the risk of endothelial cell loss and corneal graft decompensation.

For pars plana placement of glaucoma drainage device, a limbal peritomy is performed and the lateral and superior rectus muscles are engaged by 4-0 silk traction sutures. The sclera is exposed further back by elevating the conjunctiva and Tenon's capsule with blunt dissection. The plate is secured to the superotemporal sclera with 6-0 polyester sutures. Then a three-port pars plana vitrectomy is performed through sclerostomies 3.5mm from the limbus. The tube is introduced 5mm into the vitreous through the superotemporal sclerostomy. A sclera, corneal, dural or pericardial patch may be used to cover the tube and the conjunctival-Tenon flap is sutured to the limbus with 7-0 polygalactin sutures. A Pars Plana Clip (Model PC,New World M, Inc., Rancho Cucamonga, CA, USA), which can be used with any drainage device, or Hoffman elbow, which is mounted on a Baerveldt 350-mm2 implant (Advanced Medical Optics, Inc., Santa Ana, CA, USA) may be used. New pars plana Ahmed and Baeverdlt implants are also available and the procedure may be performed using even the regular glaucoma setones, preferably those with a "valve". Fluid-gas exchange provides a temporary tamponade and prevents postoperative hypotony. Pars plana vitrectomy and placement of glaucoma shunt device may be performed endoscopically in eyes with media opacity such as corneal opacity.[32] This procedure allows controlling the glaucoma first and then performing corneal surgery later to improve visual acuity. Possible unique complications for this procedure include vitreous hemorrhage, retinal detachment and choroidal detachment. Although corneal graft failure is reduced if the glaucoma drainage device is placed through the ciliary sulcus or pars plana and if the glaucoma is controlled, it should be remembered that there are other causes that may result in graft failure.

In posterior lamellar grafts, if a glaucoma shunt tube is introduced into the anterior chamber, the graft may block the tip of the tube resulting in increased IOP. It can be avoided by trimming the tip of the tube, so it will not be blocked. It is also possible to pre-plane the corneal surgery and to prepare a thin lamellar graft or perform a DMEK rather than DSAEK (Figures 4,5).[29] Tube-endothelial touch without blockage may also occur and is manifested as corneal edema. It may increase the risk for corneal graft rejection. If tube-endothelial touch or tube blockage is suspected, the diagnosis may be confirmed by direct visualization with slit lamp biomicroscopy or indirectly with UBM, Scheimpflug camera (Pentacam) or anterior segment OCT. When tube-endothelial touch or tube blockage is confirmed, the tube should be trimmed. The trimming should be performed so that the opening of the tip would not face the corneal graft, because turbulence at the tip may cause progressive loss of endothelial cells and corneal decompensation that will require a new transplant. The opening should not face the iris as well because it may be blocked. The tip may also be redirected if long and mobile enough. This can be done by retrieving the tube from the anterior chamber, creating a new passage into the chamber and suturing the old route. Just moving the tube in the existing route is usually unhelpful. If the graft is edematous at the time of managing the tube, regrafting may be performed later when the IOP is stable and the eye is quiet, if the edema has not been resolved.

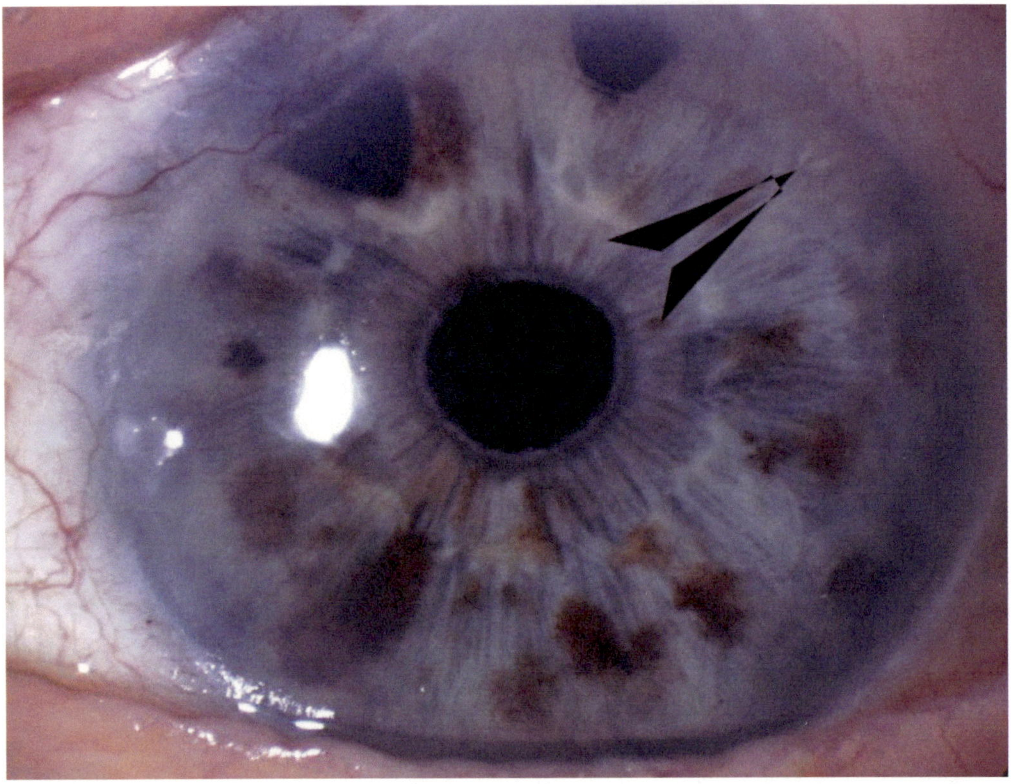

Fig. 4. Glaucoma shunt tube (arrow) in an eye after Descemet's membrane - endothelial keratoplasty (DMEK). Note the clear lamellar graft

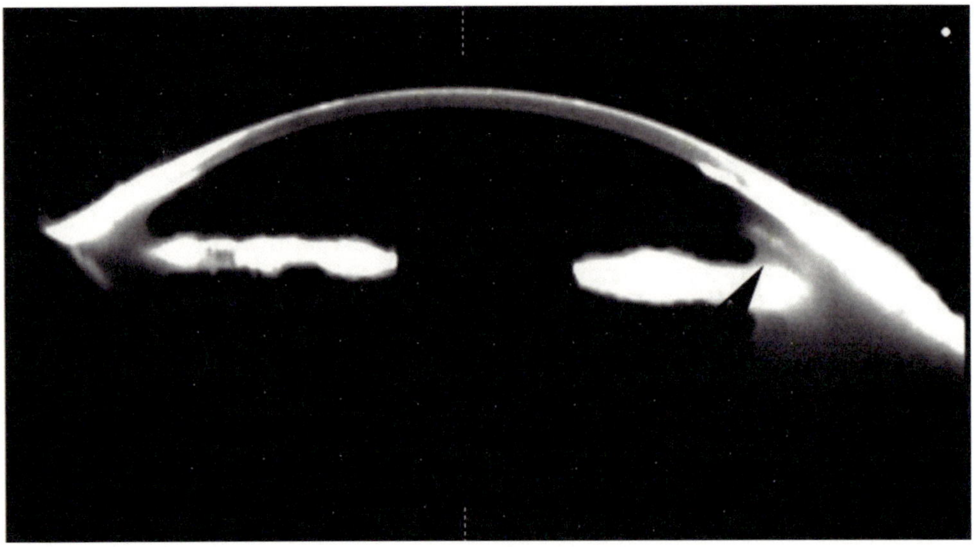

Fig. 5. Pentacam image of the same eye as in figure 4 showing the position of the tube in the anterior chamber (arrow)

Laser procedures for the angle such as selective trabeculoplasty have a limited value in the long-term treatment of secondary open angle glaucomas and therefore, were not included in the sequence of treatment. The main reason is their limited effect in this type of glaucoma. Even in primary open angle glaucoma, where it is more effective, the success rate is only 50% 5 years after the procedure.

## 10. Closed angle glaucoma

Closed angle glaucoma should be confirmed by gonioscopy or UBM or with other imaging techniques (anterior segment OCT or Scheimpflug camera). The first treatment modality, which is usually simplest, if the cornea is clear, is peripheral laser iridotomy. This is usually performed with Neodymium: Yttrium-Aluminum-Garnet (Nd:YAG) laser. After instillation of topical pilocarpine 2% or 4% and topical analgesic (e.g., oxybuprocaine HCl 0.4% or proparacaine HCl 0.5%) eye drop, a spot of 10mJ is placed over the peripheral iris. Two pulses may be used simultaneously. The size of the spot is constant depending on the instrument (50-70µm). The spot is placed at the periphery of the iris in the superior half to avoid glare and over a thin part of the iris (usually a crypt) avoiding blood vessels. If bleeding occurs, the cornea is pressed by a contact lens until bleeding ceases. The procedure may be performed with contact lens such as Abraham (+66D), Wise (+103D), CGI or without it. The advantages of a contact lens are additional magnification, focusing the beam, absorbing part of the heat, stabilizing the eye and maintaining the eyelids open. Topical glycerin may be placed over the cornea before the procedure if it is edematous. Topical apraclonidine (Iopidine®) 0.5%-1.0% or other alpha 2 agonist (e.g., brimonidine tartrate) is administered following the procedure to decrease IOP spikes and corticosteroids such as prednisolone acetate 1% qid are prescribed of a week to decrease intraocular inflammation and risk for synechiae formation. Additional anti-glaucoma medications may be added. This procedure facilitates aqueous flow from the posterior into the anterior chamber and may result in deepening of the anterior chamber and lowering the IOP. The major complication is acceleration of cataract. If Nd:YAG laser is unavailable, Argon laser iridotomy may be performed. The parameters for this procedure depend on the iris pigmentation. For brighter iris, the power is lower than for darker ones. The preparatory stretch burns are of 200-600mW, 0.2-0.6 sec, 200-500µm. The penetration burns are of 800-1000mW, 0.2 sec, 50µm. The iridotomy size should be increased to 150-500µm. The position of the Argon iridotomy in this case is preferably supero-nasal to prevent injury to the macula. The treatment before and after the procedure is identical to Nd:YAG laser iridotomy. Perforation of the iris is obtained when aqueous mixed with pigment is flowing from the posterior to the anterior chamber through the iridotomy. The lens should be visible through the iridotomy, since positive transillumination is not reliable. When laser iridotomy is not feasible, surgical peripheral iridectomy should be performed. Complications include visual disturbances such as halo and glare, development and progression of cataract, corneal burns that are usually transient, temporary increase in IOP, intraocular inflammation and rarely retinal injury, CME and malignant glaucoma.

If laser iridotomy does not result in decrease in IOP, surgical peripheral goniosynechiolysis or laser peripheral iridoplasty may be performed. This should be performed as earlier as possible and preferably if the angle closure is of less than 6 months. Otherwise, it is usually useless, because of scarring. Peripheral goniosynechiolysis is performed through a paracentesis. It may be performed under viscoelastic material or with anterior chamber maintainer. A spatula is transferred along the peripheral iris to withdraw it from the angle.

Goniosynechiolysis may be performed in a similar way with viscoelastic agent injected toward the angle to open it. However, the viscoelastic material should be removed at the conclusion of the procedure to prevent postoperative high IOP. Laser iridoplasty is performed after instillation of topical anesthetic eye drop with Argon laser, 200-400mW, 0.3-0.6 sec, 500 μm, 20-40 burns in a row with 2-beam diameter space between each spot over 360° peripheral iris avoiding blood vessels. The procedure is performed with a contact lens such as the Abraham (+66D), Wise (+103D), CGI or Goldmann three-mirror lens (through the center, non-mirror part) or without it. The preparations before and the management following the procedure are similar to this described above for Nd:YAG laser iridotomy. The procedure is aimed to contract the peripheral iris away from the angle. The contraindications for the procedure include extensive synechial closure and flat anterior chamber. The complications of the procedure include corneal burns, increased IOP, iritis, new synechiae formation and mydriasis.

If the IOP did not decrease substantially to the target level following these two procedures, medical treatment with anti-glaucoma medications including pilocarpine 2% four times a day may be added. If pilocarpine is added, it is worthwhile to have two consecutive days off this medication every month. This decreases the probability to have fixed small pupil, which may be an obstacle if cataract extraction is required.

If the IOP remained high or becoming high despite of medical treatment, other surgical procedures may be performed. The usual approach is to have trabeculectomy first. Trabeculectomy in this case may require a long tunnel (or sclerostomy) that will penetrate the peripheral cornea anterior to the peripheral anterior synechiae.

When a trabeculectomy is failed, a glaucoma shunt tube may be placed as mentioned earlier. In aphakic and pseudophakic eyes it may be placed into the ciliary sulcus.

## 11. Steroid-induced glaucoma

Steroid-induced glaucoma is defined as elevation of IOP following administration of topical and/or systemic corticosteroids that remains high after their discontinuation. Steroid responder is a patient in whom the IOP returns to normal after discontinuation of the steroids. These medications are often used after corneal transplantation to prevent or treat corneal graft rejection. They are also used to treat postoperative intraocular inflammation. Differentiation between steroid-induced glaucoma and inflammatory (uveitic) glaucoma may be performed by increasing the topical corticosteroid dosage for several days. If IOP remains high despite decreased intraocular inflammation, a corticosteroid-induced glaucoma is most reasonable.

In cases of steroid responders or steroid-induced glaucoma, discontinuation of the corticosteroids is mandatory. Patients, who are steroid responders, should be aware that they are "allergic" to steroid in the specific form that causes their IOP to increase. This should be written in their medical chart and added to a note (or a card) for the patient, specify that he should not receive this type of drug. For episodes of graft immune rejection, a combination of topical NSAID (sodium diclofenac 0.1% or ketorolac tromethamine 0.5%) and topical cyclosporine-A may be employed. Systemic cyclosporine-A or other drugs such as PO tacrolimus 0.1mg/kg/day may be added. Another option is to use IOP-sparing corticosteroids such as loteprednol etabonate 0.5% (Lotemax®) or rimexolone 1% (Vexol®). Judicious use of systemic corticosteroids instead of topical corticosteroids may be adopted if they do not cause an increase in IOP.

The treatment of steroid-induced glaucoma follows the same principles applied for primary open-angle glaucoma (see above).

## 12. Glaucoma in patients with corneal and posterior segment disorders

Glaucoma in cases of posterior segment disorders (e.g. proliferative diabetic retinopathy, neovascular glaucoma, uveitic glaucoma) along with corneal disorders are more challenging to treat. Pars plana vitrectomy may require a temporary keratoprosthesis for visualization of the posterior segment. Following which, a corneal transplantation is being performed. Otherwise, pars plana vitrectomy may be performed endoscopically. In both instances, if the glaucoma is refractory to medical treatment, a pars plana implantation of glaucoma drainage implant is advised.

Cyclodestructive procedures should be avoided if possible, because the degree of IOP reduction and intraocular inflammation are unpredictable. Excessive intraocular inflammation may cause intense pain, CME and hypotony that may result in phthisis bulbi. External inflammation may cause excessive scarring of the conjunctiva, preventing other procedures such as trabeculectomy to be performed. The corneal graft may also fail. Cyclodestructive procedures should be reserved only for painful eyes with no potential for visual rehabilitation. If cyclodestructive procedures are employed, transscleral cyclophotocoagulation (contact or non-contact, Nd:YAG or diode laser) or transcorneal ciliary processes photocoagulation should be preferred over cyclocryoablation. The former causes less postoperative pain, postoperative inflammatory reaction and phthisis bulbi than cyclocryoablation. Even when transscleral cyclophotocoagulation (contact or non-contact, Nd:YAG or diode laser) or transcorneal ciliary processes photocoagulation is being performed, it may be applied to half to two thirds of the ciliary body to prevent these complications. This book contains a chapter on controlled cyclophotocoagulation to decrease complications.

For cyclodestructive procedures, sub-Tenon, peribulbar or retrobulbar anesthesia with 2% lidocaine (or a 1:1 mixture with 0.75% bupivicaine) is used. Transscleral Nd:YAG (1064nm) may be contact or non-contact, continuous or pulsed. Eight to 25 applications of 1.5-10J are placed 2-3mm beyond the limbus over 180°. This position corresponds to the location of the ciliary body and is confirmed by transillumination. Trans scleral Diode (810nm), 10-20 applications of 5-6mJ over 180-270° is performed 2mm posterior to the limbus. Following the procedure, topical corticosteroids such as prednisolone acetate 1% qid or more and atropine sulfate 1% tid for a few weeks are warranted. Analgesia may also be required. The anti-glaucoma medications are tapered gradually according to the decrease in IOP. The success of the procedure is usually assessed 4 weeks after treatment. The complications include hyphema, corneal decompensation, chronic intraocular inflammation, CME, epiretinal membranes, chronic hypotony and even phthisis bulbi. They may be fewer with Diode laser with G-probe.[33]

## 13. Prognosis

The prognosis of preexisting glaucoma depends on its type.[17] It is usually more favorable for primary open angle glaucoma as long as precautions have been taken during the penetrating keratoplasty or the lamellar grafting. The prognosis for graft survival is also better than with other types of preexisting glaucoma, as long as the IOP is well controlled and the corneal graft has a healthy endothelium.

The prognosis for secondary open angle glaucoma is similar. If the IOP is poorly controlled, there are increased risks for corneal decompensation and development of bullous keratopathy that may require additional grafting. However, performing corneal transplantation in an eye with uncontrolled glaucoma is inadvisable. Resolution of post-keratoplasty glaucoma has been observed in chronic angle closure glaucoma after an additional corneal transplantation probably due to changes in the angle configuration by applying the above advises. In steroid responders, the IOP returns to normal following discontinuation of the corticosteroids.

With the approaches described in this chapter, it would be possible to improve the outcomes of patients with corneal transplants and coexisting glaucoma.

### 13.1 Follow-up

Patients undergoing corneal surgery and having or developing glaucoma usually have concurrent disorders and are more challenging to treat. These patients should be followed-up regularly at least every 3 months for their lifetime. If they experience ocular pain, decrease in vision or redness of the eye, they should immediately report to their ophthalmologist. It is essential not to postpone the next step in treatment if the current one is not sufficient to abolish the risk of further deterioration.

## 14. Controversies in management of glaucoma in patients with corneal grafts

Whether trabeculectomy with MMC or glaucoma drainage implant is the surgical treatment of choice for glaucoma in patients with corneal grafts is still controversial. Different authors have reported comparable results with both. At present, it is up to the decision of the surgeon according to his experience. Comparative studies are required for a definite answer. Such studies will be required also to decide whether simultaneous procedures have the same success rate as separate procedures and whether the new anterior glaucoma devices such as Solx gold shunt or iStent, will have a benefit over the posterior ones.

## 15. Glaucoma in cases of permanent keratoprosthesis

Several types of keratoprosthesis are available including one that pass through the cornea and fused eyelids (type II) and the more common ones through the cornea only (type I, e.g., Boston and osteo-odonto-keratoprosthesis) (Figures 6,7). Keratoprosthesis is usually reserved for eyes in which other corneal procedures have failed and the prognosis for additional ones is poor. A publication on repeated corneal transplantation demonstrated that as the number of repeated corneal grafts is increased, the prognosis for long-term survival of the regraft decreases.[12] Most of the regrafts do fail due to graft rejection, glaucoma and other complications. These findings have led keratoprosthesis specialists to advocate keratoprosthesis. However, the publication was intended to elaborate the importance of proper preventive measures and early and correct treatment of corneal transplantation complications of rather than to advocate the use of keratoprosthesis. With better preventive measures and treatments, it will be possible to decrease the necessity for repeated transplantation and of course to avoid keratoprosthesis.

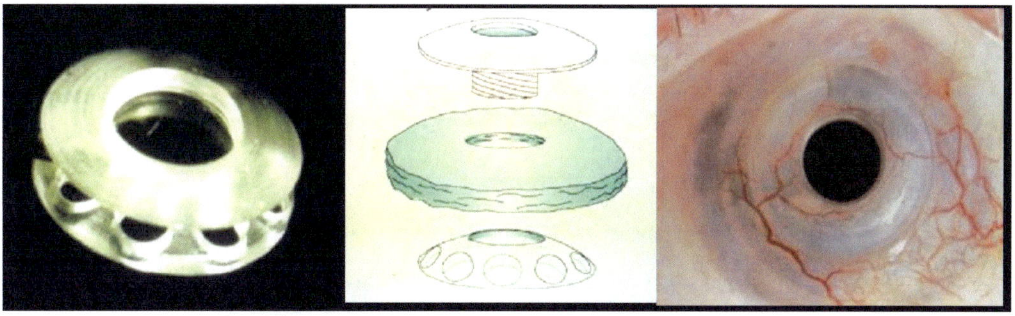

Fig. 6. Type I keratoprosthesis (courtesy of Peter Rubin, MD)

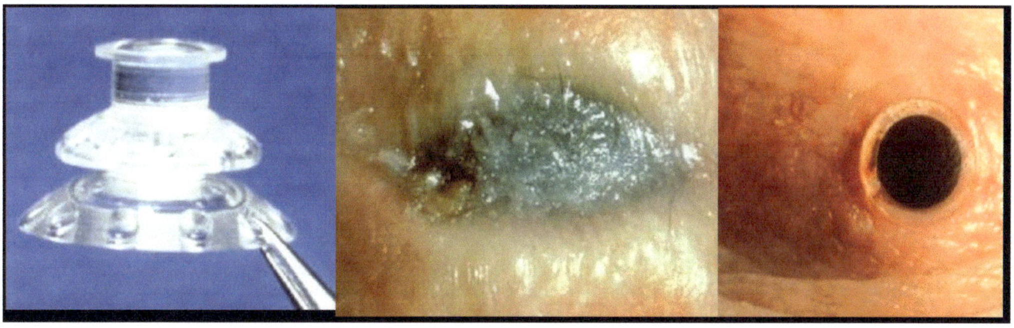

Fig. 7. Type II keratoprosthesis (courtesy of Peter Rubin, MD)

Many of the patients undergoing keratoprosthesis have multiple ocular pathologies and glaucoma is one of them. Between 36-76% of the eyes with keratoprosthesis have glaucoma.[34-39] Of these, about 2-28% develop glaucoma after the implantation of keratoprosthesis, usually because of progressive angle closure. This may be caused because of inadvertent injury to the angle and postoperative intraocular inflammation. A peripheral iridectomy may decrease the risk of postoperative angle closure. The prosthesis may also serve as a scaffold for retoprosthetic membrane that may cover the angle. The use of corticosteroids for prolonged period may also cause corticosteroid-induced glaucoma in susceptible patients.

Glaucoma is more frequent in keratopsrosthetic patients than in repeated corneal transplantation. One of the most challenging situations in the presence of keratoprosthesis is to detect and follow-up glaucoma, because it is impossible to check the IOP using the standard methods such as Goldmann applanation tonometry or Schiotz indentation tonometry. These instruments are employed through normal cornea and not through a keratoprosthesis, which cannot be indent. In many cases, visualization of the optic disc may be difficult and therefore, changes in cupping are difficult to observe or document directly, or indirectly using Heidelberg Retinal Tomography (HRT), scanning laser polarimeter (GDx) or OCT. Reliable visual fields may also be difficult to obtain and the maximal field that may be obtained is 60° with type I and 40° with type II.

It is paramount to obtain the history of glaucoma in patients with keratoprosthesis and to document it. In presence of keratoprosthesis, IOP qualitative estimation may be performed by digital palpation over the sclera. It should not be performed over the keratoprosthesis or the glaucoma shunt plate. Qualitative estimation with glass rod over the conjunctiva is

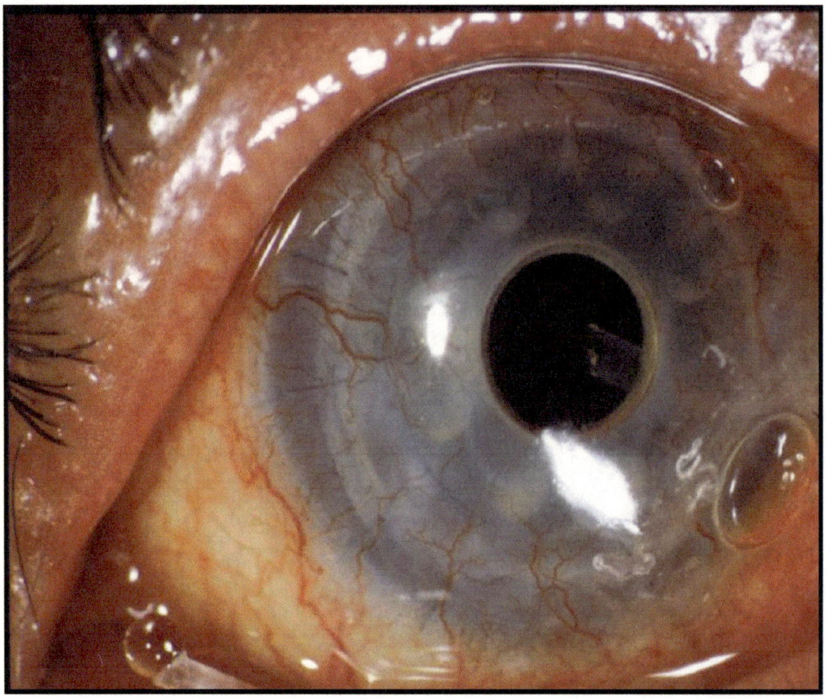

Fig. 8. The tip of Ahmed shunt tube seen through type I keratoprosthesis. It was placed into the vitreous though the pars plana (courtesy of Peter Rubin, MD)

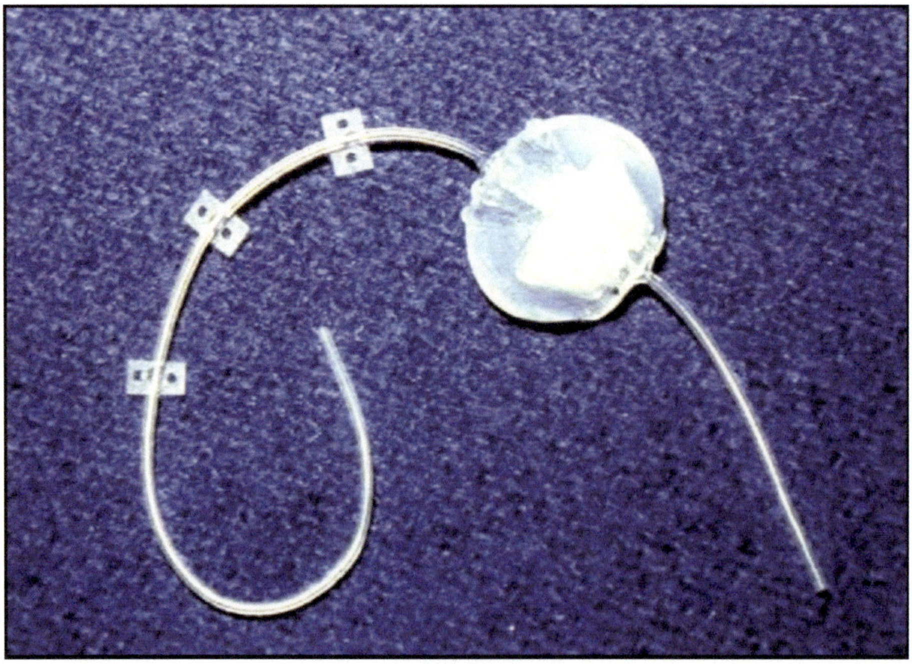

Fig. 9. A modified Ahmed closed shunt (courtesy of Peter Rubin, MD)

more challenging as quantitative estimation of the IOP by Tonopen or Schiotz indentation tonometry through the limbal area. If the IOP cannot be estimated in follow-up visits, it is also possible to follow patients by observing the optic disc and visual fields for deterioration as is done with some patients without keratoprosthesis who do not allow checking their IOP. New transducers are being developed to allow IOP measurements in patients with keratoprosthesis.

In patients who are candidate for keratoprosthesis, it is preferable to implant glaucoma drainage device and to wait for 3-6 months before placing the keratoprosthesis especially when the IOP is refractory to medical treatment or the damage to the optic disc is advanced. This period would allow the postoperative intraocular inflammation to subside and to the IOP to stabilized.

The respond to medical treatment in patients with keratoprosthesis is limited because there is no absorption area in patients with type II and limited absorption area with type I keratoprosthesis and the glaucoma is usually more severe compared with glaucoma in penetrating keratoplasty. The next step is introducing a glaucoma drainage device (Figure 8). A placement of glaucoma shunt tube into the vitreous through the pars plana may be better than into the anterior chamber that is already crowded because of the back-plate of the prosthesis. In aphakic eyes, it is mandatory to ascertain that no vitreous remains in the anterior chamber, by meticulous anterior vitrectomy. Since the patients are either aphakic or pseudophakic, the tube may be inserted through the ciliary sulcus. Recently, it was suggested to place the valved drainage tube such as Ahmed valve in the lacrimal sac, ethmoid or maxillary sinuses and to avoid the subconjunctival plate.[38,39] The shunt tube was modified for this purpose (Figure 9) and was placed into the lacrimal sac or the ethmoid sinus through an external dacryocystorhinostomy incision although it may be placed in a similar manner as a Pyrex tube in conjunctivo-dacryo-cystorhinostomy. Placement into the maxillary sinus was performed through a lower eyelid crease or subciliary incision but it is also possible to go through the inferior fornix. Penetration may be performed with intravenous catheter and the tube may be passed through it after removing the catheter hub. These procedures may decrease the failure of glaucoma shunt tube from fibrosis around the subconjunctival plate. The main risk in these cases is endophthalmitis. Therefore, I would not advocate these procedures if the lacrimal sac or the sinus is not sterile. Therefore, such a procedure should be avoided in patients with active sinusitis or history of this disorder. In one series of 37 patients, one (3%) developed endophthalmitis.[38] Cyclophotocoagulation may be employed as an adjunct treatment to glaucoma drainage implants for painful eyes with no potential for visual rehabilitation.[42,43]

## 16. References

[1] Thoft RA, Gardon JM, Dohlman CH. Glaucoma following penetrating keratoplasty. *Trans Am Acad Ophthalmol Otolaryngol* 1974;78:352-64.

[2] Polack FM. Keratoplasty in aphakic eyes with corneal edema: results in 100 cases with 10-year follow-up. *Ophthalmic Surg* 1980;11:701-7.

[3] Goldberg DB, Schanzlin DJ, Brown SI. Incidence of increased intraocular pressure after keratoplasty. *Am J Ophthalmol* 1981;92:372-7.

[4] Foulks GN. Glaucoma associated with penetrating keratoplasty. *Ophthalmology* 1987; 94:871-4.

[5] Polack FM. Glaucoma in keratoplasty. *Cornea* 1988;7:67-9.
[6] Simmons RB, Stern RA, Teekhasaenee C, Kenyon KR. Elevated intraocular pressure following penetrating keratoplasty. *Trans Am Ophthalmol Soc* 1989;87:79-91.
[7] Cowden J, Kaufman HE, Polack FM. The prognosis of keratoplasty after previous graft failures. *Am J Ophthalmol* 1974;78:523-5.
[8] Robinson CH. Indications, complications and prognosis for repeated penetrating keratoplasty. *Ophthalmic Surg* 1979;10:27-34.
[9] Insler MS, Pechous B. Visual results in repeat penetrating keratoplasty. *Am J Ophthalmol* 1986;102:371-5.
[10] MacEwen CJ, Khan ZUH, Anderson E, MacEwen CG. Corneal re-graft: indications and outcome. *Ophthalmic Surg* 1988;19:706-12.
[11] Rapuano CJ, Cohen EJ, Brady SE et al. Indications and outcomes of repeat penetrating keratoplasty. *Am J Ophthalmol* 1990;109:689-95.
[12] Bersudsky V, Blum-Hareuveni T, Rehany U, Rumelt S. The profile of repeated corneal transplantation. *Ophthalmology* 2001;108:461-9.
[13] Sugar A. An analysis of corneal endothelial and graft survival in pseudophakic bullous keratopathy. *Trans Am Ophthalmol Soc* 1989;87:762-801.
[14] Byrd S, Tayeri T. Glaucoma associated with penetrating keratoplasty. *Clin Ophthalmol* 1999;39:17-28.
[15] Rumelt S, Blum-Hareuveni T, Bersudsky V, Rehany U. Persistent epithelial defects and ulcers in repeated corneal transplantation: incidence, causative agents, predisposing factors and treatment outcomes. *Eye*, 2008;246:1139-1145.
[16] Aldave AJ, Rudd JC, Cohen EJ et al. The role of glaucoma therapy in the need for repeat penetrating keratoplasty. *Cornea* 2000, 19:772-6.
[17] Rumelt S, Bersudsky V, Blum-Hereuveni T, Rehany U. Preexisting and postoperative glaucoma in repeated corneal transplantation. *Cornea*, 2002;21:759-765.
[18] Kirkness CM. Penetrating keratoplasty, glaucoma, and silicone drainage tubing. *Dev Ophthalmol* 1987;14:161-5.
[19] Ates H, Palamar M, Yagci A, Egrilmez S. Evaluation of mini Ex-Press glaucoma shunt implantation in refractory penetrating glaucoma. *J Glaucoma* 2010;19:556-60.
[20] McDonnell PJ, Robin JB, Schanzlin DJ et al. Molteno implant for control of glaucoma in eyes after penetrating keratoplasty. *Ophthalmology* 1988;95:364-9.
[21] Kirkness CM, Ling Y, Rice NSC. The use of silicone drainage tubing to control postkeratoplasty glaucoma. *Eye* 1988;2:583-90.
[22] Beebe WE, Starita RJ, Fellman RL, Lynn JR, Gelender H. The use of Molteno implant and anterior chamber tube shunt to encycling band (ACTSEB) for treatment of glaucoma in penetrating keratoplasty. *Ophthalmology* 1990;97:1414-22.
[23] Sherwood MB, Smith MF, Driebe WT Jr et al. Drainage tube implants in the treatment of glaucoma following penetrating keratoplasty. *Ophthalmic Surg* 1993:24:185-9.
[24] Rapuano CJ, Schmidt CM, Cohen EJ, et al. Results of alloplastic tube shunt procedures before, during, oafter penetratikeratoplasty. *Cornea* 1995;14:26-32.
[25] Coleman AL, Mondino BJ, Wilson MR, Casey R. Clinical experience with the Ahmed glaucoma valve implant in eyes with prior or concurrent penetrating keratoplasties. *Am J Ophthalmol* 1997;123:54-61.

[26] Rumelt S. Rehany U. Implantation of glaucoma drainage implant tuinto the ciliary sulcuin patients with corneal transplants. *Arch Ophthalmol* 1998;116:685-7.
[27] Tello C, Espana EM, Mora R, et al. Baerveldt glaucoma implant insertion in the posterior chamber sulcus. *Br J Ophthalmol* 2007;91:739-42.
[28] Weiner A, Cohn AD, Balasubramaniam M, Weiner AJ. Glaucoma tube shunt implantation through the ciliary sulcus in pseudophakic eyes with high risk of corneal decompensation. *J Glaucoma* 2010;19:405-11.
[29] Bersudsky V, Treviño A, Rumelt S. Management of endothelial decompensation because of glaucoma shunt tube touch by Descemet membrane endothelial keratoplasty and tube revision. *Cornea* 2011;30:709-11.
[30] Gandham SB, Costa VP, Katz LJ, Wilson RP, SA, Belmont J, Smith M. Aqueous tube-shunt implantation and pars plana vitrectomy in eyes with refractory glaucoma. *Am J Ophthalmol* 1993;116:189-95.
[31] Ritterband DC, Shapiro D, Trubnik V, et al. Cornea Glaucoma Implant Study Group (COGIS). Penetrating keratoplasty with pars plana glaucoma drainage devices. *Cornea* 2007;26:1060-6.
[32] Tarantola RM, Agarwal A, Lu P, Joos KM. Long-term results of combined endoscope-assisted pars plana vitrectomy and glaucoma tube shunt surgery. *Retina* 2011; 31:275-83.
[33] Fishbaugh G. Overview and new technology in cyclodestructive procedures. *Insight* 1999;19:26-9.
[34] Netland PA, Terada H, Dohlman CH. Glaucoma associated with keratoprosthesis. *Ophthalmology* 1998;105:751-7.
[35] Zerbe BL, Belin MW, Ciolino JB. Boston Type 1 Keratoprosthesis Study Group. Results from the multicenter Boston Type 1 Keratoprosthesis Study. *Ophthalmology* 2006; 113:1779.
[36] Aldave AJ, Kamal KM, Vo RC, Yu F. The Boston type I keratoprosthesis: improving outcomes and expanding indications. *Ophthalmology* 2009;116:640-51.
[37] Bradley JC, Hernandez EG, Schwab IR, Mannis MJ. Boston type 1 keratoprosthesis: the university of California Davis experience. *Cornea* 2009;28:321-7.
[38] Chew HF, Ayres BD, Hammersmith KM, et al. Boston keratoprosthesis outcomes and complications. *Cornea* 2009;28:989-96.
[39] Rivier D, Paula JS, Kim E, Dohlman CH, Grosskreutz CL. Glaucoma and keratoprosthesis surgery: role of adjunctive cyclophotocoagulation. *J Glaucoma* 2009;18:321-4.
[40] Rubin PA, Chang E, Bernardino CR, Hatton MP, Dohlman CH. Oculoplastic technique of connecting a glaucoma valve shunt to extraorbital locations in cases of severe glaucoma. *Ophthal Plast Reconstr Surg* 2004;20:362-7.
[41] Dohlman CH, Grosskreutz CL, Chen TC, et al. Shunts to divert aqueous humor to distant epithelialized cavities after keratoprosthesis surgery. *J Glaucoma* 2010; 19:111-5.
[42] Rivier D, Paula JS, Kim E, Dohlman CH, Grosskreutz CL. Glaucoma and keratoprosthesis surgery: role of adjunctive cyclophotocoagulation. *J Glaucoma* 2009;18:321-4.

[43] Parthasarathy A, Aung T, Oen FT, Tan DT. Endoscopic cyclophotocoagulation for the management of advanced glaucoma after osteo-odonto-keratoprosthesis surgery. *Clin Experiment Ophthalmol* 2008;36:93-4.